HYPERTENSION PRIMER
SECOND EDITION

The Essentials of High Blood Pressure

Senior Editors
Joseph L. Izzo, Jr, MD, and Henry R. Black, MD

Section Editors
Theodore L. Goodfriend, MD; James R. Sowers, MD; Theodore A. Kotchen, MD;
Jeffrey A. Cutler, MD, MPH; Donald G. Vidt, MD; Sheldon G. Sheps, MD;
Domenic A. Sica, MD

From the Council on High Blood Pressure Research
American Heart Association

Editor: David Charles Retford
Managing Editor: Jennifer Ann Kullgren
Project Editor: Joan Denise C. Scullin

Copyright © 1999 American Heart Association

Dallas, Texas

Format, design, and index © 1999
Lippincott Williams & Wilkins
351 West Camden Street
Baltimore, Maryland 21210-2436 USA

Rose Treet Corporate Center
1400 North Providence Road
Building II, Suite 5025
Media, Pennsylvania 19063-2043 USA

Printed in the United States of America

First Edition, 1993

ISBN 0-87493-202-5

Library of Congress Cataloging-in-Publication Data

Hypertension primer : the essentials of high blood pressure / Joseph L. Izzo, Jr. and Henry R. Black, senior
 editors : Theodore L. Goodfriend ... [et al.], section editors. — 2nd ed.
     p.   cm.
    "From the Council on High Blood Pressure Research. American Heart Association".
    Includes bibliographical references and index.
    ISBN 0-87493-202-5.—ISBN 0-683-30706-1
    1. Hypertension.   I. Izzo, Joseph L.   II. Black. Henry R. (Henry Richard), 1942–
III. Goodfriend. Theodore L.   IV. Council for High Blood Pressure Research (American Heart
Association)
    [DNLM: 1. Hypertension. WG 340H99654 1999]
RC685.H8H923 1999
616.1'32—dc21
DNLM/DLC
for Library of Congress   98-41673
                                                CIP

To purchase additional copies of this book, call our customer service department at **(800) 638-0672** or fax orders to **(800) 447-8438.** For other book services, including chapter reprints and large quantity sales, ask for the Special Sales department.

Canadian customers should call **(800) 665-1148,** or fax **(800) 665-0103.** For all other calls originating outside of the United States, please call **(410) 528-4223** or fax us at **(410) 528-8550.**

Visit Lippincott Williams & Wilkins on the Internet: http://www.wwilkins.com or contact our customer service department at **custserv@wwilkins.com.** Lippincott Williams & Wilkins customer service representatives are available from 8:30 am to 6:00 pm, EST, Monday through Friday, for telephone access.

00 01 02
3 4 5 6 7 8 9 10

Preface

We are extremely pleased to publish the Second Edition of the Hypertension Primer. In the preface to the First Edition, we quoted Webster's where a primer was defined as a "small introductory book on a subject." Though each chapter was small and introductory, the book itself provided a comprehensive look at the science and art of understanding hypertension and treating hypertensive patients. Having received many favorable comments on the First Edition, we knew that there was strong support for this work and for this format. Though our original intention was to create an easy-to-read and focused resource for students and house officers, it has turned out that many specialists have commented that they, too, have been able to find information in specific areas of hypertension that otherwise would have escaped their notice. Because hypertension is a special area of medicine that spans the very basics of basic science, population science, diagnostics, and therapeutics (both nonpharmacological and pharmacological), perhaps we shouldn't have been surprised that our "specialist" colleagues found the primer so useful, especially in areas in which they were not experts.

Thus, we have adhered faithfully to the format developed for the First Edition but we feel that the Second Edition is substantially improved. We have taken pains to stratify information into three rather than five basic categories: basic science, population science, and clinical management. The members and fellows of the AHA Council for High Blood Pressure Research have again rallied behind the project and have provided state-of-the-art short chapters that cover an enormous variety of basic and clinical topics related to hypertension, its pathogenesis, epidemiology, impact, and management. Some new chapters have been added and all have been revised to reflect new developments in the field. Each of these chapters could be viewed as a fragment of a larger and more traditional article and one that would include the full spectrum of information on the subject. The short chapter format avoids many of the redundancies that can occur in a standard textbook and increased the number of experts whose opinions and expertise are contained in the book. The net result is that more state-of-the-art information is included and that the format of the information is more consistent. Creating this matrix arrangement has been a major editorial challenge but one that we believe has been successfully accomplished through the splendid hard work of the section editors (Drs. Theodore Goodfriend, James Sowers, Jeffrey Cutler, Theodore Kotchen, Dominic Sica, Sheldon Sheps, and Donald Vidt) and the project staff.

We have had critical support from a number of different people without whose help this project would never have been completed. Our special thanks go out to the more than 200 distinguished authors who contributed to the Primer. We are very grateful to Astra Pharmaceuticals, especially to Dr. Warren Cooper, for the unrestricted educational grant that made the Second Edition of the Primer possible. We remain deeply indebted to Drs. Jan Breslow and Martha Hill, who were the President and President-elect, respectively, of the American Heart Association when this book was planned and developed and to Dr. Rod Starke and Dr. Kathryn Taubert and the staff of the American Heart Association for their continued support of the project. The dedication of the production managers, Kathleen Jun and Julie Kostyo, has made an enormous difference in the quality and consistency of the chapters. Without these two individuals, the book would not have been possible. The assistance of Lippincott Williams & Wilkins as a publisher and the work of Jennifer Kullgren and her staff have also been exemplary and crucial to the book's success. We are also indebted to Dr. Richard Charles, who helped develop the JNC VI practice guidelines included in the front inside cover of this book.

As always, beauty is in the eye of the beholder. The impact of this work will depend largely on its ability to be helpful to our readers. We believe that many different types of trainees and healthcare providers can use this information in the format presented and all scientists and clinicians can profit from the correlation of information provided. Please let us know what you think.

Joseph L. Izzo, M.D.
Henry R. Black, M.D.
August 22, 1998

Preface from First Edition

Webster defines a primer as a "small introductory book on a subject." With several high-quality specialty journals devoted to hypertension and many excellent textbooks available, why do we need a Hypertension Primer? The answer to that question lies in several linked issues. There has been an explosion of knowledge about the basic biology and physiology of hypertension. When this information is combined with concurrent dramatic advances in molecular genetics and epidemiology and an increased number of effective antihypertensives, it has become virtually impossible for physicians, scientists, and trainees to access (let alone master) the fundamental knowledge that is relevant to hypertension. The result is a worsening of the fragmented nature of hypertension knowledge today. Despite these dramatic advances and despite the clinical importance of hypertension, which remains the most common reason why Americans visit physicians, there are few attempts to integrate clinical and scientific information. In most medical schools, hypertension is taught in a piecemeal fashion in such courses as biochemistry, physiology, pathology, pharmacology, and epidemiology, as well as in clinical medicine, pediatrics, and surgery. Such curricular fragmentation is further reinforced by organ-oriented subspecialists, who generally deal with a small part of the larger whole and who tend to view high blood pressure only in light of their particular interest. For that matter, no single author or editor can include the mass of relevant information in a single standard textbook. Thus, a primer becomes a useful tool.

Yet how can an intrinsically fragmented Primer assist in integration of information? The answer to that question lies in the matrix organization of the information presented. The Hypertension Primer has been designed to provide ready access to basic, essential information, both new and old. We capitalized on the expertise of numerous members of the Council for High Blood Pressure Research of the American Heart Association. Authors were asked to write short, concise chapters highlighting their own areas of expertise in well-defined aspects of the field. No chapter in the primer is a full review of current information; rather, each chapter represents selected key concepts about the subject assigned. Authors were asked not to reference these concepts in full but rather to suggest additional reading for those who wish to probe the subject further. Key concepts have been highlighted in each chapter's "bullet points," which summarize the key factors discussed. This condensed format engendered a continuing challenge and tension among those who wanted to provide a complete perspective in each chapter (as a standard textbook does) and those who favored presenting smaller, more digestible segments of the information for discussion. We hope our final result provides elements of both.

It is hoped that this condensed matrix format will be conducive to different styles of self-education and will be suitable for both novices and subspecialist experts who wish to gain access to information in an otherwise unfamiliar area. The Primer is organized in a three-dimensional matrix to permit access to linked fields from any part. The reader can begin with a clinical question and work backward to basic science or vice versa. The first level of organization is the five major sections: biochemistry and cell biology; pathophysiology; epidemiology and prevention; diagnosis; and treatment. Each section is further divided into subsections that represent major themes related to 41 diverse thematic concerns, including "endogenous vasodilators," "angiotensins," "stress and hypertension," and many others. Finally, each chapter is cross-referenced with other linked areas in different sections of the book to provide different "learning paths." Thus, chapters can be read in sequence, can be approached in any order, or can be read simply one at a time, so as to provide basic information on a limited subject. The index also reinforces these interchapter links by providing a grouping of chapters as well as specific pages under the key words used for indexing. The book also features extensive diagrams and tables. Perhaps the most remarkable thing about the Hypertension Primer was that it was completed in less than a year. Senior Editors and Section Editors reviewed contributions from almost 200 internationally recognized North American experts. The use of this concise format allowed relatively rapid chapter completion.

In the end, the credit for the work belongs to its authors and the section editors. Without their help and especially without the extraordinary dedication of Dr. Kathryn Taubert of the American Heart Association, who provided scientific and administrative support, the Primer never would have been completed. We are also very grateful for the efforts of Starr Wheelan, project manager, the editorial services staff, and the word processing staff at the American Heart Association and to Julieann Kostyo of the Clinical Pharmacology Program at the State University of New York at Buffalo for their enormous organizational efforts. There was consistent scientific support for the project as well, particularly from Dr. Edward Frohlich, former Chairman of the Council on High Blood Pressure Research, and Dr. Theodore Kotchen, former Chairman of the Professional Education Committee of the Council on High Blood Pressure Research, and Dr. Edward Roccella of the National High Blood Pressure Education Program. Drs. Allen Cowley, Aram Chobanian, and Patrick Mulrow as well as the Executive Committee of the Council worked closely with us during the planning and implementation phases of the project and gave us invaluable guidance and support. Finally, without the cooperation of Hoechst-Roussel Pharmaceuticals and The Upjohn Company, we would not have been able to provide this book to you. Their educational grant supported the project, but the editors, authors, and other members of the Council are totally responsible for the editorial content of the Hypertension Primer.

We hope we have succeeded in providing a "small introductory book" for medical students and students of medicine. We would be glad to receive your comments on how we might improve it in the future and whether or not we have achieved our goal of providing a readable, easy-to-use digest of both the breadth and the depth of information available in the field of high blood pressure.

Joseph L. Izzo Jr, MD
Henry R. Black, MD
October 6, 1993

Contents

Part A: BASIC SCIENCE

Vasoactive Substances

1 **Adrenergic and Dopaminergic Receptors and Actions** 3
   Kathleen H. Berecek, PhD; Robert M. Carey, MD

2 **Catecholamine Synthesis, Release, Reuptake and Metabolism** 7
   Richard Weinshilboum, MD

3 **Angiotensins: Actions and Receptors** 11
   Theodore L. Goodfriend, MD

4 **Angiotensinogen** 14
   Morton P. Printz, PhD

5 **Renin Synthesis and Release** 16
   William H. Beierwaltes, PhD

6 **Angiotensin I–Converting Enzyme** 19
   Randal A. Skidgel, PhD; Ervin G. Erdös, MD

7 **Angiotensin Formation and Degradation** 21
   Carlos M. Ferrario, MD

8 **Tissue Renin-Angiotensin Systems** 23
   M. Ian Phillips, PhD, DSc

9 **Mineralocorticoid Receptors and Actions** 25
   David J. Morris, DPhil; Charles O. Watlington, MD

10 **Aldosterone and Other Mineralocorticoid Synthesis and Regulation** 26
   Celso E. Gomez-Sanchez, MD

11 **Cardiovascular Effects of Sex Steroids** 28
   David C. Kem, MD

12 **Prostaglandins and P450 Metabolites** 30
   John C. McGiff, MD; Alberto Nasjletti, MD

13 **Lipoxygenase Products** 33
   Jerry L. Nadler, MD

14 **Cardiovascular Effects of Fatty Acids** 35
   Brent M. Egan, MD

15 **Endothelin** 36
   Ernesto L. Schiffrin, MD, PhD

16 **Vasopressin and Neuropeptide Y** 38
   Allen W. Cowley, Jr, PhD

17 **Kinins** 40
   Oscar A. Carretero, MD

18 **Endogenous Natriuretic Peptides** 42
   John C. Burnett, Jr, MD; Yorman Shenker, MD

19 **Nitric Oxide** 44
   Ferid Murad, MD, PhD; R. Clinton Webb, PhD

20 **Acetylcholine, GABA, Serotonin, Adenosine, and Endogenous Quabain** 47
   Roger J. Grekin, MD; John M. Hamlyn, PhD

21 **Adrenomedullin-Derived Peptides and CGRP** 50
   Willis K. Samson, PhD

Cell Physiology

22 **Membrane Sodium Transport** 51
   Alan B. Weder, MD

23 **Intracellular pH and Cell Volume** 53
   Bradford C. Berk, MD, PhD

24 **Cellular Potassium Transport** 56
   Jason Xiao-Jian Yuan, MD, PhD; Mordecai P. Blaustein, MD

25 **Calcium Transport and Calmodulin** 58
   David J. Triggle, PhD

26 **Signal Transduction: Receptors** 61
   Greti Aguilera, MD

27 **Signal Transduction: Guanine Nucleotide Binding Proteins** 63
   James C. Garrison, PhD

28 **Signal Transduction: Cyclic Nucleotides** 66
   Kevin J. Catt, MD, PhD; Tamas Balla, MD, PhD

29 **Signal Transduction: Inositol Phosphates** 69
   Kevin J. Catt, MD, PhD; Tamas Balla, MD, PhD

30 **Signal Transduction: Protein Phosphorylation** . . 71
   George W. Booz, PhD; Kenneth M. Baker, MD

31 **Adhesion Molecules** 76
   Willa A. Hsueh, MD

32 **Vascular Smooth Muscle Contraction and Relaxation** 78
   Anna F. Dominiczak, MD; David F. Bohr, MD

Vasoregulatory Systems

33 **Functional Neuroanatomy of Central Vasomotor Control Centers** 80
   Donald J. Reis, MD

34 **Arterial Baroreflexes** 83
   Mark W. Chapleau, PhD

35 **Cardiopulmonary Baroreflexes** 87
   Pramod K. Mohanty, MD

36 **Renal Nerves and ECF Volume Regulation** 89
   Jeffrey L. Osborn, PhD; Suzanne G. Greenberg, PhD

37 **Systemic Hemodynamics and Regional Blood Flow Regulation** 92
   Thomas G. Coleman, PhD; John E. Hall, PhD

38 **Autoregulation of Blood Flow** 95
   Richard J. Roman, PhD

Pathophysiology of Essential Hypertension

39 **Monogenic Determinants of Blood Pressure: Adrenal Steroid Disorders** 98
   Robert G. Dluhy, MD

40 **Polygenic Determinants of Blood Pressure** . . . 101
   George T. Cicila, PhD

41 **Renin-Angiotensin Genetics** 104
   James R. Sowers, MD

42 **Sympathetic Nervous System Abnormalities in Hypertension** 106
   J. Michael Wyss, PhD

43 **The Sympathetic Nervous System in Human Hypertension** 109
    Joseph L. Izzo, Jr, MD

44 **Hyperkinetic Hypertension and Vascular Hyperresponsiveness** 113
    Mark A. Creager, MD; Marie D. Gerhard, MD

45 **Hemodynamic Profiles and Responses** 115
    Fetnat Fouad-Tarazi, MD; Joseph L. Izzo, Jr, MD

46 **Obesity** 118
    Lewis Landsberg, MD

47 **Insulin Resistance and Hypertension** 121
    Helmut O. Steinberg, MD

48 **Salt Sensitivity** 123
    Myron H. Weinberger, MD

49 **Divalent Cations in Essential Hypertension** . . . 125
    Lawrence M. Resnick, MD

50 **Experimental Models of Hypertension** 128
    Donald J. DiPette, MD

Pathophysiology of Secondary Hypertension

51 **Pathophysiology of Renovascular Hypertension** 131
    Luis Gabriel Navar, PhD; David W. Ploth, MD

52 **Pathophysiology of Renal Parenchymal Hypertension** 135
    Vito M. Campese, MD

53 **Pathophysiology of Adrenal Cortical Hypertension** 138
    Burl R. Don, MD; Morris Schambelan, MD

54 **Pathophysiology of Pheochromocytoma** 141
    William M. Manger, MD, PhD

55 **HTN Caused by Thyroids and Parathyroid Abnormalities and Acromegaly** 143
    Yoram Shenker, MD

56 **Coarctation of the Aorta** 146
    Albert P. Rocchini, MD

57 **Pathophysiology of Sleep Apnea** 148
    Barbara J. Morgan, PhD

58 **Affective Illness and Hypertension** 150
    Wayne L. Creelman, MD, MMM, FAPA

59 **Pathophysiology of Preeclampsia** 152
    Ellen W. Seely, MD; Marshall D. Lindheimer, MD

60 **Hypertension and Transplantation** 155
    Stephen C. Textor, MD

Mechanisms of Target Organ Damage

61 **Mechanisms of Vascular Hypertrophy** 157
    Paul R. Standley, PhD

62 **Arterial Stiffness and Hypertension** 160
    Michael F. O'Rourke, MD, DSc

63 **Oxidative Stress and Hypertension** 163
    David G. Harrison, MD; Zorina Galis, PhD; Sampath Parthasarathy, PhD; Kathy K. Griendling, PhD

64 **Endothelial Dysfunction** 167
    James R. Sowers, MD; Joseph L. Izzo, Jr, MD

65 **Atherogenesis** 170
    John P. Cooke, MD, PhD

66 **Microvascular Regulation and Dysregulation** 173
    Andrew S. Greene, PhD

Sequelae of Hypertension

67 **Pathogenesis of Coronary Artery Disease** 175
    Charles K. Francis, MD

68 **Pathogensis of Left Ventricular Hypertrophy and Diastolic Dysfunction** 177
    Joseph L. Izzo, Jr, MD

69 **Pathogenesis of Congestive Heart Failure** 180
    Edmund H. Sonnenblick, MD; Thierry H. LeJemtel, MD

70 **Pathogenesis of Stroke** 183
    Patrick Pullicino, MD, PhD

71 **Pathogenesis of Acute Hypertensive Encephalopathy** 186
    Donald D. Heistad, MD; William J. Lawton, MD

72 **Pathogenesis of Vascular Disease and Mixed Dementia** 188
    Linda A. Hershey, MD, PhD

73 **Pathogenesis of Hypertensive Renal Damage** . . 190
    Sharon Anderson, MD

74 **The Eye in Hypertension** 194
    Robert N. Frank, MD

Part B: **POPULATION SCIENCE**

Cardiovascular Risk and Hypertension

75 **Cardiovascular Risk Factors and Hypertension** 199
    William B. Kannel, MD; Peter W.F. Wilson, MD

76 **Cerebrovascular Risk** 203
    Philip A. Wolf, MD

77 **Left Vertricular Hypertrophy Prognosis** 208
    Daniel Levy, MD

78 **Renal Risk** 211
    Michael J. Klag, MD, MPH

79 **Peripheral Arterial Disease and Hypertension** 215
    Michael H. Criqui, MD, MPH; Julie O. Denenberg, MA; Robert D. Langer, MD, MPH; Arnost Fronek, MD, PhD; Gloria Bensussen, MD, MPH

80 **Genetics and Family History of Hypertension** 218
    Steven C. Hunt, PhD; Roger R. Williams, MD

81 **Gene-Enviroment Interactions** 222
    Anne E. Kwitek-Black, PhD; Howard J. Jacob, PhD

Impact of Hypertension: Globally and Special Populations

82 **Geographic Patterns of Hypertension: A Global Perspective** 224
Richard S. Cooper, MD

83 **Geographic Patterns of Hypertension in the United States** 226
W. Dallas Hall, MD

84 **Gender and Blood Pressure** 229
David A. Calhoun, MD; Suzanne Oparil, MD

85 **Blood Pressure in Children** 233
Alan R. Sinaiko, MD

86 **The Elderly Patient with Hypertension** 236
William B. Applegate, MD, MPH

87 **Ethnicity and Socioeconomic Status in Hypertension** 239
John M. Flack, MD, MPH; Beth A. Staffileno, DNSc;
Carla Yunis, MD, MPH

88 **Socioeconomic Status and Blood Pressure** . . . 242
Daniel W. Jones, MD

Lifestyle Factors and Blood Pressure

89 **Overall Dietary Patterns and Blood Pressure** 244
Frank M. Sacks, MD

90 **Salt and Blood Pressure** 247
Norman M. Kaplan, MD

91 **Potassium and Blood Pressure** 250
Paul K. Whelton, MD, MSc

92 **Calcium, Magnesium, and Blood Pressure** 253
Lawrence J. Appel, MD, MPH

93 **Obesity, Body Fat Distribution, and Insulin Resistance: Clinical Relevance** 256
Steven M. Haffner, MD

94 **Physical Activity, Fitness, and Blood Pressure** 259
Denise G. Simons-Morton, MD, PhD

95 **Alcohol Use and Blood Pressure** 263
William C. Cushman, MD

96 **Psychosocial Stress and Blood Pressure** 266
Thomas G. Pickering, MD, DPhil

Prevention and Control

97 **Trends in Blood Pressure Control and Mortality** 268
Thomas J. Thom, BA; Edward J. Roccella, PhD, MPH

98 **Hypertension: A Worldwide Epidemic** 271
Patrick J. Mulrow, MD

99 **Prevention of Hypertension** 274
Jeffrey A. Cutler, MD, MPH; Jeremiah Stamler, MD

100 **Treatment Trials: Morbidity and Mortality** 279
Bruce M. Psaty, MD, PhD; Curt D. Furberg, MD, PhD

101 **Antihypertensive Treatment Trials: Quality of Life** 283
Richard H. Grimm, Jr, MD, PhD

102 **Economic Impact of Blood Pressure** 286
William B. Stason, MD, MSc

103 **Economic Considerations in the Management of Hypertension** 289
William J. Elliott, MD, PhD

Part C: CLINICAL MANAGEMENT

General Diagnostic Aspects

104 **Blood Pressure Measurement** 295
Carlene M. Grim, RN, MSN, SpDN; Clarence E. Grim, MS, MD

105 **Initial Workup of the Hypertensive Patient** . . . 299
Marvin Moser, MD

106 **Out of Office Blood Pressure Monitoring** 302
William B. White, MD

107 **Genetic Profiling in Hypertension** 306
Haralambos Gavras, MD

Evaluation of Target Organs

108 **Neurological Evaluation in Hypertension** 308
Stephen J. Phillips, MBBS, FRCPC; Irene Meissner, MD, FRCPC

109 **Basic Cardiac Evaluation: Physical Examination, Electrocardiogram, and Chest Radiograph** . . . 311
Clarence Shub, MD; John A. Rumberger, PhD, MD

110 **Cardiac Imaging** 313
Clarence Shub, MD; John A. Rumberger, PhD, MD

111 **Exercise Stress Testing** 317
Michael F. Wilson, MD; Mofid N. Khalil Ibrahim, MD, PhD

112 **Evaluation of Renal Parenchymal Disease** 320
Michael A. Moore, MD

113 **Evaluation of the Peripheral Circulation** 323
Jeffrey W. Olin, DO

114 **Evaluation of Arterial Compliance** 327
Gary E. McVeigh, MD, PhD

115 **Evaluation of Aortocarotid Baroreflexes** 330
Addison Taylor, MD, PhD

Principles of Management

116 **Approach to Treatment of the Hypertensive Patient** 333
Ray W. Gifford, Jr, MD

117 **Treatment Goals in the Hypertensive Patient** 337
Kenneth Jamerson, MD

118 **Lifestyle Modifications** 339
Theodore A. Kotchen, MD; Jane Morley Kotchen, MD, MPH

xi

119 **Dose-Response Relationship and Dose Adjustments** 342
Domenic A. Sica, MD; Todd W.B. Gehr, MD

120 **Variability in Individual Responses to Antihypertensive Drugs** 345
Joseph L. Izzo, Jr, MD

121 **Adherence to Antihypertensive Therapy** 348
Martha N. Hill, RN, PhD

122 **When to Refer Patients for Hypertensive Consultation** 352
Gary L. Schwartz, MD

123 **Managment of Patients with Refractory Hypertension** 354
Henry R. Black, MD

Antihypertensive Drugs

124 **Diuretics** 358
Jules B. Puschett, MD

125 **Beta Adrenergic Blockers** 362
William H. Frishman, MD

126 **Alpha Adrenergic Blockers** 366
Richard H. Grimm, Jr, MD, PhD

127 **Alpha-Beta Adrenergic Blockers** 368
Mahboob Rahman, MD, MPH; Jackson T. Wright, Jr, MD, PhD

128 **Central and Peripheral Sympatholytics** 370
Barry J. Materson, MD, MBA

129 **Angiotensin-Converting Enzyme Inhibitors** ... 372
Domenic A. Sica, MD; Elizabeth Ripley, MD

130 **Angiotensin II Receptor Blockers** 377
Michael A. Weber, MD

131 **Dihydropyridine Calcium Antagonists** 379
Matthew R. Weir, MD

132 **Non-Dihydropyridine Calcium Antagonists** ... 382
T. Barry Levine, MD; Domenic A. Sica, MD

133 **Direct Vasodilators** 385
C. Venkata S. Ram, MD

134 **Other Agents: Potassium Channel Openers, Serotonin-Related Agents, Dopamine Agonists, Renin Inhibitors, Imidazolines, Neutral Endopeptidase Inhibitors, and Endothelin-Receptor Antagonists** 388
William J. Elliott, MD, PhD

Managing Hypertension (Target Organ Damage)

135 **Management of Orthostatic Hypotension, Hypertension, and Tachycardia** 390
David H.P. Streeten, MB, DPhil, FRCP

136 **Management of Baroreflex Failure** 393
David Robertson, MD

137 **Management of Hypertensive Patients with Cerebrovascular Disease** 396
Robert D. Brown, Jr, MD

138 **Management of Hypertensive Patients with Ischemic Heart Disease** 398
Jay M. Sullivan, MD, Charles K. Francis, MD

139 **Management of Hypertensive Patients with Left Ventricular Hypertrophy and Diastolic Dysfunction** 402
Edward D. Frohlich, MD

140 **Management of Hypertensive Patients with Dilated Cardiomyopathy (Systolic Dysfunction)** 405
Jay N. Cohn, MD

141 **Management of Hypertensive Patients with Chronic Renal Insufficiency** 407
Marc A. Pohl, MD

142 **Management of Hypertensive Patients with Peripheral Arterial Disease** 410
Jeffrey W. Olin, DO

Management of Special Populations

143 **Management of Minority Patients with Hypertension** 413
Keith C. Ferdinand, MD

144 **Management of the Obese Hypertensive Patient** 415
Efrain Reisen, MD

145 **Management of the Hypertensive Patient with Lipid and Lipoprotein Abnormalities** 418
Michael D. Cressman, DO

146 **Treatment of Hypertensive Patients with Diabetic Nephropathy** 421
George L. Bakris, MD

147 **Management of Hypertensive Children and Adolescents** 424
Bonita Falkner, MD

148 **Management of Pregnant Hypertensive Patients** 427
Phyllis August, MD

149 **Management of Hypertension in Older Persons** 430
Henry R. Black, MD

150 **Management of Borderline Hypertension** 433
Stevo Julius, MD

151 **Management of Hypertensive Emergencies and Urgencies** 437
Donald G. Vidt, MD

152 **Workplace Management of Hypertension** 441
Michael H. Alderman, MD

Management of Secondary Hypertension

153 **Management of Renovascular Hypertension** 443
Joseph V. Nally, Jr, MD

154 **Management of Pheochromocytoma** 446
William F. Young, Jr, MD; Sheldon G. Sheps, MD

155 **Management of Hypercortisolism and Hyperaldosteronism** 449
Emmanuel L. Bravo, MD

156 **Management of Thyroid and Parathyroid Disorders** 454
William F. Young, Jr, MD

157 **Management of Sleep Apnea** 456
Paul D. Levinson, MD; Richard P. Millman, MD

158 **Management of Drug-Induced and Iatrogenic Hypertension** 458
Ehud Grossman, MD; Franz H. Messerli, MD

Index 463

Contributors

Greti Aguilera, MD
Chief, Section on Endocrine Physiology
Developmental Endocrinology Branch
National Institutes of Child Health and Human Development
National Institutes of Health
Bethesda, Maryland

Michael H. Alderman, MD
Professor of Medicine and Epidemiology and Social Medicine
Albert Einstein College of Medicine
Department of Epidemiology and Social Medicine
Bronx, New York

Sharon Anderson, MD
Professor of Medicine
Associate Head, Division of Nephrology
Oregon Health Sciences University
Portland, Oregon

Lawrence J. Appel, MD, MPH
Associate Professor of Medicine, Epidemiology, and International Health
Johns Hopkins Medical Institutions
Baltimore, Maryland

William B. Applegate, MD, MPH
Professor and Chairman of Preventive Medicine
University of Tennessee, Memphis
Memphis, Tennessee

Phyllis August, MD
Department of Medicine
Chief, Hypertension Division
Cornell University Medical College
New York, New York

Kenneth M. Baker, MD
Professor of Cellular and Molecular Physiology and Medicine
Penn State College of Medicine
Weis Center for Research
Danville, Pennsylvania

George L. Bakris, MD
Associate Professor of Preventive and Internal Medicine
Vice Chairman, Department of Preventive Medicine
Director, Rush Hypertension Program and Clinical Research Center
Rush Presbyterian/St. Luke's Medical Center
Chicago, Illinois

Tamas Balla, MD, PhD
Senior Investigator, Endocrinology and Reproduction Research Branch
NICHD, National Institutes of Health
Bethesda, Maryland

William H. Beierwaltes, PhD
Associate Professor of Medicine
Senior Staff Scientist, Hypertension and Vascular Research Division
Henry Ford Hospital and Health Sciences Center
Case Western Reserve Detroit Medical Campus
Detroit, Michigan

Gloria E. Bensussen, MD, MPH
Clinical Research Associate, Venous Study
University of California, San Diego
La Jolla, California

Kathleen H. Berecek, PhD
Professor of Physiology and Biophysics
Associate Scientist, Vascular Biology
 and Hypertension Research Center
Senior Scientist, Cell Adhesion and Matrix Research Center
University of Alabama at Birmingham
Birmingham, Alabama

Bradford C. Berk, MD, PhD
Paul Yu Professor of Medicine
Chief, Cardiology Unit
Director, Cardiovascular Research Center
University of Rochester School of Medicine and Dentistry
Rochester, New York

Henry R. Black, MD
Charles J. and Margaret Roberts Professor and Chairman,
Department of Preventive Medicine
Professor, Internal Medicine
Rush-Presbyterian-St. Luke's Medical Center
Chicago, Illinois

Mordecai P. Blaustein, MD
Professor and Chairman, Department of Physiology
University of Maryland School of Medicine
Baltimore, Maryland

David F. Bohr, MD
Professor, Physiology
University of Michigan Medical School
Ann Arbor, Michigan

George W. Booz, PhD
Assistant Professor of Cellular and Molecular Physiology
Penn State College of Medicine
Weis Center for Research
Danville, Pennsylvania

Emmanuel L. Bravo, MD
Staff, Department of Nephrology and Hypertension
Division of Internal Medicine
Cleveland Clinic Foundation
Cleveland, Ohio

Robert D. Brown, Jr, MD
Consultant, Department of Neurology, Mayo Clinic
Associate Professor of Neurology, Mayo Medical School
Rochester, Minnesota

John C. Burnett, Jr, MD
Professor of Medicine and Physiology
Director of Cardiorenal Research Laboratory
Mayo Clinic
Rochester, Minnesota

David A. Calhoun, MD
Assistant Professor of Medicine
University of Alabama at Birmingham
Birmingham, Alabama

Vito M. Campese, MD
Professor of Medicine
Associate Chief, Division of Nephrology
University of Southern California
Los Angeles, California

Robert M. Carey, MD
James Carroll Flippin Professor of Medical Science
Dean, School of Medicine
University of Virginia
Charlottesville, Virginia

Oscar A. Carretero, MD
Division Head, Hypertension and Vascular Research Division
Henry Ford Health Sciences Center
Professor of Medicine,
Henry Ford Health Sciences Center/Case Western Reserve University
Detroit, Michigan

Kevin J. Catt, MD, PhD
Chief, Endocrinology and Reproduction
Research Branch
National Institute of Child Health and Human Development
National Institutes of Health
Bethesda, Maryland

Mark W. Chapleau, PhD
Associate Professor, Internal Medicine
University of Iowa
Research Health Science Specialist
Veterans Affairs Medical Center
Iowa City, Iowa

George T. Cicila, PhD
Assistant Professor, Physiology and Molecular Medicine
Medical College of Ohio
Toledo, Ohio

Jay N. Cohn, MD
Professor of Medicine
University of Minnesota Medical School
Minneapolis, Minnesota

Thomas G. Coleman, PhD
Professor Emeritus, Physiology and Biophysics
University of Mississippi Medical Center
Jackson, Mississippi

John P. Cooke, MD, PhD
Associate Professor and Director, Section of Vascular Medicine
Stanford University School of Medicine
Stanford, California

Richard S. Cooper, MD
Professor and Chair
Preventive Medicine and Epidemiology
Loyola University, Chicago
Maywood, Illinois

Alan W. Cowley, Jr, PhD
Professor and Chairman
Department of Physiology
Medical College of Wisconsin
Milwaukee, Wisconsin

Mark A. Creager, MD
Associate Professor of Medicine, Harvard Medical School
Cardiovascular Division, Brigham & Women's Hospital
Boston, Massachusetts

Wayne Lewis Creelman, MD, MMM, FAPA
Corporate Medical Director/COO
Brylin Hospitals
Buffalo, New York

Michael D. Cressman, DO
Associate Professor of Medicine
University of Pittsburgh School of Medicine
Director, Clinical Trials Program
Center for Clinical Pharmacology
Pittsburgh, Pennsylvania

Michael H. Criqui, MD, MPH
Professor, Departments of Family and Preventive Medicine and Medicine
Director, Preventive Cardiology Academic Award
University of California, San Diego
La Jolla, California

William C. Cushman, MD
Professor of Preventive Medicine and Medicine
University of Tennessee College of Medicine
Memphis, Tennessee

Jeffrey A. Cutler, MD, MPH
Director, Clinical Applications and Prevention Program
Division of Epidemiology and Clinical Applications
National Heart, Lung, and Blood Institute
Bethesda, Maryland

Julie O. Denenberg, MA
Staff Research Associate II
Department of Family and Preventive Medicine
School of Medicine
University of California, San Diego
San Diego, California

Donald J. DiPette, MD
Professor of Medicine
Director, Division of General Internal Medicine
Vice Chair for Inpatient Clinical Affairs
University of Texas Medical Branch
Galveston, Texas

Robert G. Dluhy, MD
Professor of Medicine
Harvard Medical School
Senior Physician
Brigham and Women's Hospital
Boston, Massachusetts

Anna F. Dominiczak, MD
British Heart Foundation Professor of Cardiovascular Medicine
University of Glasgow
Scotland, United Kingdom

Burl R. Don, MD
Associate Professor of Medicine
Medical Director, University of California Renal Center
San Francisco, California

Brent M. Egan, MD
Professor of Pharmacology and Medicine
Medical University of South Carolina
Charleston, South Carolina

William J. Elliott, MD, PhD
Associate Professor of Preventive Medicine
Rush Medical College of Rush University
Rush-Presbyterian-St. Luke's Medical Center
Chicago, Illinois

Ervin G. Erdös, MD
Professor, Departments of Pharmacology and Anesthesiology
University of Illinois, College of Medicine
Chicago, Illinois

Bonita Falkner, MD
Professor of Medicine and Pediatrics
Allegheny University of the Health Sciences
Philadelphia, Pennsylvania

Keith C. Ferdinand, MD, FACC
Medical Director, Heartbeats Life Center
Associate Professor of Clinical Pharmacology
Xavier University College of Pharmacy
New Orleans, Louisiana

Carlos M. Ferrario, MD
Director, Hypertension and Vascular Disease Center
Professor of Surgery, Nephrology and Physiology/Pharmacology
Dewitt Cordell Professor of Surgical Research
Wake Forest University School of Medicine
Winston-Salem, North Carolina

John M. Flack, MD, MPH
Associate Chairman, Department of Internal Medicine
Director, Cardiovascular Epidemiology and Clinical Applications Program
Professor of Medicine and Community Medicine
Wayne State University Medical School and the Detroit Medical Center
Detroit, Michigan

Fetnat H. Fouad-Tarazi, MD
Department of Cardiology/Imaging Section
Head, Syncope Clinic
Hemodynamic-Neuroregulatory Lab
Cleveland Clinic Foundation
Cleveland, Ohio

Charles K. Francis, MD
Professor of Clinical Medicine
College of Physicians & Surgeons
Columbia University
Director, Department of Medicine
Head, Urban Health Institute
Harlem Hospital Center
New York, New York

Robert N. Frank, MD
Professor of Ophthalmology
Professor of Anatomy and Cell Biology
Kresge Eye Institute
Wayne State University School of Medicine
Detroit, Michigan

William H. Frishman, MD
Professor and Chairman, Department of Medicine
Professor of Pharmacology, New York Medical College
Director of Medicine, Westchester Medical Center
Valhalla, New York

Edward D. Frohlich, MD
Vice President for Academic Affairs
Alton Ochsner Distinguished Scientist
Alton Ochsner Medical Foundation
New Orleans, Louisiana

Arnost Fronek, MD, PhD
Professor, Department of Surgery and Bioengineering
University of California, San Diego
La Jolla, California

Curt D. Furberg, MD, PhD
Professor and Chair, Department of Public Health Sciences
Wake Forest University School of Medicine
Winston-Salem, North Carolina

Zorina S. Galis, PhD
Assistant Professor of Medicine and Biology
Emory University School of Medicine and
Georgia Institute of Technology
Atlanta, Georgia

James C. Garrison, PhD
Professor and Chair
Department of Pharmacology
University of Virginia School of Medicine
Health Sciences Center
Charlottesville, Virginia

Haralambos Gavras, MD
Professor of Medicine
Chief, Hypertension and Atherosclerosis Section
Director, Specialized Center of Research in Molecular Genetics
    of Hypertension
Boston University School of Medicine
Boston, Massachusetts

Todd W.B. Gehr, MD
Associate Professor of Internal Medicine
Virginia Commonwealth University
Richmond, Virginia

Marie D. Gerhard, MD
Vascular Clinical Center
Associate Physician
Brigham & Women's Hospital
Harvard Medical School
Boston, Massachusetts

Ray W. Gifford, Jr, MD
Consultant, Department of Nephrology &
    Hypertension
Cleveland Clinic Foundation
Cleveland, Ohio
Professor of Internal Medicine
Ohio State University
Columbus, Ohio

Celso E. Gomez-Sanchez, MD
Professor of Internal Medicine
Harry S Truman Memorial Veterans Hospital
University of Missouri–Columbia
Columbia, Missouri

Theodore L. Goodfriend, MD
Professor of Medicine and Pharmacology
University of Wisconsin
Associate Chief of Staff for Research
William S. Middleton Veterans Hospital
Madison, Wisconsin

Andrew S. Greene, PhD
Professor of Physiology
Medical College of Wisconsin
Milwaukee, Wisconsin

Suzanne G. Greenberg, PhD
Assistant Professor, Obstetrics and Gynecology
University of Cincinnati
Cincinnati, Ohio

Roger J. Grekin, MD
Associate Chief of Staff for Research
Veterans Affairs Medical Center
Professor of Internal Medicine
University of Michigan
Ann Arbor, Michigan

Kathy K. Griendling, PhD
Associate Professor of Medicine
Emory University School of Medicine
Atlanta, Georgia

Carlene Minks Grim, BSN, MSN, SpDN
President, Shared Care Research and Education
Los Angeles, California
Research
Medical College of Wisconsin
Milwaukee, Wisconsin

Clarence E. Grim, MS, MD
Professor of Cardiovascular Medicine
Hypertension Research Program
Medical College of Wisconsin
Milwaukee, Wisconsin

Richard H. Grimm, Jr, MD, PhD
Director, Berman Center for Outcomes and Clinical
    Research
Hennepin County Medical Center
Professor of Medicine and Epidemiology
University of Minnesota
Minneapolis, Minnesota

Ehud Grossman, MD
Associate Professor of Medicine
Head, Internal Medicine Department
The Chaim Sheba Medical Center
Affiliated to the Tel-Aviv University
Tel-Hashomer, Israel

Steven Haffner, MD
Professor of Medicine
University of Texas Health Science Center
San Antonio, Texas

John E. Hall, PhD
Professor and Chairman
Physiology and Biophysics
University of Mississippi Medical Center
Jackson, Mississippi

W. Dallas Hall, MD, MACP
Professor of Medicine Emeritus
Emory University School of Medicine
Atlanta, Georgia

John M. Hamlyn, PhD
Associate Professor, Department of Physiology
University of Maryland at Baltimore
Baltimore, Maryland

David G. Harrison, MD
Professor of Medicine
Division of Cardiology
Emory University School of Medicine
Atlanta, Georgia

Donald D. Heistad, MD
Distinguished Professor, Internal Medicine and
    Pharmacology
Deputy Director, Iowa Cardiovascular Research Center
University of Iowa
Iowa City, Iowa

Linda A. Hershey, MD, PhD
Professor, Neurology and Pharmacology
Neurology Manager, VA WNY Healthcare System
State University of New York at Buffalo
Buffalo, New York

Martha N. Hill, RN, PhD
Professor
Johns Hopkins University School of Nursing
Baltimore, Maryland

Willa Hsueh, MD
Professor of Medicine
Chief, Division of Endocrinology, Diabetes and Hypertension
University of California, Los Angeles
Los Angeles, California

Steven C. Hunt, PhD
Professor of Medicine
University of Utah School of Medicine
Salt Lake City, Utah

Mofid N. Khalil Ibrahim, MD, PhD
Senior Cardiology Fellow
Department of Cardiovascular Medicine
CGF—Millard Fillmore Division
Buffalo, New York

Joseph L. Izzo, Jr, MD
Professor, Medicine and Pharmacology
Chief, Clinical Pharmacology
State University of New York at Buffalo
Buffalo, New York

Howard J. Jacob, PhD
Associate Professor
Department of Physiology, Medical College of Wisconsin
Milwaukee, Wisconsin

Kenneth A. Jamerson, MD
Associate Professor of Internal Medicine
University of Michigan Medical School
Ann Arbor, Michigan

Daniel W. Jones, MD
Professor of Medicine
Director, Division of Hypertension
Vice Chairman for Primary Care
University of Mississippi Medical Center
Jackson, Mississippi

Stevo Julius, MD, ScD
Professor of Medicine and Physiology
Frederick G.L. Huetwell Professor of Hypertension
University of Michigan Medical School
Ann Arbor, Michigan

William B. Kannel, MD, MPH, FACC
Professor of Medicine and Public Health
Boston University School of Medicine
Boston, Massachusetts

Norman M. Kaplan, MD
Professor of Internal Medicine
University of Texas–Southwestern Medical School
Dallas, Texas

David C. Kem, MD
Professor, Internal Medicine
Chief, Section of Endocrinology, Metabolism, and Hypertension
University of Oklahoma and VA Medical Center
Oklahoma City, Oklahoma

Michael J. Klag, MD, MPH
David M. Levine Professor, Medicine
Director, Division of General Internal Medicine
Johns Hopkins University School of Medicine
Baltimore, Maryland

Theodore A. Kotchen, MD
Professor and Chairman
Department of Medicine
Medical College of Wisconsin
Milwaukee, Wisconsin

Jane Morley Kotchen, MD, MPH
Professor, Division of Epidemiology
Medical College of Wisconsin
Milwaukee, Wisconsin

Anne E. Kwitek-Black, PhD
Research Scientist, Laboratory of Genetics Research
Department of Physiology
Medical College of Wisconsin
Milwaukee, Wisconsin

Lewis Landsberg, MD
Irving S. Cutter Professor and Chairman,
Department of Medicine
Physician-in-Chief
Northwestern University Medical School
Northwestern Memorial Hospital
Chicago, Illinois

Robert D. Langer, MD, MPH
Associate Professor, Family and Preventive Medicine
University of California–San Diego
La Jolla, California

William J. Lawton, MD
Associate Professor, Division of Nephrology
Medical Director, Renal Dialysis Treatment Center
Department of Internal Medicine
University of Iowa College of Medicine
Iowa City, Iowa

Thierry H. LeJemtel, MD
Professor of Medicine
Albert Einstein College of Medicine
Bronx, New York

T. Barry Levine, MD
Director, Michigan Institute for Heart Failure and
Transplant Care
Botsford General Hospital
Farmington Hills, Michigan
Professor of Medicine, University of Michigan
Ann Arbor, Michigan

Paul D. Levinson, MD
Associate Professor of Medicine
Endocrinology Division
Brown University School of Medicine
Providence, Rhode Island

Daniel Levy, MD
Director, Framingham Heart Study
National Heart, Lung, and Blood Institute
Framingham, Massachusetts

Marshall D. Lindheimer, MD, FACP, FRCOG
Professor, Departments of Medicine, Obstetrics and Gynecology, and Clinical
Pharmacology
University of Chicago
Chicago, Illinois

William Muir Manger, MD, PhD
Professor of Clinical Medicine, NYU Medical Center
Chairman of The National Hypertension
Association
Lecturer in Medicine, Columbia Medical Center
New York, New York

Barry J. Materson, MD, MBA
Professor of Medicine
University of Miami School of Medicine
Miami, Florida

John C. McGiff, MD
Professor and Chairman
Department of Pharmacology
New York Medical College
Valhalla, New York

Gary E. McVeigh, MD, PhD
Associate Professor of Medicine
University of Minnesota
Minneapolis, Minnesota

Irene Meissner, MD, FRCP(C)
Associate Professor of Neurology
Mayo Graduate School of Medicine
Mayo Clinic
Rochester, Minnesota

Franz H. Messerli, MD
Medical Director, Division of Research
Alton Ochsner Medical Foundation
New Orleans, Louisiana

Richard P. Millman, MD
Professor of Medicine
Brown University School of Medicine
Director, Sleep Disorders Center of Lifespan Hospitals
Rhode Island Hospital
Providence, Rhode Island

Pramod K. Mohanty, MD
Professor of Medicine, Virginia Commonwealth
    University
Chief, Cardiology Division, McGuire VA Medical Center
Richmond, Virginia

Michael A. Moore, MD
Nephrologist, Danville Urologic Clinic
Danville, Virginia
Associate Clinical Professor of Medicine
Wake Forest University School of Medicine
Winston-Salem, North Carolina

Barbara J. Morgan, PhD
Associate Professor, Department of Surgery
University of Wisconsin–Madison
Madison, Wisconsin

David J. Morris, DPhil
Professor of Pathology, Brown University School of Medicine
Director of Chemistry, The Miriam Hospital
Providence, Rhode Island

Marvin Moser, MD
Clinical Professor of Medicine, Yale University School of
    Medicine
Senior Medical Advisor, National High Blood Pressure Education
    Program
National Heart, Lung, and Blood Institute
Bethesda, Maryland

Patrick J. Mulrow, MD
Secretary General, World Hypertension League
Professor Emeritus, Medical College of Ohio
Toledo, Ohio

Ferid Murad, MD, PhD
Professor and Chairman
Department of Integrative Biology and Pharmacology
University of Texas–Houston Medical School
Houston, Texas

Jerry L. Nadler, MD
Director, Department of Diabetes and Endocrinology
City of Hope Medical Center
Duarte, California

Joseph V. Nally, Jr, MD
Staff Nephrologist
Department of Nephrology and Hypertension
Cleveland Clinic Foundation
Cleveland, Ohio

Alberto Nasjletti, MD
Professor of Medicine
New York Medical College
Valhalla, New York

L. Gabriel Navar, PhD
Professor and Chairman, Department of Physiology
Tulane University School of Medicine
New Orleans, Louisiana

Jeffrey W. Olin, DO
Chairman, Department of Vascular Medicine
Cleveland Clinic Foundation
Cleveland, Ohio

Suzanne Oparil, MD
Director, Vascular Biology and Hypertension Program of th
    Division of Cardiovascular Disease
Professor of Medicine
University of Alabama at Birmingham
Birmingham, Alabama

Michael F. O'Rourke, DSc, MD
Professor of Medicine, University of New South Wales
Cardiologist, St. Vincents Hospital
Sydney, Australia

Jeffrey L. Osborn, PhD
Associate Professor of Physiology
Director, MCW Center for Science Education
Medical College of Wisconsin
Milwaukee, Wisconsin

Sampath Parthasarathy, PhD
Professor of Gynecology and Obstetrics and Professor of Medicine
Emory University
Atlanta, Georgia

M. Ian Phillips, PhD, DSc
Professor and Chairman
University of Florida
Gainesville, Florida

Stephen J. Phillips, MBBS, FRCPC
Associate Professor of Medicine, Dalhousie University
Director, Acute Stroke Service
Queen Elizabeth II Health Sciences Centre
Halifax, Nova Scotia, Canada

Thomas G. Pickering, MD, DPhil
Professor of Medicine, Hypertension Center
New York Presbyterian Hospital
New York, New York

David W. Ploth, MD
A.V. Williams Jr Professor of Medicine
Director, Division of Nephrology
Medical University of South Carolina
Charleston, South Carolina

Marc A. Pohl, MD
Department of Nephrology and Hypertension
Cleveland Clinic Foundation
Cleveland, Ohio

Morton P. Printz, PhD
Professor, Department of Pharmacology
Director, Program in Genetics of Hypertension and Receptor Mechanisms
University of California at San Diego
La Jolla, California

Bruce M. Psaty, MD, PhD
Co-Director, Cardiovascular Health Research Unit
Professor, Medicine, Epidemiology, Health Services
University of Washington
Seattle, Washington

Patrick Pullicino, MD, PhD
Professor, Neurology
State University of New York at Buffalo
Buffalo, New York

Jules B. Puschett, MD
Professor and Chairman, Department of Medicine
Tulane University Medical Center
New Orleans, Louisiana

Mahboob Rahman, MBBS, MS
Assistant Professor of Medicine
Case Western Reserve University, School of Medicine
Cleveland, Ohio

C. Venkata S. Ram, MD
Clinical Professor of Internal Medicine
University of Texas Southwestern Medical Center
Director of Continuing Medical Education
St. Paul Medical Center/Texas Heatlh Resources
Medical Director, Hypertension Center of Dallas
Dallas, Texas

Donald J. Reis, MD
Cotzias Distinguished Professor of Neurology and Neuroscience
Cornell University Medical College
New York, New York

Efrain Reisin, MD
Professor of Medicine
Louisiana State University
New Orleans, Louisiana

Lawrence M. Resnick, MD
Professor of Medicine
Director of Hypertension
Wayne State University Medical Center
Detroit, Michigan

Elizabeth B.D. Ripley, MD
Assistant Professor, Division of Nephrology
Medical College of Virginia Campus of Virginia Commonwealth University
Richmond, Virginia

David Robertson, MD
Elton Yates Professor of Medicine, Pharmacology, and Neurology
Autonomic Dysfunction Center
Vanderbilt University
Nashville, Tennessee

Edward J. Roccella, PhD, MPH
Coordinator, National High Blood Pressure Education Program
National Heart, Lung, and Blood Institute
Bethesda, Maryland

Albert P. Rocchini, MD
Director of Pediatric Cardiology
Professor of Pediatrics
University of Michigan Health Systems
Ann Arbor, Michigan

Richard J. Roman, PhD
Professor, Department of Physiology
Medical College of Wisconsin
Milwaukee, Wisconsin

John A. Rumberger, PhD, MD
Diagnostic Cardiovascular Consultants
Columbus, Ohio

Frank M. Sacks, MD
Associate Professor in Nutrition, Harvard School of Public Health
Associate Professor of Medicine, Harvard Medical School
Boston, Massachusetts

Willis K. Samson, PhD
Professor and Chair of Physiology
University of North Dakota School of Medicine
Grand Forks, North Dakota

Morris Schambelan, MD
Professor of Medicine
University of California, San Francisco
Chief, Division of Endocrinology
Director, General Clinical Physiology Center
San Francisco General Hospital
San Francisco, California

Ernesto L. Schiffrin, MD, PhD, FRCPC, FACP
Professor of Medicine, University of Montreal
Director, MRC Multidisciplinary Research Group on Hypertension
Clinical Research Institute of Montreal
Montreal, Quebec, Canada

Gary L. Schwartz, MD
Assistant Professor of Medicine
Mayo Medical School
Chair, Division of Hypertension
Mayo Clinic
Rochester, Minnesota

Ellen W. Seely, MD
Assistant Professor of Medicine
Harvard Medical School
Director of Clinical Research
Endocrine-Hypertension Division
Brigham and Women's Hospital
Boston, Massachusetts

Yoram Shenker, MD
Associate Professor of Medicine
Head (Interim), Section of Endocrinology, Diabetes, and
Metabolism
University of Wisconsin, Madison
VA Hospital
Madison, Wisconsin

Sheldon G. Sheps, MD
Emeritus Professor of Medicine
Mayo Clinic
Mayo Foundation and Mayo Medical School
Rochester, Minnesota

Clarence Shub, MD
Professor of Medicine, Mayo Medical School
Consultant in Cardiovascular Diseases
Mayo Clinic
Rochester, Minnesota

Domenic A. Sica, MD
Professor, Medicine and Pharmacology
Chairman, Clinical Pharmacology and Hypertension
Medical College of Virginia
Virginia Commonwealth University
Richmond, Virginia

Denise G. Simons-Morton, MD, PhD
Leader, Prevention Scientific Research Group
National Heart, Lung, and Blood Institute
Bethesda, Maryland

Alan R. Sinaiko, MD
Professor, Department of Pediatrics
University of Minnesota
Minneapolis, Minnesota

Randal A. Skidgel, PhD
Associate Professor
Departments of Pharmacology and
Anesthesiology
University of Illinois at Chicago
Chicago, Illinois

Edmund H. Sonnenblick
Edmond J. Safra Professor of Medicine
Division of Cardiology
The Albert Einstein College of Medicine
Bronx, New York

James R. Sowers, MD
Professor of Medicine and Physiology
Wayne State University School of Medicine
Detroit, Michigan

Beth A. Staffileno, DNSc
Assistant Professor
Department of Internal Medicine
Wayne State University
Detroit, Michigan

Jeremiah Stamler, MD
Professor Emeritus
Department of Preventive Medicine
Northwestern University Medical School
Chicago, Illinois

Paul R. Standley, PhD
Assistant Professor, Physiology
Midwestern University
Glendale, Arizona

William B. Stason, MD
Senior Vice President
Medical Scientists, Inc.
Boston, Massachusetts

Helmut O. Steinberg, MD
Assistant Professor of Medicine
Indiana University School of Medicine
Indianapolis, Indiana

David H.P. Streeten, MB, DPhil, FRCP, FACP
Professor of Medicine Emeritus
SUNY Health Science Center
Syracuse, New York

Jay M. Sullivan, MD
Professor of Medicine
Chief, Division of Cardiovascular Diseases
University of Tennessee
Memphis, Tennessee

Addison A. Taylor, MD, PhD
Professor of Medicine and Pharmacology
Chief, Section on Hypertension and Clinical Pharmacology
Associate Dean of Clinical Research
Baylor College of Medicine
Houston, Texas

Stephen C. Textor, MD
Professor of Medicine, Mayo Medical School
Division of Hypertension
Mayo Clinic
Rochester, Minnesota

Thomas J. Thom, BA
Statistician
National Heart, Lung, and Blood Institute
National Institutes of Health
Bethesda, Maryland

David J. Triggle, PhD
University Distinguished Professor
Dean, Graduate School
State University of New York
Buffalo, New York

Donald G. Vidt, MD
Senior Physician
Department of Nephrology and Hypertension
Cleveland Clinic Foundation
Cleveland, Ohio
Professor of Medicine
Ohio State University
Columbus, Ohio

Charles O. Watlington, MD, PhD
Emeritus Professor of Medicine
Endocrine Division of the Department of Internal Medicine
Medical College of Virginia/VCU
Richmond, Virginia

R. Clinton Webb, PhD
Professor, Department of Physiology
University of Michigan
Ann Arbor, Michigan

Michael A. Weber, MD
Chairman, Department of Medicine
The Brookdale University Hospital and Medical Center
Professor of Medicine
State University of New York
Health Science Center at Brooklyn
Brooklyn, New York

Alan B. Weder, MD
Professor of Internal Medicine
University of Michigan
Ann Arbor, Michigan

Myron H. Weinberger, MD
Professor of Medicine
Director, Hypertension Research Center
Indiana University School of Medicine
Indianapolis, Indiana

Richard M. Weinshilboum, MD
Professor of Pharmacology and Medicine
Mayo Medical School
Rochester, Minnesota

Matthew R. Weir, MD
Professor of Medicine
Director, Division of Nephrology and Clinical Research Unit
University of Maryland School of Medicine
Baltimore, Maryland

Paul K. Whelton, MD, MSc
Professor of Epidemiology and Dean
Tulane University School of Public Health and Tropical Medicine
New Orleans, Louisiana

William B. White, MD
Professor of Medicine
Chief, Section of Hypertension and Clinical Pharmacology
Department of Medicine
University of Connecticut School of Medicine
Farmington, Connecticut

Roger R. Williams, MD
Professor of Medicine (Cardiology)
Director, Cardiovascular Genetics Research Clinic
University of Utah School of Medicine
Salt Lake City, Utah

Peter W.F. Wilson, MD
Director of Laboratories
Framingham Heart Study
National Heart, Lung, and Blood Institute
Framingham, Massachusetts

Michael F. Wilson, MD, FACC, FACP
Professor, Medicine and Nuclear Medicine, SUNY at Buffalo
Director, Cardiovascular Medicine,
CGF Health System, Millard Fillmore Division
Buffalo, New York

Philip A. Wolf, MD
Professor of Neurology
Boston University School of Medicine
Boston, Massachusetts

Jackson T. Wright, Jr, MD, PhD
Professor of Medicine
Director, Clinical Hypertension Program
University Hospitals of Cleveland
Chief, Hypertension Section
Cleveland VAMC
Cleveland, Ohio

J. Michael Wyss, PhD
Professor of Cell Biology
Professor of Medicine
University of Alabama at Birmingham
Birmingham, Alabama

William F. Young, Jr, MD
Associate Professor of Medicine
Consultant, Division of Hypertension and Endocrinology and Metabolism
Mayo Clinic
Rochester, Minnesota

Jason Xiao-Jian Yuan, MD, PhD
Associate Professor, Medicine and Physiology
University of Maryland School of Medicine
Baltimore, Maryland

Carla Yunis, MD, MPH
Associate Professor of Surgical Sciences and Public Health Sciences
Medical Director of "Health on Wheels"
The Hypertension and Vascular Disease Center
Wake Forest University School of Medicine
Winston-Salem, North Carolina

Part A

BASIC SCIENCE

Section Editors: *Theodore L. Goodfriend, MD*
James R. Sowers, MD

Vasoactive Substances
Cell Physiology
Vasoregulatory Systems
Pathophysiology of Essential Hypertension
Pathophysiology of Secondary Hypertension
Mechanisms of Target Organ Damage
Sequelae of Hypertension

Chapter 1

Adrenergic and Dopaminergic Receptors and Actions

Kathleen H. Berecek, PhD; Robert M. Carey, MD

KEY POINTS

- There are 10 different adrenergic receptor subtypes in 3 main classes, α_1, α_2, and β, and 5 dopaminergic receptor subtypes in 2 main classes, D_1-like and D_2-like.

- Adrenergic and dopaminergic receptors are coupled to G proteins and affect cells by altering intracellular calcium, cyclic nucleotides, inositol phosphates, and protein phosphorylation.

- Receptor desensitization and downregulation reduce responses of cells to continuous exposure to catecholamines.

- Alterations in adrenergic and dopaminergic receptors and their functions may play a role in hypertension, cardiac ischemia, congestive heart failure, nocturnal asthma, and obesity.

See also Chapters 2, 26, 125, 126, 127

Adrenergic Receptors

Norepinephrine (NE) and epinephrine, the endogenous catecholamines released by postganglionic sympathetic nerve terminals and the adrenal gland, interact with cell surface receptor molecules in many diverse target organs. This interaction begins a cascade of membrane and intracellular events culminating in cellular changes and regulation of virtually every organ system **(see Table 1.1).**

Characteristics of Adrenergic Receptor Subtypes

Classically, peripheral adrenergic receptors (ARs) have been divided into 2 principal types: α and β. New synthetic compounds that stimulate or inhibit adrenergic targets have allowed further differentiation of ARs into the subtypes α_1, α_2, β_1, and β_2. The most recent methods involving molecular biology have uncovered several additional AR subtypes, leading to the current division of 10 AR subtypes in 3 families: $\alpha_{1A,B,C}$, $\alpha_{2A,B,C,D}$, and $\beta_{1,2,3}$. ARs are members of a large superfamily of receptors that mediate their activities through interaction with one of a series of guanosine nucleotide–binding regulatory proteins (G proteins).

Each type of AR preferentially couples to a different major subfamily of G_α proteins: α_1-AR to $G_{q\alpha}$, α_2-AR to $G_{i\alpha}$, and β-AR to $G_{s\alpha}$. Each of the G_α proteins can be linked to ion channels or other effector molecules, although most target cells have preferred linkages. Thus, α_1-ARs are preferentially linked by G_q to activation of phospholipases, especially phospholipase C_2, and in some tissues to activation of Ca^{2+} channels, activation of Na^+-H^+ and Na^+-Ca^{2+} exchange, and activation or inhibition of K^+ channels. Receptors of the α_2 subtype are linked by G_i to inhibition of adenylyl cyclase and in some tissues to regulation of K^+ and Ca^{2+} channels. β-Adrenergic receptors are linked by G_s to activation of adenylyl cyclase and Ca^{2+} channels in some tissues. Each of these linkages leads to changes in intracellular concentrations of second messengers, such as cAMP, Ca^{2+}, diacylglycerol, and 1,4,5-trisphosphate, which regulate the phosphorylated states of cellular proteins by modifying the activity of a variety of protein kinases.

Structural features of ARs are shared by all G protein–coupled receptors. They have an extracellular amino terminal with sites for N-linked glycosylation, 7 α-helical domains that span the plasma membrane, and intracellular carboxy terminals containing amino acid sequences that are probable sites of phosphorylation by one or more protein kinases. Through various interactions with ion channels and second messengers, different AR subtypes enable NE and epinephrine to have a broad range of physiological actions.

AR subtypes, their tissue distributions, and the responses that they mediate are shown in Table 1. Also included in Table 1 are the pharmacological agents that stimulate or inhibit various receptor subtypes. As shown in this table, individual AR subtypes are not restricted to a single cell. Moreover, most tissues contain more than one subtype. The response of a cell will depend on the concentration of NE and epinephrine in the tissue, the subtypes and kinetics of the receptors on the cell, and the second messenger system(s) altered by occupancy of the receptors.

Pharmacology and Function of ARs

Receptors of the α_1-subtype are located on postsynaptic cells in smooth muscle, heart, vas deferens, and brain. They are stimulated by methoxamine and phenylephrine and inhibited by antagonists such as prazosin, phentolamine, and corynanthine.

Many α_2-ARs are autoreceptors localized on the postganglionic presynaptic nerve terminals that synthesize NE. When activated by catecholamines, presynaptic α_2-ARs inhibit further NE release. Activation of brain α_2-ARs reduces systemic sympathetic outflow, whereas blockade of this receptor subtype facilitates release of NE from sympathetic nerve terminals. These receptor subtypes are stimulated by clonidine, guanfacine, and α-methyl NE (formed from α-methyldopa) and inhibited by yohimbine and rauwolscine. Post-

Table 1.1. Tissue Distribution, Responses, and Pharmacology of Adrenergic Receptor Subtypes

RECEPTOR	PHYSIOLOGY		PHARMACOLOGY	
	TISSUE	RESPONSE	AGONISTS	ANTAGONISTS
$\alpha_{1,A,B,C}$	Smooth muscle: vascular, iris, radial ureter, pilomotor, uterus, sphincters (gut, bladder)	Contraction	Methoxamine	Prazosin Terazosin Doxazosin
	Smooth muscle (gut)	Relaxation		Corynanthine
	Heart	Positive inotropic ($\beta_1 \gg \alpha_1$), cell growth, hypertrophy		Phentolamine
	Salivary gland	Secretion		Phenoxybenzamine
	Adipose tissue	Glycogenolysis		
	Sweat glands	Secretion		
	Kidney (proximal tubule)	Gluconeogenesis, Na$^+$ reabsorption		
$\alpha_{2A,B,C,D}$	Presynaptic autoreceptor on sympathetic nerve endings	Inhibition of norepinephrine release	Guanfacine Clonidine	Yohimbine Piperoxan
	Platelets	Aggregation, granule release	α-Methyl-NE	Rauwolscine
	Endocrine pancreas	Inhibition of insulin release	Tramazoline	Phentolamine
	Adipose tissue	Inhibition of lipolysis	Xylazine	Phenoxybenzamine
	Vascular smooth muscle	Contraction	Guanadrel	
	Kidney	Inhibition of renin release (?)	Oxymetazoline	
β_1	Heart	Positive inotropic effect, positive chronotropic effect, cell growth, hypertrophy	Isoproterenol Prenaterol	Propranolol Betaxolol
	Adipose tissue	Lipolysis	Dobutamine	Atenolol
	Kidney	Renin release		Practolol Metoprolol
β_2	Liver	Glycogenolysis, gluconeogenesis	Isoproterenol	Propanolol
	Skeletal muscle	Glycogenolysis, lactate release	Terbutaline	Butoxamine
	Smooth muscle: bronchi, uterus, gut, vascular (skeletal muscle), detrusor	Relaxation	Salbutamol Rimiterol Albuterol	High concentration of β_1-antagonists
	Endocrine pancreas	Insulin secretion (?)		
	Salivary gland	Amylase secretion		
β_3	Adipose tissue	Lipolysis	BRL 37344	
	Striated muscle	Thermogenesis		

synaptic α_2-receptors also occur, and diverse cell types, such as endothelium and platelets, manifest α_2-receptors as well.

Activation of β_1-ARs stimulates the rate and strength of cardiac contraction, lipolysis in fat cells, and renin release from the kidneys. This receptor is stimulated by isoproterenol, dobutamine, and prenaterol and inhibited by β-blockers such as propranolol and betaxolol. The β_2-AR relaxes smooth muscle cells in bronchi, vasculature, uterus, gut, and bladder and is stimulated by isoproterenol, terbutaline, albuterol, salbutamol, and rimiterol and inhibited by IPS 339 and ICI 118,551. The order of potency for stimulation of β_1-ARs by catecholamines is isoproterenol>epinephrine=NE. For the β_2-ARs, the order of potency is isoproterenol>epinephrine>NE.

Normal and Abnormal Regulation of ARs

After stimulation, both α- and β-ARs decrease target organ responses to further stimulation, ie, they "desensitize" rapidly and are downregulated after prolonged exposure. Regulation of β-AR function involves modifications at several loci, including the gene itself. One cascade that decreases β-adrenergic responses includes phosphorylation of agonist-occupied receptors, uncoupling of the receptors from G proteins, and internalization of receptors from the membrane into the cy-

toplasm. Immediately after agonist presentation, β-AR kinase catalyzes phosphorylation of consensus sequences near the carboxy terminus (cytoplasmic domain) of the receptor. Subsequent events cause internalization of the receptor, after which the receptor can either be degraded or reinserted into the plasma membrane.

In addition to desensitization and downregulation induced by the agonist itself (homologous desensitization), β-ARs display heterologous desensitization. In this case, β-ARs become less responsive to agonists after stimulation of the same cell by a nonadrenergic cyclase activator, such as another neurotransmitter. Heterologous desensitization is associated with cAMP activation of protein kinases and subsequent phosphorylation and desensitization of the β-ARs.

Long-term regulation of β-ARs is controlled principally at the gene level. The β_1-, β_2-, and β_3-AR subtypes are encoded on human chromosomes 10, 5, and 8, respectively. Stimulation of β-ARs modifies both the transcription rate and the steady-state level of β-AR messenger RNA. cAMP-responsive elements in the promoter region of the gene, as well as exposure of cells to several humoral agents (ie, glucocorticoids and thyroid hormone), modify the expression of β-ARs.

Regulation of α-ARs has been less completely examined. α_1-ARs are divided into 3 subtypes based on structure, location, and pharmacological properties. The genes for both the α_{1A}- and α_{1B}-subtypes are located on human chromosome 5, and that for the α_{1C}-AR is located on human chromosome 8. The genes for α_2-AR subtypes α_{2A}, α_{2B}, and α_{2C}, are located on human chromosomes 10, 2, and 4, respectively.

Increased expression of ARs in myocardial ischemia and hypertension and decreased expression of β-ARs in congestive health failure have been reported as well as genetic polymorphisms in β_2-ARs in patients with asthma and β_3-ARs in patients with morbid obesity.

Dopaminergic Receptors

Dopamine (DA) is an endogenous catecholamine that serves as a precursor of NE and epinephrine and as a neurotransmitter in its own right. DA is released by postganglionic sympathetic neurons and dopaminergic neurons and is synthesized by and released from proximal renal tubule cells of gastrointestinal epithelium. The vast majority of circulating DA derives from the kidney. DA modulates a variety of physiological functions, including behavior, movement, nerve conduction, hormone synthesis and release, ion transport, vascular tone, and blood pressure.

Characteristics of Dopaminergic Receptors

Peripheral dopaminergic receptors (DRs) **(as shown in Table 1.2)** have been divided into 2 major types: D_1-like and D_2-like. Recently, molecular studies have revealed 5 major subtypes (D_1 through D_5). D_1-like receptors include D_1 and D_5. D_2-like receptors include D_2, D_3, and D_4 receptors. DRs contain the 7 transmembrane domains that characterize the other G protein–coupled receptors. The D_1-like receptors have no introns and are encoded by a single exon, whereas the D_2-like family is encoded by a mosaic of exons and contains introns within its protein-coding regions. Therefore, it is likely that the D_1- and D_2-like receptors derive from 2 different gene families.

The D_1- and D_2-like receptors induce 2 different types of signal transduction. One of these, the adenylyl cyclase pathway, is obligatory for all cell systems. D_1-like receptors are associated with stimu-

lation and D_2-like receptors with inhibition of adenylyl cyclase. The other pathways are cell-specific and are different for different cells. These other pathways include activation of calcium or potassium channels and stimulation of phosphoinositide hydrolysis.

In peripheral tissues, DRs are distributed in the sympathetic nervous system, the pituitary gland, the cardiovascular system, kidney, and adrenal cortex. Molecular studies suggest that the peripheral D_1- and D_2-like receptors are identical to those in the central nervous system.

Pharmacology and Function of DRs

D_1-like DRs are located postsynaptically in the heart (atrial and ventricular myocardium and coronary vessels), arterial blood vessels (vascular smooth muscle cells), adrenal cortex (zona glomerulosa cells), and kidney (proximal tubule, thick ascending loop of Henle, cortical collecting duct, and vascular smooth muscle).

Selective stimulation of D_1-like receptors by fenoldopam, a selective D_1-like DR agonist, leads to vasodilation (renal and systemic), diuresis, natriuresis, and a decrease in systemic blood pressure without postural hypotension or increased plasma renin activity. The natriuresis is caused by an increase in renal blood flow and a decrease in renal tubule sodium reabsorption. These effects occur at doses of fenoldopam that do not increase plasma renin activity. In proximal tubule cells, inhibition of sodium transport from the tubule lumen is mediated by stimulation of adenylyl cyclase, increased protein kinase A activity, and inhibition of Na^+/K^+ antiport activity at the brush border membrane. In the medullary thick ascending loop of Henle, DA acts through D_1-like receptors to increase cAMP-dependent protein kinase, which phosphorylates a protein, DARPP-32 (DA-related phosphoprotein), which phosphorylates basolateral membrane Na^+/K^+ ATPase, causing inactivation of this enzyme. D_1-selective antagonists include SCH-23390, SCH-39166, and SKF-83566.

DA synthesized in and released from renal proximal tubule cells is thought to act as a paracrine substance (cell-to-cell mediator)

Table 1.2. Classification of Dopamine Receptors

	PHARMACOLOGICAL CLASS				
	D_1-LIKE GROUP		D_2-LIKE GROUP		
Molecular biological class	D_1	D_5	D_2	D_3	D_4
Effector	G_s	G_s	G_i/G_0	G_i/G_0	G_i/G_0
	+AC/PLC	+AC	−AC	−AC	−AC
			+K^+ channel	+K^+ channel?	+K^+ channel
			−Ca^{2+} channel	−Ca^{2+} channel	−Ca^{2+} channel
Group selective agonists	Fenoldopam*		Bromocriptine†		
Group selective antagonists	SCH 23390*, SCH 39166*, SKF 83566*		YM-09151†		
Sybtype selective agonists	None	None	NO437	PD128907 Quinpirole Quinelorane	None
Subtype selective antagonist	None	None	Eticlopride	Nafadotride UH 232‡ U-99, 194A	U-101958 L-745,870 L-741,742 NGD·94

AC indicates adenylyl cyclase; PLC, phospholipase C; ?, not established; +, stimulatory; and −, inhibitory.
*Selective for D_1-like but cannot distinguish D_1 from D_5; †selective for D_2-like but cannot distinguish subtypes; ‡partial agonist.

stimulating D_1-like DR on these cells to inhibit sodium reabsorption in tonic fashion. A defect in the proximal tubule D_1-like DR is present in spontaneously hypertensive rats and in human hypertension. This tubule DR defect promotes renal sodium reabsorption and may contribute to the development of hypertension.

D_2-like DRs in the periphery are distributed both presynaptically and postsynaptically in the sympathetic nervous system. Presynaptic D_2-like DRs inhibit NE release from sympathetic neurons. Postsynaptic and nonneuronal D_2-like DRs are present in the endothelial and adventitial layers of blood vessels, on pituitary lactotrophs (where they inhibit prolactin secretion in response to DA), and in the adrenal zona glomerulosa (where they inhibit aldosterone secretion). D_3 receptors, one of the D_2-like DR group, have been identified in the glomeruli, proximal tubules, and blood vessels of the kidney, and a novel D_2-like receptor (the D_{2K} receptor) has been described in inner medullary collecting duct cells. The functions of the D_3 and D_{2K} receptors are unknown. Aside from inhibition of NE, prolactin, and aldosterone secretion, the physiological role of peripheral D_2-like DRs is not established,

and it is unclear whether these receptors have a role in the pathophysiology of cardiovascular disease.

Bromocriptine and domperidone are selective agonists at D_2-like receptors. Although there are no specific agonists for D_3 receptors, quinpirole has a higher affinity for D_3 than for D_2 receptors.

SUGGESTED READING

1. Insel PA. Adrenergic receptors: evolving concepts and clinical applications. *N Engl J Med.* 1996;334:580–585.
2. Graham RM, Perez DM, Hwa J, Piascik MT. α_1-Adrenergic receptor subtypes: molecular structure, function, and signaling. *Circ Res.* 1996;78:737–749.
3. Rockman HA, Koch WJ, Lefkowitz RJ. Cardiac function in genetically engineered mice with altered adrenergic receptor signaling. *Am J Physiol.* 1997;272(*Heart Circ Physiol* 41):H1553-H1559.
4. Carey RM. Dopamine, hypertension and the potential for agonist therapy. In: Laragh JH, Brenner DM, eds. *Hypertension: Pathophysiology, Diagnosis and Management.* 2nd ed. New York, NY: Raven Press Ltd; 1995:2937–2952.
5. Jose PA, Felder RA. What can we learn from the selective manipulation of dopaminergic receptors about pathogenesis and treatment of hypertension? *Curr Opin Nephrol Hypertens.* 1996;5:447–451.

Chapter 2

Catecholamine Synthesis, Release, Reuptake, and Metabolism

Richard Weinshilboum, MD

KEY POINTS

- Catecholamines are synthesized from the amino acid tyrosine by a series of enzymatic steps.

- Catecholamines are stored in vesicles in adrenergic neurons and adrenal chromaffin cells and are released by exocytosis in response to nerve or adrenal chromaffin cell stimulation.

- Catecholamine neurotransmitter action is terminated predominantly by reuptake into the presynaptic nerve terminal.

- Catecholamines are metabolized within the adrenergic neuron by monoamine oxidase and outside the neuron by monoamine oxidase, catechol *O*-methyltransferase, and phenol sulfotransferase.

See also Chapters 1, 54, 154

The catecholamines dopamine, norepinephrine, and epinephrine play an important role in cardiovascular function, both as a result of direct actions on the heart and blood vessels and as a result of actions in the central nervous system (CNS). Included among processes that occur within the presynaptic adrenergic nerve terminal are catecholamine biosynthesis, vesicular storage, release into the synapse, and reuptake into the nerve terminal, followed by metabolism and/or restorage in vesicles (**Figure 2.1**). Catecholamine metabolism also occurs outside the neuron. Drugs have been developed that can interfere with each of these processes, and many of those drugs are used to treat hypertension.

Catecholamine Biosynthesis

Catecholamines are synthesized by a series of enzymatic steps (**Figure 2.2**), beginning with the conversion of the amino acid tyrosine to dihydroxyphenylalanine (L-dopa) by the enzyme tyrosine hydroxylase (TH, Figure 2, reaction 1). The reaction catalyzed by TH is usually the rate-limiting step in catecholamine biosynthesis. Therefore, this enzyme is a logical point for pharmacological "attack" on catecholamine biosynthesis, and an inhibitor of TH, α-methyl-*p*-tyrosine, is used to treat patients with metastatic pheochromocytoma. α-Methyl-*p*-tyrosine inhibits catecholamine biosynthesis within the pheochromocytoma, thus preventing the cardiovascular and other effects of catecholamines released from the tumor.

The second step in catecholamine biosynthesis is catalyzed by aromatic L-amino acid decarboxylase (AAAD), also referred to as "dopa decarboxylase" (Figure 2, reaction 2). Unlike TH, which is localized within adrenergic neurons and the adrenal medulla, AAAD is a cytoplasmic enzyme that is present in many tissues. Although potent inhibitors of AAAD are available, these drugs are not useful for the treatment of hypertension. However, AAAD inhibitors, such as carbidopa, that do not cross the blood-brain barrier are used to inhibit the peripheral metabolism of L-dopa when that drug is used to treat patients with Parkinson's disease.

The third enzyme involved in catecholamine biosynthesis is dopamine β-hydroxylase (DBH, Figure 2, reaction 3). DBH is a copper-containing enzyme that is localized to catecholamine storage vesicles in adrenergic nerve terminals and the adrenal medulla. Because copper is essential for the enzymatic activity of DBH, agents that chelate copper can inhibit this enzyme. An example of such a compound is disulfiram (Antabuse), a drug used to inhibit the enzyme aldehyde dehydrogenase during the "aversion therapy" of alcoholic patients. Although inhibitors of DBH have been tested as antihypertensive agents, none are currently used to treat patients with elevated blood pressure.

The final enzyme involved in catecholamine biosynthesis is phenylethanolamine N-methyltransferase (PNMT, Figure 2, reaction 4). PNMT is localized to the adrenal medulla and a small number of neurons in the CNS that synthesize epinephrine as a neurotransmitter. Although PNMT inhibitors have also been tested for use in the treatment of hypertension, none are currently used in clinical practice.

Regulation of Catecholamine Biosynthesis

The activities of the enzymes involved in catecholamine biosynthesis are subject to both short- and long-term regulation. The activity of TH increases rapidly in response to nerve stimulation. That increase is thought to be caused by decreased catecholamine concentrations within the nerve terminal, which decreases the feedback inhibition of TH by catecholamines. A second mechanism for short-term increase in TH activity is phosphorylation of the enzyme that occurs in response to nerve stimulation. Long-term increases in the rate of nerve firing also result in sustained increases in neuronal levels of both TH and DBH. In the adrenal medulla, PNMT is induced by glucocorticoids from the adrenal cortex, and the activity of this enzyme falls to nearly undetectable levels after hypophysectomy, with its associated decline in glucocorticoid synthesis. Therefore, both neural and humoral mechanisms participate in the regulation of catecholamine biosynthesis.

Catecholamine Vesicular Storage

Catecholamines in adrenergic nerve terminals and in adrenal chromaffin cells are stored within vesicles. These vesicles contain high concentrations of catecholamines together with ATP and storage proteins

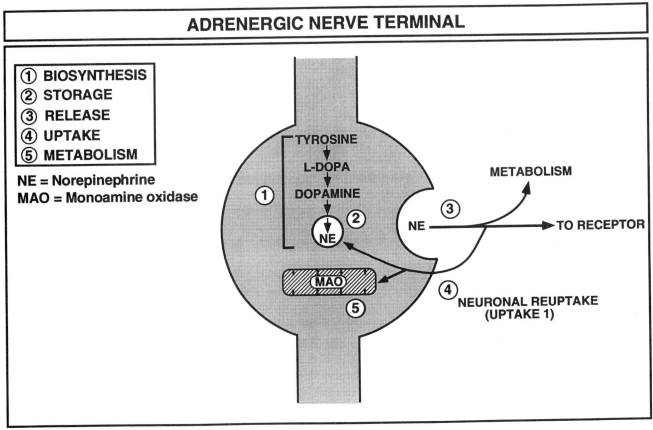

Figure 2.1.   Adrenergic nerve terminal catecholamine biosynthesis, vesicular storage, release, reuptake, and metabolism.

that are referred to collectively as "chromogranins." Because DBH is localized within the vesicle, dopamine must be taken up into vesicular storage sites (Figure 1, process 2) before the β-hydroxylation reaction that converts it to norepinephrine. Vesicular uptake is a two-step process that requires the ATP-dependent transport of hydrogen ions into the vesicle, followed by the exchange of hydrogen ions for biogenic amines. This second step involves a vesicular monoamine transporter that is distinct from the separate uptake process that occurs at the neuronal membrane, also known as uptake-1 or neuronal reuptake (Figure 1, process 4). Neuronal reuptake involves a separate transport protein that is inhibited by different drugs from those that inhibit vesicular uptake. The vesicular monoamine transporter consists of 12 hydrophobic transmembrane-spanning domains and shows amino acid sequence homology to several other transport proteins. However, it has very little sequence similarity to the neural membrane monoamine transporters.

The antihypertensive drug reserpine inhibits the vesicular uptake of catecholamines. Reserpine blocks the vesicle membrane amine–hydrogen ion exchange mechanism and, as a result, depletes vesicular stores of catecholamines, as well as those of serotonin and other biogenic amines that are stored in vesicles. The antihypertensive drugs guanethidine and guanadrel also inhibit the vesicular storage of catecholamines, probably by interference with the amine–hydrogen ion exchange mechanism.

Catecholamine Release

Catecholamines are released by exocytosis after the stimulation of sympathetic nerves and chromaffin cells (Figure 1, process 3).

This calcium-dependent process involves discharge of the contents of the vesicle through an opening in the cell membrane. Catecholamines, ATP, chromogranins, and a small amount of DBH are simultaneously released to the exterior of the cell during exocytosis. Therefore, both DBH and chromogranins can be found circulating in blood.

Exocytotic release of catecholamines can be regulated by neurotransmitter and hormone receptors located on the presynaptic adrenergic nerve terminal. Perhaps the most important of these presynaptic receptors is the α_2-adrenergic receptor, which, when stimulated, inhibits neurotransmitter release. Therefore, intrasynaptic norepinephrine can decrease subsequent exocytotic release through a negative feedback process mediated by presynaptic α_2-adrenergic receptors.

In addition to release by exocytosis, catecholamines can also be released from adrenergic nerve terminals by an indirect mechanism. Amphetamines and tyramine, a monoamine found in certain cheeses and red wines, stimulate the release of catecholamines into the synaptic cleft by a nonexocytotic process. That fact, as discussed subsequently, is particularly important in patients who have been treated with inhibitors of the catecholamine-metabolizing enzyme monoamine oxidase (MAO).

Catecholamine Reuptake

The neurotransmitter actions of catecholamines are terminated principally by reuptake into the nerve terminal, so-called uptake-1 (Figure 1, process 4). This process should not be confused with

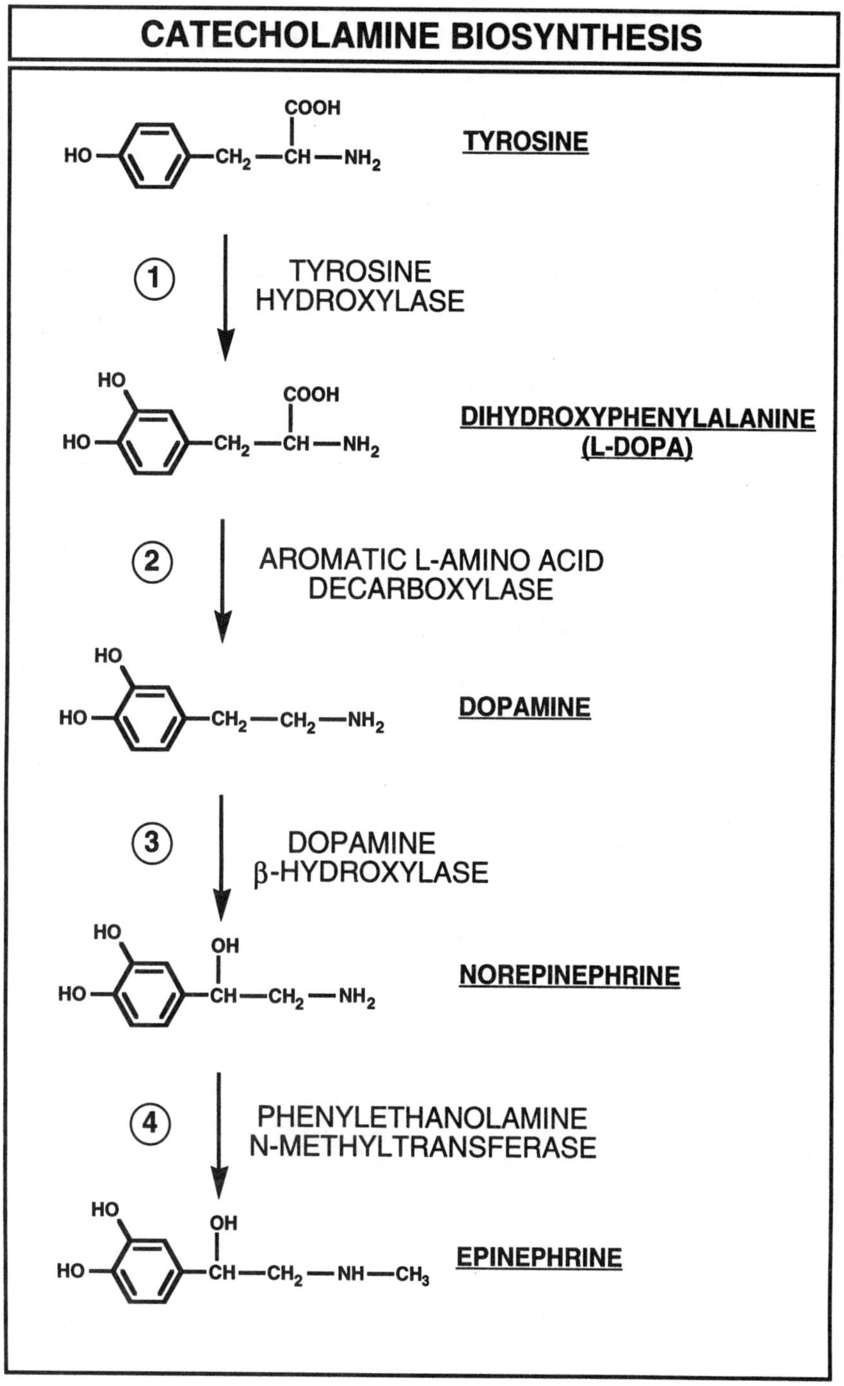

CATECHOLAMINE BIOSYNTHESIS

Figure 2.2. Catecholamine biosynthesis.

the uptake of catecholamines into vesicles within the neuron (Figure 1, process 2). Specific and separate membrane transporters for norepinephrine and dopamine have been cloned. Neural membrane transporters require the Na$^+$ gradient across the cell membrane that is maintained by Na$^+$, K$^+$-ATPase. These transporters, like the vesicular monoamine transporter, have 12 membrane-spanning domains, but their amino acid sequences differ from that of the vesicular transporters, ie, they are different proteins. Catecholamine reuptake into the neuron is inhibited by tricyclic antidepressant medications, such as imipramine, and by cocaine.

Catecholamine Metabolism

Catecholamines are metabolized primarily by three enzymes: MAO, catechol O-methyltransferase (COMT), and phenol sulfotransferase (PST). MAO is a mitochondrial membrane enzyme present in many cells, including the adrenergic nerve terminal. MAO catalyzes the oxidative deamination of catecholamines (**Figure 2.3, reaction 1**) in the adrenergic nerve terminal and also plays a role in the metabolism of catecholamines outside of vesicles. There are two MAO isoforms, MAO A and MAO B, which differ in their substrate specificity

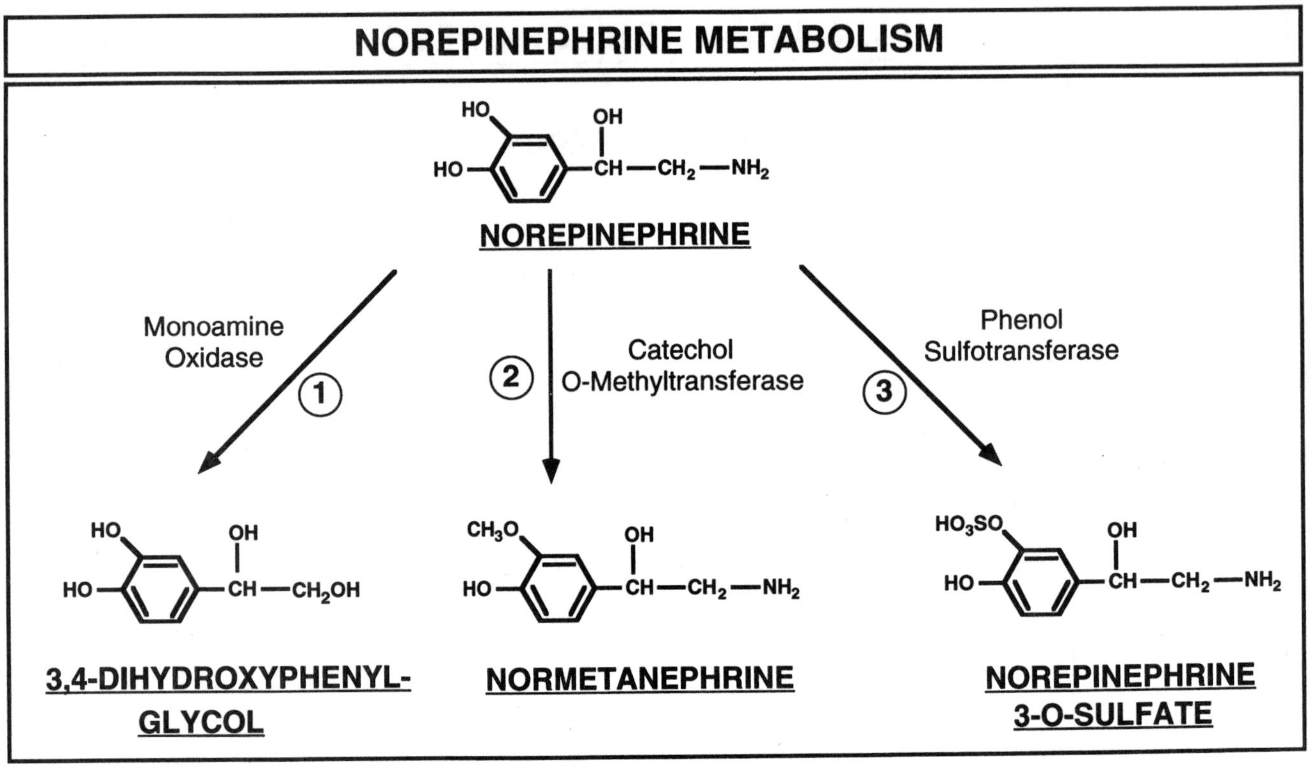

NOREPINEPHRINE METABOLISM

Figure 2.3. Norepinephrine metabolism.

and inhibitor sensitivity. The type A enzyme preferentially catalyzes the metabolism of norepinephrine and serotonin, whereas MAO B preferentially oxidizes phenylethylamine; both forms metabolize dopamine. Inhibitors of MAO are used to treat both hypertension and depression and are thought to achieve their clinical effect through increased CNS synaptic levels of neurotransmitter. The MAO B inhibitor selegiline (deprenyl) is also used as an adjunct to L-dopa therapy of Parkinson's disease. Clinical use of MAO inhibitors has been limited because of the possibility of life-threatening hypertensive crises in patients treated with these agents who ingest compounds like tyramine that are metabolized by MAO and can indirectly release catecholamines.

COMT is a widely distributed cytoplasmic enzyme that, unlike MAO, is not found in adrenergic nerve terminals. COMT catalyzes the ring O-methylation of catechols (Figure 3, reaction 2) and plays an important role in the metabolism of catecholamines after their escape from the adrenergic synapse. Because L-dopa is metabolized by COMT, inhibitors of COMT are used clinically to enhance treatment effects in patients with Parkinson's disease who are on therapy with L-dopa.

PST is a cytoplasmic enzyme that catalyzes the sulfate conjuga-

tion of catecholamines (Figure 3, reaction 3). From 95% to 99% of the circulating dopamine in humans and $\approx$70% of the circulating epinephrine and norepinephrine are sulfate conjugated. No inhibitors of PST are used clinically at present.

Catecholamine metabolites are measured clinically, primarily in the urine, to help diagnose pheochromocytomas. The metabolites most commonly measured are vanillylmandelic acid, a product of the sequential metabolism of norepinephrine and epinephrine by MAO and COMT, or metanephrine and normetanephrine, which are O-methylated products, respectively, of epinephrine and norepinephrine.

SUGGESTED READING

1. Norepinephrine and epinephrine. In: Cooper JR, Bloom FE, Roth RG, eds. *The Biochemical Basis of Neuropharmacology.* 7th ed. New York, NY: Oxford University Press; 1996:226–292.
2. Hoffman BB, Lefkowitz RJ, Taylor P. Neurotransmission: the autonomic and somatic motor nervous systems. In: Hardman JG, Limbird LE, Molinoff PB, Ruddon RW, Gilman A, eds. *The Pharmacological Basis of Therapeutics.* 9th ed. New York, NY: McGraw-Hill; 1996:105–139.
3. Povlock SL, Amara SG. The structure and function of norepinephrine, dopamine, and serotonin transporters. In: Reith MEA, ed. *Neurotransmitter Transporters: Structure, Function and Regulation.* Totowa, NJ: Humana Press; 1997:1–28.

Chapter 3

Angiotensins: Actions and Receptors

Theodore L. Goodfriend, MD

KEY POINTS

- Angiotensin II stimulates aldosterone secretion and affects the heart, vessels, and kidneys in ways that raise arterial blood pressure within minutes to hours.

- Angiotensin II stimulates growth of some cell types in the heart and vessels.

- Angiotensin peptides affect several functions of the brain that regulate plasma volume and blood pressure.

- There are at least two major receptor subtypes for angiotensins, of which the AT1 subtype mediates pressor effects of angiotensins by increasing intracellular calcium and protein phosphorylation in target cells.

See also Chapters 4, 5, 6, 7, 8, 41, 51, 130

Angiotensins are the products of a series of proteolytic reactions, starting with the cleavage of angiotensinogen by renin **(Figure 3.1)**. The peptide with the broadest known range of activities and the highest potency in the cardiovascular system is angiotensin II (Ang II).

Angiotensins

The angiotensins smaller than Ang II, such as angiotensin 2–8 (also called angiotensin III), angiotensin 3–8 (also called angiotensin IV), and angiotensin 1–7, are weak vasoconstrictors but may be important hormones at other sites, especially the brain. The amino acid sequences of these peptides and the pathways of their formation are depicted in Chapter 7.

Biological Actions

The best-established biological effects of the angiotensins are listed in the **Table 3.1**, and some are depicted in the Figure. Most of the rapid actions of Ang II can be viewed as a concerted response that supports the circulation when it is threatened by shrinkage of intravascular volume. These pressor actions include (1) vasoconstriction to reduce the capacity of the vascular tree, (2) increased aldosterone secretion to retain salt, (3) increased thirst and release of antidiuretic hormone to conserve water, (4) increased strength of myocardial contraction to maintain cardiac output, and (5) potentiation of sympathetic nervous system activity to synergize with the vasoconstrictor and inotropic actions of angiotensin. Platelet agglutination might also be considered a volume-conserving response to hemorrhage, and the effect of Ang II on the gut would reduce intestinal volume loss. Other acute effects of the angiotensins, such as stimulation of glycogenolysis in the liver and inhibition of prolactin release from the pituitary, do not fit neatly into our understanding of a response to decreased intravascular volume, and their significance remains to be established.

In addition to the acute effects described above, Ang II experimentally administered for days or weeks can cause trophic changes in animals, even at doses that do not acutely affect blood pressure. These changes include hyperplasia of vascular smooth muscle and myocardium, deposition of extracellular matrix, and sensitization of the vessels to low concentrations of vasoconstrictors. These could be viewed as part of a slow, structural remodeling of the cardiovascular system to compensate for prolonged volume contraction. Because prolonged volume contraction is not a common problem for humans, the trophic effects of angiotensins are more likely to be pathogenic than protective. Reversal of the trophic effects of angiotensin may help explain why angiotensin receptor blockers lower blood pressure progressively during the first few weeks of therapy and why ACE inhibitors ameliorate a wide variety of cardiovascular diseases.

Receptor Subtypes

Angiotensin, like other peptide hormones, interacts with receptors at the surface of its target cells. Three subtypes of receptor have been described, designated AT_1, AT_2, and AT_4. Virtually all the well-known actions of Ang II and III are mediated by the first type of receptor, AT_1. AT_2 has relatively high affinity for Ang III, and AT_4 for Ang IV.

The AT_1 receptor is a member of the superfamily of peptide hormone receptors, with seven membrane-spanning regions linked to G proteins. In all organs in which they have been studied, occupancy of AT_1 receptors by Ang II activates phospholipase C, which hydrolyzes phosphoinositide to form inositol trisphosphate (IP_3) and diacylglycerol. These second messengers, and possibly other mechanisms, increase intracellular calcium concentration and activate protein kinases. AT_1 receptors do not increase, and may decrease, intracellular cAMP.

The AT_2 subtype is much more prevalent in fetuses than in adults. This and other facts suggest that the AT_2 receptor affects growth and remodeling of organs. It is commonly believed that AT_2 antagonizes, attenuates, or modulates pressor and growth-promoting effects of Ang II that would otherwise compromise the fetus if renin activity were to increase. Similar reasoning may pertain to some situations in adults, especially injury to skin, heart, or blood vessels. It has also been proposed that apoptosis is affected by AT_2 receptor activation. AT_2 receptors are also present in adult brain, gut, and adrenal medulla. In rat intestine, AT_2 receptors mediate sodium reabsorption.

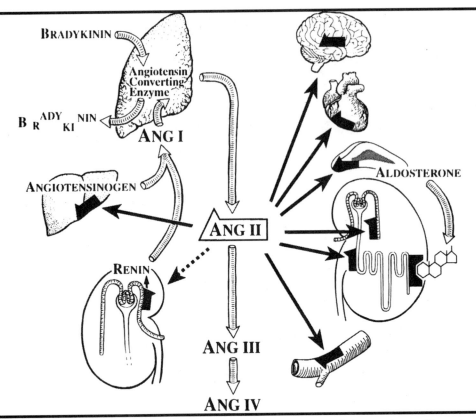

Figure 3.1. Schematic of renin-angiotensin-aldosterone system (RAAS). Tubular arrows on left show pathway of formation of Ang II and degradation of bradykinin by enzymes in blood and lung. Arrows in center show cascade of proteolytic cleavages that form smaller congeners of Ang II. Solid arrows indicate stimulatory actions of Ang II, and dashed arrow shows its principal inhibitory action: to reduce release of renin. Solid symbols at end of solid arrows indicate angiotensin receptors. Except for brain, which has three subtypes, all receptors in this figure are AT$_1$ subtype. Three actions of Ang II on kidney are depicted: inhibition of renin release, stimulation of proximal tubular sodium reabsorption, and constriction of efferent glomerular arterioles. Also shown is formation of aldosterone by adrenal glomerulosa under stimulus of Ang II and mineralocorticoid receptor on distal renal tubule. Not shown is formation of Ang (1–7) or synthesis of angiotensin within tissues independent of blood-borne RAAS.

Table 3.1. Angiotensin Targets and Actions

TARGET ORGAN OR CELL	ACTION (STIMULATORY, AND MEDIATED BY THE AT$_1$ RECEPTOR SUBTYPE UNLESS INDICATED)
Vascular smooth muscle	Vasoconstriction, hypertrophy, hyperplasia
Vascular endothelim	Prostaglandin, NO, endothelin production
Vascular connective tissue	Extracellular matrix synthesis
Myocardium	Strength of contraction, hypertrophy
Platelets	Aggregation by catecholamines
Monocytes	Adhesion to vessel wall
Adrenal glomerulosa	Aldosterone secretion
Adrenal medulla	Catecholamine release
Adrenal fasciculata	Cortisol secretion
Anterior pituitary	Inhibit prolactin release
Posterior pituitary	ADH release
Ovarian granulosa	Unknown (AT$_2$ receptors)
Kidney	Embryogenesis (AT$_1$ and AT$_2$)
Juxtaglomerular cells	Inhibit renin release
Mesangial cells	Contraction
Proximal tubule	Sodium reabsorption
Sympathetic neurons	Norepinephrine release
Brain	Pressor center activation, baroreceptor blunting, ADH synthesis, thirst, prostaglandin relase (Ang 1–7), unknown actions mediated by AT$_4$
Intestine	Salt and water absorption (AT$_2$)
Liver	Glycogenolysis, angiotensinogen synthesis

Receptor Regulation and Interactions

In addition to AT$_2$ receptors, other mechanisms attenuate Ang II action. Repeated exposure to Ang II reduces the responsiveness of most target organs (except the adrenal glomerulosa). This "tachyphylaxis" is principally a result of receptor "downregulation," a process that includes internalization of the hormone-receptor complex, and other postreceptor events. Autacoids released from Ang II targets modulate or amplify its actions. Prostaglandins released by Ang II and angiotensin (1–7) probably protect some vital organs, such as the kidney and brain, from ischemia that might otherwise ensue when renin levels rise. Angiotensins also induce formation of nitric oxide, which antagonizes vasoconstriction. By contrast, Ang II stimulates formation of endothelin, which amplifies its vascular actions, and various growth factors, which participate in the trophic changes caused by angiotensins.

SUGGESTED READING

1. deGasparo M, et al. Proposed update of angiotensin receptor nomenclature. *Hypertension*. 1995;25:924–927.
2. Goodfriend TL, Elliott ME, Catt KJ. Angiotensin receptors and their antagonists. *N Engl J Med*. 1996;334:1649–1654.
3. Inagami T, et al. Molecular biology of angiotensin II receptors: an overview. *J Hypertens*. 1994;12:S83–S94.
4. Robertson JIS, Nicholls MG, eds. *The Renin-Angiotensin System*. London, UK: Gower Medical Publishing; 1993.
5. Wright JW, et al. The angiotensin IV system: functional implications. *Front Neuroendocrinol*. 1995;16:23–52.

Chapter 4

Angiotensinogen

Morton P. Printz, PhD

KEY POINTS

- Angiotensinogen is the protein from which angiotensins are formed by proteolytic cleavage reactions.

- Angiotensinogen synthesis is under complex control by hormones and autocoids.

- Angiotensinogen levels in plasma affect blood pressure.

See also Chapters 3, 5, 6, 7, 8, 41, 51

Angiotensinogen is the only known precursor protein for the family of angiotensin peptides, angiotensin I, II, III (des-Asp^1-angiotensin II), IV (des-Asp^1-Arg^2-angiotensin II), and angiotensin$_{1-7}$ (des-Phe^8-angiotensin II). Thus, angiotensinogen may be a limiting factor in the activity of systemic (or tissue) renin-angiotensin systems. Systemic angiotensinogen appears to derive primarily from hepatocytes while the prohormone is also synthesized in the central nervous system, heart, vasculature, kidney, and fat cells.

Biochemistry, Physiology, and Pathophysiology

Preproangiotensinogen is processed and glycosylated in a species- and tissue-dependent manner. Hepatic angiotensinogen is the substrate for active renin, which is the prime determinant of the physiological activity of the circulating renin-angiotensin system. Genetic models, however, suggest that plasma concentrations of angiotensinogen contribute as well. Mice engineered to carry zero to four copies of the angiotensinogen gene have parallel plasma angiotensinogen concentrations and resting arterial pressure.

Angiotensinogen releases angiotensin after cleavage by a variety of enzymes. Cleavage of the N-terminal decapeptide angiotensin I by renin occurs in the circulation. While renin mRNA has been identified in some extraneural tissues, alternative modes of enzymatic processing of tissue angiotensinogen are likely to occur. Tissue angiotensinogen may be a substrate for cathepsin G, tonin, and chymase.

Plasma angiotensinogen exhibits complex and varying degrees of glycosylation. Evidence for an independent brain angiotensinogen system is the structural dissimilarity of angiotensinogen in these different pools. The role of the attached carbohydrate moieties on angiotensinogen-renin kinetics is a question now under reexamination.

A high-molecular-weight form of human systemic angiotensinogen appears during pregnancy, with increased levels found in pregnancy-induced hypertension. The origin and physiological significance of these unique molecular forms of angiotensinogen remain to be established. Another area of potential clinical significance is the recently discovered adipose tissue angiotensinogen. Adipose angiotensinogen mRNA is upregulated by insulin and downregulated by β-adrenergic agonists.

In contrast to renin, the half-life of plasma angiotensinogen is quite long, up to 16 hours. The steady-state level of systemic angiotensinogen is determined primarily by the rate of synthesis and secretion of the prohormone from hepatocytes. Cleavage by renin accounts for only 5% to 10% of the total rate of elimination of angiotensinogen from the circulation. Angiotensinogen constitutes an extremely small fraction of the total serum protein pool but comprises up to 2% of cerebrospinal fluid protein.

Control of Angiotensinogen Release

Hepatocyte angiotensinogen is constitutively secreted with little if any intracellular storage. Plasma levels of angiotensinogen are the result of transcriptional regulation (into mRNA), mRNA lifetime, and protein lifetime in the circulation. Glucocorticoids, estrogens, thyroid hormone, insulin, and selected cytokines exert transcriptional control via specific regulatory DNA sequences of the angiotensinogen gene. Angiotensin II may exert positive feedback regulation via the AT$_1$ receptor.

Several lines of evidence suggest that angiotensinogen contributes to the hypertensive phenotype. Studies using antisense nucleotide sequences to inhibit angiotensinogen mRNA translation, transgenic constructs, and homologous recombination have shown that plasma angiotensinogen levels affect arterial pressure. CNS administration of antisense sequences against the mRNA encoding angiotensinogen lowers arterial pressure in the spontaneously hypertensive rat. Rats made transgenic with human angiotensinogen have been found to be hypertensive. Mice with different numbers of copies of the gene have proportionately different blood pressures. These studies strengthen the association of angiotensinogen levels with arterial pressure and may imply direct involvement with hypertension but have not yet established a "causal" association with the human disease.

Molecular Genetics

The angiotensinogen gene has been cloned and sequenced. There is one copy of the angiotensinogen gene in the mammalian genome, 11 800 bases in length. The gene has five exons that encode for the protein separated by four introns. From the DNA sequence, it is evident that exon 1 codes for the 5′ nontranslated portion of the mRNA for angiotensinogen, while the signal peptide and the coding region for angiotensin I are encoded by exon 2. The other three exons contain the balance of information for the protein and the 3′ nontranslated region. Most of the reported physiological or pathophysiological factors that affect systemic angiotensinogen synthesis and secretion operate through transcriptional regulation. The 3′ nontranslated sequences of angiotensinogen mRNA contain recognition sequences for cytosolic proteins that stabilize the mRNA. This places angiotensinogen in a growing list of proteins that are regulated partly through mRNA stability.

Polymorphisms within the angiotensinogen gene have been genetically linked with familial hypertension in some human populations, but these findings are not consistent across all groups.

SUGGESTED READING

1. Brasier AR, Li J. Mechanisms for inducible control of angiotensinogen gene transcription. *Hypertension.* 1996;27:465–475.
2. Corvol P, Soubrier F, Jeunemaitre X. Molecular genetics of the renin-angiotensin-aldosterone system in human hypertension. *Pathol Biol (Paris).* 1997;45: 229–239.
3. Kim HS, Krege JH, Kluckman KD, Hagaman JR, Hodgin JB, Best CF, Jennette JC. Genetic control of blood pressure and the angiotensinogen locus. *Proc Natl Acad Sci U S A.* 1995;92:2735–2739.
4. Klett CP, Printz MP, Bader M, Ganten D, Eggena P. Angiotensinogen messenger RNA stabilization by angiotensin II. *J Hypertens Suppl.* 1996;14:S25–S36.
5. Wielbo D, Sernia C, Gyurko R, Phillips MJ. Antisense inhibition of hypertension in the spontaneously hypertensive rat. *Hypertension.* 1995;25:314–319.

Chapter 5

Renin Synthesis and Release

William H. Beierwaltes, PhD

KEY POINTS

- Renin is the rate-limiting step in the formation of the vasoconstrictor angiotensin II.

- The juxtaglomerular cells are the site of renin synthesis, storage, and release, initiated by formation of first a preprorenin, then inactive prorenin, which is deposited in storage granules and cleaved to form the active enzyme.

- Secretion of active renin occurs in response to four regulatory mechanisms: the renal baroreceptor, the macula densa, β_1-receptor stimulation by renal nerves, and humoral factors.

See also Chapters 3, 4, 6, 7, 8, 36, 41, 51

Renin Synthesis in Juxtaglomerular Cells

Renin catalyzes the rate-limiting step in a cascade that forms angiotensin II and its congeners (**see Figure 5.1**). Renin is an aspartyl proteolytic enzyme whose substrate is angiotensinogen, a 60,000-Da peptide formed within the liver and released into the general circulation. The target bond of renin action is located between leucine in position 10 and valine in position 11, between the body of the angiotensinogen molecule and its amino-terminal decapeptide. The decapeptide released from the substrate is angiotensin I, which in turn is changed by ACE into the potent vasoactive hormone angiotensin II. Because renin catalyzes the critical rate-limiting step in the formation of angiotensin II, renin activity is generally used as an index of the endogenous formation of angiotensin II and reflects the importance of the signals that control renin synthesis and release.

The juxtaglomerular (JG) cells are the locus for renin synthesis, storage, and release. The initial step in renin synthesis is the formation of preprorenin by renin messenger RNA. This is an intermediate form, which is transported into the rough endoplasmic reticulum. The 23-amino-acid "pre" sequence is cleaved, leaving prorenin, an inactive form of the enzyme (47,000 Da), which is passed through the Golgi apparatus, glycosylated, and deposited in lysosomal granules. There, the carboxyl-terminal 43-amino-acid "pro" sequence is cleaved to form the enzymatically active form of renin (40,000 Da). It is thought that cleavage and activation within the granules are initiated by the enzyme cathepsin B. Once the pro sequence is removed, unmasking the active aspartyl residues of the molecule, secretion or release of active renin occurs in response to various regulatory stimuli (discussed below). Renin-storing granules migrate to the cellular surface, where they release active enzyme by exocytosis into the vascular lumen and possibly into the renal interstitium. There is basal (or constitutive) release of active renin into the circulation, accounting for basal plasma renin activity and circulating levels of angiotensin II.

Prorenin release and its presence in the circulation, which under basal conditions is 2-fold to 5-fold greater than circulating active renin, are not regulated by acute control mechanisms and may only reflect synthesis. Any other significance of circulating prorenin is unknown. When active renin secretion is stimulated, circulating inactive renin tends to be diminished, presumably as more prorenin is channeled into granular storage or activated.

In most mammals, the kidney is the primary source of synthesis and secretion of active renin, although prorenin has been found in a number of extrarenal sources, including the adrenal glands, the pituitary, and the submandibular glands. These extrarenal ("tissue") renin-angiotensin systems are discussed in chapter 8.

Renal renin is synthesized, stored, and released by the JG cells, which are derived from vascular smooth muscle and located in the vascular wall near the terminus of the afferent arteriole, where they abut the glomerulus and macula densa. In response to chronic sodium deprivation, there is a unique "recruitment" of non-JG afferent arteriolar cells upstream, which become renin-positive as renin secretion and plasma renin activity increase under these conditions. Renin gene expression is mediated by hormones through hormone-response elements for androgens and thyroxine. Sodium restriction also leads to renin expression in the JG cell, as do chronic increases in cAMP, whereas angiotensin has been proposed as a negative (feedback) regulator of renin gene expression.

Physiological Regulation of Renin Release

Release of active renin is regulated by the renal baroreceptor, the macula densa, renal nerves, and humoral factors. The renal baroreceptor is an intrarenal vascular receptor in the afferent arteriole that stimulates renin secretion in response to reduced renal perfusion pressure and attenuates it as renal perfusion is elevated. The renal baroreceptor is perhaps the most powerful regulator of renin release. Chronic stimulation of the renal baroreceptor contributes to the hyperreninemic phase of renovascular hypertension, and chronic activation can lead to both increased renin release and renin synthesis.

The macula densa is a modified plaque of cells in the distal tubule of the nephron, located at the end of the loop of Henle and adjacent to the afferent arteriole, the JG cells, and extraglomerular mesangium. All of these components make up the JG apparatus, which sends a feedback signal when the macula densa senses a decrease in distal

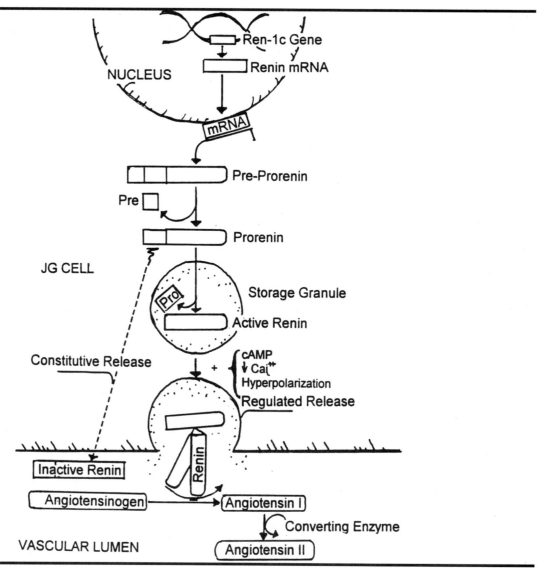

Figure 5.1. Cascade of renin synthesis, activation, and release in juxtaglomerular (JG) cell in afferent arteriole, leading to enzymatic formation of angiotensin II.

tubular salt delivery. This signal initiates a series of steps that ultimately stimulates renin secretion. While the specific nature of the feedback signal remains a topic of considerable interest, adenosine is the substance most often implicated, although many other factors, including prostaglandin E_2 and nitric oxide, may be involved. The macula densa mechanism is most likely a chronic adaptive system for regulating renin rather than an acute mediator.

JG cells are directly innervated by sympathetic nerves. Direct stimulation of the renal nerves causes an increase of renin from the JG cells through a β_1-adrenergic–mediated mechanism. The renal nerves are stimulated via a pathway that involves cardiac mechanoreceptors, aortocarotid pressoreceptors, chemoreceptors, and vagal afferent fibers. Several central neural reflex pathways mediate stimulation of efferent sympathetic renal nerve traffic and the subsequent stimulation of renin secretion. Renal nerve–mediated renin secretion constitutes an acute pathway by which rapid activation of the renin-angiotensin system is provoked by such stimuli as stress and posture.

Although the three pathways discussed above are the "classic" regulators of renin release, a series of humoral factors has also been implicated. The primary stimulatory intracellular "second messenger" for renin release is the cyclic nucleotide cAMP, which is probably the second messenger for stimulation by β-adrenergic nerves and E-series prostaglandins.

Unlike most secretory responses, renin release is inhibited, not stimulated, by increased intracellular calcium. This occurs via a calmodulin-mediated process. In other words, there is an inverse relationship between intracellular calcium concentration and renin release. Electrical depolarization of the JG cell permits calcium entry and inhibits renin release. Conversely, hyperpolarization leads to decreased JG cell calcium and increased renin release. Among the depolarizing, inhibitory humoral factors are vasoconstrictors, such as angiotensin, α-adrenergic agonists, thromboxane (or the endoperoxide prostaglandin H_2), adenosine A_1 agonists, and endothelin.

The cyclic nucleotide cGMP may act as another inhibitory second messenger. Factors that stimulate guanylate cyclase, such as atrial natriuretic factor and nitric oxide, inhibit renin release. It is also possible that some of these inhibitory hormones stimulate phospholipase C, leading to release of intracellular calcium from sequestered stores.

Humoral agents such as prostacyclin, endothelium-derived hyperpolarizing factor, and nitric oxide may hyperpolarize vascular smooth muscle cells and JG cells, leading to decreased influx of calcium across cell membranes. Integration of these humoral mechanisms into the more classic pathways of renin stimulation remains the focus of considerable investigation.

SUGGESTED READING

1. Hsueh WA, Baxter JD. Human prorenin. *Hypertension.* 1991;17:469–477.
2. Keeton TK, Campbell WB. The pharmacologic alteration of renin release. *Pharmacol Rev.* 1980;32:81–227.
3. Navar LG, Inscho EW, Majid SA, Imig JD, Harrison-Bernard LM, Mitchell KD. Paracrine regulation of the renal microcirculation. *Physiol Rev.* 1996;76: 425–536.
4. Sigmund CD, Gross KW. Structure, expression, and regulation of the murine renin genes. *Hypertension.* 1991;18:446–457.

Chapter 6

Angiotensin I–Converting Enzyme

Randal A. Skidgel, PhD; Ervin G. Erdös, MD

KEY POINTS

- Angiotensin I–converting enzyme (ACE) hydrolyzes inactive angiotensin I to form the active pressor angiotensin II and also inactivates the vasodilator bradykinin.

- ACE is found on endothelial cells, especially in the lung, retina, and brain. It is also present in the choroid plexus, proximal tubules of the kidney, and testes.

See also Chapters 3, 4, 5, 7, 8, 41, 51, 129, 130

Angiotensin I–converting enzyme (ACE) converts the inactive decapeptide angiotensin I to the active octapeptide angiotensin II by releasing the C-terminal histidyl-leucine dipeptide. The enzyme is not specific for angiotensin, because it cleaves a variety of other peptides, including bradykinin, luteinizing hormone–releasing hormone, enkephalins, and substance P. On the basis of enzyme kinetics, ACE is a better "kininase" than "converting enzyme" or "enkephalinase" because of the very low K_m of bradykinin. Thus, ACE activates the vasoconstrictor angiotensin while it inactivates the vasodilator bradykinin **(Figure 6.1)**. ACE inhibitors interfere with both reactions, prolonging the half-life of bradykinin while inhibiting the formation of angiotensin II. Some of the beneficial cardiac actions of ACE inhibitor therapy may be attributable to potentiating and prolonging the effects of bradykinin. ACE is a metalloenzyme that always requires zinc as cofactor and also needs chloride ions to cleave most substrates; angiotensin I conversion is absolutely chloride dependent, whereas bradykinin hydrolysis is less affected.

Distribution and Properties

Human ACE has a molecular weight of 150 000 to 180 000, of which 146.6 kD is protein and the balance is carbohydrate. The majority of ACE is membrane-bound and is present on the plasma membrane of various cell types **(Figure 6.2)**. ACE is inserted into the membrane by a 17-amino-acid hydrophobic region near the C-terminus. Proteolytic cleavage near the C-terminus results in the release of ACE from the plasma membrane, which happens normally in vivo. ACE can be detected in many body fluids **(Figure 6.2)**.

In vascular beds, ACE is bound to the plasma membrane of endothelial cells, where it cleaves circulating peptides such as angiotensin I or bradykinin. Vessels of the lung, retina, and brain are especially rich in ACE; epithelial cells in general have a higher concentration of ACE than do endothelial cells. The human kidney contains 5 to 6 times more ACE per wet weight than the lung; the proximal tubular brush border is a major site of kidney ACE. Other microvillar structures of epithelial linings in the small intestine, choroid plexus, and placenta are also very rich in ACE **(Figure 6.2)**. ACE is concentrated in some other regions of the brain in addition to the choroid plexus, such as the subfornical organ, area postrema, substantia nigra, and locus ceruleus.

Primary Structure

The primary structure of ACE was first determined by cloning and sequencing of its complementary DNA from a human endothelial cell complementary DNA library. The sequence unexpectedly revealed the presence of two putative active centers **(Figure 6.2)** located within two highly homologous domains, which probably evolved through gene duplication. Testicular ACE contains only one of these domains and therefore may represent the ancestral, nonduplicated form of the enzyme.

Endothelial ACE contains two zinc ions and two inhibitor binding sites per molecule, indicating the presence of two functional active sites. The K_m values for the classic substrates (angiotensin I or bradykinin) do not differ between the active centers on the N- and C-domains, but the turnover number (K_{cat}) with the C-domain is higher *in vitro*. However, some other physiological peptide substrates are preferentially cleaved by the N-domain active site. The rates of

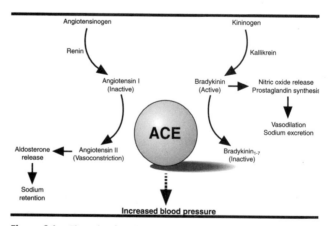

Figure 6.1. The role of angiotensin I–converting enzyme (ACE) in the metabolism of vasoactive peptides. ACE can contribute to the elevation of blood pressure by converting the inactive peptide angiotensin I to the active vasoconstrictor angiotensin II and by inactivating the vasodilator bradykinin. By blocking vasoconstriction and promoting sodium excretion, ACE inhibitors can lower blood pressure. Modified with permission from Skidgel RA, Erdös EG. Biochemistry of angiotensin I converting enzyme. In: Robertson JIS, Nichols MG, eds. *The Renin Angiotensin System.* London, UK: Gower Medical Publishing; 1993.

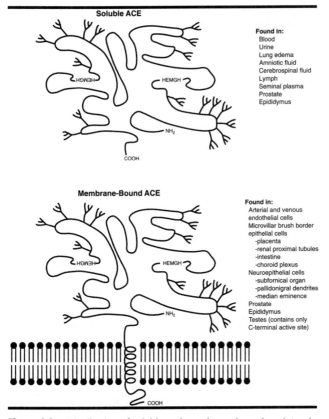

Soluble ACE

Found in:
Blood
Urine
Lung edema
Amniotic fluid
Cerebrospinal fluid
Lymph
Seminal plasma
Prostate
Epididymus

Membrane-Bound ACE

Found in:
Arterial and venous
 endothelial cells
Microvillar brush border
 epithelial cells
  -placenta
  -renal proximal tubules
  -intestine
  -choroid plexus
Neuroepithelial cells
  -subfornical organ
  -pallidonigral dendrites
  -median eminence
Prostate
Epididymus
Testes (contains only
 C-terminal active site)

Figure 6.2. Distribution of soluble and membrane-bound angiotensin I–converting enzyme (ACE). ACE is widely distributed in tissues, cells, and body fluids. Membrane-bound ACE, shown in schematic, is attracted to lipid bilayer by a C-terminal hydrophobic anchor peptide, whereas soluble ACE has been shown to lack this portion of the molecule. The HEMGH (His-Glu-Met-Gly-His) sequence represents the zinc-binding motif in the two active-site domains of ACE, and branched structures denote potential glycosylation sites.

dissociation of ACE inhibitors from the active centers in the two domains differ, so the duration of their inhibition also differs.

Studies on the structure of the human ACE gene revealed an insertion (I)/deletion (D) polymorphism in the noncoding region, corresponding to the presence or absence of a 287-bp sequence in intron 16. Individuals homozygous for the insertion polymorphism (II) have lower levels of ACE in plasma than do those with the DD genotype. The effects of this polymorphism in cardiovascular and renal diseases have been the subject of many studies. Some investigations suggest an association of the D allele with an increased risk for myocardial infarction or diabetic nephropathy.

SUGGESTED READING

1. Ehlers MRW, Riordan JR. Angiotensin-converting enzyme: biochemistry and molecular biology. In: Laragh JH, Brenner BM, eds. *Hypertension: Pathophysiology, Diagnosis, and Management.* 2nd ed. New York, NY: Raven Press Ltd; 1990: 1217–1231.

2. Erdös EG, Skidgel RA. Metabolism of bradykinin by peptidases in health and disease. In: Farmer SG, ed. *The Kinin System: Handbook of Immunopharmacology.* London, UK: Academic Press; 1997:112–141.

3. Linz W, Wiemer G, Gohlke P, Unger T, Schölkens BA. Contribution of kinins to the cardiovascular actions of angiotensin-converting enzyme inhibitors. *Pharmacol Rev.* 1995;47:25–49.

4. Ramchandran R, Kasturi S, Douglas JG, Sen I. Metalloprotease-mediated cleavage secretion of pulmonary ACE by vascular endothelial and kidney epithelial cells. *Am J Physiol.* 1996;271:H744–H751.

5. Soubrier F, Wei L, Hubert C, Clauser E, Alhenc-Gelas F, Corvol P. Molecular biology of the angiotensin I-converting enzyme, II: structure-function: gene polymorphism and clinical implications. *J Hypertens.* 1993;11:599–604.

6. Minshall RD, Tan F, Nakamura F, Rabito SF, Becker RP, Marcic B, Erdös EG. Potentiation of the actions of bradykinin by angiotensin I converting enzyme (ACE) inhibitors. The role of expressed human bradykinin B2 receptors and ACE in CHO cells. *Circul Res* 1997;81:848–856.

7. Wei I, Clauser E, Alhenc-Gelas F, Corvol P. The two homolgous domains of human angiotensin I-converting enzyme interact differently with competitive inhibitors. *J Biol Chem* 1992;267:13398–13405.

Chapter 7

Angiotensin Formation and Degradation

Carlos M. Ferrario, MD

KEY POINTS

- A family of angiotensins is derived from angiotensin (Ang) I through the action of converting enzyme, chymase, aminopeptidases, and neutral endopeptidase.

- Ang-(1–7), a naturally occurring competitive inhibitor of Ang II produced by neutral endopeptidases and increased during ACE inhibition, may have vasodepressor function and Ang-(2–8) and –(3–8) may also affect blood pressure regulation and other functions.

- Chymases (angiotensin convertases) and other alternate routes exist to degrade Ang I to other effectors of the renin-angiotensin system and their inactive fragments.

- Blockade of angiotensin-converting (ACE) enzymes initially reduces Ang II levels; Ang II levels may increase during chronic therapy, probably because of tissue chymases.

See also Chapters 3, 4, 5, 6, 8, 41, 51, 129, 130

In mammalian systems, the net concentration of a hormone such as angiotensin (Ang) II is controlled at its receptor by numerous factors, including those that influence its synthesis, secretion, and removal. Major mechanisms by which peptides are removed include enzymatic degradation by peptidases, hemodynamic factors, and sequestration by endocytosis of the ligand-receptor complex.

Metabolic Pathways

The **Figure 7.1** illustrates the enzymatic pathways leading to the production and metabolism of the active angiotensins. Ang I, the prohormone of the system, is processed into Ang II primarily by ACE and into the heptapeptide Ang-(1–7) by tissue endopeptidases. A chymase (angiotensin convertase) has recently been recognized as an alternative pathway for the production of Ang II.

Three endopeptidases can form Ang-(1–7) from Ang I: prolyl endopeptidase (EC 3.4.21.26), neutral endopeptidase (NEP) 24.11 (EC 3.4.24.11), and NEP 24.15 (EC 3.4.24.15). NEP 24.11 can also cleave Ang II into two inactive tetrapeptides.

Of all the enzymes that degrade angiotensin, the most active in vivo are aminopeptidases. Glutamyl aminopeptidase (EC 3.4.11.7) cleaves Ang II to Ang III [Ang-(2–8)], and arginyl aminopeptidase (EC 3.4.11.6) cleaves Ang III to Ang IV [Ang-(3–8)].

Although Ang II is the major pressor and trophic factor of the renin-angiotensin system, Ang-(3–8) increases cGMP production and may have effects on learning and memory. Ang-(3–8) probably binds to a specific receptor different from those that bind Ang II.

The amino-terminal heptapeptide Ang-(1–7) ([des-Phe[8]]-Ang II) can stimulate release of vasopressin, act as an excitatory neurotransmitter, augment synthesis and release of vasodilator prostaglandins, potentiate the actions of bradykinin, and release nitric oxide.

The major determinants of the duration of action of angiotensin peptides are enzymatic degradation and endocytosis. AT_1 receptors are the primary mediators of intracellular transport of Ang II, but the internalization of the ligand-receptor complex may also be influenced by the AT_2 receptor subtype.

The possibility of forming two different active angiotensin peptides [Ang II and Ang-(1–7)] from a common substrate, Ang I, could allow cells to regulate selective production of one or the other product. Further processing of these two active peptides into smaller fragments may add another kind of specificity to the signaling process.

Functions of Alternative Pathways

Inhibition of ACE initially increases the concentration of Ang I and decreases Ang II and aldosterone. However, plasma levels of Ang II may not remain suppressed during chronic therapy with ACE inhibitors, even though blood pressure remains controlled. Dissociation of the therapeutic effects of ACE inhibitors and the levels of plasma Ang II may indicate incomplete blockade of the enzyme. Furthermore, ACE-inhibitor–induced increases in renin and circulating Ang I may exceed the inhibitory capacity of the drugs in plasma or tissues. Chymase, which is unaffected by ACE inhibitors, provides another route for the formation of Ang II during ACE-inhibitor therapy. The relative importance of alternative pathways in counteracting the antihypertensive effects of ACE inhibitors is currently the subject of debate.

Chronic inhibition of ACE also raises plasma concentration of Ang-(1–7) in both humans and animals. Ang-(1–7) is an endogenous competitive inhibitor of native Ang II; blockade of Ang-(1–7) activity or synthesis reverses the antihypertensive effects of ACE inhibition. Ang-(1–7) can be degraded to the inactive product Ang-(1–5) by ACE with a catalytic affinity (K_{cat}) comparable to that of bradykinin, so ACE inhibitors have two actions that can increase levels of Ang-(1–7). These findings suggest an

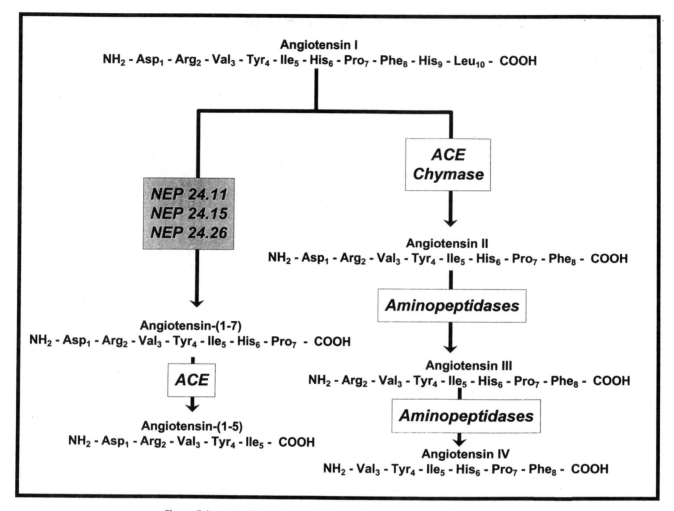

Figure 7.1.   Proteolytic pathways linking angiotensin I to its smaller products.

important role of ACE in regulating the opposing actions of Ang II and Ang-(1–7). The role of ACE and other peptidases in regulating the balance between constriction (Ang II) and dilation (Ang-[1–7] and bradykinin) in peripheral tissues may be important in the regulation of blood pressure and the structural changes associated with hypertension.

SUGGESTED READING

1. Ferrario CM, Chappell MC, Tallant EA, Brosnihan KB, Diz DI. Counterregulatory actions of angiotensin-(1–7). *Hypertension.* 1997;30:535–541.

2. Harding JW, Wright JW, Swanson GN, Hanesworth JM, Krebs LT. AT4 receptors: specificity and distribution. *Kidney Int.* 1994;46:1510–1512.

3. Iyer SN, Chappell MC, Averill DB, Diz DI, Ferrario CM. Vasodepressor actions of angiotensin-(1–7) unmasked during combined treatment with lisinopril and losartan. *Hypertension.* 1998;31:699–705

4. Luque M, Martin P, Martell N, Fernandez C, Brosnihan KB, Ferrario CM. Effects of captopril related to increased levels of prostacyclin and angiotensin-(1–7) in essential hypertension. *J Hypertens.* 1996;14:799–805.

5. Urata H, Nishimura H, Ganten D. Chymase-dependent angiotensin II forming system in humans. *Am J Hypertens.* 1996;9:277–284.

6. Chappell MC, Pirro NT, Sykes A, Ferrario CM. Metabolism of Angiotensin-(1–7) by Angiotensin-Converting enzyme. *Hypertension.* 1998;31:362–367.

Chapter 8

Tissue Renin-Angiotensin Systems

M. Ian Phillips, PhD, DSc

KEY POINTS

- Many tissues can synthesize angiotensin II independent of circulating renin.

- Brain and testes contain significant amounts of angiotensin II despite the barriers that separate these tissues from the blood.

- Locally formed angiotensins can act as growth factors, neurotransmitters, and smooth muscle constrictors.

See also Chapters 3, 4, 5, 6, 7, 41, 51, 129, 130

The classic renin-angiotensin system (RAS), consisting of renin produced by the kidney, renin substrate (angiotensinogen) produced by the liver, and ACE localized in the vasculature and lungs, is not the only source of angiotensin II (Ang II) in the body. There are independent Ang II–generating systems in the brain, aorta, arteries, ventricles, adrenal glands, kidneys, adipocytes, leukocytes, ovaries, testes, uterus, spleen, and skin.

Brain

Except for specialized periventricular areas (such as the area postrema), the brain is separated from the blood-borne RAS by the blood-brain barrier. Therefore, Ang II in the brain itself must come from angiotensin-synthesizing cells within the brain. Angiotensinogen mRNA is abundant in glial cells and is also expressed in some neurons. Renin mRNA is present in brain but in low abundance. ACE is widely distributed in the brain; because ACE is an ectoenzyme, the synthesis of Ang II is transcellular between glia and neurons.

Ang II can be cleaved by aminopeptidases to form the heptapeptide Ang III or the hexapeptide angiotensin 3–8 (Ang IV), both of which can exert physiological effects in the brain. The highest concentrations of angiotensins in the brain are found in the hypothalamus and brainstem, with lesser amounts in the spinal cord, cerebellum, cortex, and amygdala.

AT_1 receptors are clustered on the hypothalamic neurons that synthesize vasopressin and in the nucleus of the tractus solitarius. AT_2 receptors are found in the locus coeruleus and the inferior olivary nucleus, which synthesize catecholamines. Ang IV receptors are in the hippocampus. Ang 1–7 receptors are on vasopressin-forming neurons. AT_1 receptors in the brain are increased in hypertensive rats, and reducing or inhibiting brain AT_1 receptors reduces hypertension.

Ang II injected directly into the brain causes drinking behavior, increased blood pressure, and increased sodium appetite. The blood pressure response to Ang II results from combined effects of vasopressin release, sympathetic nervous system activation, and inhibition of baroreflexes. Increases of hypothalamic Ang II in the early part of the female reproductive cycle suggest that the peptide is a neurotransmitter that participates in the surge of luteinizing hormone essential for ovulation.

Pituitary

Ang II levels per gram of tissue are higher in the anterior pituitary than in the brain. Renin mRNA is present in the pituitary in the anterior and intermediate lobes but not in the posterior lobe. Ang II is concentrated in the gonadotrophs of the anterior pituitary and is colocalized with renin mRNA in the cells that produce luteinizing hormone. Thus, Ang II may modulate increased estrogen production in females and testosterone production in males. Ang II also inhibits prolactin release from lactotrophs.

Blood Vessels

All the components needed for the formation of Ang II are present in vessels. However, much of the angiotensinogen mRNA is expressed in the adventitial layers and in the fatty tissue surrounding blood vessels. Because of the differences in distribution and the fact that renin can be taken up from plasma, it is not certain whether vascular tissue angiotensin formation is independent of the blood-borne RAS.

Heart

All the components of the RAS have also been demonstrated in cardiac tissue. Angiotensin receptors are widely distributed within the heart, particularly on the valves and the myocardium. The atria contain higher levels of angiotensinogen than the ventricles, and the ventricles contain higher levels of renin than the atria. ACE has been found only in the left ventricle. Cardiac fibroblasts possess all the components of the RAS.

Cardiac RAS activity is increased by glucocorticoids, estrogen, thyroid hormone, and high-sodium diet, all of which increase angiotensinogen mRNA. Pressure overload on the heart is associated with a rise in ACE content and angiotensinogen mRNA.

Adrenal Glands

The adrenal glands contain the highest levels of tissue Ang II that have been measured. The majority of Ang II produced by the adrenal gland is localized in the cortex, within the zona glomerulosa and zona fasciculata, where it may stimulate aldosterone and corticosteroid synthesis. Levels of renin in the rat adrenal cortex are independent of plasma renin levels.

Kidney

In addition to releasing renin into the circulation, the kidney contains all of the elements for local production of angiotensin. ACE is present in tubular epithelial cells. Ang II is found in the proximal tubule cells and mesangial cells. Intrarenal Ang II constricts afferent and efferent arterioles and directly increases sodium reabsorption from the tubules. In addition, Ang II is a renal growth promoter, and excessive amounts of Ang II may contribute to nephrosclerosis.

Testes

Because the testes have a blood-tissue barrier, circulating renin, angiotensinogen, and Ang II would not be expected to accumulate in testicular cells. Nevertheless, Ang I, II, and III have been measured in testes, and AT_1 receptors are found on Leydig cells and sperm tails. The testis has a unique form of ACE that is found in the luminal wall of the epididymus. Testicular Ang II may have a growth-regulating role in spermatogenesis.

Ovaries

There is a high rate of production of renin and its precursor, prorenin, in human ovarian cells. All the components of the RAS have been demonstrated in human ovarian follicular fluid. Ovarian angiotensin receptors are also present, exclusively in follicular granulosa cells. Granulosa and theca cells, which secrete estrogen, contain renin and angiotensin. In contrast to the testes, the ovary secretes large amounts of prorenin and renin. Prorenin is secreted continuously by the ovary during pregnancy, and its presence implies a function for the ovarian RAS in normal pregnancy.

Adipose Tissue

The major source of angiotensinogen mRNA in blood vessels is the adipose tissue surrounding them. In obesity, highly vascularized fatty tissue may be a site at which locally formed Ang II causes vasoconstriction, raises systemic vascular resistance, and promotes hypertension.

Skin

Ang II and angiotensinogen mRNA are expressed in rat and human skin fibroblasts. The local concentration of Ang II is greatly elevated after injury, even though plasma levels are unchanged. For this reason, Ang II has been suggested to contribute to wound healing, perhaps by stimulating release of growth factors and promoting vascular smooth muscle cell growth.

Overview

Local RAS systems producing tissue Ang II independent of the blood-borne system may allow local adjustment of blood flow. In contractile cells, such as vascular smooth muscle, mesangium, cardiocytes, and sperm tails, Ang II stimulates contraction. In these and many other cells, Ang II also stimulates growth factor secretion. Ang II may be formed in tissue by the enzymatic activity of renin or by proteases such as tonin, chymase, and cathepsins. Ang II synthesized in one cell can act on a neighboring cell, a paracrine action. Excess tissue Ang II can contribute to ventricular hypertrophy, renal sclerosis, vessel stenosis, and high blood pressure.

SUGGESTED READING

1. Dostal DE, Baker KM. Evidence for a role of an intracardiac renin-angiotensin system in normal and failing hearts. *Trends Cardiovasc Med.* 1993;3:67–74.
2. Dzau VJ, Burt DW, Pratt RE. Molecular biology of the renin-angiotensin system. *Am J Physiol.* 1988;255:F563–F573.
3. Harding HW, Wright JW, Swanson GN, Hanesworth JM, Krebs LT. AT_4 receptors: specificity and distribution. *Kidney Int.* 1994;46:1510–1512.
4. Phillips MI. Antisense inhibition and adeno-associated viral vector delivery for reducing hypertension. *Hypertension.* 1997;29:177–187.
5. Phillips MI, Speakman EA, Kimura B. Levels of angiotensin and molecular biology of the tissue renin angiotensin system. *Regul Pept.* 1993;43:1–20.
6. Unger T, Gohlke P. Tissue renin-angiotensin systems in the heart and vasculature: possible involvement in the cardiovascular actions of converting enzyme inhibitors. *Am J Cardiol.* 1990;65:3I–10I.

Chapter 9

Mineralocorticoid Receptors and Actions

David J. Morris, DPhil; Charles O. Watlington, MD

KEY POINTS

- Mineralocorticoid specificity depends on a combination of receptor specificity and degree of oxidation of competing glucocorticoids.

- In patients who cannot oxidize cortisol, the continued mineralocorticoid receptor occupancy causes abnormal sodium retention and the syndrome of apparent mineralocorticoid excess. Licorice mimics this syndrome.

- Mineralocorticoids affect electrolyte balance by inducing and activating proteins in epithelial cells.

See also Chapters 10, 11, 53, 155

The principal mineralocorticoids in humans are aldosterone and deoxycorticosterone. The principal steroid receptors are the mineralocorticoid receptor (MR, or steroid receptor type 1) and the glucocorticoid receptor (GR, or steroid receptor type 2). Both are members of the steroid/vitamin D/retinoic acid superfamily of transcriptional regulators. The MR and the GR have high amino acid homology to each other and relatively high homology and overlap of action with the progesterone and androgen receptors, thus comprising a four-member subfamily. The superfamily members share a COOH-terminal ligand-binding domain, a short zinc finger, and a highly conserved DNA binding domain. GRs seem to exist in every cell, mediating diverse metabolic, immunogenic, and neurological actions.

Mineralocorticoids bind to MRs in epithelial cells located along discrete portions of the renal tubule, parotid gland, and colon. Mineralocorticoids stimulate Na^+ uptake and K^+ and H^+ secretion into the tubule fluid in the cortical and medullary collecting duct of the mammalian kidney. These mineralocorticoid actions most likely result from (1) activation or synthesis of ouabain-sensitive Na^+, K^+-dependent ATPase pump activity in the serosal membrane of the target cell, and (2) activation of Na^+ channels in the luminal side. Mineralocorticoids also bind to MRs in vascular smooth muscle and in discrete areas of the brain and heart.

Mineralocorticoid Receptor Specificity

Because of the higher circulating levels of glucocorticoids relative to mineralocorticoids, it was always presumed that MRs bind only, mineralocorticoids. However, it is now known that both glucocorticoids and mineralocorticoids bind to MRs with equal affinity. Specificity is conferred by 11β-hydroxysteroid dehydrogenase (HSD), an enzyme that oxidizes cortisol to inactive cortisone. Biochemical studies of children with the rare syndrome of apparent mineralocorticoid excess have revealed that cortisol is the cause of their excessive salt retention, hypertension, and hypokalemia; their renin-angiotensin-aldosterone system is suppressed. These children have mutations of the 11β-HSD isoform 2 (11β-HSD2), which is the major isoform present in human kidney. Because their 11β-HSD2 can-

not inactivate cortisol to cortisone (and protect kidney MRs from this glucocorticoid), cortisol acts excessively as a mineralocorticoid.

The glucocorticoids cortisol and corticosterone can also act as mineralocorticoids in patients after excessive ingestion of licorice. The active ingredient, glycyrrhetinic acid, potently inhibits renal 11β-HSD2, permitting these steroids to act as ligands for the MR and causing excessive sodium and water retention, hypertension, and hypokalemic alkalosis. In this circumstance, the synthesis of aldosterone and the renin-angiotensin system are also suppressed. These experiments of nature have strengthened the belief that coexpression of 11β-HSD2 with MRs in tissues confers specificity of MRs toward mineralocorticoids.

Mineralocorticoid Effects

The sequence of steroid action on living cells begins when steroid molecules enter the cell by diffusion and bind to avid, specific receptor proteins in the cytoplasm and/or nucleus and activate them. The steroid-receptor complex alters transcription of certain target genes. Steroid binding to the COOH terminal of the receptor causes disassociation of heat shock proteins. The receptor then undergoes conformational changes to allow dimerization, with high-affinity binding of the dimer to the regulatory end of specific target genes, called hormone-responsive elements. It is thought that several phosphorylation steps contribute to activation of the receptor. The active receptor-DNA complex activates recruitment and stabilization of other transcriptional factors at the target gene's promoter, initiates new mRNA synthesis, and thus directs coding for proteins required for hormone action.

SUGGESTED READING

1. Arriza JL, Wienberger C, Cerelli G, Glaser TM, Handelin BL, Housman DE, Evans RM. Cloning of human mineralocorticoid receptor complementary DNA: structural and functional kinship with the glucocorticoid receptor. *Science.* 1987;237:268–275.
2. Brann DW, Hendry LB, Mahesh VB. Emerging diversities in the mechanism of action of steroid hormones. *J Steroid Biochem Molec. Biol.* 1995; 52:113–133.
3. Pearce D. A mechanistic basis for distinct mineralocorticoid and glucocorticoid receptor transcriptional specificities. *Steroids.* 1994; 59:153–159.

Chapter 10

Aldosterone and Other Mineralocorticoid Synthesis and Regulation

Celso E. Gomez-Sanchez, MD

KEY POINTS

- Aldosterone is produced in the zona glomerulosa of the adrenal cortex and is regulated primarily by angiotensin II and potassium.

- The adrenal also synthesizes weaker sodium-retaining steroids, including deoxycorticosterone (DOC), 18-oxycortisol, 18-hydroxydeoxycorticosterone, and 19-nordeoxycorticosterone.

- Adrenal adenomas often produce weaker mineralocorticoids instead of aldosterone.

See also Chapters 9, 11, 53, 155

Mineralocorticoids are steroids that act on renal and other epithelia to enhance sodium reabsorption and excretion of potassium and hydrogen ions. Water is retained along with sodium, leading to expanded extracellular volume. Mineralocorticoids also act in the brain to influence blood pressure levels. Aldosterone is the most important mineralocorticoid, but other adrenal corticosteroids also have variable mineralocorticoid activity, including deoxycorticosterone (DOC), 18-oxycortisol, 19-nordeoxycorticosterone (19-nor-DOC), and 18-hydroxydeoxycorticosterone (18-OH-DOC).

Synthesis

The adrenal cortex behaves as if it were 2 different glands. The outermost layer, the zona glomerulosa, synthesizes aldosterone and is involved in salt metabolism. The zona fasciculata-reticularis, between the zona glomerulosa and the adrenal medulla, synthesizes cortisol (corticosterone in some species), the most important glucocorticoid, as well as androgens. The same enzymes are required for most of the steps in the synthesis of both cortisol and aldosterone, but the enzymes and regulation of terminal conversions differ.

Cortisol biosynthesis occurs in the zona fasciculata of the adrenal cortex. The synthesis is the same up to the synthesis of pregnenolone. In the fasciculata, cytochrome P450–17α-hydroxylase hydroxylates pregnenolone to 17α-hydroxypregnenolone, which is then 21-hydroxylated to 11-deoxycortisol. 11-Deoxycortisol moves passively back into the mitochondria, where the cytochrome P450–11β-hydroxylase transforms it to cortisol. Smaller amounts of corticosterone are also synthesized from DOC in the zona fasciculata in some species, including humans (**Figure 10.1**).

The biosynthesis of aldosterone occurs in 3 consecutive phases. First, cholesterol is transported from intracellular lipid droplets to the outer mitochondrial membrane, then to the inner mitochondrial membrane, where it is converted to pregnenolone by cytochrome P450 side-chain cleavage enzyme. The rate-limiting step is the transfer of cholesterol from the cytosol to the inner mitochondrial membrane. This transfer occurs at intermembrane contact sites and involves steroidogenic acute regulator protein (StAR).

The second phase of aldosterone synthesis is the conversion within the endoplasmic reticulum of pregnenolone to progesterone by the 3β-hydroxysteroid dehydrogenase 4,5-isomerase enzyme, followed by 21-hydroxylation of progesterone by the cytochrome P450–21-hydroxylase to form DOC. The final phase involves passive transfer of DOC back into the mitochondria, where the cytochrome P450 aldosterone synthase on the inner mitochondrial membrane catalyzes 3 successive hydroxylations, converting DOC to corticosterone (11-hydroxylation), corticosterone to 18-hydroxycorticosterone (18-OH-B), and 18-OH-B to aldosterone.

In humans, 2 cytochrome P450–11β-hydroxylases are described, classic 11β-hydroxylase and aldosterone synthase, with genes located on chromosome 8q21-q22 separated by ≈40 kb. The 2 genes have 9 exons spread over 7 kb of DNA and a sequence homology of 95% in the coding region and 90% in the introns.

Regulation

ACTH, which stimulates the first step in all steroid pathways, is the primary regulator of cortical synthesis. Aldosterone regulation is primarily under the control of angiotensin II and extracellular fluid potassium. ACTH stimulates aldosterone secretion acutely, but continued ACTH stimulation does not result in a sustained response. Changes in vascular volume or sodium ingestion affect aldosterone secretion by altering levels of angiotensin II.

Other Mineralocorticoids

Although the zona glomerulosa expresses only aldosterone synthase, not the 11β-hydroxylase, adrenal adenomas usually express both enzymes, as well as the 17α-hydroxylase, and are able to synthesize cortisol. In aldosterone-producing adenomas, 11-deoxycortisol can be metabolized by aldosterone synthase to generate the aldosterone analogues 18-hydroxycortisol and 18-oxocortisol.

18-Oxycortisol. Patients with aldosterone-producing adenomas and with glucocorticoid-remediable aldosteronism produce excessive amounts of 18-oxocortisol. This steroid has ≈2% of the mineralocorticoid activity of aldosterone and can produce hypertension when

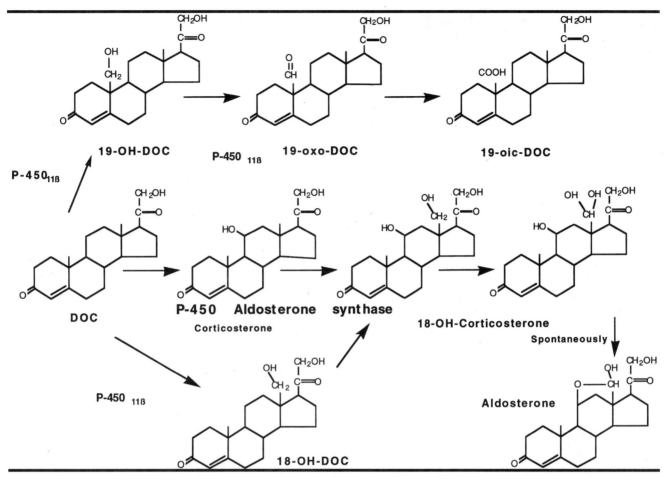

Figure 10.1. Pathways of synthesis of the mineralocorticoids, starting with the common precursor deoxycorticosterone (DOC).

injected into rats or sheep. Its quantitative contribution to the hypertension in the conditions in which it is secreted in excess remains unclear.

Deoxycorticosterone and 18-hydroxydeoxycorticosterone. DOC is synthesized from progesterone by microsomal 21-hydroxylase. Under normal situations, it is only an intermediate in the synthesis of other steroids, but in cases of 11β-hydroxylase deficiency, it is present in sufficient quantities to act as a mineralocorticoid. 18-Hydroxy-DOC is produced by the 11β-hydroxylase in the zona fasciculata or aldosterone synthase in the zona glomerulosa. In normal humans, concentrations of this steroid are relatively low, but in unusual circumstances, elevations of this steroid occur, by unclear mechanisms. It is a weak mineralocorticoid that has been associated with some cases of hypertension.

19-Nordeoxycorticosterone. The steroid 19-norDOC was initially identified in the urine from rats undergoing adrenal regeneration and was found to be a potent mineralocorticoid. 19-NorDOC is formed extra-adrenally, probably in the kidney, from the adrenal precursor 19-oicDOC. This steroid has been found to be elevated in some rat models of genetic hypertension and in rare cases of adrenal hypertension, including rare aldosterone-producing adenomas. Another 19-nor steroid, 19-noraldosterone, has also been shown to be synthesized and is excreted in excessive amounts in patients with

primary aldosteronism. Its mineralocorticoid properties are similar to or slightly greater than those of aldosterone, but its production rates are significantly lower. It is likely that this steroid plays a minor or unimportant role in sodium metabolism or hypertension.

Extra-Adrenal Synthesis of Steroids

Steroid transformations can occur outside steroid-producing glands, including the brain, which can synthesize estradiol, 5α-dihydrotestosterone, pregnenolone, progesterone, and 5α-derivatives. Corticosterone and aldosterone can be formed in vascular tissue and in the brain, in which all the steroidogenic enzymes present in the adrenal are also expressed in very small amounts. It is likely that corticosterone and aldosterone formed in vascular and brain tissue play a paracrine or autocrine role, because their contribution to circulating steroid levels seems to be negligible.

SUGGESTED READING

1. Melby JC, Griffing GT, Gomez-Sanchez CE. 19-Nor-deoxycorticosterone (19-nor-DOC) in genetic and experimental hypertension in rats and in human hypertension. In: Biglieri EG, Melby JC, eds. *Endocrine Hypertension.* New York, NY: Raven Press Ltd; 1990:183–194.

2. White PC. Inherited forms of mineralocorticoid hypertension. *Hypertension.* 1996;28:927–936.

Chapter 11

Cardiovascular Effects of Sex Steroids

David C. Kem, MD

KEY POINTS

- Sex steroids produce different effects on the cardiovascular system depending on dosage, duration, and other factors.

- High dosages of estrogens and androgens result in sodium retention, alter circulating vasopressor and depressor hormones, increase vascular reactivity, and may elevate blood pressure.

- Low-dose estrogens lower blood pressure in postmenopausal women, probably by increasing vasodilator responsiveness to endothelial factors, including nitric oxide.

See also Chapters 9, 10, 53, 64, 155

Hypertension and alterations in cardiovascular function have been associated with excessive production or administration of estrogen, androgens and progestins. The view that sex steroids primarily alter blood pressure (BP) by enhancing or diminishing sodium and water metabolism has been supplemented by recent evidence indicating that these hormones also alter vascular tone and cardiac function.

Estrogens

Elevation of basal BP or exacerbation of preexisting hypertension was observed shortly after the introduction of estrogen therapy. These studies, using relatively high dosages of estrone, estradiol, and synthetic progestins, produced evidence for sodium retention and a high incidence of hypertension (5% to 18%). With lower estrogen dosages (eg, 50 to 100 μg/d), the incidence of hypertension is less than 5%. Studies of estradiol dosages less than 50 μg/d have shown no significant rise in BP in otherwise normotensive women. Hypertension in patients receiving relatively high dosages by injection or by mouth is rarely encountered.

The hypertension caused by high estrogen dosages has been attributed to sodium and water retention, but volume retention alone cannot explain all of the BP effects of estrogens. Estrogens increase angiotensinogen and possibly circulating levels of Angiotensin II. Direct effects of estrogen on the vasculature are also suspected. Estrogens increase dopamine hydroxylase activity, suggesting activation of the sympathetic nervous system.

There is increasing evidence that low-dosage estrogen replacement in postmenopausal females lowers BP or blunts age-related BP increase. Low-dose estrogen directly blunts the vasoconstrictive effects of norepinephrine but not angiotensin II. This effect may involve induction of nitric oxide synthase in endothelial cells. Estrogen replacement also lowers sympathetic nervous system activity.

Results with selective estrogen-receptor modulator compounds, which mimic some but not all estrogen actions, support a dissociation between pressor and nonvascular effects of estrogen. In a recent trial of the drug raloxifene, there was no change in BP.

Progestins

Progesterone has significant antimineralocorticoid activity and may have a direct vasodilator effect on the vasculature. The rise in progesterone concentration during pregnancy is protective against the mineralocorticoid effect of the increased plasma levels of estrogens and aldosterone. A similar blocking effect is observed when progesterone is coadministered with estrogens or mineralocorticoids. Oral contraceptives that use C-17α progesterone derivatives do not exhibit this antimineralocorticoid effect and in themselves cause sodium retention. In early contraceptives, the combination of C-17α progesterone derivatives with high estrogen dosages appeared to predispose recipients to elevations of BP. This problem has been markedly diminished since introduction of low-dose formulations. Furthermore, the newer subcutaneous depo-progestin contraceptives, which are not C-17α derivatives, have not been reported to exacerbate hypertension.

Androgens

Although testosterone and the weak androgens dehydroepiandrosterone and androstenedione have been associated with some hypertensive states, the precise role of androgens in BP elevation is not clear. Hypertension and increased androgenic activity occur in Cushing's syndrome, adrenal virilizing tumors, and polycystic ovary syndrome. Androgens may have a direct effect on the vasculature, or may be converted by peripheral aromatase enzyme to estrogens, a route that may contribute significantly to production of estrone in postmenopausal women. The role of androgens and weak estrogens in the syndrome of polycystic ovaries is controversial. There is some evidence that the androgen and pressure changes are associated with insulin resistance.

The combination of high-dose testosterone or its analogues and sodium loading in experimental animals produces hypertension. In humans, androgen administration to enhance athletic performance has been associated with increased BP and adverse effects on HDL cholesterol and triglycerides. The cumulative effects of androgens on lipids and BP may account for increased stroke and myocardial events in androgen abusers.

SUGGESTED READING

1. Carr BR, Ory H. Estrogen and progestin components of oral contraceptives: relationship to vascular disease. *Contraception.*. 1997;55:267–272.

2. Hanes DS, Weir MR, Sowers JR. Gender considerations in hypertension pathophysiology and treatment. *Am J Med.* 1996;101:10S–21S.

3. Hutchison SJ, Sudhir K, Chou TM, Sievers RE, Zhu BQ, Sun YP, Deedwania PC, Glantz SA, Parmley WW, Chatterjee K. Testosterone worsens endothelial dysfunction associated with hypercholesterolemia and environmental tobacco smoke exposure in male rabbit aorta. *J Am Coll Cardiol.* 1997;29:800–807.

4. Kaplan NM. Hypertension with pregnancy and the pill. In: Kaplan NM, ed. *Clinical Hypertension.* 7th ed. Baltimore, Md: Williams & Wilkins;1998: 323–344.

5. Li P, Ferrario CM, Ganten D, Brosnihan KB. Chronic estrogen treatment in female transgenic (mRen2)27 hypertensive rats augments endothelium-derived nitric oxide release. *Am J Hypertens.* 1997;10:662–670.

6. Sudhir K, Esler MD, Jennings GL, Komesaroff PA. Estrogen supplementation decreases norepinephrine-induced vasoconstriction and total-body norepinephrine spillover in perimenopausal women. *Hypertension.* 1997;30:1538–1543.

Chapter 12

Prostaglandins and P450 Metabolites

John C. McGiff, MD; Alberto Nasjletti, MD

KEY POINTS

- Prostaglandins and other eicosanoids are produced by the action of tissue oxygenases on arachidonic acid.

- Prostacyclin (PGI_2) and prostaglandin E_2 (PGE_2) are vasodilators that counteract the pressor effects of norepinephrine and angiotensin II and stimulate diuresis and natriuresis.

- Thromboxane A_2 (TxA_2), prostaglandin H_2 (PGE_2), and 20-HETE are vasoconstrictors that influence renal salt excretion.

See also Chapters 13, 14, 63, 65

Arachidonic acid (AA) is liberated from tissue phospholipids by hormone-regulated phospholipases **(Figure 12.1)**. Once free, AA is processed by cyclooxygenases (COX), cytochrome P450 (CYP) oxygenases, or lipoxygenases to an abundance of eicosanoids capable of affecting vascular and renal functions.

COX-Derived Eicosanoids and Blood Pressure Regulation

The constitutive form of COX, COX-1, is expressed in most tissues, including blood vessels, kidney, and platelets, whereas the inducible form of COX, COX-2, is usually undetectable but can be expressed in response to cytokines and growth factors. COX catalyzes the metabolism of AA to prostaglandin H_2 (PGH_2), which subsequently is converted to thromboxane A_2 (TxA_2) by thromboxane synthase, to prostaglandin I_2 (PGI_2, or prostacyclin) by prostacyclin synthase, or to prostaglandins E_2 (PGE_2), D_2 (PGD_2), or $F_{2\alpha}$ ($PGF_{2\alpha}$) by specific isomerases **(Figure 12.1)**.

PGE_2 and PGI_2 dilate resistance blood vessels, reduce release of norepinephrine from sympathetic nerves, attenuate the vasoconstrictor responsiveness to angiotensin II and other constrictor hormones, and facilitate renal excretion of salt and water. Inhibition of COX augments vascular resistance, increases vascular responsiveness to angiotensin II and other constrictor hormones, increases antidiuretic responsiveness to vasopressin, and blunts the pressure-natriuresis response. Collectively, these observations support the concept that PGE_2 and PGI_2 serve as counterregulatory influences to pressor mechanisms mediated by the renin-angiotensin system, the sympathetic nervous system, and perhaps vasopressin. Conversely, PGE_2 and PGI_2 stimulate renin secretion, and COX inhibitors reduce plasma renin activity.

Prohypertensive mechanisms may be subserved by TxA_2 and its immediate precursor, PGH_2. These eicosanoids stimulate contraction of vascular smooth muscle directly via activation of shared receptors and indirectly by facilitating sympathetic activity. In the kidney, activation of TxA_2/PGH_2 receptors produces renal vasoconstriction and salt and water retention. Long-term systemic infusion of a synthetic agonist for TxA_2/PGH_2 receptors produces sustained elevation of blood pressure (BP), part of which is attributable to activation of central pressor mechanisms. Treatment with inhibitors of

thromboxane synthase lowers BP in some models of experimental hypertension in rats. PGH_2 may mediate endothelium-dependent vasoconstriction.

BP can increase, decrease, or remain unaffected during treatment with inhibitors of COX. This variability in BP response is not unexpected, because COX-derived eicosanoids subserve both antihypertensive and prohypertensive mechanisms. In general, COX inhibitors have little effect on BP but are more likely to increase BP in hypertensive than in normotensive states. Pressor responses are usually accompanied by deterioration of renal function. On the other hand, COX inhibitors can decrease BP in normotensive and hypertensive conditions in which the renin-angiotensin system is stimulated. The net BP response to inhibition of COX thus seems to reflect the sum of alterations in BP regulatory mechanisms having a prostaglandin component.

CYP-Derived Eicosanoids and BP Regulation

The wide distribution of the CYP monooxygenases in the vasculature and transporting epithelia and the diverse circulatory and renal functional effects of CYP-derived AA products suggest their possible participation in BP regulation. CYP catalyzes transformation of AA by three types of oxidative reactions:

1. Epoxidation of AA forms four epoxyeicosatrienoic acids (EETs) characterized by the position of unsaturated bonds: 5,6-, 8,9-, 11,12-, and 14,15-EETs **(Figure 12.2)**. The 5,6-EET is the most important, having the greatest vasoactivity and the most potent effects on salt and water metabolism. The vasodilator also known as endothelium-derived hyperpolarizing factor appears to be 5,6-EET or a related eicosanoid. Although 5,6-EET is labile, its stable metabolite, the 5,6-diol (5,6-DHT) can be measured **(Figure 12.2)**. Dietary salt loading increases EET excretion by 20-fold, the greatest increase being in 5,6-EET measured as 5,6-DHT. Inhibition of epoxygenase in salt-loaded normal rats increases BP and makes the rat salt-sensitive.

2. Allylic oxidation of AA forms hydroxyeicosatetraenoic acids (HETEs) **(Figure 12.2)**, one of which, 12(R)-HETE, is a potent inhibitor of Na^+,K^+-ATPase and exists in high levels in the vasculature in response to ischemic insults.

3. ω-Hydroxylation of AA forms 20-HETE, which exhibits several properties that may affect BP control: it is vasoactive, affects ion movement, and has mitogenic capabilities. 20-HETE also is a com-

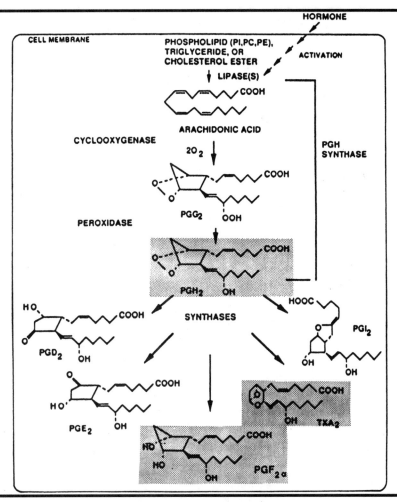

Figure 12.1.   Formation of prostaglandins by the cyclooxygenase pathway. Shading indicates prostanoids that are prohypertensive. From Smith WL. *Prostanoid biosynthesis and mechanisms of action. Am J Physiol.* 1992;263:F181–F191. Reproduced with permission.

ponent of tubuloglomerular feedback and autoregulation of renal and cerebral blood flow and favors Cl⁻ reabsorption.

The subterminal HETEs 16-, 17-, 18-, and 19-HETEs are generated in large quantities in the kidney and are released into urine and renal venous blood. They possess biological profiles that indicate a significant potential for participation in renal regulatory systems modulating vasomotion and ion transport.

There are several features of CYP-AA metabolites that distinguish them from prostaglandins:

1. After formation, both EETs and HETEs can be esterified into the Sn-2 position of phospholipids, from which storage site they can be released by hormonal stimulation of phospholipases to act as intracellular and intercellular messengers. Furthermore, incorporation of CYP-AA products into phospholipids affects membrane characteristics, such as permeability and the activity of membrane-bound enzymes. In contrast, prostaglandins are not stored.

2. Transcellular metabolism of 20-HETE and 5,6-EET via COX **(Figure 12.2)** is essential to the expression of their vasoactivity in most blood vessels.

3. There are multiple forms of CYP: more than 200 CYP genes have been isolated. The multiplicity of CYPs is complicated further by the diversity of mechanisms by which the isoforms are regulated. The rat

renal CYP 4A isoforms (4A1, 2, 3, and 8), which generate a common product, 20-HETE, may act in antihypertensive or prohypertensive mechanisms, based on differential distribution of the 4A isoforms among tubular segments and vasculature of the kidney. 20-HETE constricts preglomerular arterioles and also modulates ion movement in the medullary thick ascending limb of the loop of Henle (mTAL), each site presumably served by a different ω-hydroxylase isoform that is subject to different regulatory factors.

Increased Cl⁻ transport in the mTAL is critical to BP elevation in the Dahl salt-sensitive rat and results from deficient production of 20-HETE, which can modulate the Na⁺-K⁺-2Cl⁻ cotransporter responsible for Cl⁻ reabsorption. Induction of more 4A ω-hydroxylase with clofibrate normalizes BP in the Dahl salt-sensitive rat.

Conversely, during the period of most rapid elevation of BP in the SHR, 20-HETE production is increased. In the preglomerular microvasculature, 20-HETE may elevate BP by vasoconstriction, which reduces glomerular filtration rate and facilitates salt and water reabsorption by decreasing renal interstitial pressure. The elevation of BP in the young SHR can be prevented by induction with either cobalt or tin chloride of heme oxygenase, which catabolizes CYP.

20-HETE also acts as a second messenger for the renal tubular and vascular actions of endothelins. The dependency of the renal

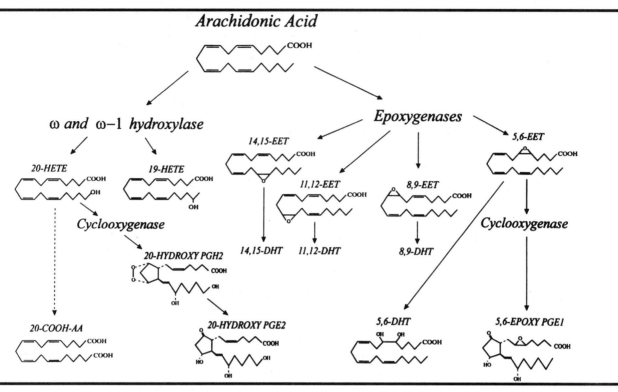

Figure 12.2.   Pathways of AA metabolism catalyzed by CYP enzymes. 20-HETE and 5,6-EET can be metabolized via cyclooxygenase to 5,6-EET and 20-COOH-AA prostaglandin analogues as shown.

functional effects of endothelins on generation of 20-HETE was shown in a mineralocorticoid/salt-induced hypertensive model in rats. The appearance of severe renal injury and rapid elevation of BP coincided with increased production of endothelins and 20-HETE. The pressor response and proteinuria were markedly attenuated by inhibition of CYP450-AA metabolism.

SUGGESTED READING

1. Keen HL, Brands MW, Smith MJ Jr, Shek EW, Hall JE. Thromboxane is required for full expression of angiotensin hypertension in rats. *Hypertension.* 1997;29:310–314.

2. Makita K, Takahashi K, Karara A, Jacobson HR, Falck JR, Capdevila JH. Experimental and/or genetically controlled alterations of the renal microsomal cytochrome P450 epoxygenase induce hypertension in rats fed a high salt diet. *J Clin Invest.* 1994;94:2414–2420.

3. McGiff JC. Cytochrome P-450 metabolism of arachidonic acid. *Annu Rev Pharmacol Toxicol.* 1991;31:339–369.

4. Nasjletti A. Arthur C. Corcoran Memorial Lecture: The role of eicosanoids in angiotensin-dependent hypertension. *Hypertension.* 1997;31:194–200.

5. Omata K, Abraham NG, Schwartzman ML. Renal cytochrome P450-arachidonic acid metabolism: localization and hormonal regulation in SHR. *Am J Physiol.* 1992;262:F591–F599.

6. Oyekan AO, McGiff JC. Cytochrome P-450-derived eicosanoids participate in the renal functional effects of ET-1 in the anesthetized rat. *Am J Physiol.* 1998;274: R52–R61.

7. Quilley J, Bell-Quilley CP, McGiff, JC. *Hypertension: Pathophysiology, Diagnosis, and Management.* New York, NY: Raven Press Ltd; 1995.

8. Roman RJ, Ma Y-H, Frohlich B, Markham B. Clofibrate prevents the develop-ment of hypertension in Dahl salt-sensitive rats. *Hypertension.* 1993;21: 985–988.

9. Sacerdoti D, Escalante B, Abraham NG, McGiff JC, Levere RD, Schwartzman ML. Treatment with tin prevents the development of hypertension in spontaneously hypertensive rats. *Science.* 1989;243:388–390.

Chapter 13

Lipoxygenase Products

Jerry L. Nadler, MD

KEY POINTS

- Three lipoxygenase enzymes oxidize arachidonic acid to short-lived, potent autacoids.

- Hydroperoxy and hydroxyl radicals can be added to arachidonic acid at position 5, 12, or 15. The 5-position derivatives can be metabolized further to leukotrienes.

- Arachidonic acid derivatives oxidized at position 5, 12, or 15 may affect vascular smooth muscle contraction and growth, renin release, aldosterone secretion, and oxidizability of low-density lipoprotein.

See also Chapters 12, 14

On stimulation of cells by hormones or inflammatory mediators, free arachidonic acid is released from membrane phospholipids by a variety of phospholipases, then oxidized (**Figure 13.1**) by cyclooxygenase and cytochrome P450 pathways, as described in chapter A12. Lipoxygenase enzymes, a related group of iron-containing proteins that oxidize arachidonic acid, are named for their ability to insert molecular oxygen at the 5-, 12-, or 15-carbon positions of arachidonic acid.

Anti-inflammatory agents block various steps in these cascades. Glucocorticoids inhibit phospholipases and thereby reduce the release of arachidonic acid. Aspirin and other nonsteroidal anti-inflammatory agents block the cyclooxygenase pathway. Currently, no inhibitors of the 12- or 15-lipoxygenase enzymes are available for clinical use.

The 5-lipoxygenase pathway converts arachidonic acid to 5-hydroperoxyeicosatetraenoic acid (5-HPETE, Figure). Another intermediate product of this pathway is leukotriene A_4 (LTA$_4$). LTA$_4$ hydrolase converts LTA$_4$ to LTB$_4$, which is a potent chemoattractant substance that causes polymorphonuclear cells to bind to vessel walls and may play a role in vascular pathology. Alternatively, LTA$_4$ can be converted to LTC$_4$, LTD$_4$, or LTE$_4$. These three leukotrienes together, formerly known as the "slow-reacting substance of anaphylaxis" (SRS-A), are potent vasoconstrictors in several vascular beds that also cause increased microvascular permeability. Leukotrienes are synthesized primarily by mast cells, eosinophils, neutrophils, and macrophages. Vascular endothelium and smooth muscle cells themselves have little capacity to produce leukotrienes, but they may convert intermediate products to leukotrienes under certain conditions.

The biological role of products of the 12- and 15-lipoxygenase pathways has become clear only over the past several years. Both enzymes produce unstable endoperoxides or HPETEs, which are subsequently converted to a variety of products, including more stable hydroxyeicosatetraenoic acids (HETEs) (**Figure 13.1**). 12- and 15-HETE production has been shown in vascular tissues, including cultured vascular smooth muscle cells, endothelial cells, aorta, and coronary arteries. These vascular cells have the capacity to incorporate these HETEs into cell lipids and to produce additional metabolites. Furthermore, 12-HETE is a major product of platelets, adrenal glomerulosa cells, and certain sites within the renal cortex, including

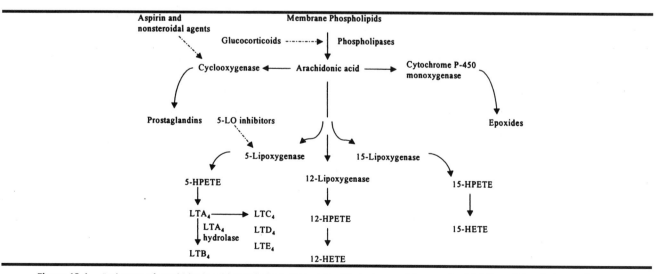

Figure 13.1. Pathways of arachidonic acid metabolism. Broken line illustrates possible areas for inhibition. Abbreviations as in text.

**Table 13.1. Potential Roles of the 12- and
15-Lipoxygenase Pathway in
Cardiovascular Disorders**

Inhibition of renin release (particularly 12-lipoxygenase pathway)

Inhibition of prostacyclin synthesisDirect vasoconstriction of certain
  vascular beds

Mediation of angiotensin II action in blood vessels and adrenal
  glomerulosa (particularly 12-lipoxygenase pathway)

Growth-promoting effect on vascular smooth muscle cells

May be involved in oxidative modification of low-density lipoprotein

Can lead to monocyte binding to human endothelium

mesangial cells and the glomerulus. Stimulation of monocytes by interleukin 4 also produces 15-HETE. Growth factors such as angiotensin II and platelet-derived growth factor can increase 12-lipoxygenase expression and activity.

The Table lists examples of potential biological effects of the 12- and 15-lipoxygenase products of arachidonic acid. The 15-lipoxygenase enzyme is found in macrophage-rich atherosclerotic areas in the human blood vessel wall, raising speculation about a role in atherogenesis. Angiotensin II has recently been shown to increase 12-lipoxygenase products and to activate transcription of the 12-lipoxygenase gene in human adrenal glomerulosa and cultured human aortic smooth muscle.

There are several possible mechanisms by which the lipoxygenase products can produce their biological effects, including increased intracellular free calcium levels and activation of protein kinase C. Arachidonic acid–derived products of the 12-lipoxygenase pathway have been shown to activate mitogen-activated protein kinase and stress-activated kinases, suggesting a role in cell proliferation and inflammation.

In summary, lipoxygenase enzymes in human vascular, inflammatory, and adrenal cells have the capacity to produce products that are highly active and may be involved in hypertension, inflammation, and atherosclerosis.

SUGGESTED READING

1. Folcik V, Nivar-Aristy R, Krajewskih L, Cathcart M. Lipoxygenase contributes to the oxidation of lipids in human atherosclerotic plaques. *J Clin Invest.* 1995;96:504–510.

2. Kim JA, Gu JL, Natarajan R, Esteban J, Berliner JA, Nadler JL. A leukocyte-type of 12-lipoxygenase is expressed in human vascular and mononuclear cells: evidence for upregulation by angiotensin II. *Arterioscler Thromb Vasc Biol.* 1995;15:942–948.

3. Lewis RA, Austen KF, Soberman RJ. Leukotrienes and other products of the 5-lipoxygenase pathway: biochemistry and relation to pathobiology of human diseases. *N Engl J Med.* 1990;323:645–655.

4. Natarajan R, Gu JL, Rossi J, et al. Elevated glucose and angiotensin II increase 12-lipoxygenase activity and expression in porcine aortic smooth muscle cells. *Proc Natl Acad Sci U S A.* 1993;90:4947–4951.

5. Rao GN, Alexander RW, Runge MS. Linoleic acid and its metabolites, hydroperoxyocatadecadienoic acids, stimulate c-fos, c-jun, and c-myc mRNA expression, mitogen-activated protein kinase activation and growth in rat aortic smooth muscle cells. *J Clin Invest.* 1995;96:842–847.

6. Scheidegger K, Butler S, Witztum J. Angiotensin II increases macrophage-mediated modification by low density lipoprotein via the lipoxygenase pathway. *J Biol Chem.* 1997;272:1609–1615.

7. Sigal E. The molecular biology of mammalian arachidonic acid metabolism. *Am J Physiol.* 1991;260:L13–L28.

8. Spector AA, Gordon JA, Moore SA. Hydroxyeicosatetraenoic acids (HETEs). *Prog Lipid Res.* 1988;27:271–323.

9. Yamamato S. Mammalian lipoxygenase: molecular structure and functions. *Biochim Biophys Acta.* 1992;1128:117–131.

10. Wen Y, Scott S, Liu Y, Gonzales N, Nadler JL. Evidence that angiotensin II and lipoxygenase products activate the c-Jun NH2-terminal kinase. *Circ Res.* 1997;81:651–655.

Chapter 14

Cardiovascular Effects of Fatty Acids

Brent M. Egan, MD

KEY POINTS

- Abdominal obesity is linked to increased concentration and turnover of nonesterified fatty acids (NEFAs).

- NEFAs may play a role in hypertension and accelerated vascular disease by enhancing vasoconstriction sensitivity to norepinephrine and vascular remodeling in response to angiotensin II.

- NEFAs stimulate protein kinase C and extracellular signal–regulated kinases, promoting mitogenesis.

See also Chapters 12, 13, 32

Several lines of evidence suggest a role for fatty acids in vascular pathophysiology and blood pressure regulation. Raising plasma nonesterified fatty acids (NEFAs) in minipigs with an infusion of intralipid and heparin acutely elevates vascular resistance and blood pressure. Infusing oleic acid into the portal vein of rats induces hypertension. Obese hypertensive patients have elevated plasma NEFAs, including oleic acid, the most abundant fatty acid in plasma. The elevated NEFAs in obese hypertensive patients are resistant to suppression by insulin and correlate with blood pressure independently of hyperinsulinemia and insulin-mediated glucose disposal. The Paris Prospective Study observed that plasma NEFAs measured under fasting conditions and after an oral glucose load were positively and strongly related to the increase in blood pressure over time.

Fatty Acids and Vascular α₁-Adrenergic Receptor Reactivity

The elevated NEFAs in abdominally obese hypertensive patients may contribute to their increased vascular α_1-adrenergic reactivity and tone by direct effects on blood vessels. Infusion of fatty acids into the dorsal hand veins of normal volunteers to concentrations approximating those observed in obese hypertensives increased by 3-fold the venoconstrictor sensitivity to phenylephrine, an α_1-adrenergic receptor agonist. Infusion of fatty acids also enhanced the magnitude and duration of the reflex venoconstrictor response to thigh cuff inflation and augmented systemic pressor sensitivity to phenylephrine in lean, normotensive volunteers. These studies raise the possibility that the elevated NEFAs in obese hypertensive patients contribute directly to their increased vascular α_1-adrenergic reactivity and tone by effects on α_1-adrenergic receptors.

Fatty acids affect endothelial and vascular smooth muscle cell (VSMC) function in vitro as well as vascular reactivity in vivo. The cellular actions of NEFAs include effects on membrane fluidity, Na^+, K^+-ATPase, Na^+ and K^+ channels, and Ca^{2+} currents. *Cis*-unsaturated NEFAs, such as oleic acid, directly activate protein kinase C (PKC), especially the calcium-independent isoforms, with EC_{50} values of ≈ 5 μmol/L, the estimated intracellular NEFA concentration.

Fatty Acids and Endothelial Function

Oleic and linoleic acids suppress NOS activity in endothelial cells and blunt endothelium-dependent relaxation in vessel rings. Raising circulating levels of NEFAs impairs regional endothelium-dependent dilator responses to methacholine in the lower extremities of healthy volunteers. These observations raise the possibility that elevated NEFAs in obese or insulin-resistant subjects contribute to endothelial dysfunction and associated vascular changes.

Fatty Acids and VSMCs

Oleic acid induces a concentration-dependent activation of PKC-dependent thymidine incorporation and increases cell number and extracellular signal–regulated kinases (ERKs) in primary cultures of VSMCs. Oleic acid but not elaidic or stearic acids, which are weak activators of PKC, increases the mitogenic response, which is blocked by inhibition of PKC. Activation of ERK has been linked to cell growth as well as VSMC migration and vasoconstriction. Thus, activation of PKC and subsequently ERK by oleic acid could link elevated NEFAs to the functional and structural changes observed in subjects with coronary risk and elevated NEFA levels.

In addition to elevated plasma levels of oleic acid, obese hypertensive patients have increased plasma renin activity. Oleic acid and angiotensin together induce a synergistic mitogenic response in cultured VSMCs, as measured by increases of thymidine uptake and cell number. The synergy between oleic acid and angiotensin requires the AT_1 receptor, PKC, and ERK. Thus, fatty acids alone and in concert with other mediators may contribute to accelerated vascular disease.

SUGGESTED READING

1. Egan BM, Stepniakowski KT. Evidence linking fatty acids, the risk factor cluster, and vascular pathophysiology: implications for the diabetic hypertensive patient. In: Sowers JR, ed. *Diabetes and Vascular Disease.* Tocowa, NJ: Humana Press; 1996:157–172.

2. Peiris A, Sothmann M, Hoffmann R, Hennes M, Wilson CR, Gustafson AB, Kissebah AH. Adiposity, fat distribution, and cardiovascular risk. *Ann Intern Med.* 1989;110:867–872.

3. Reaven GM, Lithell H, Landsberg L. Hypertension and associated metabolic abnormalities: the role of insulin resistance and the sympathoadrenal system. *N Engl J Med.* 1996;334:374–381.

Chapter 15

Endothelin

Ernesto L. Schiffrin, MD, PhD

KEY POINTS

- Endothelin-1 (ET-1) is a potent 21-amino-acid vasoconstrictor peptide produced by the endothelium.

- ET-1 may be overexpressed in blood vessels in salt-sensitive and severe forms of hypertension in experimental animals and in humans.

- Action of ET-1 depends on the tissue proportion of ET_A receptors (contraction, hypertrophy) and ET_B receptors (dilation).

See also Chapters 64, 134

Formation of Endothelins

Three mammalian endothelins (ET-1, ET-2, and ET-3) are 21-amino-acid peptides that were discovered originally in vascular endothelial cells but have since been found in many cells in different organs **(Figure 15.1)**. They are important regulators of cardiovascular and noncardiovascular functions, including those of airway smooth muscle, the digestive tract, endocrine glands, the renal and genitourinary system, and the nervous system.

Endothelial cells produce proendothelin (183 residues) from a 203-residue precursor, preproendothelin. Proendothelin is converted to big endothelin (39 amino acids) by endothelin-converting enzyme, a neutral metalloendopeptidase. Endothelin-converting enzyme cleaves big endothelin to form the mature 21-residue endothelin inside or outside of endothelial cells. The main endothelin secreted by endothelium is ET-1, and it is released in response to stimulation by pressure, low shear stress (high shear inhibits ET-1 production), angiotensin II, vasopressin, catecholamines, and transforming growth factor-β. ET-1 produced by endothelial cells is secreted primarily abluminally. Plasma endothelin, which results from spillover from the vascular wall, probably does not reliably reflect production, particularly by endothelium.

Actions of Endothelin

ET-1 secreted toward underlying smooth muscle cells acts on ET_A and ET_B receptors to induce contraction, proliferation, and cell hypertrophy **(Figure 15.2)**. ET-1 may also act on endothelial ET_B receptors, inducing release of nitric oxide and prostacyclin, which explains its bifunctional constrictor and relaxant properties. The predominant effect depends on the vascular bed; in the coronary arteries, which lack endothelial ET_B receptors, endothelins act only as vasoconstrictors.

In the heart, ET_A receptors are present in cardiomyocytes and fibroblasts. Endothelins have a chronotropic and inotropic effect on cardiac muscle and may induce cell hypertrophy. In the kidney, endothelin receptors, predominantly of the ET_A subtype, are present primarily in blood vessels and in glomerular mesangial cells. In distal tubular cells, ET_B receptors mediate a natriuretic effect.

The role of the endothelin system in development has been emphasized by gene disruption experiments. Inactivation of the ET-1 or the ET_A receptor genes in mice results in branchial arch abnormalities, inducing malformations of the mandibula, upper airway, and aortic arch (resembling the Pierre Robin syndrome), with hypoxia and hypercapnia. The slight blood pressure elevation found in this model is probably the result of the hypoxia and hypercapnia, acting through sympathetic activation. Inactivation of the ET-3 or the ET_B receptor gene results in pigmentary abnormalities and aganglionic megacolon, underlining the role of these receptors in migration of neural crest cells (melanocytes and neurons of the myenteric plexus). In humans, mutations in the ET_B receptor gene have been discovered in some of the familial and sporadic forms of Hirschsprung's disease.

Endothelin Receptors

ET-1 is the main ligand of the ET_A receptor, and ET-3 is the main ligand of the ET_B receptor. Endothelin receptors (ET_A and ET_B) have seven transmembrane domains with <70% sequence homology and are encoded by genes on different chromosomes. They are G

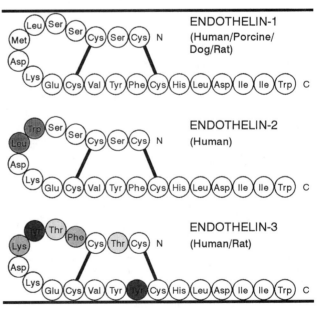

Figure 15.1. Structure of endothelins 1, 2, and 3. N and C indicate N-terminal and C-terminal ends, respectively.

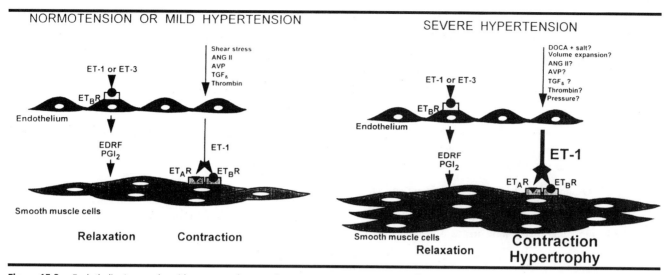

Figure 15.2. Endothelin-1 may play either a vasorelaxant role or a vasoconstrictor role in different vascular beds in normotension and in mild hypertension (left). In moderate to severe hypertension, enhanced expression of endothelin-1 produces a predominant vasoconstrictor effect associated with enhanced growth, resulting in a contribution to elevated blood pressure. Growth of vascular wall is accentuated and contributes both to further elevation of blood pressure and to complications of hypertension.

protein–coupled receptors, signaling through activation of phospholipase C, intracellular calcium mobilization, and protein kinase C activation, the latter contributing to stimulation of the Na^+/H^+ antiporter and intracellular alkalinization. Calcium influx, activation of phospholipases D and A_2, and stimulation of tyrosine kinases are other pathways that participate in intracellular signaling by endothelin receptors. Mitogen-activated protein kinase (MAPK) stimulation of immediate early genes such as c-*jun*, c-*myc*, and c-*fos* may participate in the mitogenic and hypertrophic effects of endothelins, whereas activation of apoptosis may limit endothelin-induced growth.

Endothelins in Hypertension

The endothelin system has been shown to be activated in salt-dependent models of hypertension, such as the deoxycorticosterone acetate–salt hypertensive rat and the Dahl salt-sensitive rat, which overexpress ET-1 in the endothelium of blood vessels and respond to endothelin antagonism with blood pressure lowering. In these models, severe hypertrophic remodeling of small arteries regresses during endothelin antagonist treatment. In stroke-prone spontaneously hypertensive rats and in rats infused with angiotensin II (a known stimulant of ET-1 production), vascular ET-1 expression is increased. Chronic administration of endothelin antagonists lowers blood pressure and reduces vascular smooth muscle hypertrophy. In many hypertensive models, plasma levels of endothelin are normal, emphasizing the abluminal direction of endothelin secretion from vascular endothelium, even in the presence of a significant increase in ET-1 production.

In healthy humans, the acute intravenous administration of an endothelin receptor antagonist results in slightly lower blood pressure, suggesting a role of endothelin in vascular tone. In mild essential hypertension, one study found blood pressure lowering by an ET_A/ET_B receptor antagonist similar to that found with 20 mg of enalapril. Expression of the ET-1 gene is enhanced in small arteries from subcutaneous biopsies from humans with moderate to severe essential hypertension. Other forms of human hypertension in which endothelins may be involved include rare cases of hemangioendothelioma producing endothelin, chronic renal failure, erythropoietin- and cyclosporine-induced hypertension, pheochromocytoma, and pregnancy-induced hypertension. Severity of blood pressure elevation and salt sensitivity may be common denominators for activation of the vascular endothelin system in both humans and experimental animals, but the definitive place of endothelins in the pathophysiology of hypertension is still unclear.

Figure 2 summarizes one view of the potential implication of ET-1 in blood pressure elevation and vascular hypertrophy in moderate to severe hypertension. Activation of the endothelin system may contribute to progression of atherosclerosis, cardiac hypertrophy, nephrosclerosis, and stroke. ET receptor antagonists may prove useful in many cardiovascular diseases.

SUGGESTED READING

1. Lüscher TF, Oemar BS, Boulanger CM, Hahn AWA. Molecular and cellular biology of endothelin and its receptors, parts I and II. *J Hypertens.* 1993;11:7–11, 121–126.
2. Schiffrin EL. Endothelin: potential role in hypertension and vascular hypertrophy. *Hypertension.* 1995;25:1135–1143.
3. Schiffrin EL, Intengan HD, Thibault G, Touyz RM. Clinical significance of endothelin in cardiovascular disease. *Curr Opin Cardiol.* 1997;12:354–367.
4. Yanagisawa M, Kurihara H, Kimura S, Tomobe Y, Kobayashi M, Mitsui Y, Yazaki Y, Goto K, Masaki T. A novel potent vasoconstrictor peptide produced by vascular endothelial cells. *Nature.* 1988;332:411–415.

Chapter 16

Vasopressin and Neuropeptide Y

Allen W. Cowley, Jr, PhD

KEY POINTS

- Vasopressin is a potent vasoconstrictor as well as a stimulus to water retention; it plays a significant role in normalizing blood pressure during conditions of acute hypotension; its long-term effect on blood pressure depends on water intake and counterregulatory mechanisms.

- There is evidence that elevated levels of vasopressin may contribute to hypertension in a subset of human subjects.

- Neuropeptide Y accentuates the vasoconstrictor effects of sympathetic nerves and pressor hormones; its role in short- and long-term regulation of blood pressure remains to be established.

See also Chapter 21

Arginine Vasopressin

Arginine vasopressin (AVP), also known as antidiuretic hormone (ADH), is a nonapeptide released from the posterior pituitary gland in response to reduced cardiopulmonary blood volume, decreased arterial blood pressure, or increased plasma osmolality. Stimulation of AVP release is elicited by sudden decreases in cardiac stretch with cardiac mechanoreceptor "unloading" and aortic and carotid baroreflex stimulation. AVP release is also mediated directly by receptors in the hypothalamus, which senses osmotic changes of <1%. An increase from normal concentrations of 3 pg/mL plasma AVP to only 9 pg/mL reduces renal medullary blood flow and exerts powerful antidiuretic effects by increasing water permeability of renal collecting ducts. These effects make AVP the major determinant of the rate of renal water excretion. High concentrations of plasma AVP (20 to 400 pg/mL) can be attained during volume depletion and hypotension.

Vasopressin Receptors

AVP interacts with at least two types of receptors, V_1 and V_2. The V_{1a} receptor gene is expressed in blood vessels from a wide variety of organs, including the kidneys. The V_{1a} receptor–mediated vasoconstrictor responses of blood vessels and the glycogenolytic response of hepatocytes is linked to membrane phosphatidylinositol turnover, phospholipase C stimulation, and increased cytosolic free Ca^{2+}. V_{1a} receptors in distal segments of the mammalian nephron also promote prostaglandin E_2 generation.

The most important response to V_2 receptor stimulation is adenylyl cyclase–coupled stimulation of increased water permeability of the luminal membrane of the cortical and medullary tubules. V_2 receptors in cells of the ascending limb of the loop of Henle also stimulate Na^+-K^+-Cl^- cotransport at this site. Vasodilation is observed in some parts of the systemic circulation in response to selective vasopressin V_2 agonists, but V_2 receptor mRNA and proteins have not been found in blood vessels. Vasodilation after V_2 stimulation is probably mediated through the release of paracrine hormones from the interstitial or parenchymal cells surrounding the vessels.

Physiological Role

AVP circulates normally at very low concentrations, ranging from 1 to 3 pg/mL (10 to 12 mol/L). AVP is one of the most potent vasoactive peptides circulating in the blood, and concentrations that are well within the physiological range (10 to 20 pg/mL) can produce significant vasoconstriction and blunt the pressure-diuresis-natriuresis relationship. Constrictive effects of AVP on skin, kidneys, and splanchnic and coronary beds are offset by vasodilation in skeletal muscle, contributing to variable effects on systemic BP.

AVP enhances the sympathoinhibitory influence of the arterial baroreflex and the central nervous system, which further buffers this powerful vasoconstrictor substance. As a result of these forces, only slight elevations of arterial pressure are normally observed with elevations of plasma AVP, which allows the antidiuretic action of AVP to occur without the offsetting effects of pressure-induced diuresis. In the absence of autonomic reflex mechanisms, the pressor activity of vasopressin is increased 9000-fold.

Hypertension

AVP is elevated in many forms of experimental hypertension, but the contribution of AVP to the elevated pressure in these models is unclear. After rapid hemorrhage in dogs, AVP release can bring about a rapid 70% compensation of arterial pressure in the absence of the autonomic reflexes and renin release. Yet long-term elevation of AVP does not result in sustained hypertension in rats, dogs, or humans. In contrast, infusion of a selective vasopressin V_1 agonist, either intravenously or into the medullary interstitial space of the rat, lowers renal blood flow and produces sustained hypertension. The difference between this pressor action and that of AVP itself is probably accounted for by the lack of a depressor V_2 effect from the selective V_1 agonist.

The contribution of AVP to the maintenance of arterial hypertension in humans is unclear. Plasma AVP levels are significantly elevated (5 to 20 pg/mL) in nearly 30% of male hypertensive patients and are directly correlated with systolic and diastolic blood pressure in men. By contrast, as few as 7% of female hypertensive subjects exhibit elevated plasma AVP. It is unknown whether changes in AVP concentrations in essential hypertension are primary or secondary. Plasma AVP levels can be higher ($>$20 pg/mL) in the malignant phase of hypertension or in congestive heart failure. AVP elevations of this magnitude could contribute to chronic redistribution of cardiac output and influence regional blood flow, body fluid volume status, and autonomic reflex mechanisms. Plasma AVP levels are higher in blacks than in whites, and selective vasopressin V_1 receptor inhibition was shown to lower mean arterial pressure in blacks (28 mm Hg) but not in whites.

The plasma AVP levels usually found in hypertensive humans are lower than those needed to produce pressor responses in normal subjects. However, sustained plasma levels of 10 to 20 pg/mL could result in fluid retention, volume expansion, and a rise of arterial pressure. The extent to which this occurs depends on the level of daily water intake. If hypertension does occur, as observed with chronic intravenous infusion of AVP with a fixed water intake, significant elevations of pressure are sustained for only 1 to 2 weeks because of the phenomenon known as "vasopressin escape." Escape from the fluid-retaining effects of AVP results from pressure-induced diuresis similar to that observed in patients with the syndrome of inappropriate ADH (SIADH).

Neuropeptide Y

Neuropeptide Y (NPY) is a 36-amino-acid peptide that has been implicated in numerous physiological processes, including thirst, appetite, and control of blood pressure. It is one of the most abundant peptides in the mammalian brain, where it found mainly in interneurons. It is also found in norepinephrine-containing neurons in the hypothalamus, the ventrolateral medulla, and the locus coeruleus. In the peripheral nervous system, NPY is found mainly in sympathetic ganglia, where it is manufactured, and in sympathetic terminals, where it is colocalized and coreleased with norepinephrine and ATP. NPY-containing sympathetic fibers innervate blood vessels, mainly small arteries, as well as the heart and the kidney.

Receptors and Actions

Of the three proposed NPY receptor subtypes, Y_1 and Y_2 are believed to be the most relevant for control of vascular tone. Y_1 receptors are postsynaptic, coupled to the inhibition of adenylate cyclase, and increase intracellular calcium. Y_2 receptors are predominantly presynaptic, and they decrease intracellular calcium by inhibiting N-type calcium channels in nerve terminals. NPY receptors at presynaptic sites in the vasculature, heart, and kidney mediate inhibition of transmitter release. At postsynaptic sites at neurovascular junctions, NPY can cause direct vasoconstriction or potentiate the vasoconstrictor effects of norepinephrine, angiotensin, or serotonin in some vessels.

NPY is released from nerve cells in the central and peripheral nervous system at sites at which important cardiovascular control mechanisms are known to be controlled. Administration of NPY into the nucleus tractus solitarii or caudal ventrolateral medulla lowers blood pressure and heart rate.

In contrast to the antidiuretic effects of most vasoconstrictor neurotransmitters and hormones, NPY enhances diuresis and natriuresis in vivo in anesthetized animals. NPY has been reported to reduce renin release, elevate plasma atrial natriuretic peptide, and directly modify Na,K-ATPase activity on renal proximal tubules.

Hypertension

NPY release may be enhanced in some animal models of hypertension and in a subset of patients with essential hypertension. In the brain of the spontaneously hypertensive rat (SHR), a reduced NPY content has been observed by a number of investigators. A selective NPY receptor blocker failed to change blood pressure or heart rate in SHRs; however, elevated plasma NPY levels have been found in patients with essential hypertension in several studies, including one on hypertensive children and adolescents. In summary, it appears that NPY release may be somewhat enhanced in some animal models of hypertension and in a subset of patients with essential hypertension, but the importance of this peptide in normal physiology and in hypertension remains to be determined.

SUGGESTED READING

1. Cowley AW Jr, Liard JF. Cardiovascular actions of vasopressin. In: Gash DM, Boer GJ, eds. *Vasopressin: Principles and Properties.* New York, NY: Plenum Press; 1987: 389–433.
2. Cowley AW Jr, Roman RJ. Role of the kidney in hypertension. *JAMA.* 1996;275: 1581–1589.
3. Bakris G, Bursztzen M, Gavras I, Bresnahan M, Gavras H. Role of vasopressin in essential hypertension: racial differences. *J Hypertens.* 1997;15:545–550.
4. Crofton JT, Ota M, Shore L. Role of vasopressin, the renin-angiotensin system and sex in Dahl salt-sensitive hypertension. *J Hypertens.* 1993;11:1031–1038.
5. Michel MC, Rascher W. Neuropeptide Y: a possible role in hypertension. *J Hypertens.* 1995;13:385–395.
6. Zhao XH, Sun XY, Edvinsson L, Hedner T. Does the neuropeptide Y Y1 receptor contribute to blood pressure control in the spontaneously hypertensive rat? *J Hypertens.* 1997;15:19–27.
7. McCauley MA, Chen X, Westfall TC. Central cardiovascular actions of neuropeptide Y. In: Colmers WF, Wahlestedt C, eds. *The Biology of Neuropeptide Y and Related Peptides.* Clifton, NJ: Humana Press; 1993:389–418.

Chapter 17

Kinins

Oscar A. Carretero, MD

KEY POINTS

- Kinins are potent vasodilators cleaved from kininogens by kallikreins that stimulate release of nitric oxide and prostaglandins.
- Kinin formation increases with stimulation of secretory activity in some glands and with inflammation in some cases.
- Kinins are natriuretic and diuretic.

See also Chapter 19

Kinins are vasodepressor autacoids that play an important role in the regulation of cardiovascular and renal function. In mammals, the main kinins are bradykinin and lysyl-bradykinin (kallidin). They are released from substrates known as kininogens by serine protease enzymes known as kininogenases (**Figure 17.1**). The main kininogenases are plasma and tissue (glandular) kallikrein. These are separate enzymes that differ in function and are encoded by different genes.

Kallikrein-Kinin Bioregulation

There are two main kininogens, high-molecular-weight kininogen and low-molecular-weight kininogen, both synthesized in the liver and found in very high concentrations in plasma. They are encoded by a single gene, but their messenger RNAs are generated by different splicing of the gene transcript. Plasma kallikrein releases kinins only from high-molecular-weight kininogen. Kininogens also inhibit thiol proteases such as cathepsin M and H and calpains.

Kinins are destroyed by enzymes known as kininases, located mainly in the endothelial cells of the capillaries of the lungs and other tissues. The best-known kininases are ACE (also known as kininase II), neutral endopeptidases 24.11 and 24.15, aminopeptidases, and carboxypeptidases (**Figure 17.1**). However, even after inhibition of most of these enzymes, the half-life of kinins in vivo is <15 seconds, suggesting that other peptidases are important in the metabolism of these peptides.

Functions

Kinins act mainly as local autocrine and paracrine hormones via two different types of receptors, B_1 and B_2. B_1 receptors are expressed primarily during administration of lipopolysaccharides (such as endotoxin) and in inflammation. Most of the known effects of kinins are mediated by B_2 receptors. This receptor belongs to a family of peptide hormone receptors with seven membrane-spanning regions linked to G proteins. Prostaglandins, nitric oxide, endothelium-derived hyperpolarizing factor, and tissue plasminogen activator mediate some of the effects of kinins.

In some organs, kinins appear to play an important role in the regulation of blood flow to match metabolic demands. In rat submandibular salivary glands, kallikrein secretion and vasoconstriction are increased by sympathetic nerve stimulation. After stimulation, vasodilation is mediated by kinins. This vasodilation is greatly magnified by blocking kinin hydrolysis with ACE inhibitors. Because other glands of the gastrointestinal tract contain kallikrein, it is possible that after a meal, kallikrein is secreted and kinins mediate part of the resultant vasodilation. Similarly, eccrine (sweat) glands contain a kallikrein-like enzyme, and kinins may participate in regulation of sweat formation and vasodilation during sweating.

Kinins may also mediate part of the vasodilation and edema observed during inflammation. Kininogenase, low-molecular-weight and high-molecular-weight kininogens, and neutral endopeptidase are present in leukocytes. Kinins can also stimulate release of cytokines such as interleukin-1 from monocytes.

Renal Kallikrein-Kinin System

Renal kallikrein is located in the connecting cells of the tubules; kinin receptors are present in the collecting duct. Kinins play a role in regulation of the renal microcirculation and water and sodium excretion. The natriuretic and diuretic effects of kinins are mediated in part by prostaglandin E_2. In vitro, stimulation of the release of nitric oxide from endothelial cells by bradykinin or acetylcholine increases cGMP and inhibits sodium reabsorption by cortical collecting duct cells. In vivo, bradykinin causes natriuresis and diuresis without affecting the glomerular filtration rate.

The diuretic and natriuretic effects of neutral endopeptidase 24.11 inhibitors are due in part to inhibition of kinin and atrial natriuretic factor hydrolysis. These two peptides act in synergy to inhibit water and sodium transport in the nephron; inhibition of either peptide blocks the natriuretic and diuretic effects of endopeptidase inhibitors.

Relationship to Hypertension

Decreased activity of the kallikrein-kinin system may play a role in hypertension. Low urinary kallikrein excretion in children is one of the major genetic markers associated with a family history of essential hypertension, and children with high urinary kallikrein excretion have less probability of a genetic background of hypertension. Urinary kallikrein excretion is decreased in various models of genetic hypertension. A restriction fragment length polymorphism for the kallikrein gene family in spontaneously hypertensive rats is linked to high blood pressure. Urinary and arterial tissue kallikrein are also decreased in renovascular hypertension. Mice in which the bradykinin B_2 receptor is deleted by homologous recombination (gene knockout) develop hypertension when fed a high-sodium diet. Thus, low kinin activity may be involved in the development and maintenance of salt-sensitive high blood pressure. In mineralocorticoid hypertension, however, circulating kinin levels and urinary kallikrein excretion are increased.

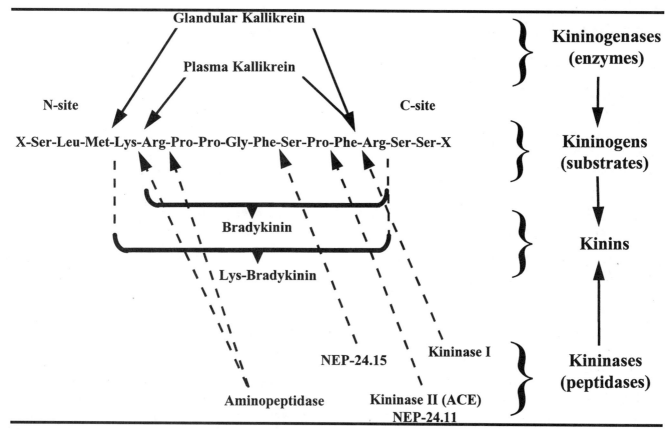

Figure 17.1. Sites of kininogen cleavage (solid arrows) by main kininogenases (glandular and plasma kallikrein). Broken arrows indicate sites of kinin cleavage by kininases (kininase I, kininase II [ACE], neutral endopeptidases [NEP] 24.11 and 24.15, and aminopeptidases).

Role of Kinins in the Antihypertensive Effect of ACE Inhibitors

Increased tissue kinin concentrations and potentiation of their effect may be involved in the therapeutic effect of ACE inhibitors. This hypothesis is supported by the following facts.

1. ACE is one of the main peptidases that hydrolyze kinins.
2. Tissue and urinary kinins increase after treatment with ACE inhibitors, possibly promoting vasodilation and increased sodium and water excretion.
3. Inhibition of the kallikrein-kinin system with kinin antagonists partially blocks the acute but not the chronic hypotensive effects of ACE inhibitors.
4. In kininogen- and kinin-deficient Brown Norway rats with experimental renovascular hypertension, the acute antihypertensive effect of ACE inhibitors is significantly reduced compared with rats with normal kinins.

Cardiac, Vascular, and Hemostatic Influence of Kallikrein-Kinin System

Components of the kallikrein-kinin system, especially tissue kallikrein, are present in the heart, arteries, and veins. Kinins are found in the venous effluent of isolated perfused hearts, and their release is rapidly increased during ischemia. Kinin release after administration of ACE inhibitors may help to protect the myocardium from damage during subsequent ischemic episodes ("preconditioning").

ACE inhibitors reverse cardiac remodeling and improve cardiac function in experimental heart failure due to myocardial infarction in rats. The benefit of ACE inhibitors in this model can be reversed by a kinin antagonist, suggesting that kinins have a cardioprotective effect.

The bradykinin cascade intersects with the hemostatic system in several ways. Plasma kallikrein, high-molecular-weight kininogen, and Hageman factor are involved in the intrinsic pathway of blood clotting and in fibrinolysis. Kinins induce formation of nitric oxide and prostaglandin I_2, which inhibit platelet aggregation. Kinins are also potent stimulators of the release of tissue plasminogen activator and may promote fibrinolysis. These effects may help explain some of the beneficial properties of ACE inhibitors in patients with heart disease.

SUGGESTED READING

1. Bhoola KD, Figueroa CD, Worthy K. Bioregulation of kinins: kallikreins, kininogens, and kininases. *Pharmacol Rev.* 1992;44:1–80.
2. Carretero OA, Scicli AG. The kallikrein-kinin system. In: Fozzard HA, et al, eds. *The Heart and Cardiovascular System: Scientific Foundations.* New York, NY: Raven Press; 1991;2:1851–1874.
3. Liu YH, Yang XP, Sharov VG, Nass O, Sabbah HN, Peterson E, Carretero OA. Effects of angiotensin-converting enzyme inhibitors and angiotensin II type 1 receptor antagonists in rats with heart failure: role of kinins and angiotensin II type 2 receptors. *J Clin Invest.* 1997;99:1926–1935.
4. Margolius HS. Tissue kallikreins and kinins: regulation and roles in hypertensive and diabetic diseases. *Annu Rev Pharmacol Toxicol.* 1989;29:343–364.
5. Nasjletti A, Malik KU. The renal kallikrein-kinin and prostaglandin systems interaction. *Annu Rev Physiol.* 1981;43:597–609.
6. Yang XP, Liu YH, Scicli GM, Webb CR, Carretero OA. Role of kinins in the cardioprotective effect of preconditioning: study of myocardial ischemia/reperfusion injury in B_2 kinin receptor knockout mice and kininogen-deficient rats. *Hypertension.* 1997;30:735–740.

Chapter 18

Endogenous Natriuretic Peptides

John C. Burnett, Jr, MD; Yoram Shenker, MD

KEY POINTS

- ANP (atrial natriuretic peptide) and BNP (brain natriuretic peptide) are released from myocardium when it is stretched; CNP is released from endothelium.

- ANP and BNP induce sodium diuresis by a direct effect on the kidney; they also inhibit renin release and aldosterone secretion.

- Natriuretic peptides relax vascular smooth muscle by activating two types of receptors that generate cGMP; a third type of receptor helps clear the peptides from the circulation.

See also Chapters 36, 134

Types of Natriuretic Peptides

It is now well established that the heart is an endocrine organ that synthesizes and releases the peptide hormone atrial natriuretic peptide (ANP), one of three structurally related natriuretic and vasoactive peptides. The actions of ANP (**Table 18.1**) include natriuresis, inhibition of the renin-angiotensin-aldosterone system, modulation of the sympathetic nervous system, selective increases in capillary permeability, arterial vasodilation, and inhibition of vascular smooth muscle cell proliferation.

ANP is normally synthesized in atrial myocytes and is released from the heart in response to atrial stretch. Examples of situations that cause stretch and release are intravascular volume expansion and atrial pressure overload. The ANP prohormone contains 126 amino acids and is cleaved in cardiac tissue into two fragments; the C-terminal 28-amino-acid peptide (proANP 99–126) is the biologically active circulating hormone. The sequence proANP 95–126, known as urodilatin, has been isolated from human urine and may arise by alternative processing of proANP in the kidney.

Brain natriuretic peptide (BNP) complements ANP and exerts similar biological actions (**Table 18.1**). BNP has a different sequence but is structurally related to ANP. It is synthesized and stored in central nervous tissue and atrial cells. BNP normally circulates at lower concentrations than ANP, but in hypertension and congestive heart failure it may circulate at levels that exceed those of ANP. The increase in circulating ANP and BNP in chronic cardiovascular disease states follows recruitment of ventricular myocardium to synthesize peptides. This underscores the potential importance of the ventricle as well as the atrium as endocrine organs.

The third member of this family of peptides is CNP. In contrast to ANP and BNP, CNP is a product of endothelial cells and is not of cardiac origin. CNP is a potent vasoactive peptide (**Table 18.1**) that dilates both veins and arteries. In addition, CNP is antimitogenic. Unlike ANP and BNP, CNP is only minimally natriuretic and does not inhibit the renin-angiotensin-aldosterone system. CNP probably functions in a paracrine manner, acting locally on vascular smooth muscle cells, whereas ANP and BNP function as circulating hormones.

Natriuretic Peptide Receptors

There are three different natriuretic peptide receptors. Two of these, ANPR-A and ANPR-B, are guanylyl cyclases with identical extracellular domains. The C-terminal intracellular sequences of these two receptors are guanylyl cyclase catalytic domains. Both ANP and BNP bind to the A-receptor, whereas CNP binds exclusively to the B-receptor. This binding results in formation of cGMP. The ANPR-A receptor is highly expressed in vascular endothelial cells and in renal epithelial cells, whereas the ANPR-B receptor is highly expressed in vascular smooth muscle cells.

The ANPR-C receptor is homologous to the two other natriuretic peptide receptors in its extracellular domain but lacks any intracellular domain or guanylyl cyclase activity. ANPR-C may act as a "clearance" receptor that removes natriuretic peptides from the circulation.

Physiological Significance

The natriuretic peptides could be viewed as a "mirror image" of the renin-angiotensin-aldosterone system. ANP and BNP are secreted in response to volume expansion and pressure overload in the heart. Not only do they inhibit renin and aldosterone release, but they also oppose the actions of angiotensin II and aldosterone through their effects on vascular tone and cell growth and renal sodium reabsorption.

Administration of an antagonist of ANPR-A and ANPR-B impairs the natriuretic response to an acute intravenous volume load in rats. Mice that lack the ANP gene have higher blood pressure than controls, but they are able to cope with a sustained increase in dietary sodium. These results suggest that ANP and BNP contribute to blood pressure regulation but are not essential for chronic sodium and water homeostasis.

Clinical Significance

CNP is present in human plasma, but its role in cardiovascular disease states remains undefined. ANP and BNP are elevated in long-standing hypertension and congestive heart failure, but their levels appear inappropriately low for the degree of atrial pressure and volume overload. Thus, these disease states may represent relative natriuretic peptide deficiency states.

Therapeutic strategies are emerging that amplify the biological

Table 18.1. Biological Actions of the Natriuretic Peptides

Atrial natriuretic peptide (ANP) and brain natriuretic peptide (BNP)

Natriuresis
Arterial vasodilation
Inhibition of the renin-angiotensin-aldosterone system
Inhibition of sympathetic function
Inhibition of endothelin
Increase in capillary permeability
Antimitogenesis

C-type natriuretic peptide (CNP)

Venous and arterial vasodilation
Inhibition of endothelin
Antimitogenesis
Minimal natriuresis

actions of ANP and BNP. The effects of these peptides are limited by their removal by the clearance receptor (ANPR-C) and their degradation by neutral endopeptidase. ANPR-C receptor blockade and neutral endopeptidase inhibition both potentiate the biological actions of endogenous ANP and BNP, and these inhibitors have shown therapeutic utility in the treatment of experimental hypertension and congestive heart failure.

Another use for these peptides may be in clinical diagnosis. Raised levels of ANP or BNP are good reflections of failing cardiac function and may serve as a guide for treatment, helping to titrate the dose of medications. There are also early indications that plasma levels of ANP or other fragments of proANP may predict mortality in elderly patients.

SUGGESTED READING

1. Koller KJ, Goeddel DV. Molecular biology of the natriuretic peptides and their receptors. *Circulation.* 1992;86:1081–1088.
2. Lainchbury JG, Espiner EA, Frampton CM, Richards AM, Yandle TG, Nicholls MG. Cardiac natriuretic peptides as predictors of mortality. *J Intern Med.* 1997;241: 257–259.
3. Margulies KB, Burnett JC Jr. Neutral endopeptidase 24.11: a modulator of natriuretic peptides. *Semin Nephrol.* 1993;13:71–77.
4. Tikkanen I, Metsarinne K, Fyhrquist F, Leidenius R. Plasma atrial natriuretic peptide in cardiac disease and during infusion in healthy volunteers. *Lancet.* 1985;:66–69.
5. Wilkins MR, Redondo J, Brown LA. The natriuretic-peptide family. *Lancet.* 1997; 349:1307–1310.

Chapter 19

Nitric Oxide

Ferid Murad, MD, PhD; R. Clinton Webb, PhD

KEY POINTS

- Nitric oxide is formed from endogenous arginine by nitric oxide synthase or from exogenous nitrovasodilators such as nitroglycerin and stimulates guanylate cyclase, forming cyclic GMP.

- Nitric oxide synthase activity is affected by many hormones and drugs.

- The nitric oxide/cyclic GMP system causes smooth muscle relaxation in blood vessels and other hollow organs and affects platelets, nerves, macrophages, and other cells.

- Molecular effects of nitric oxide unrelated to cyclic GMP can be seen on enzymes containing iron, other free radicals, protein modification (through nitrosylation and ADP ribosylation), and DNA synthesis reactions.

See also Chapters 17, 63, 64, 65

Nitric oxide (NO) is a reactive free radical that can act as an intracellular or extracellular regulatory substance. Its half-life in biological systems is 3 to 5 seconds. It freely diffuses through cell membranes and can function as a neurotransmitter, an autacoid, or a paracrine substance. NO has diverse physiological effects including vascular and nonvascular smooth muscle relaxation.

Endogenous NO Production

Most cells and tissues can oxidize the guanidino nitrogen of arginine to form citrulline and NO. The enzyme that catalyzes this reaction is called NO synthase, which has multiple isoforms. The enzyme uses reduced nicotinamide adenine dinucleotide phosphate, flavin adenine dinucleotide, flavin mononucleotide, and tetrahydrobiopterin as cofactors; heme is its prosthetic group (**Figure 19.1**). Some isoforms of NO synthase are calcium and calmodulin dependent. Hormones and drugs that alter intracellular calcium can thereby increase NO synthase activity and formation of NO, which mediates some of the effects of those hormones or drugs (**Figure 19.2**). The effects of acetylcholine, insulin, and other vasodilators are mediated through endothelial cell formation of "endothelium-derived relaxing factor" (EDRF), also known as NO (**Figure 19.2**).

Endotoxin and a variety of cytokines can induce the synthesis of NO synthase in cells and tissues including vascular smooth muscle, macrophages, and liver. The inducible isoenzyme is calcium independent. The severe vasodilation seen in sepsis and endotoxin shock may result from formation of excessive amounts of NO.

Cyclic GMP, the Second Messenger for NO

The intracellular mechanism most commonly described as mediating the actions of NO in vascular smooth muscle cells involves the second messenger cyclic GMP (see the figures. NO binds to the heme-containing enzyme guanylate cyclase, which converts GTP to cyclic GMP. Intracellular levels of cyclic GMP rise within seconds of exposure of smooth muscle cells to NO. The increased level of cyclic GMP leads to activation of protein kinase G, which phosphorylates several proteins involved in the relaxation and antiproliferative responses of vascular smooth muscle. Inhibitors of cyclic GMP production and action such as methylene blue block most of the effects of NO, while analogues of cyclic GMP mimic NO.

Metabolic Interactions

The NO/cyclic GMP signal-transduction pathway can be potentiated or interrupted by a variety of mechanisms. These include hormones and receptor antagonists, agents that can affect NO synthase cofactors or can oxidize NO to an inactive metabolite, agents that alter calcium and/or calmodulin, arginine analogues and substrate-based inhibitors of synthases, agents like hemoglobin that scavenge NO, and phosphodiesterase inhibitors that increase cyclic GMP levels. Some forms of NO synthase can also be acylated with fatty acids and/or phosphorylated by various protein kinases.

Actions of NO

The NO/cyclic GMP signal-transduction system is quite ubiquitous. In addition to vascular and nonvascular smooth muscle relaxation, this pathway can regulate platelet function, ganglionic neurotransmission, neuronal long-term potentiation and memory, insulin secretion, penile erection, macrophage-induced cytotoxicity, and atherogenesis. The list of processes regulated by the NO/cyclic GMP signal-transduction pathway continues to grow significantly (**Table 19.1**).

Cyclic GMP–Dependent Vasodilator Actions

The following cyclic GMP–dependent actions contribute to the relaxation of vascular smooth muscle cells in response to NO: (1) inhibition of calcium channels and calcium release from intracellular stores, causing a fall in cytosolic calcium levels; (2) stimulation of sodium-potassium ATPase; (3) stimulation of plasma membrane-associated calcium ATPase; (4) inhibition of phospholipase C, causing decreased turnover of phosphoinositides; and (5)

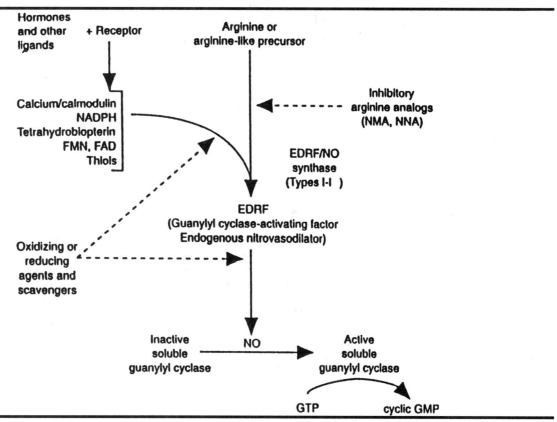

Figure 19.1. Nitric oxide (NO)/cyclic GMP signal-transduction pathway. The NO formed from the oxidation of the guanidino nitrogen of arginine can act as an intracellular or intercellular messenger to regulate cyclic GMP synthesis. EDRF indicates endothelium-derived relaxing factor; NMA, N^G-methyl-L-arginine; NNA, N^ω-nitro-L-arginine; NADPH, reduced nicotinamide adenine dinucleotide phosphate; FMN, flavin mononucleotide; FAD, flavin adenine dinucleotide. Dashed lines indicate inhibitory effect.

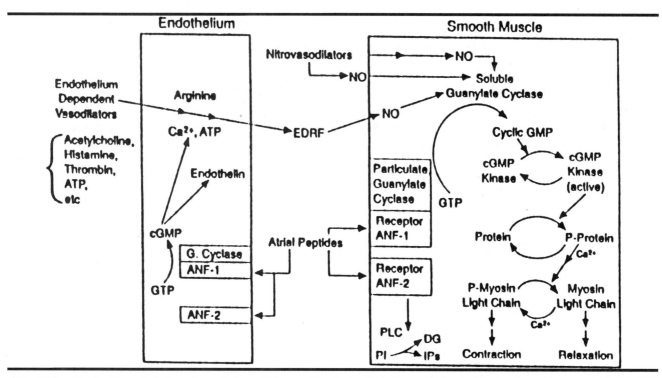

Figure 19.2. Effects of the endothelium-dependent vasodilators and the direct-acting nitrovasodilators and natriuretic peptides on cyclic GMP (cGMP) synthesis and vascular relaxation. NO indicates nitric oxide; EDRF, endothelium-derived relaxing factor; ANF, atrial natriuretic factor; PLC, phospholipase C; PI, phosphoinositide; IP, inositol phosphates; DG, diacylglycerol.

Table 19.1. Biological Targets or Processes Regulated by Nitric Oxide or Cyclic GMP

Enzymes and macromolecules

  Guanylyl cyclase
  Cyclic nucleotide protein kinases
  Cyclic nucleotide phosphodiesterases
  Cyclooxygenase (COX II)
  Heme proteins (iron center and thiol groups)
  DNA modifications and repair
  Glutamate (NMDA) receptor regulation*
  Phospholipase C

Processes

  Smooth, cardiac* and skeletal* muscle relaxation
  Retinal phototransduction
  Intestinal secretion and ion transport
  Renal tubular-glomerular feedback*
  Endothelial permeability*
  Smooth muscle proliferation
  Platelet adhesion and aggregation
  Insulin secretion*
  Hormone production and secretion*
  Neurotransmission
  Long-term potentiation and memory*
  Transcriptional regulation*
  Tissue injury and inflammation
  Pathogen cytotoxicity
  Tumor cytotoxicity
  Calcium transport and redistribution

In some cases the effects of nitric oxide and/or cyclic GMP are well substantiated. However, some of the effects can be considered interesting but preliminary and are designated with an asterisk.

phosphorylation of regulatory and contractile proteins by protein kinase G.

Cyclic GMP–Dependent Antiproliferative Actions

Cyclic GMP, via protein kinase G, alters the activity of several enzymes that participate in growth responses of vascular smooth muscle cells. Tyrosine phosphatase opposes the effect of tyrosine kinases and thereby inhibits early G1 cell-cycle events. Cyclic GMP also influences growth responses of smooth muscle cells by inhibiting protein synthesis. The concentrations of NO required to inhibit DNA synthesis and proliferation of cultured smooth muscle cells are in the range of 10^{-5} to 10^{-3} mol/L, which are two to three orders of magnitude greater than those required for smooth muscle relaxation.

Actions of NO Independent of Cyclic GMP

NO influences the contractile state of vascular smooth muscle by a number of actions that do not require an elevation in intracellular cyclic GMP levels. NO directly inhibits calcium-activated potassium efflux, leading to vasodilation. Another potentially important action of NO stems from its ability to alter the activity of enzymes containing iron. Two such enzymes known to produce vasoactive metabolites from arachidonate are cyclooxygenase and cytochrome P450. NO modifies several proteins through nitrosylation and ADP-ribosylation reactions. NO also causes strand breaks in DNA and inhibits DNA synthesis by binding to the iron-containing enzyme ribonucleotide reductase.

NO and the Vascular Changes in Hypertension

In hypertension, the reduced production and/or bioavailability of NO may lead to cellular events that promote acute or chronic vasoconstriction, reduce vasodilation, and contribute to structural damage in the vasculature. A decrease in cyclic GMP as a result of impaired NO would also result in augmented vascular wall growth.

SUGGESTED READING

1. Dattilo JB, Makhoul RG. The role of nitric oxide in vascular biology and pathobiology. *Ann Vasc Surg.* 1997;11:307–314.
2. Ferro CJ, Webb DJ. Endothelial dysfunction and hypertension. *Drugs.* 1997;53(suppl 1):30–41.
3. Haller H. Endothelial function: general considerations. *Drugs.* 1997;53(suppl 1):1–10.
4. Ignarro L, Murad F. Nitric oxide: biochemistry, molecular biology, and therapeutic implications. *Advances in Pharmacology.* New York, NY: Academic Press; 1995.
5. Murad F. Cyclic GMP: synthesis, metabolism, and function: introduction and some historical comments. *Adv Pharmacol.* 1994;26:1–5.
6. Murad F. The 1996 Albert Lasker Medical Research Awards. Signal transduction using nitric oxide and cyclic guanosine monophosphate. *JAMA.* 1996;276: 1189–1192.
7. Murad F. The nitric oxide–cyclic GMP signal transduction system for intracellular and intercellular communication. *Recent Prog Horm Res.* 1994;49:239–248.

Chapter 20

Acetylcholine, GABA, Serotonin, Adenosine, and Endogenous Ouabain

Roger J. Grekin, MD; John M. Hamlyn, PhD

KEY POINTS

- Acetylcholine, through muscarinic receptors, dilates blood vessels and slows the heart; through nicotinic receptors in autonomic ganglia, it vasoconstricts.

- Serotonin, through central and peripheral 5-HT$_1$ receptors, vasodilates; through 5-HT$_2$ receptors, it vasoconstricts.

- Adenosine is a direct vasodilator.

- GABA has tonic central depressor effects.

- Endogenous ouabain is a novel steroidal cardiac glycoside of probable adrenocortical origin. It inhibits the sodium-potassium pump.

- Endogenous ouabain circulates in elevated amounts in many patients with essential hypertension. Its prohypertensive effects may be mediated by the central nervous system.

See also Chapters 32, 134

Acetylcholine

Acetylcholine, a neurotransmitter with widespread cardiovascular and noncardiovascular actions, is synthesized in nerve terminals by active uptake of choline followed by acetylation. Acetylcholine is stored in vesicles and released into synapses in response to electrical stimulation. It is rapidly degraded by acetylcholinesterase, an enzyme that is present in large amounts in neural tissue.

Acetylcholine serves as the primary neurotransmitter for (1) postganglionic parasympathetic neurons, (2) sympathetic and parasympathetic ganglion cells and the adrenal medulla innervated by preganglionic autonomic fibers, (3) motor end plates in skeletal muscle, and (4) some neurons within the central nervous system.

Muscarinic Effects

Postganglionic parasympathetic effects are mediated by muscarinic receptors. Three functional subtypes of muscarinic receptors have been identified. M$_2$ receptors mediate the cardiac and coronary artery effects of acetylcholine, and M$_3$ receptors mediate endothelium-dependent vascular responses. M$_1$ and M$_3$ receptors also mediate direct smooth muscle–constrictive effects. These effects are blocked by atropine. Cardiovascular effects mediated by muscarinic receptors include vasodilation and negative chronotropic and inotropic effects. The vasodilatory effects of acetylcholine are mediated through endothelial M$_3$ receptors, which results in endothelial release of nitric oxide. Acetylcholine also stimulates release of an endothelium-derived hyperpolarizing factor that contributes to vasodilation of arterial smooth muscle. To date, there is no evidence that either neurally derived or circulating acetylcholine is a signifi-

cant regulator of vascular tone in vivo, and administration of atropine has minimal effects on systemic vascular resistance.

Tonic vagal release of acetylcholine is a predominant regulator of heart rate, particularly in young, healthy individuals. Atropine administration often increases heart rate by 30 to 40 bpm.

Nicotinic Effects

Autonomic ganglionic neurotransmission is mediated by nicotinic cholinergic receptors. Ganglionic blocking agents result in inhibition of both sympathetic and parasympathetic postganglionic neurons. Inhibition of adrenergic tone results in both arterial and venous vasodilation with increased flow and decreased venous return. Postural hypotension is a particularly prominent response. Two ganglionic blockers, trimethophan and mecamylamine, have been used as antihypertensive agents in the past. Because vagal effects usually predominate in the regulation of heart rate, ganglionic blockers commonly cause tachycardia.

Serotonin

Serotonin, or 5-hydroxytryptamine (5-HT) (**Figure 20.1**) is synthesized in a two-step process involving hydroxylation of tryptophan to 5-hydroxytryptophan followed by decarboxylation. Serotonin is present in the enterochromaffin cells of the gastrointestinal tract, in the central and peripheral nervous systems, and in platelets. Within neural cells, serotonin is stored in granular vesicles similar to those of catecholamines. De novo synthesis occurs only in the enterochromaffin cells and the nervous system. Serotonin released from enterochromaffin cells is metabolized almost entirely in liver. The remainder of intestinal and neurally derived

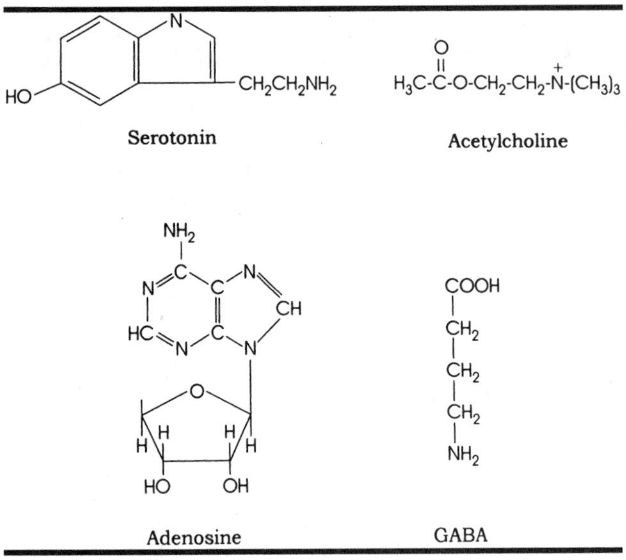

Figure 20.1. Structures of serotonin, acetylcholine, adenosine, and GABA.

serotonin is taken up by high-affinity uptake systems in platelets and nerves. As a result, circulating concentrations of serotonin are extremely low.

Within the cardiovascular system, serotonin has a complex set of actions. Serotonin causes vasoconstriction in most vascular beds, including renal, splanchnic, and cerebral circulations. By contrast, vasodilatory effects of serotonin predominate in skeletal muscle and skin, particularly at lower concentrations. Serotonin is also a potent venoconstrictor. Direct cardiac effects of serotonin include increased inotropic and chronotropic activity. Serotonin-containing neurons in the central nervous system affect arterial pressure. Discrete groups of nerves in the midbrain and medulla elicit pressor responses, whereas other serotonin-containing nerves in the medulla mediate depressor responses.

The complexity of vascular responses to serotonin is a result of its effects on nerve endings, endothelial cells, and smooth muscle cells. These effects are mediated by at least 13 different 5-HT receptors. 5-HT type 1 receptors have been divided into four subgroups, as outlined in the Table. 5-HT$_{1c}$ receptors mediate endothelium-dependent vasodilatory responses, 5-HT$_{1B}$ receptors inhibit neuronal release of norepinephrine and acetylcholine, and central administration of serotonin causes vasodepressor effects mediated through 5-HT$_{1A}$ receptors in the ventral medulla. 5-HT$_2$ receptors are responsible for direct vasoconstrictive effects, increases in local concentrations of norepinephrine, and augmented vasoconstrictive effects of norepinephrine and other pressor agents.

Blood pressure changes after intravenous serotonin are variable. Commonly, a brief depressor phase mediated by 5-HT$_3$ receptors is followed by a 1- to 2-minute pressor response due to direct effects of serotonin on cardiac output and peripheral resistance. Thereafter, a more prolonged fall in blood pressure occurs, probably due to vasodilation in skeletal muscle.

Studies with a 5-HT$_2$ serotonin antagonist, ketanserin, suggest a role for endogenous serotonin in the maintenance of arterial blood pressure. Ketanserin lowers blood pressure both acutely and chroni-

cally. Although ketanserin has α_1-adrenergic blocking properties, its hypotensive effects derive in part from its ability to inhibit 5-HT$_2$ receptors.

Adenosine

Adenosine is composed of adenine and D-ribose. When combined with phosphate, it forms AMP, ADP, and ATP. Adenosine itself is distributed throughout all body tissues and is formed by breakdown of adenine nucleotides and by hydrolysis of adenosylmethionine and adenosylhomocysteine. Adenosine production is increased during periods of tissue ischemia, and through its vasodilatory actions it probably serves to ameliorate the effects of ischemia. Adenosine is rapidly metabolized with a half-life of 1 to 7 seconds. Plasma levels are in the range of 1.5×10^{-7} mol/L in healthy individuals.

Adenosine suppresses sinus node automaticity and AV nodal conduction and decreases inotropy. Adenosine has direct vasodilatory effects in both coronary and systemic vascular beds and causes hypotension in anesthetized individuals. Adenosine administration has minor effects on blood pressure in conscious individuals but results in decreased vagal tone and reflex activation of the sympathetic nervous system. Adenosine is commonly used in the treatment of supraventricular tachycardias and as a test agent for coronary artery disease. By inducing coronary vasodilation, it produces a "steal" effect, revealing areas of coronary ischemia.

Four types of adenosine receptors have been characterized. A$_1$ receptors inhibit adenylate cyclase and activate K$^+$ channels. A$_{2A}$ and A$_{2B}$ receptors stimulate adenylate cyclase. Cardiac effects are largely mediated through A$_1$ receptors, whereas vasodilation is primarily an A$_2$ receptor effect.

GABA

γ-Aminobutyric acid (GABA) is an inhibitory amino acid neurotransmitter distributed throughout the central nervous system. Tonic release of GABA by neurons in the posterior hypothalamus and ventral medulla plays a role in blood pressure homeostasis. Administration of GABA into these brain regions decreases blood pressure, and GABA antagonists increase blood pressure. Spontaneously hypertensive rats have no response to hypothalamic injection of GABA antagonists, suggesting that these animals may have a deficiency in tonic GABA-ergic input.

Endogenous "Ouabain"

Endogenous "ouabain" (EO) is a novel mammalian steroidal counterpart that is isomeric with the plant glycoside ouabain (**Figure 20.2**). Structural differences between the mammalian and plant-derived compounds are under investigation. Human EO is a

Table 20.1. Cardiovascular Actions Mediated by Serotonin Receptor Subtypes

5-HT$_{1A}$	Centrally mediated hypotension
5-HT$_{1B}$	Decreased acetylcholine and norepinephrine release
5-HT$_{1C}$	Endothelium-dependent vasodilation
5-HT$_2$	Direct arterial and venous constriction
5-HT$_3$	Transient bradycardia and hypotension

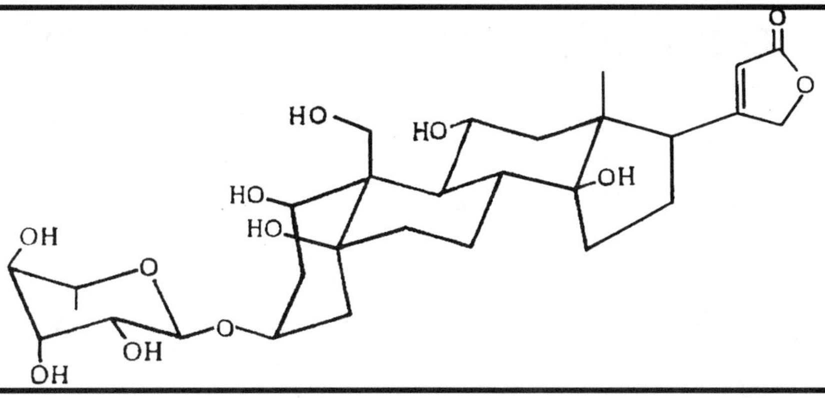

Figure 20.2.   Structure of ouabain. The A/B and C/D rings are both *cis*-fused. A five-member lactone ring is attached at C_{17} in the β-orientation. The deoxy-L-sugar rhamnose is linked to C_3. The steroid nucleus of ouabain is heavily oxygenated (positions 1, 3, 5, 14, and 19). In endogenous ouabain, the position and orientation of at least two of the steroidal oxygen atoms may differ, but the precise details are not yet known.

high-affinity, reversible, and specific inhibitor of Na,K-ATPase and has inotropic and vasopressor activity. The primary site of EO production is thought to lie within the adrenal zona glomerulosa. Secretion of EO is stimulated by ACTH and angiotensin II AT_2 receptors. The latter receptors specifically activate EO secretion via a signal transduction pathway distinct from that involved in secretion of aldosterone. There is conservation of the binding site for EO on the sodium pump and evidence that the circulating level is maintained by de novo synthesis from an adrenocortical source, suggesting that EO is a hormone.

The physiological role and pathological significance of EO may relate to its ability to regulate cellular responsivity to stimulation, especially in key neuronal circuits involved in long-term arterial pressure and electrolyte homeostasis. In the rat, sustained plasma levels of ouabain ranging from 1 to 5 nmol/L have a slow pressor effect that induces hypertension with normal plasma renin activity. The severity of the hypertension is dose-dependent and influenced by genetic factors and renal function.

Approximately 30% to 45% of whites with essential hypertension and hypertensive individuals with certain adrenocortical tumors have elevated circulating levels of EO that correlate with blood pressure. Elevated plasma EO has also been described in patients with congestive heart failure. These and related observations suggest that EO has a significant influence on cardiovascular function.

SUGGESTED READING

1. Appenzeller O. *The Autonomic Nervous System.* Amsterdam, Netherlands: Elsevier Publishing Co; 1982.
2. Blaustein MP. The physiological effects of endogenous ouabain: control of cell responsiveness. *Am J Physiol.* 1993;264:C1367–C1387.
3. Chalmers J, Arnolda L, Llewellyn-Smith I, Minson J, Pilowsky P, Suzuki S. Central neurons and neurotransmitters in the control of blood pressure. *Clin Exp Pharmacol Physiol.* 1994;21:819–829.
4. Eglen RM, Hegde SS, Watson N. Muscarinic receptor subtypes and smooth muscle function. *Pharmacol Rev.* 1996;48:531–565.
5. Hamlyn JM, Hamilton BP, Manunta P. Endogenous ouabain, sodium balance and blood pressure: a review and an hypothesis. *J Hypertens.* 1996;14:151–167.
6. Hindle AT. Recent developments in the physiology and pharmacology of 5-hydroxytryptamine. *Br J Anaesth.* 1994;73:395–407.
7. Pelleg A, Porter RS. The pharmacology of adenosine. *Pharmacotherapy.* 1990;10:157–174.

Chapter 21

Adrenomedullin-Derived Peptides and CGRP

Willis K. Samson, PhD

KEY POINTS

- Adrenomedullin (AM) exerts potent hypotensive actions via activation of vascular nitric oxide production and via direct diuretic and natriuretic actions in kidney.

- Proadrenomedullin N-20 terminal peptide (PAMP), derived from the same prohormone as AM, exerts its vasodilatory effects via presynaptic inhibition of sympathetic terminals innervating the vasculature. Both AM and PAMP also inhibit aldosterone secretion.

- Calcitonin gene–related peptide (CGRP) shares structural homology with AM and exerts many similar actions (eg, vasodilation); however, unique CGRP receptors have been identified.

See also Chapters 2, 16

Adrenomedullin (AM) and Proadrenomedullin N-20 Terminal Peptide (PAMP)

The 52-amino-acid AM and the 20-amino-acid PAMP are products of the same gene, and are produced by posttranslational processing of a larger preprohormone. The adrenomedullin gene is expressed primarily in the vasculature and also in brain and kidney. Adrenomedullin is structurally similar to CGRP, but exerts its effects via at least one unique G protein–linked AM receptor that activates adenylate cyclase and phospholipase C.

Adrenomedullin exerts its potent hypotensive action via activation of nitric oxide synthase (NOS) in endothelial cells. PAMP, on the other hand, does not activate NOS but activates potassium channels and exerts presynaptic inhibition of sympathetic nerves innervating blood vessels. Thus, the adrenomedullin gene encodes at least two peptides with shared biological activity but unique mechanisms of action.

Adrenomedullin circulates in low (pg/mL) levels in normal humans. The metabolic clearance rate is 27.4 mL/kg per minute. In humans, AM has a plasma half-life of 22 minutes and a volume of distribution of approximately 900 mL/kg. Infusion of low doses of AM (2 and 8 ng/kg per minute) in healthy volunteers results in significant reductions in mean arterial pressure with no activation of the sympathetic nervous system, alteration in renin secretion, or change in renal function. Thus, the vascular actions of AM may have a lower threshold than do the extravascular effects.

Elevations of circulating AM levels have been reported in hypertension complicated by renal failure, in heart failure, liver disease with ascites, acute asthma, and septic shock. Vascular production of AM is potently activated by pro-inflammatory cytokines (eg, tumor necrosis factor, interleukin-1), leading to the hypothesis that the hypotension of sepsis is due, at least in part, to excessive AM in the vasculature. Shear stress also elevates vascular production of AM. High circulating AM levels may be caused by the disease state itself or by compensatory mechanisms activated by the disease.

Potentially important extravascular actions of one or both peptides have been reported. AM increases renal blood flow even in the face of reductions in arterial pressure, has tubular effects to stimulate sodium excretion and prevent water reabsorption, and can directly stimulate renin secretion. Renal effects of PAMP have not been reported.

In the adrenal gland, both AM and PAMP inhibit angiotensin II and potassium-stimulated aldosterone secretion (PAMP being more potent). PAMP can inhibit nicotine-stimulated catecholamine release. In the pituitary gland, both AM and PAMP inhibit ACTH secretion. AM can inhibit water drinking and salt appetite by direct effects on the brain. In sum, AM acts in a variety of sites to compensate for increased plasma volume by decreasing venous return, increasing urine volume, decreasing aldosterone, and decreasing fluid and salt intake.

Recently, direct positive inotropic and chronotropic effects of AM have been demonstrated, and both AM and PAMP have been shown to act within the brain to stimulate sympathetic function. Thus, the volume-unloading effects may be balanced by sympathostimulatory and positive cardiac actions ensuring cardiac output. The ability of AM to increase cerebral blood flow may protect against cerebral hypoperfusion. AM has also been demonstrated to exert antimitogenic effects in vascular tissue and kidney. Of all its effects, only the role of AM in salt appetite has been demonstrated to be unequivocally physiologically relevant.

Calcitonin Gene–Related Peptide (CGRP)

CGRP is an alternative product of calcitonin gene expression. The peptide is found predominantly in peripheral and CNS neurons, often colocalized with acetylcholine. Like AM, CGRP is a potent hypotensive agent. Some of AM's vasodilatory effects may result from binding to the CGRP receptor; however, the AM receptor apparently does not recognize CGRP. Central and peripheral levels of CGRP are elevated in a variety of pathological states. CGRP may play a role in the genesis of migraine, and there is potential for its use in the treatment of Raynaud's phenomenon.

SUGGESTED READING

1. Nakamura M, Yoshida H, Makita S, Arakawa N, Niiuma H, Hiramori K. Potent and long-lasting vasodilatory effects of adrenomedullin in humans: comparisons between normal subjects and patients with chronic heart failure. *Circulation.* 1997;95:1214–1221.

2. Samson WK. A novel vascular hormone: adrenomedullin. In: Sowers JRP, ed. *Endocrinology of the Vasculature.* Totowa, NJ: Humana Press; 1997:269–281.

3. Lainchbury JG, Cooper GJ, Coy DH, Jiang NH, Lewis LK, Yandle TG, Richards AM, Nicholls MG. Adrenomedullin: a hypotensive hormone in man. *Clin Sci.* 1997;92:467–472.

4. Brain SD, Cambridge H. Calcitonin gene-related peptide: vasoactive effects and potential therapeutic role. *Gen Pharmacol.* 1996;27:607–611.

Chapter 22

Membrane Sodium Transport

A.B. Weder, MD

KEY POINTS

- Na$^+$,K$^+$-ATPase establishes a gradient of sodium ions across cell membranes that can power other ion movements.

- Measurement of sodium fluxes in cells of the blood may reveal genetic abnormalities of ion transport linked to hypertension.

See also Chapters 23, 124

Types of Transport

Most mammalian cells pump out Na$^+$ ions in exchange for extracellular K$^+$ ions **(Figure 22.1)** by the action of Na$^+$,K$^+$-ATPase. This process is called active Na$^+$ transport because energy is expended in creating electrochemical gradients for Na$^+$ and K$^+$. Numerous "passive" or "secondarily active" Na$^+$ transporters use the energy of the electrochemical sodium and potassium gradients generated by Na$^+$,K$^+$-ATPase. Passive transporters permit controlled transmembrane movements of Na$^+$ down its electrochemical gradient, often in conjunction with the movement of calcium or other ions or molecules. When Na$^+$ ion transport is coupled to the movement of another ion or molecule in the same transmembrane direction, the process is referred to as cotransport or symport; when the movement of Na$^+$ ions and the coupled substance are directionally opposite, the process is called countertransport or antiport.

Na$^+$ channels are membrane-spanning proteins that permit passive downhill movements of Na$^+$ ions not linked to the movement of other ions or molecules; the flow of ions through such pathways is often referred to as a "leak" flux **(Figure 22.1)**.

Disorders of Active Na$^+$ Transport and Cellular Na$^+$ Content

The red and white blood cells of some patients with essential hypertension have been shown to have increased Na$^+$ content, which has been ascribed to a deficiency in pump activity. One proposal is that the Na$^+$ pump is inhibited by circulating ouabain or a ouabain-like substance, which inhibits active Na$^+$ transport. Partial membrane depolarization produced by inhibition of the Na$^+$ pump would be expected to activate voltage-dependent Ca^{2+} channels, enhance Ca^{2+} influx into myocardial and vascular smooth muscle cells, and promote increased cardiac output and peripheral vasoconstriction. Alternatively, Na$^+$ pump inhibition could raise cellular Na$^+$ content and decrease the inward transmembrane Na$^+$ gradient sufficiently to decrease the energy available for the coupled countertransport of extracellular Na$^+$ ions for intracellular Ca^{2+} ions (Na$^+$-Ca^{2+} exchange). Inhibition of the Na$^+$-Ca^{2+} exchange could result in decreased Ca^{2+} extrusion and increased intracellular Ca^{2+} concentrations, again promoting cardiac and vascular muscle contraction. Either mechanism or both could raise blood pressure.

Disorders of Passive Na$^+$ Transport

Suppression of active Na$^+$ transport may not explain the abnormalities of passive Na$^+$ transport that have been observed in animal and human hypertension, as described below.

Na$^+$-Li$^+$ Countertransport

Na$^+$-Li$^+$ countertransport is a quantitatively minor Na$^+$ transport pathway in red blood cells, the activity of which is increased in some hypertensive patients. There is, however, considerable overlap between hypertensive and normotensive individuals. The activity of the red cell Na$^+$-Li$^+$ countertransporter is genetically transmitted and may be controlled by a single genetic determinant. These qualities make red cell Na$^+$-Li$^+$ countertransport an interesting candidate marker for a genetic basis of human essential hypertension. Unfortunately, the transport protein itself has not been isolated and characterized, nor is it clear what physiological role Na$^+$-Li$^+$ exchange plays.

Na$^+$-H$^+$ Exchange

Na$^+$-H$^+$ exchange is a function widely distributed in mammalian cells and is mediated by a family of Na$^+$-H$^+$ exchangers, differentially expressed in different cell types. The main physiological role of these transporters seems to be to respond to intracellular acid loads, particularly those produced by metabolic activation. The best studied Na$^+$-H$^+$ antiporter (NHE-1) is a target of various growth factors, and activation of Na$^+$-H$^+$ exchange may be part of the cellular response to many vasoactive substances, including angiotensin II. Increased activity of the Na$^+$-H$^+$ exchanger has been consistently demonstrated in human essential hypertension, as well as in some genetic animal models. A genetic linkage study has excluded the *NHE-1* gene as a cause of human hypertension. The phenotype of increased Na$^+$-H$^+$ exchange persists in immortalized lymphoblasts derived from hypertensives, suggesting that a genetically fixed disorder of intracellular signal transduction could contribute to enhanced Na$^+$-H$^+$ exchange and hypertension.

Na$^+$-K$^+$ (+2Cl$^-$) Cotransport

Na$^+$-K$^+$ (+2Cl$^-$) cotransport is inhibited by loop-active diuretics, such as furosemide and bumetanide. There are geographic and ethnic variations in cotransport activity, and there appears to be a subgroup of hypertensive persons with abnormal cotransport.

Cellular Sodium Transport Pathways in Essential Hypertension

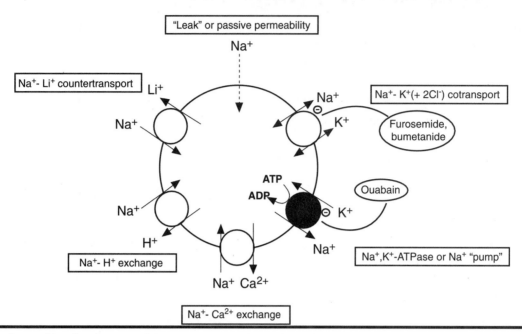

Figure 22.1. Abnormalities of one or more of the Na^+ transport pathways depicted are thought to contribute to development of essential hypertension. Active transport is shaded, passive transports are unshaded. Inhibitors are indicated in ovals.

Passive Na⁺ Transport

Na^+ leak flux, a passive Na^+ transport not attributable to the above systems, may flow through Na^+ channels in the membrane. A subset of persons with essential hypertension with increased leak fluxes has been described.

Some of the cellular disturbances produced by passive transport abnormalities (decreased Na^+-K^+ cotransport, increased Na^+ leak) could in theory contribute to increased cell Na^+ content, whereas others (increased Na^+-H^+ exchange) could alter other important cellular physiological functions, such as cell pH. It is also possible that a disorder of pas-

sive cellular Na^+ transport in a specialized tissue, such as the renal tubular epithelium, could alter physiological processes such as Na^+ reabsorption and renal Na^+ retention, which could cause hypertension.

SUGGESTED READING

1. Doris PA. Endogenous inhibitors of the Na,K pump. *Miner Electrolyte Metab* 1996;22:303–310.
2. Lijnen P. Alterations in sodium metabolism as an etiological model for hypertension. *Cardiovasc Drugs Ther* 1995;9:377–399.
3. Siffert W, Dusing R. Sodium-proton exchange and primary hypertension: an update. *Hypertension* 1995;26:649–655.

Chapter 23

Intracellular pH and Cell Volume

Bradford C. Berk, MD, PhD

KEY POINTS

- Anion and cation transporters and exchangers regulate intracellular pH and cell volume.

- Na^+-H^+ exchange is abnormal in some hypertensive humans and some animal models.

- Abnormal Na^+-H^+ exchange can cause cell swelling, sensitivity to pressors, and cell hypertrophy.

See also Chapters 22, 124

Cells maintain a homeostatic balance that requires regulation of both volume and intracellular pH (pH_i) around "set points." Both pH_i and cell volume are regulated by ion transport systems that include the HCO_3^--Cl^- exchangers and the Na^+-H^+ exchangers.

Regulation of pH_i

Vascular smooth muscle cells (VSMCs) maintain vessel tone by altering their contractile state and maintain vessel structure by altering their growth rate. Intracellular pH plays a critical role in both functions. Regulation of pH_i is due to both "buffering" and transport of H^+ (or OH^-) across membranes. Intracellular buffering is complex and includes physicochemical buffering by the interaction of H^+ with cellular proteins, compartmentalization, and metabolic consumption.

Three ion transport mechanisms participate in pH_i homeostasis: (1) Na^+-H^+ exchange, (2) Na^+-dependent HCO_3^--Cl^- exchange, and (3) cation-independent HCO_3^--Cl^- exchange (**Figure 23.1**). Na^+-H^+ exchange is an electroneutral transport process that under physiological conditions exchanges one intracellular H^+ for one extracellular Na^+. The Na^+-H^+ exchanger participates in multiple cellular functions, including regulation of pH_i and transport of salt and water. It is now known that Na^+-H^+ exchange is mediated by a family of at least six related Na^+-H^+ exchanger gene products (NHE-1 through NHE-6). These have unique tissue distribution and sensitivity to inhibition by pharmacological agents. The NHE-1 isoform appears to be ubiquitous and is dominant in VSMCs. The primary function of NHE-1 is to regulate pH_i, as evidenced by the pH_i dependence of the rate of transport. Basal NHE-1 activity maintains normal VSMC pH_i at 0.3 to 0.5 pH units above the Donnan equilibrium for H^+. Rapid increases in Na^+/H^+ exchange activity occur upon exposure to growth factors and vasoconstrictors. This stimulation is characterized by a change in affinity for intracellular H^+ and extracellular Na^+.

At normal pH_i (7.4), the Na^+-H^+ exchanger is inactive, but it is greatly stimulated when the cell is acidified, indicating the existence of an intracellular H^+ sensor. The sensitivity of this intracellular site can be shifted to more acid pH_i by depletion of ATP or to more alkaline pH_i by growth factor stimulation or cell shrinkage. The efficiency of Na^+-H^+ exchange in restoring pH_i of an acid-loaded cell is inversely proportional to the buffering power (β): only a few exchanges are required to induce a large pH recovery when β is low.

In the absence of CO_2-HCO_3^-, as might occur with decreased blood flow, the Na^+-H^+ exchanger is the dominant pH_i regulator. In the presence of CO_2-HCO_3^-, the Na^+-dependent HCO_3^--Cl^- exchanger is dominant. This transporter normally exchanges extracellular Na^+ and HCO_3^- for intracellular Cl^- (and probably H^+), with stoichiometry for Na^+/Cl^-/acid-base equivalents of 1:1:2. It can be distinguished from Na^+-H^+ exchange by its sensitivity to stilbene derivatives and resistance to amiloride.

The cation-independent HCO_3^--Cl^- exchanger transports anions across the cell membrane with a stoichiometry of 1:1 and is electroneutral. Like Na^+-H^+ exchange, HCO_3^--Cl^- exchange has been shown to be mediated by a multigene family of transporters (AE1 through AE3). At normal intracellular Cl^- and HCO_3^- concentrations, net transport of the exchanger would be one intracellular HCO_3^- for one extracellular Cl^-, producing intracellular acidification. Thus, as shown in Figure 1, HCO_3^--Cl^- exchange will lower pH_i in alkaline-loaded cells. There is no alkaline pH_i regulatory mechanism in the absence of HCO_3^--CO_2 except for transporters that normally extrude H^+ working in reverse.

Regulation of Cell Volume

Cells regulate their volume by unloading excess water if swollen or by taking on water if shrunken. Usually, cell volume is corrected by altering the number of osmotically active particles in the cytoplasm, thereby causing obligate water movement. The volume-sensing mechanisms are unknown, but possibilities include changes in cytoplasmic electrolyte concentrations (eg, protons and membrane potential), changes in cell shape (eg, cytoskeleton-membrane interactions), or alterations in kinases that regulate shape (such as the myosin light chain kinase). Volume regulation is particularly important in VSMCs, because they undergo rapid transient volume changes during contraction and slower sustained volume changes during hypertrophy.

Two mechanisms have been described that regulate volume in VSMCs: (1) Na^+-H^+ exchange and Cl^--HCO_3^- exchange–coupled transport and (2) Na^+-K^+-$2Cl^-$ cotransport and Na^+, K^+-AT-Pase–coupled transport (**Figure 23.2**). Na^+-H^+ and Cl^--HCO_3^-

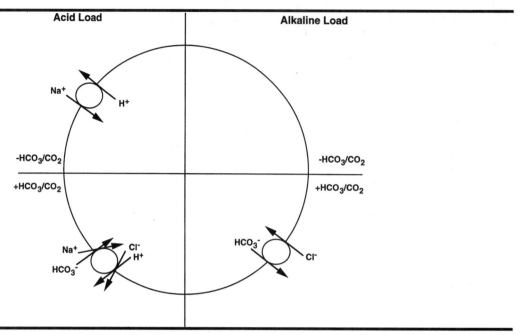

Figure 23.1.   Regulation of intracellular pH. Shown are pH regulatory ion transport mechanisms in response to an acid load (left) or an alkaline load (right). Nature of transport is also influenced by bicarbonate (bottom) or absence of bicarbonate (top). There is no regulatory ion transport process for alkaline loads in absence of bicarbonate, and cell relies on intracellular generation of protons.

are functionally coupled with pH_i, because H^+ regulates Na^+-H^+ exchange and also determines the concentration of HCO_3^-. As an example of the link between pH_i and volume, consider the situation after a sudden intracellular acidification. Because the buffering power is not infinitely large, a finite amount of time will be required for Na^+-H^+ exchange to restore pH_i to the basal level. The time required will be dependent on the buffering power and the rate of Na^+-H^+ exchange. Cell volume changes because Na^+-H^+ exchange is activated, resulting in an increased influx of Na^+ and water. H^+ ions are generated by intracellular metabolism "fueling" the exchange. If Cl^--HCO_3^- exchange is also present, the initial rate of pH recovery will be faster, because intracellular Cl^- is exchanged for extracellular HCO_3^-, which raises pH_i. Although the loss of intracellular Cl^- will initially cause a decrease in cell volume, this will be followed by coupled Na^+/H^+ and Cl^--HCO_3^- exchange. The result of this coupling is the inward movement of Na^+ by Na^+-H^+ exchange and of Cl^- by Cl^--HCO_3^- exchange. The H^+ and HCO_3^- transported out of the cell in exchange for Na^+ and Cl^- are converted into H_2O and CO_2, increasing cell volume **(Figure 23.2)**. Key to this increase in cell volume are the facts that H^+ is generated from cell metabolism (and hence "created" de novo) and the $Na^+-K^+-2Cl^-$ cotransporter can mediate a net influx of Cl^- with increases in Na^+ and K^+. The changes in Na^+ activate the Na^+,K^+-ATPase, which works to maintain transcellular gradients for Na^+ and K^+. The net result is obligate inward movement of water and cell volume increase.

Regulation of the Na^+/H^+ Exchanger: Implications for Vascular Smooth Muscle Function in Hypertension

The abnormalities of vessel tone and growth seen in hypertension may be, in part, the result of changes in the regulation of cell vol-

ume and pH_i. A large number of studies suggest that increased NHE-1 activity is prevalent in hypertension. Alterations in Na^+-H^+ exchange in hypertension can theoretically be divided into three categories: mutation in the gene, increased expression of the gene product, and altered posttranslational regulation of existing exchangers.

By restriction fragment length polymorphism analysis, there is no linkage between the human Na^+-H^+ exchanger gene and essential hypertension. There also does not appear to be any alteration in NHE-1 mRNA or protein expression in the spontaneously hypertensive rat. However, there is clearly an increase in both NHE-1 phosphorylation and cell growth in cells derived from the hypertensive rats and human hypertensive patients. These findings support the simple concept that increased activity of an NHE-1 kinase (or decreased activity of an NHE-1 phosphatase) is responsible for increased basal activity of the exchanger in tissues of hypertensive persons and animals. Alternatively, an NHE-1 regulatory protein whose activity is modulated by phosphorylation may be altered in hypertension. Studies with mutated or deleted NHE-1 proteins indicate that modulation of NHE-1 by phosphorylation shifts the pH range over which the "pH_i sensor" of the exchanger regulates ion exchange. Thus, the primary alteration in Na^+/H^+ exchange in VSMCs in hypertension is likely to involve a change in phosphorylation of an NHE-1 regulatory protein or NHE-1 itself.

The Na^+/H^+ exchanger may play a pathogenic role in hypertension **(Figure 23.3)** by modifying pH_i and altering signal transduction pathways by which vasoactive agents regulate vascular tone and VSMC growth. The effect of increased Na^+/H^+ exchange on growth would most likely be an enhanced sensitivity to mitogens. Increased activity of the Na^+/H^+ exchanger could lead to increased vascular tone by two mechanisms. First, increased Na^+ entry would activate

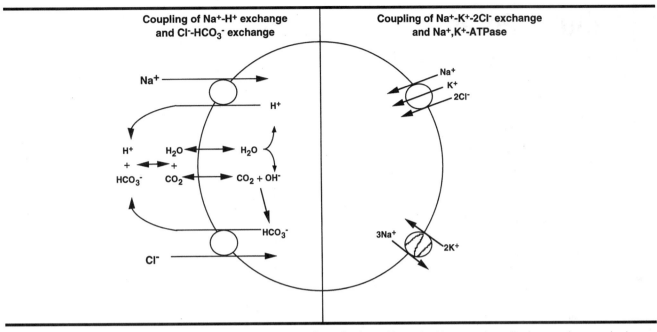

Figure 23.2. Coupling of several exchangers and sodium pump to regulate cell volume. Change in pH may regulate cell volume, and conversely, changes in cell volume may alter intracellular pH as discussed in text.

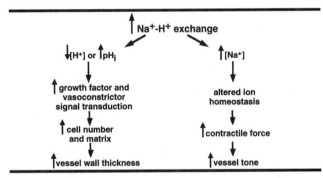

Figure 23.3. Effect of Na^+-H^+ exchange on VSMC growth and tone. Increased activity leads to alterations in concentrations of H^+ and Na^+ that secondarily modulate signal transduction and contractile force. Chronic changes mediated by these alterations may lead to fixed structural abnormalities, such as medial hypertrophy and smooth muscle hyperplasia.

Na^+/Ca^{2+} exchange, leading to increased intracellular calcium. Second, increased pH_i would enhance the calcium sensitivity of the contractile apparatus, leading to an increase in contractility for a given intracellular calcium concentration. Due to the activation of the Na^+/H^+ exchanger by both hyperplastic and hypertrophic agents, it has been proposed that abnormal function of this protein may be involved in the pathophysiology of hypertension. Evidence for dysfunction of the Na^+/H^+ exchanger in hypertension includes obser-

vations that its activity is increased in skeletal muscle, VSMCs, lymphocytes, platelets from spontaneously hypertensive rats, and platelets from hypertensive patients.

SUGGESTED READING

1. Berk BC. Regulation of the Na^+/H^+ exchanger in vascular smooth muscle. In: Fliegel L, Austin RG. *The Na +/H+ Exchanger.* Landes Co Austin, TX; 1996:47–67.
2. Berk BC, Vallega G, Muslin AJ, Gordon HM, Canessa M, Alexander RW. Spontaneously hypertensive rat vascular smooth muscle cells in culture exhibit increased growth and Na^+/H^+ exchange. *J Clin Invest.* 1989;83:822–829.
3. Chamberlin ME, Strange K. Anisosmotic cell volume regulation: a comparative view. *Am J Physiol.* 1989;257:C159–C173.
4. Lifton RP, Hunt SC, Williams RR, Pouyssegur J, Lalouel JM. Exclusion of the Na^+-H^+ antiporter as a candidate gene in human essential hypertension. *Hypertension.* 1991;17:8–14.
5. Orlov SN, Tremblay J, Hamet P. Cell volume in vascular smooth muscle is regulated by bumetanide-sensitive ion transport. *Am J Physiol.* 1996;270: C1388–C1397.
6. Orlowski J, Grinstein S. Na^+/H^+ exchangers of mammalian cells. *J Biol Chem.* 1997;272:22373–22376.
7. Rosskopf D, Dusing R, Siffert W. Membrane sodium-proton exchange and primary hypertension. *Hypertension.* 1993;21:607–617.
8. Siczkowski M, Davies JE, Ng LL. Na^+-H^+ exchanger isoform 1 phosphorylation in normal Wistar-Kyoto and spontaneously hypertensive rats. *Circ Res.* 1995;76: 825–831.
9. Wakabayashi S, Fafournoux P, Sardet C, Pouyssegur J. The Na^+/H^+ antiporter cytoplasmic domain mediates growth factor signals and controls "H^+-sensing." *Proc Natl Acad Sci U S A.* 1992;89:2424–2428..

Chapter 24

Cellular Potassium Transport

Jason Xiao-Jian Yuan, MD, PhD; Mordecai P. Blaustein, MD

KEY POINTS

- The activity of K^+ channels governs membrane potential in vascular smooth muscle cells and is a major determinant of cytosolic free Ca^{2+} concentration and vascular tone.

- Multiple types of K^+ channels are expressed in VSMCs: voltage-gated, Ca^{2+}-activated, and ATP-sensitive K^+ channels.

- Endothelium-derived relaxing factors regulate vascular tone by affecting K^+ channel activity.

- Dysfunction of K^+ channels in VSMCs is associated with membrane depolarization, increased cytosolic free Ca^{2+}, and arterial hypertension.

See also Chapters 25, 91, 134

The membrane potential (E_m) in vascular smooth muscle cells (VSMCs) is a function of the Na^+, K^+, and Cl^- concentration gradients across the plasma membrane and the relative ion permeabilities (P) as given by: $E_m \approx 58 \log [(P_{Na}[Na^+]_{out} + P_K[K^+]_{out} + P_{Cl}[Cl^-]_{cyt})/(P_{Na}[Na^+]_{cyt} + P_K[K^+]_{cyt} + P_{Cl}[Cl^-]_{out})]$, where *out* and *cyt* refer to the extracellular and cytosolic ion concentrations. In resting VSMCs, membrane potential is controlled primarily by K^+ permeability and gradient, because $P_K > P_{Cl} > P_{Na}$. K^+ permeability is directly related to the whole-cell K^+ current ($I_K = NiP_o$, where N is the number of membrane K^+ channels, i is the single-channel current, and P_o is the open-state probability of a K^+ channel). When K^+ channels close, P_K and I_K decrease, and cell membrane potential becomes less negative (ie, depolarizes).

At least four types of K^+ current have been described in VSMCs: voltage-gated K^+ currents [$I_{K(V)}$], Ca^{2+}-activated K^+ currents [$I_{K(Ca)}$], ATP-sensitive K^+ currents [$I_{K(ATP)}$], and inward rectifier K^+ currents [$I_{K(IR)}$]. These currents are carried by three corresponding K^+ channels: voltage-gated channels (K_V), Ca^{2+}-activated channels (K_{Ca}), and inward rectifier channels (K_{IR}). Voltage-gated and Ca^{2+}-activated channels are composed of two structurally distinct types of subunits: large pore-forming α subunits, and small cytoplasmic β subunits. The kinetics and gating of the K^+ channels encoded by certain α subunits can be dramatically affected by their associated β subunits. Different K^+ channel subunits (α and β) can coassociate in vivo to yield a large number of functionally distinct K^+ channels.

Voltage-Gated K+ Channels

The voltage-gated K^+ (K_V) channels of VSMCs carry a rapidly inactivating A-type current, a slowly inactivating delayed rectifier current, and a noninactivating delayed rectifier current. These are activated in the voltage range of resting E_m in VSMCs; the unitary conductance is 5 to 65 pS. 4-Aminopyridine (4-AP) is a potent blocker of K_V channels. Functionally, the noninactivating or slowly inactivating delayed rectifier K_V channels are the major determinants of resting E_m and thus intracellular Ca^{2+} concentration and tonic tension in VSMCs. Inhibition of K_V channels (eg, by 4-AP, or hy-

poxia in pulmonary VSMCs) depolarizes the cells, induces Ca^{2+}-dependent action potentials, raises $[Ca^{2+}]_{cyt}$, and causes vasoconstriction. In contrast, activation of K_V channels by agents including nitric oxide hyperpolarizes VSMCs, closes voltage-gated Ca^{2+} channels, and causes vasodilation.

Native K_V channels are homomultimers or heteromultimers composed of four identical or similar α subunits and perhaps four β subunits. The α subunit consists of six transmembrane domains (S1 through S6), a pore-forming region (H5, located in the loop between the S5 and S6 domains), and cytoplasmic N- and C-termini. Segment S4 is the voltage sensor. There are at least 11 subfamilies of K_V channel α subunits (K_V1 through K_V9, K_VLQT, and *eag*). Four (K_V5, K_V6, K_V8, and K_V9) are electrically silent modulatory α subunits, while the remainder are functional α subunits. There are three subfamilies of β subunits: $K_V\beta1$ through $K_V\beta3$.

Ca2+-Activated K+ Channels

Ca^{2+}-activated K^+ (K_{Ca}) channels are the major Ca^{2+}-regulated channels. By opening when Ca^{2+} enters cells, these channels may contribute to negative-feedback regulation of membrane potential and vascular tone. There are three types of K_{Ca} channels: small-conductance (4 to 14 pS; SK channels), intermediate-conductance (100 to 200 pS; IK channels), and large-conductance (200 to 285 pS; BK or maxi-K channels). Apamin blocks SK channels but negligibly affects BK and IK channels. BK channels are very sensitive to charybdotoxin (from scorpion venom) and tetraethylammonium. Voltage and Ca^{2+} gating for K_{Ca} channels are synergistic; therefore, K_{Ca} channels play a critical role in coupling changes in $[Ca^{2+}]_{cyt}$ to changes in E_m. K_{Ca} channels are half-maximally activated between -12 and $+30$ mV, and most are closed in VSMCs under resting conditions, where $E_m = -60$ to -40 mV and $[Ca^{2+}]_{cyt} = 50$ to 100 nmol/L. Toxins that inhibit K_{Ca} channels enhance evoked membrane depolarization and elevation of $[Ca^{2+}]_{cyt}$ in stimulated VSMCs. Normally, K_{Ca} channels control E_m and vascular tone by negative-feedback regulation of the degree of membrane depolarization caused by myogenic factors and vasoactive substances.

The α subunit of the large-conductance K_{Ca} channel is encoded by the slowpoke gene (*Slo*), first identified in *Drosophila*. The channel protein shares extensive homology with the K_V channels of the Shaker (K_V1) subfamily. Recently, the small-conductance, apamin-sensitive K_{Ca} channel was also cloned; it has a membrane topology similar to those of K_V and the large-conductance K_{Ca} channels.

Inward Rectifier K+ Channels

Rectifiers conduct current in one direction only. K_{IR} channels conduct inward K^+ current but little outward current. K_{IR} channels are blocked by intracellular Mg^{2+} and Cs^+ and external Ba^{2+}. K_{IR} channels in VSMCs set the resting E_m, prevent membrane hyperpolarization by the electrogenic Na^+, K^+-ATPase, mediate K^+-induced vasodilation, and minimize loss of cell K^+. In contrast to K_V and K_{Ca} channels, K_{IR} channels contain only two transmembrane domains (M1 and M2). Heteromultimeric combinations of different K_{IR} channel subunits form distinct K^+ channels; for example, the acetylcholine-sensitive, G-protein–gated K^+ channel (I_{KACh}) is a heteromultimer composed of two distinct types of K_{IR} subunits, $K_{IR}3.1$ and $K_{IR}3.4$.

ATP-Sensitive K+ Channels

K_{ATP} channels are inhibited by intracellular ATP and activated by ADP. They fall into two categories: low-conductance (10 to 50 pS) and large-conductance (≈130 pS) K_{ATP} channels. Electrophysiological studies demonstrate that $I_{K(ATP)}$ is voltage independent. Sulfonylureas such as glibenclamide are selective blockers of K_{ATP} channels. In coronary and cerebral arteries, metabolic regulation of basal tone and blood flow involves modulation of K_{ATP} channels. During hypoxia or ischemia, ATP falls and ADP rises. This activates K_{ATP} channels, hyperpolarizes VSMCs, and contributes to vasodilation. K_{ATP} channels are heteromultimers: four $K_{IR}6.2$ (pore-forming) subunits and four SUR1 subunits are required to form a K_{ATP} channel. $K_{IR}6.2$ also serves as the ATP sensor, while SUR1 confers sensitivity to sulfonylureas, channel openers like diazoxide, and ADP.

Role of K+ Channels in Regulating E_m, $[Ca^{2+}]_{cyt}$, and Vascular Tone

Owing to the voltage dependence of sarcolemmal voltage-gated Ca^{2+} channels, E_m plays an important role in regulating intracellular Ca^{2+} in VSMCs. Closure or inactivation of K^+ channels lowers E_m (depolarizes), which increases $[Ca^{2+}]_{cyt}$ by opening voltage-gated Ca^{2+} channels. This influx of Ca^{2+} causes vasoconstriction. In contrast, opening or activation of K^+ channels hyperpolarizes VSMCs, closes voltage-gated Ca^{2+} channels, and causes vasodilation. Many vasodilators activate K^+ channels, including β-adrenergic agonists, muscarinic agonists, and nitroglycerin. Endothelium-derived relaxing factors (eg, NO and prostacyclin) open K_V and K_{Ca} channels in pulmonary and systemic vessels. Antihypertensive drugs such as diazoxide and cromakalim also open K_{ATP} channels.

Dysfunctional K+ Channels and Hypertension

Defective K^+ channels have been implicated in some types of essential hypertension and pulmonary hypertension. In systemic (renal and mesenteric) VSMCs from spontaneously hypertensive rats, voltage-activated and cromakalim-activated K^+ channels are significantly decreased compared with those in normotensive rats. In pulmonary VSMCs from patients with primary pulmonary hypertension, voltage-activated K^+ current is significantly attenuated compared with that in control cells. Hypoxia and the anorexic agent fenfluramine can cause pulmonary hypertension. In pulmonary VSMCs, both hypoxia and fenfluramine reduce the 4-AP–sensitive K^+ current, depolarize E_m, and increase cytoplasmic Ca^{2+}. These observations fit the view that dysfunctional K^+ channels in pulmonary and systemic VSMCs may play an etiological role in the development of pulmonary and systemic arterial hypertension.

SUGGESTED READING

1. Carl A, Lee HK, Sanders KM. Regulation of ion channels in smooth muscles by calcium. *Am J Physiol.* 1996;271:C9–C34.
2. Cook NS. The pharmacology of potassium channels and their therapeutic potential. *Trends Pharmacol Sci.* 1988;9:21–28.
3. Nelson MT, Patlak JB, Worley JF, Standen N. Calcium channels, potassium channels, and voltage dependence of arterial smooth muscle tone. *Am J Physiol.* 1990;259:C3–C18.
4. Nelson MT, Quayle JM. Physiological roles and properties of potassium channels in arterial smooth muscle. *Am J Physiol.* 1995;268:C799–C822.
5. Yuan X-J, Tod ML, Rubin LJ, Blaustein MP. NO hyperpolarizes pulmonary artery smooth muscle cells and decreases the intracellular Ca^{2+} concentration by activating voltage-gated K^+ channels. *Proc Natl Acad Sci U S A.* 1996;93:10489–10494.
6. Yuan X-J. Voltage-gated K^+ currents regulate resting membrane potential and $[Ca^{2+}]_i$ in pulmonary arterial myocytes. *Circ Res.* 1995;77:370–378.

Chapter 25

Calcium Transport and Calmodulin

David J. Triggle, PhD

KEY POINTS

- Intracellular calcium is regulated by pumps, channels, and storage sites associated with both plasma and intracellular membranes and organelles. Regulation of intracellular calcium concentrations defines key cellular functions, including excitation-contraction and stimulus-secretion coupling.

- There are at least six classes of voltage-gated calcium channels associated with the cell membranes, two of which, L-type and T-type channels, are particularly important to cardiovascular function and are blocked by drugs.

- Ligand-gated calcium channels open in response to hormones, second messengers, or exogenous agents such as ryanodine.

- Calcium regulation of intracellular effectors is mediated through its binding to calmodulin and related calcium-binding proteins to control protein phosphorylation.

See also Chapters 32, 49, 131, 132

Intracellular Calcium

Calcium is a cation of critical significance to cellular control mechanisms. Calcium serves as a second messenger and, in excitable cells, as a current-carrying ion. Both roles serve to link events at the plasma membrane with cellular effector responses, including muscle contraction and hormone and neurotransmitter release. During excitation, the intracellular Ca^{2+} concentration rises either by entry through the plasma membrane or by release from intracellular stores. Ca^{2+} sensors that control the activities of pumps, enzymes, and other targets detect these increased Ca^{2+} levels.

In resting states, the free ionized concentration of cellular Ca^{2+} is maintained at $\leq 5 \times 10^{-8}$ mol/L despite extracellular concentrations that exceed the millimolar range. During stimulation, the intracellular Ca^{2+} concentration rises significantly, to $\geq 10^{-5}$ mol/L. Elevated intracellular Ca^{2+} concentrations are coupled to cellular responses through a homologous group of Ca^{2+} binding proteins, including calmodulin.

The changes in intracellular Ca^{2+} concentrations are both temporally and spatially heterogeneous, and localized "hot spots" or "sparks" of Ca^{2+} are observed, together with "waves" of Ca^{2+} propagated through the cell. These oscillations may represent a graded signal being converted into digital signals or the sequential activation of Ca^{2+}-demanding processes that require different timing or concentrations of Ca^{2+}. This heterogeneity of Ca^{2+} mobilization may protect the cell against the detrimental consequences of persistently elevated Ca^{2+} levels.

Ca^{2+} movements are tightly regulated. Various Ca^{2+} regulatory processes are depicted in the **Figure 25.1.** These processes are not of equal importance in every cell type, but all cells maintain mechanisms that permit Ca^{2+} influx, efflux, storage, and mobilization and that generate overall Ca^{2+} homeostasis. Of particular importance in the cardiovascular system are the various Ca^{2+} channels of both voltage- and ligand-gated classes. Defects in Ca^{2+} storage, mobilization, or movement may contribute to a variety of pathological states, including the hyperreactivity of vascular smooth muscle in hypertension, cell death from ischemia, myocardial stunning, and impaired cellular energy control.

Calmodulin

Expression of the Ca^{2+} signal requires the presence of intracellular sensors or receptors. Calmodulin and other members of this homologous protein family bind Ca^{2+} with micromolar affinity and undergo conformational changes linked to effector regulation. These proteins share a common structural motif: the EF hand, a helix-loop-helix structure that binds Ca^{2+}. Calmodulin, a 17-kDa protein that binds four Ca^{2+} ions, contains two of these structures separated by a solvent-exposed straight helix. There are >160 members of this EF-hand family. Calmodulin is found in all smooth muscle and nonmuscle cells, where it regulates broad families of intracellular Ca^{2+}-dependent enzymes, including cyclic nucleotide phosphodiesterase, adenylyl cyclase, Ca^{2+}-ATPase, phosphorylase kinase, and phospholipase A2. Additional targets include nitric oxide synthase, voltage-gated L-type channels, inositol 1,4,5,-triphosphate (IP_3) and ryanodine receptors, and proteins like synapsin that regulate neurotransmitter release.

Calmodulin regulation is achieved through activation of both specific and multifunctional calmodulin-dependent (CaM) kinases. Multifunctional CaM kinase (type II CaM kinase, or simply CaM kinase) is the general kinase of Ca^{2+} signaling systems and is a particularly widespread enzyme. CaM kinases comprise four distinct classes, each encoded by a separate gene. The α- and β-classes are restricted to neurons, but the γ- and δ-classes are widely distributed. In smooth muscle, the major pathway of control of contractility is through the phosphorylation of myosin light-chain kinase via a dedicated CaM kinase. Other pathways include CaM kinase–dependent phosphorylation of calponin and caldesmon, major smooth muscle proteins that interact with thin filaments. In the heart, Ca^{2+} binding to troponin C is the key event in the initiation and control of myocardial contraction.

CaM kinase shows complex autoregulatory behavior in which au-

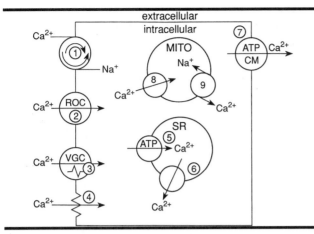

Figure 25.1. Regulation of cellular Ca^{2+}. 1, Na^+-Ca^{2+} exchanger; 2, receptor-operated channels (ROC); 3, voltage-gated channels (VGC); 4, "leak" and nonselective channels; 5, ATP-dependent Ca^{2+} uptake into sarcoplasmic reticulum (SR); 6, Ca^{2+} release channel in sarcoplasmic reticulum; 7, ATP-dependent pump across the plasma membrane (CM indicates cell membrane); 8 and 9, mitochondrial (MITO) transport processes. From *Cleveland Clin J Med.* 1992;59:617–627. Reproduced with permission.

tophosphorylation increases the affinity of the enzyme for calmodulin by a factor of several hundred. This traps calmodulin on the phosphorylated enzyme for prolonged periods of time and has the effect of maintaining kinase activation beyond the duration of the original Ca^{2+} signal.

Calcium Pumps

The two principal pumps involved in the control of poststimulus cytosolic Ca^{2+} levels are located in the sarcoplasmic reticulum and plasma membrane **(Figure 25.1)**. The calmodulin-dependent Ca^{2+}-ATPase of plasma membranes is widely distributed in eukaryotic cells. Its mechanism is similar to that of other P-type ion pumps and involves Ca^{2+}-dependent phosphorylation and Ca^{2+} transport with a Ca^{2+}:ATP stoichiometry of 1:1. The pump is also modulated by acidic phospholipids and polyunsaturated fatty acids, notably phosphatidylinositol and its phosphorylated derivatives. Calcium activation of the pump provides a link between Ca^{2+}-mobilizing processes and the processes that lower poststimulus Ca^{2+} levels.

Calcium Channels

Two sources of Ca^{2+} are used in cellular signaling: release from intracellular stores in the sarcoplasmic reticulum or equivalent structures and entry across the plasma membrane. Ca^{2+} mobilization through these routes can give rise to "elementary calcium events" representing the opening of as little as one channel. These elementary events can be visualized as "sparks" and "puffs" in dye-loaded cardiac and vascular smooth muscle.

Intracellular Calcium Release

Intracellular release of calcium is controlled by two classes of channels: the IP_3, controlled by angiotensin II and other peptides, and the ryanodine receptors. These channels are structurally related but exist in multiple subclasses that are expressed in tissue-specific

manner. Both types of channels show a biphasic sensitivity to cytosolic concentration of Ca^{2+}: at low concentrations, Ca^{2+} mediates release, and at higher concentrations, it inhibits release. The low-dose stimulatory effect of Ca^{2+} underlies the phenomenon of "calcium-induced calcium release" and is of critical importance in translating "digital" spike signals of Ca^{2+} into "analog" graded signals.

Mitochondrial Calcium Transport

Mitochondria also possess at least three Ca^{2+} transport systems, including uniporter-mediated influx down an electrochemical gradient, efflux through an Na^+:Ca^{2+} exchanger, and Na^+-independent efflux. Mitochondria can buffer cellular Ca^{2+} by accumulating it. Mitochondrial Ca^{2+} transport systems link cytosolic Ca^{2+} levels to the level of oxidative metabolism.

Cell Membrane Channels

At least six major classes of voltage-gated Ca^{2+} channels exist in the plasma membrane: T, L, N, P, Q, and R. They are distinguished by electrophysiological characteristics including conductance and voltage ranges of activation and inactivation, by localization, by function, and by their pharmacological characteristics. The N, P, Q, and R channels are specific to the central and peripheral nervous system. T and L channels play important roles in the cardiovascular system, including contraction, pacemaker activity, and neurohormone control **(Table 25.1)**. These channels have a heteromeric subunit organization, with the principal protein, the α_1-subunit, bearing the drug-binding sites that control the functional gating and permeation machinery of the channel. These properties, as well as the expression of the channels, are substantially modified by other subunits.

The L-type channel is the site of action of verapamil, diltiazem, and the 1,4-dihydropyridines. This heterogeneous group of drugs interacts at structurally distinct sites on the major subunit of the channel. Mibefradil is a Ca^{2+} antagonist with L-channel activity that exhibits selectivity for the T-type channel.

Table 25.1. Properties of L- and T-Type Calcium Channels

	T=TYPE	L=TYPE
Electrophysiology		
Conductance	Low (small)	High (large)
Voltage for activation	Low	High
Inactivation rate	Fast	Slow
Function	Fast	Slow
	Pacemaker	...
	S-S coupling	S-S coupling
	VSM contraction	VSM contraction
	...	Cardiac contraction
Distribution		
VSM	+	++
Sinus node	+++	+
Myocardium	+/−	+++
Pharmacology		
Verapamil	+	−
Diltiazem	+	−
Nifedipine	+	−
Mibefradil	+	+

VSM indicates vascular smooth muscle.

Finally, there are voltage-independent Ca^{2+} channels associated with the plasma membrane. Their properties and structures are ill defined, but they represent Ca^{2+} channels opened by agonist-receptor–mediated processes, notably, but not exclusively, G protein–coupled receptors. No drugs currently available block these channels.

SUGGESTED READING

1. Bootman MD, Berridge MJ. The elemental principles of calcium signaling. *Cell.* 1995;83:675–678.

2. Braun AP, Schulman H. The multifunctional calcium/calmodulin-dependent protein kinase: from form to function. *Annu Rev Physiol.* 1995;57:417–445.

3. Brown EM, Vassilev PM, Hebert SC. Calcium ions as extracellular messengers. *Cell.* 1995;83:679–682.

4. Clementi E, Meldolesi J. Pharmacological and functional properties of voltage-independent Ca^{2+} channels. *Cell Calcium.* 1996;19:269–279.

5. Gill DL, Waldron RT, Rys-Sikora KE, Ufret-Vincenty CA, Graber MN, Favre CJ, Alfonso A. Calcium pools, calcium entry, and cell growth. *Biosci Rep.* 1996;16:139–157.

6. Jiang H, Stephens NL. Calcium and smooth muscle contraction. *Mol Cell Biochem.* 1994;135:1–9.

7. Meissner G. Ryanodine receptor/Ca^{2+} release channels and their regulation by endogenous effectors. *Annu Rev Physiol.* 1994;56:485–508.

8. Orlov SN, Li JM, Tremblay J, Hamet P. Genes of intracellular calcium metabolism and blood pressure control in primary hypertension. *Semin Nephrol.* 1995;15:569–592.

9. Rios E, Stern MD. Calcium in close quarters: microdomain feedback in excitation-contraction coupling and other cell biological phenomena. *Annu Rev Biophys Biomol Struct.* 1997;26:47–82.

Chapter 26

Signal Transduction: Receptors

Greti Aguilera, MD

KEY POINTS

- Receptors are protein complexes that recognize specific hormones and translate extracellular hormone levels into intracellular events.

- The guanyl nucleotide protein–coupled receptor superfamily is the largest group of plasma membrane receptors.

- Hormone-ligand binding activates the receptors, usually downregulates receptor number or affinity, and reduces tissue sensitivity.

See also Chapters 1, 27, 28, 29, 30

Cell communication, an essential component of integrated physiological function in multicellular organisms, is mediated largely through informational molecules, such as hormones and neurotransmitters. These molecules, or first messengers, are recognized by specific receptor proteins in the target cell, which are of two types. Type 1 includes receptors for growth factors, catecholamines, cytokines, and prostaglandins located in the plasma membrane. Type 2 receptors, including receptors for steroids and iodothyronines, are located in the cytoplasm or nucleus of the cell. Receptors have two major functions: (1) recognition of a specific hormone ligand and (2) intracellular transmission of information leading to modification of cell function. Modified hormone analogues capable of binding the receptor without activating transduction mechanisms act as receptor antagonists.

Receptor Binding Properties

The use of radiolabeled ligands has made possible the identification and measurement of receptors for steroids, peptide hormones, and neurotransmitters in their target tissues. In general, each ligand-receptor interaction is rapid and reversible, consistent with the time course of the biological effects of hormones. Binding kinetics depend on the rates of association and dissociation of the ligand receptor complexes, which are affected by temperature and pH. The ratio between association and dissociation rates determines the association constant (K_a). The reciprocal of the association constant is the dissociation constant (K_d), which is usually expressed as the ligand concentration necessary to saturate the binding sites.

Receptor-ligand binding exhibits high affinity, which allows for significant binding despite low circulating levels of hormones. Receptor binding is always saturable, indicating a limited number of binding sites. Receptor affinity usually correlates well with the tissue sensitivity to the biological effect of the hormone, but in a number of systems, full biological response is achieved with only partial receptor occupancy. The presence of excess or "spare" receptors may be important to maintain biological effects of hormones in physiological or pathological conditions involving alterations of receptor number.

Transduction Mechanisms

In general, a requisite for a receptor molecule is the ability to communicate information to effector molecules inside the cell. The informational transduction can be carried out by the receptor itself or through activation of intermediary signaling molecules. Intracellular receptors, such as steroid and thyroid hormone receptors, are dimeric proteins consisting of a hormone-binding subunit and a regulatory subunit. After ligand (first-messenger) binding, the regulatory subunit dissociates from the complex and the activated hormone-binding subunit interacts with DNA, influencing gene transcription. Activated receptors interact with DNA-responsive elements in the form of homodimers. Receptor-DNA binding activity can be modulated through formation of heterodimers with other cellular proteins or transacting factors.

In contrast to intracellular receptor systems, interaction of hormones or neurotransmitters with cell surface receptors leads to modification of cell function through a chain of events involving the generation of second-messenger molecules. Cell surface receptors can be categorized into two major groups: (1) receptors with intrinsic enzymatic or ion channel activity and (2) receptors coupled to cellular effector molecules through a transduction protein. Molecular cloning and characterization of these receptors show that they are anchored to the cell membrane through one or several hydrophobic amino acid sequences. In general, the structure of these receptors consists of an extracellular domain, transmembrane regions, and one or more intracellular regions responsible for catalytic activity or coupling to intermediary proteins.

Receptors With Intrinsic Activity

Growth-factor and insulin receptors include a tyrosine kinase domain, and one or more tyrosine phosphorylation sites are a structural part of the receptor molecule. Ligand interaction with these receptors results in receptor autophosphorylation, leading to binding of the phosphorylated receptor domains to signaling molecules such as phosphatidylinositol kinase, GTPase-activating factor, phospholipase C, *sarc*, or serine kinases. Receptor-gated ion channels, in which the receptor is a structural component of the ion channel, also exhibit intrinsic activity. Examples of this type are γ-aminobutyric acid (GABA)$_A$ receptors associated with Cl^- and HCO_3^- transport; nicotinic acetylcholine receptors associated with Na^+, K^+, and Ca^{2+} transport; N-methyl-D-aspartate (NMDA) and non-NMDA glutamate receptors associated with Na^+, K^+, and Ca^{2+} transport; 5-hydroxytryptamine (HT)$_3$ receptors associated with Na^+ and K^+ transport; and channel-opening ATP receptors associated with Ca^{2+}, Na^+, and Mg^{2+} transport.

Receptors Without Intrinsic Activity

A second group of cell-surface receptors lacks intrinsic activity and uses an intermediary protein such as adenylate cyclase, phospholipase C, ion channels, or tyrosine kinases for coupling to effectors. Two major types belong to this group: (1) the cytokine receptor superfamily, including growth hormone and prolactin receptors, which activate tyrosine kinases of the JAK family, and (2) the guanyl nucleotide–binding protein (G-protein) receptor superfamily (GPCR). Guanylnucleotide binding proteins are located on the intracellular side of the plasma membrane, where they can interact with the receptor as well as an effector signaling system. G proteins consist of three subunits, α, β, and τ, of which α has GTP binding and GTPase activity properties. Occupancy of the receptor by its ligand causes conformational changes in the associated G protein, allowing binding of the α-subunit to GTP and dissociation from the β/τ-complex. The activated α-subunit activates an effector molecule, such as adenylyl cyclase or phospholipase C. This process is rapidly reversible upon degradation of bound GTP by the intrinsic GTPase activity of the α-subunit. Although ligand binding is responsible for hormonal activation of receptors, there is evidence that unligated GPCRs exist in at least two states, an inactive conformation and a constitutively active conformation, which has affinity for the G protein in the absence of agonist. Inverse agonists are ligand analogues, which preferentially stabilize the receptor in the inactive conformation, decreasing basal receptor activity in the absence of ligand.

Receptor Regulation

The effectiveness of a hormone depends on hormone concentration, the number and affinity of receptors in the target tissue, and postreceptor events. For a given set of conditions, changes in receptor number result in changes in sensitivity in tissues containing spare receptors or changes in the magnitude of the response in tissues in which receptor number is limiting. Although peptide hormone receptors undergo changes in number and affinity when exposed to their ligand (homologous regulation), the binding and activity of many receptors can be regulated by heterologous hormones.

Increased hormone levels usually result in receptor loss and desensitization of the biological responses to the hormone. Mechanisms leading to receptor downregulation include negative cooperativity, in which partial receptor occupancy decreases the binding affinity of the remaining receptors (insulin receptor); internalization and lysosomal degradation of hormone-receptor complexes (epidermal growth factor, human chorionic gonadotropin, gonadotropin-releasing hormone [GnRH], insulin); and receptor phosphorylation, which can be heterologous (by second messenger–dependent kinases) or homologous (phosphorylation of agonist-occupied receptor by G-protein receptor kinases). Guanyl nucleotides have been shown to reduce high-affinity binding in membrane preparations of a number of G protein–coupled receptors, probably through conformational changes in the receptor protein. Some peptide hormone receptors, such as the adrenal angiotensin II, prolactin, and GnRH receptors, have been shown to undergo upregulation after exposure to increased hormone levels.

In a number of conditions, receptor regulation can contribute to the sensitivity of the target tissue to a hormone. For example, downregulation of AII receptors could account for the low pressor responses to the peptide during sodium restriction and other clinical states of high renin secretion. Conversely, upregulation of angiotensin II receptors may contribute to the increases in sensitivity of the adrenal glomerulosa to AII during sodium restriction.

SUGGESTED READING

1. Ferguson SS, Barak LS, Zhang J, Caron M. G-protein-coupled receptor kinases and arrestins. *Can J Pharmacol.* 1996;74:1095–1110.
2. Freedman NJ, Lefkowitz RJ. Desensitization of G-protein-coupled receptors. *Recent Prog Horm Res.* 1996;51:319–351.
3. Ihle JN, Nosaka T, Thierfelder W, Quelle FW, Shimoda K. Jaks and Stats in cytokine signaling. *Stem Cells.* 1997;1(15 suppl):105–112.
4. Kahn RC, Smith RJ, Chin WW. Mechanism of action of hormones that act at the cell surface. In: Wilson JD, Foster DW, eds. *Williams Textbook of Endocrinology.* Philadelphia, Pa: WB Saunders; 1992.
5. Koshland DE. The structural basis of negative cooperativity: receptors and enzymes. *Current Opin Struct Biol.* 1996;6:757–761.
6. Rodbell M. The complex regulation of receptor-coupled G-proteins. *Adv Enzyme Regul.* 1997;37:427–435.
7. Wess J. G-protein coupled receptors: molecular mechanisms involved in receptor activation and selectivity of G-protein recognition *FASEB J.* 1997;11:346–354.

Chapter 27

Guanine Nucleotide Binding Proteins

James C. Garrison, PhD

KEY POINTS

- A large family of seven transmembrane receptors regulates intracellular processes via guanine nucleotide binding proteins ("G proteins").

- G proteins communicate the signal of ligand binding by regulating the activity of intracellular effectors such as adenylyl cyclase, phospholipase C-β, and ion channels.

- Changes in the activity of these effectors regulate the levels of second messengers, such as cAMP, inositol phosphates, diacylglycerol, and K^+ or Ca^{2+} ions in the cytoplasm.

- Changes in the levels of these second messengers regulate the differentiated activity of the target cells.

See also Chapters 26, 28, 29, 30

Receptors

A large number of cell-surface receptors regulate intracellular effectors through a family of signal-transducing proteins called guanine nucleotide binding proteins, or G proteins. G proteins, effectors, and second messengers described are common to virtually all cells. The specificity of response in a given tissue is achieved by differential expression of the receptors that activate the signaling process and the nature of the intracellular substrates for the various kinases. These receptors are responsible for monitoring signals from neurotransmitters, hormones, autacoids, chemokines, light, and other sensory stimuli in the extracellular environment. Surprisingly, >60% of these receptors are involved in smell, vision, and taste. In the cardiovascular system, G protein–linked receptors are found for acetylcholine (muscarinic receptors), serotonin, catecholamines, angiotensin, vasopressin, endothelin, histamine, bradykinin, and adenosine.

G protein–coupled receptors are monomeric proteins of the rhodopsin family with molecular weights ranging from 35 000 to 70 000 kDa. G protein–coupled receptors share a characteristic structure composed of seven membrane-spanning domains with four intracellular loops that are responsible for direct interaction with the G proteins. The intracellular segments most responsible for recognition of the G proteins include the third intracellular loop between helices V and IV and the carboxyl-terminal domain.

G protein–coupled receptors can form complex regulatory networks in which one receptor may couple to multiple G proteins and generate a variety of signals in a given cell. Conversely, multiple receptor subtypes may interact with a single member of the G protein family and generate the same signal. The best-studied effectors regulated by this mechanism are adenylyl cyclase, cGMP, phosphodiesterase, phospholipase C-β, phospholipase A_2, and the calcium, sodium, and potassium channels.

The G Protein Family

The heterotrimeric G proteins themselves are composed of three subunits: α-subunits with molecular weights of 39 to 45 kDa, β-subunits with molecular weights of 35 to 40 kDa, and γ-subunits with molecular weights of 6 to 8 kDa. The α-subunits can bind 1 mol GTP or GDP/mol α-subunit. The β- and γ-subunits form a functional unit, called the βγ-dimer, that cannot be dissociated without loss of activity. There is significant diversity in the subunits making up the heterotrimer. Currently, 17 genes are known to encode α-subunits, 5 to encode β-subunits, and 11 to encode γ-subunits. Alternative splicing of some genes yields ≈21 different α-, 7 β-, and 11 γ-proteins. Although some sensory cells express only a limited subset of α- and βγ-proteins, most cells can express the majority of the known proteins that compose the heterotrimer (**Table 27.1**). Both the α- and γ-subunits are posttranslationally modified with lipids, causing the heterotrimer to reside at the inner surface of the plasma membrane.

The G-protein heterotrimers are grouped into four families with overall stimulatory or inhibitory function according to the similarity in their amino acid sequences and/or the function of their α-subunits (**Table 27.1**). Members of the G_s (stimulatory) family include the G_s and G_{olf} proteins, which stimulate adenylyl cyclase to produce the second messenger cAMP. Members of the G_i (inhibitory) family are more diverse and include the G_t, G_{i1}, G_{i2}, G_{i3}, G_o, G_z, and G_g proteins. These α-subunits inhibit adenylyl cyclase, regulate the gating of ion channels, and stimulate the cGMP phosphodiesterases involved in the senses of vision and taste. The G_q family includes G_q, G_{11}, G_{14}, G_{15}, and G_{16}. These α-subunits stimulate phospholipase C-β to hydrolyze phosphatidylinositol 4,5-biphosphate, leading to formation of the second messengers inositol trisphosphate (IP_3) and diacylglycerol (DAG). The G_{12} family includes the G_{12} and G_{13} α-subunits.

Activation of G Proteins by Receptors

The basal state of this signaling system consists of the receptor α-GDP-βγ complex. When an agonist ligand binds to the receptor, a conformational change in the receptor causes the α-subunit to release the bound GDP. The binding site becomes occupied with GTP from the cytoplasm, causing a conformational change in the

Table 27.1. **Properties of G Protein α-Subunits**

α-SUBUNIT	TISSUE DISTRIBUTION	EFFECTOR (ACTION)	EFFECT ON MESSAGE
G_s family			
G_s*	Wide	Adenylyl cyclase (↑)	Increase cAMP
		Ca^{2+} channels (↑)	Increase Ca^{2+} Current
G_{olf}	Olfactory tissue	Adenylyl cyclase (↑)	Increase cAMP
G_i family			
G_{i1}	Wide	Adenylyl cyclase (↓)	Decrease cAMP
G_{i2}	Wide	Adenylyl cyclase (↓)	Decrease cAMP
G_{i3}	Wide	Adenylyl cyclase (↓)	Decrease cAMP
G_o*	Neuronal	Ion channels (↓)	Decrease Ca^{2+} Current
G_i and G_o via βγ		K^+ channels (↑)	Increase K^+ Current
		Phospholipase C-β (↑)	Increase IP_3, DAG
		Ca^{2+} channels (↓)	Decrease Ca^{2+} Current
G_t	Rod and cone cells	cGMP phosphodiesterase (↑)	Decrease cGMP
G_g	Tongue	cGMP phosphodiesterase (↑)	Decrease cGMP
G_z	Brain	Adenylyl cyclase (↓)	Decrease cAMP
		(Others?)	
G_q family			
G_q	Wide	Phospholipase C-β (↑)	Increase IP_3, DAG
G_{11}	Wide	Phospholipase C-β (↑)	Increase IP_3, DAG
G_{14}	Wide	Phospholipase C-β (↑)	Increase IP_3, DAG
G_{15}	Hematopoietic cells	Phospholipase C-β (↑)	Increase IP_3, DAG
G_{16}	Hematopoietic cells	Phospholipase C-β (↑)	Increase IP_3, DAG
G_{12} family			
G_{12}	Wide	Rho GTP exchange factor, cyclase (?)	Activate Rho targets
G_{13}	Wide	Rho GTP exchange factor, Na^+/H^+ antiporter (?)	Activate Rho targets

*The G_s and G_o α-subunits have multiple splice variants.

α-subunit, a reduction in its affinity for the βγ-subunit, and generates two active signaling molecules, the α-GTP complex and the βγ-dimer. Both of these signals can activate effectors (**Figure 27.1**). The activated α-GTP complex regulates effectors such as adenylyl cyclase, the cGMP phosphodiesterase in the visual system, phospholipase C-β, or ion channels. Most of these interactions lead to an increase in the level of a second messenger in the cell (eg, an increase in adenylyl cyclase activity causing a rise in cAMP levels).

As receptor occupancy increases, a greater number of α-subunits are activated, causing a larger cellular response. βγ-subunits also play an active regulatory role on adenylyl cyclase, phospholipase C-β, ion channels, the muscarinic K^+ channel in the atrium, and inhibition of the L- and N-type Ca^{2+} channels in neural tissue. Because of the high concentrations of G_i and G_o in the plasma membrane, it is thought that the βγ-dimers released from these α-subunits may play important regulatory roles. Thus, receptors coupled to G_i or G_o may regulate certain cell functions via the βγ-dimer and others via the α-subunit.

The G-protein signal is terminated by the intrinsic GTPase activity of the α-subunit. This activity spontaneously hydrolyzes bound GTP to GDP (which remains bound to the α-subunit) and converts the α-subunit from the active to the inactive form. When the bound GTP is hydrolyzed, the affinity of the α-subunit for the βγ-dimer increases, and the GDP-bound form of the α-subunit sequesters the β,γ-subunit. These two events return the system to the basal state.

Regulation of Effectors

The effects of the α-GTP complex and the βγ-dimer initiate complex signaling patterns with certain common features. The activation of effectors by both the α-GTP complex and the βγ-dimer appears to occur by direct protein-protein interactions, causing the effector to shift to a more active state. Activation of these proteins changes the concentration of intracellular messengers such as cAMP, DAG, IP_3, Ca^{2+}, or K^+ ions. Adenylyl cyclase and phospholipase C-β are important effectors found in virtually all cells and regulate the response of organ systems to a large number of hormones, neurotransmitters, and autacoids. An important example of activation of adenylyl cyclase in the cardiovascular system is the β-adrenergic stimulation of cardiac rate and force of contraction. β-Adrenergic receptors activate adenylyl cyclase and increase the level of cAMP in all cardiac tissues. The rise in cAMP activates protein kinases, which increase both cardiac rate and force of contraction.

Phospholipase C-β plays a very important role in regulating the contraction of smooth muscle by controlling the level of Ca^{2+} in the cytoplasm of these cells. The $α_1$-adrenergic receptor that regulates vascular tone is coupled to the G_q α-subunit. Activation of this receptor by norepinephrine produces an active G_q–α-GTP complex that markedly stimulates phospholipase C-β, leading to increases in IP_3, DAG, intracellular Ca^{2+} levels, and contraction of the smooth muscle.

Adenylyl cyclase activity can also be inhibited by receptors coupled to the G_i α-subunit in most cells. Examples of cardiovascular

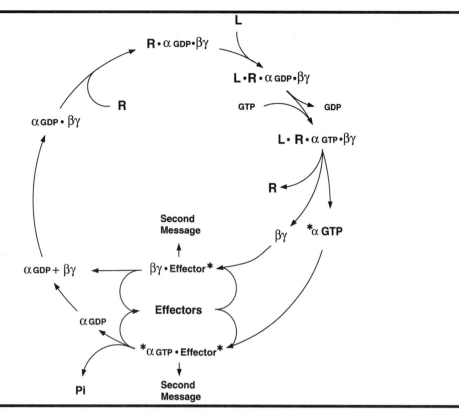

Figure 27.1.   Sequence of activation and inactivation of G protein–coupled systems. Binding of hormone or other ligand (L) to its receptor (R) causes dissociation of GDP and binding of GTP to α-subunit of G-protein trimer. Ligand-receptor binding also causes dissociation of G-protein subunits. GTP α-subunit and βγ-subunit are regulators (*) of various effectors. Hydrolysis of GTP to GDP and inorganic phosphate (Pi) terminates participation of G-protein subunits and leads to their reassociation into the inactive heterotrimer.

receptors that inhibit cyclase include the muscarinic m_2, α_2-adrenergic, adenosine A_1, and angiotensin AT_1 receptors.

In many cases, the second messengers generated by receptor activation lead to stimulation of protein kinases that produce a cellular response by increasing the phosphorylation state of important regulatory proteins in the target cells. This is the case for cAMP, Ca^{2+}, and DAG, which activate the cAMP-dependent protein kinase, Ca^{2+}/calmodulin-dependent protein kinase, and protein kinase C, respectively.

Counterregulatory Effects

In many tissues, it is common to find two or more receptors acting to regulate important functions via opposing effects. In the sinoatrial node in cardiac tissues, activity of the cardiac pacemaker cells is stimulated by norepinephrine acting on β_1-adrenergic receptors, which in turn stimulates adenylyl cyclase via the activated G_s α-subunit. This raises the level of cAMP in the cells and increases pacemaker activity. However, the muscarinic potassium channel in the sinoatrial node directly opposes the actions of norepinephrine, inhibiting pacemaker activity by two mechanisms. The muscarinic m_2 receptor couples to the G_i protein to produce the G_i–α-GTP complex and the βγ-dimer. The activated G_i complex inhibits adenylyl cyclase (lowering cAMP), and the βγ-dimer directly activates the K^+ channel. Both the decrease in cAMP and the increase in K^+ conductance slow the heart and oppose the effects of norepinephrine.

SUGGESTED READING

1. Hamm HE. The many faces of G protein signaling. *J Biol Chem.* 1998;273:669–672.
2. Neer EJ. Heterotrimeric G proteins: organizers of transmembrane signals. *Cell.* 1995;80:249–257.
3. Sprang SR. G protein mechanisms: insights from structural analysis. *Annu Rev Biochem.* 1997;66:639–678.

Chapter 28

Signal Transduction: Cyclic Nucleotides

Kevin J. Catt, MD, PhD; Tamas Balla, MD, PhD

KEY POINTS

- Guanine nucleotide (G) protein–coupled receptors regulate the activities of plasma membrane enzymes (adenylyl cyclase and phospholipase C) that produce the intracellular messengers cyclic AMP, inositol trisphosphate, and diacylglycerol (DAG).

- Cyclic AMP and DAG activate protein kinases A and C, respectively, which phosphorylate regulatory proteins in the plasma membrane, cytoplasm, and nucleus.

- Cyclic GMP is produced by guanylate cyclases that are activated by atrial natriuretic peptide and nitric oxide, and it stimulates protein phosphorylation by protein kinase G.

See also Chapters 26, 27, 29, 30

The actions of numerous hormones, neurotransmitters, and growth factors on their target cells are mediated by highly specific receptors in the plasma membrane. Many of these are coupled through guanine nucleotide regulatory proteins (G proteins) to enzymes (adenylyl cyclases and phospholipases) that produce intracellular signaling molecules, or second messengers. These molecules include cyclic AMP (cAMP), inositol phosphates, diacylglycerol (DAG), and arachidonic acid. cGMP is produced by intrinsic guanylyl cyclases of membrane receptors for natriuretic factors and by soluble guanylyl cyclases that are activated by nitric oxide.

Numerous G protein–coupled receptors are coupled through G_s to the activation of adenylyl cyclase and the formation of cAMP, which acts predominantly through cAMP-dependent protein kinase (PKA) to control multiple aspects of cell function through phosphorylation of protein substrates. The cGMP that is formed by activated guanylyl cyclases has a more restricted range of actions that are expressed through protein phosphorylation mediated by cGMP-dependent protein kinase.

Adenylyl Cyclases

Several structurally related types of adenylyl cyclase have been identified in animal cells; in general, they contain two hydrophobic domains composed of six transmembrane helices that are associated with the plasma membrane. Type I adenyl cyclase is expressed in neural tissues, type II in brain and lung, type III in olfactory tissue, type IV in the brain and elsewhere, and types V and VI in heart, brain, and other tissues. All six enzymes are stimulated by G_{sa} and forskolin, and types I and III are also activated by Ca^{2+}-calmodulin (CaM). The latter adenylyl cyclases are abundant in neural tissue and are sensitive to transmitter-induced changes in cytoplasmic calcium concentration. In several cell types, Ca^{2+} exerts a direct inhibitory effect on the activity of the type VI enzyme. Because Ca^{2+}-mobilizing hormones usually act through stimulation of phosphoinositide hydrolysis, G_q is indirectly responsible for regulating the activities of the Ca^{2+}- and CaM-sensitive adenylyl cyclases.

In addition to being regulated by G_s or G_i α-subunits that activate or inhibit enzyme activity, some of the adenylyl cyclases are also controlled by βγ-subunits. The type I enzyme, when stimulated by $α_s$ or Ca^{2+}-CaM, is inhibited by βγ. Conversely, stimulation of the type II and type IV enzymes by $α_s$ is potentiated by βγ-subunits. The βγ-subunits that modulate adenylyl cyclase activity are probably derived from G_i and G_o, which are abundant in the brain and elsewhere. The basal and $α_s$-stimulated activities of the type II enzyme are also increased by calcium-dependent protein kinase (PKC) during activation of G_q by calcium-mobilizing hormones. Thus, the activation of adenylyl cyclases by G_s can be potentiated or inhibited by other receptor-mediated pathways that operate through G_i, G_o, or G_q in the same cell type.

Cyclic Nucleotide Phosphodiesterases

The cyclic nucleotides produced in agonist-stimulated cells are rapidly inactivated by phosphodiesterases (PDEs) and are released to a variable extent into the extracellular fluid. Intracellular cyclic nucleotide levels are usually governed by changes in their rates of formation, but in some tissues (eg, the retina), activation of PDEs is the major determinant of their concentration. Another important function of PDEs is to coordinate the activities of the cyclic nucleotide and phosphoinositide signaling pathways, largely through the regulatory action of Ca^{2+}-CaM on PDE activity.

Mammalian cells contain ≈20 PDEs that are classified into five main types according to their physical and functional properties. All possess a central catalytic domain and an N-terminal regulatory domain that binds Ca^{2+}-CaM and also contains binding sites for cGMP. Type I PDEs are stimulated by Ca^{2+}-CaM and are activated by calcium-mobilizing agonists and inhibited by methylxanthines. Type II PDEs are stimulated by cAMP and are activated by atrial natriuretic peptides (ANPs). Type III PDEs are inhibited by cGMP, which competes with cAMP at the catalytic site, and are regulated by insulin, glucagon, and dexamethasone. Type IV PDEs are specific for cGMP and are activated by cAMP-stimulating agonists. Type V PDEs are specific for cGMP and include rod and cone isoforms that are activated by transducin. Agonist-induced increases in cAMP are accompanied by increased activity of the cGMP-inhibited PDEs as a result of their cAMP-dependent phosphorylation and by a transient decrease in the activity of the Ca^{2+}-CaM–dependent PDEs. Several hormones that stimulate cAMP production also increase the expression of the high-affinity cAMP-specific PDEs.

cAMP-Dependent Protein Kinases

PKAs are present in all eukaryotic cells and are the major mediators of the effects of cAMP on cellular function. Cyclic nucleotide–dependent protein kinases are rapidly activated by the micromolar concentrations of cAMP or cGMP that occur in hormone-stimulated cells. The cyclic nucleotides bind to specific regulatory sites on the enzymes, which share several common structural features. In PKA, the regulatory and catalytic domains are expressed as two separate molecules that associate to form an inactive complex. In the cGMP-dependent enzyme (PKG), these domains are present in a single molecule.

The inactive form of PKA is a tetramer ($R_2 \cdot C_2$) composed of two regulatory (R) subunits and two catalytic (C) subunits. In the absence of cAMP, the subunits bind to each other with high affinity, and sequences in the regulatory subunits interact with the catalytic site and maintain the holoenzymes in their basal inactive state. Binding of cAMP to the regulatory subunits dissociates the inactive holoenzyme and releases catalytic subunits that phosphorylate intracellular substrates **(Figure 28.1)**. The regulatory subunits released by

cAMP-induced dissociation of protein kinase remain as an R_2 dimer and later undergo reassociation with free catalytic subunits. This sequence can be represented by the equation $R_2 \cdot C_2 + 4\ cAMP \rightleftharpoons R_2 \cdot cAMP_4 + 2\ C$. The catalytic subunit is common to both major forms of PKA, but the regulatory subunits show several differences. Two forms of protein kinase are present in most tissues, but their proportions vary in each cell type. The holoenzymes are generally similar in subunit composition ($R_2 \cdot C_2$) and molecular mass (≈ 170 kDa). The regulatory subunits differ in their molecular masses, R_1 being smaller (49 kDa) and more uniform in size than R_2 (52 to 56 kDa).

The R_1 and R_2 subunits exist in α- and β-isoforms that differ in size and tissue distribution. The α-isoforms are expressed constitutively in many tissues, but the β-isoforms have a more limited distribution and are most abundant in the nervous system. The selective regulation of these isoforms during differentiation and hormonal stimulation could mediate specific responses to the cAMP pathway. In some tissues, free R_1 and R_2 subunits are present in excess over the catalytic subunit and interact with other cellular proteins or structures. Selective increases in the R_2 subunit occur in several tissues during cAMP-induced differentiation. The catalytic subunits are also encoded by multiple genes, giving rise to α-, β-, and γ-isoforms. Because each regulatory subunit can associate with any of the C subunits, a wide variety of $R_2 \cdot C_2$ holoenzymes could exist in various tissues. The presence of at least 12 forms of PKA provides for a considerable degree of diversity in the tissue-specific expression, intracellular localization, and activation properties of the individual enzymes.

Nuclear Signaling by the cAMP/PKA Pathway

The receptor-mediated activation of adenylyl cyclase activity is often followed by cAMP-mediated stimulation of gene transcription. This results from the phosphorylation by PKA of transcriptional regulatory proteins that bind to cAMP-responsive enhancer elements (CREs) located in the promoter regions of cAMP-regulated genes. The CRE-binding (CREB) proteins that mediate transcriptional activation during stimulation of cAMP production include both activators and inhibitors of gene expression. The CREB proteins belong to a superfamily of transcription factors that are characterized structurally as basic region leucine zipper (bZip) proteins. Such proteins interact via their leucine zipper domains to form specific homodimers and heterodimers with other family members. In some CREBs, the phosphorylation of a specific serine residue by PKA promotes their transcriptional activation potential and stimulates gene expression. The same residue is also phosphorylated by Ca^{2+}-CaM–dependent protein kinases and thus serves to integrate signals from two distinct signaling pathways **(Figure 28.1)**.

An important subset of the CREB family are called CRE modulator (CREM) proteins, which are derived from a single gene by a variety of transcriptional and translational processes. CREM proteins possess specific activator or inhibitory functions and tissue localizations and are important mediators of physiological and neuroendocrine responses. CREMs are phosphorylated by PKA and Ca^{2+}-CaM–dependent kinases at the same serine residue as CREB, as well as by PKC and the mitogen-activated S6 kinase. The CREM proteins are thus responsive to multiple signal transduction pathways, including those responsible for mitogen-induced gene expression.

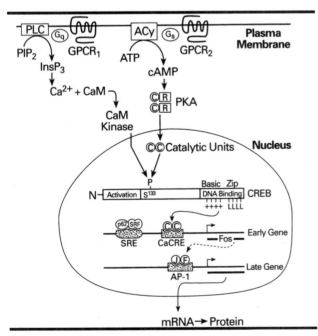

Figure 28.1. Receptor-mediated activation of cAMP and inositol phosphate signaling pathways. Diagram also illustrates manner in which both pathways converge on phosphorylation and activation of nuclear transcription factor, cAMP-responsive enhancer element–binding (CREB) protein. Activated CREB protein binds to CRE located in promoter of *fos* and other early-response genes. Increase in *fos* and formation of *fos-jun* heterodimers activates AP1 sites that promote expression of intermediate- and late-response genes.

Guanylyl Cyclase

cGMP is a major physiological regulator of vasodilatation induced by ANPs, which activate membrane-associated guanylyl cyclase in smooth muscle, kidney, endothelial cells, and adrenal glands. Several hormones that stimulate phospholipid turnover also increase cGMP production, probably reflecting the activation of guanylyl cyclase by PKC and/or arachidonic acid metabolites. The resulting increases in cGMP production are responsible for smooth muscle relaxation and vasodilation via activation of PKG and phosphorylation of specific proteins involved in the contractile mechanism.

In vertebrates, cGMP serves as the intracellular messenger mediating visual transduction by modulating the activity of a cation channel in the plasma membrane of rod photoreceptors of the retina. The guanylyl cyclases that catalyze the formation of cGMP from GTP are present in most mammalian cells as membrane-associated and soluble forms. The membrane-associated enzymes are located within the cytoplasmic regions of cell-surface receptors with a single transmembrane domain and an extracellular hormone-binding domain. These receptors are activated by ANPs, heat-stable *Escherichia coli* enterotoxin, and sea urchin egg peptides that stimulate sperm motility. The three major forms of receptor guanylyl cyclase (called GC-A, GC-B, and GC-C) contain a cysteine-rich extracellular domain for ligand binding and an intracellular catalytic domain that is highly conserved in guanylyl and adenylyl cyclases. The ANPs produced in the heart and brain act on GC-A and GC-B receptors, and enterotoxin probably acts on the GC-C receptor.

Soluble guanylyl cyclases are present in most tissues and are abundant in lung and smooth muscle. They contain no membrane-spanning domains and are activated by nitric oxide, which interacts with a potential heme-binding region of the molecule. This effect of nitric oxide is responsible for the vasodilator actions of nitroglycerin and related compounds. It also accounts for the actions of endogenous vasodilators, such as acetylcholine, bradykinin, and substance P, which stimulate nitric oxide synthesis in endothelial cells. The gaseous messenger diffuses into the adjacent cells and activates soluble guanylate cyclase, leading to activation of PKG and smooth muscle relaxation.

PKGs are abundant in invertebrates but have a more limited distribution in mammalian tissues. Whereas PKAs regulate the activities of major metabolic pathways, including lipolysis, glycogenolysis, and steroidogenesis, the cGMP-dependent enzymes are involved in the control of gene expression, neuronal function, vascular tone, and platelet aggregation. Because PKGs are monomeric molecules, their activation does not involve the subunit dissociation that is typical of the cAMP-dependent enzyme. There are marked amino acid sequenced homologies between cGMP- and cAMP-dependent protein kinases, suggesting that the two enzymes have evolved from an ancestral phosphotransferase.

SUGGESTED READING

1. Della Fazia MA, Servillo G, Sassone-Corsi, P. Cyclic AMP signalling and cellular proliferation: regulation of CREB and CREM. *FEBS Lett.* 1997;410:22–24.
2. Divecha N, Irvine RF. Phospholipid signaling. *Cell.* 1995;80:269–278.
3. Exton JH. Cell signalling through guanine-nucleotide-binding regulatory proteins (G proteins) and phospholipases. *Eur J Biochem.* 1997;243:10–20.
4. Lincoln TM, Cornwell TL, Komalavilas P, Boerth N. Cyclic GMP-dependant protein kinase in nitric oxide signaling. *Methods Enzymol.* 1996;269:149–166.
5. Montminy M. Transcriptional regulation by cyclic AMP. *Annu Rev Biochem.* 1997;66:807–822.

Chapter 29

Signal Transduction: Inositol Phosphates

Kevin J. Catt, MD, PhD; Tamas Balla, MD, PhD

KEY POINTS

- The receptor-mediated hydrolysis of plasma-membrane phosphoinositides by phospholipase C is a major signaling system that operates in virtually all cells.

- Inositol trisphosphate binds to receptor channels in the endoplasmic reticulum and stimulates calcium release from intracellular stores.

See also Chapters 26, 27, 28, 30

The main substrate of phospholipase C action is phosphatidylinositol 4,5-bisphosphate (PIP_2), a minor component of the membrane phospholipid pool that is synthesized from phosphatidylinositol (PI) via phosphatidylinositol 4-phosphate (PIP). In agonist-stimulated cells, PIP_2 is rapidly hydrolyzed by phospholipase C to form two second messengers, inositol 1,4,5-trisphosphate [$Ins(1,4,5)P_3$] and diacylglycerol (DAG) (**Figure 29.1**).

$Ins(1,4,5)P_3$ binds to specific receptors in the endoplasmic reticulum to release stored calcium into the cytoplasm. The resulting "calcium transient" initiates cellular responses such as exocytosis, contraction, and neurotransmission. However, the endogenous calcium transient must be supplemented by entry of calcium from the extracellular fluid to maintain cellular responses during continued agonist stimulation. This calcium influx occurs through plasma-membrane calcium channels that are activated either directly or indirectly by $Ins(1,4,5)P_3$, which thus serves to both initiate and maintain specific cellular responses. After exerting its action on calcium mobilization, $Ins(1,4,5)P_3$ is rapidly degraded to lower inositol phosphates [$Ins(1,4)P_2$, $Ins(4)P$] and then to inositol, which is subsequently reincorporated into the biosynthetic pathway to form PI, PIP, and PIP_2.

Thus, agonist stimulation causes increased turnover of the phosphoinositide cycle, with concomitant generation of two powerful but transitory messenger molecules, $InsP_3$ and DAG. In addition to being catabolized to inositol, $Ins(1,4,5)P_3$ is also phosphorylated to form $Ins(1,3,4,5)P_4$, which may also participate in calcium regulation and contributes to a minor degree to the formation of higher inositol phosphates ($InsP_5$ and $InsP_6$), which are present in many cell types. The DAG formed by phospholipase C activation acts as a co-messenger with the $Ins(1,4,5)P_3$-induced rise of intracellular calcium to activate protein kinases, particularly protein kinase C (PKC), that phosphorylate numerous key proteins, receptors, ion channels, and enzymes in the cytoplasm and nucleus.

Phospholipase C

Multiple forms of phospholipase C have been identified in various tissues. These have been designated as α, β, γ, and δ, and they contain conserved regions within their generally dissimilar amino acid sequences. One such domain is the catalytic site of the enzyme, and another, called SH2, has homology with the *src* oncogene and binds to phosphotyrosine residues in proteins. Phospholipase C-β is activated by receptors of the G protein–coupled variety, which possess a rhodopsin-like structure with seven transmembrane domains and mediate the actions of numerous hormones and neurotransmitters. In contrast, phospholipase C-γ is activated by receptors for growth factors, such as platelet-derived growth factor and epidermal growth factor, that undergo tyrosine phosphorylation and thus bind to the SH2 domain of phospholipase C-γ and other signaling molecules.

Within the calcium-phosphoinositide signaling system, phospholipases β and γ appear to be the major enzymes responsible for generating the important second messengers that activate cell responses to hormones and growth factors. The β-isozyme of phospholipase C exists in three forms, two of which ($β_1$ and $β_3$) are activated by G protein α-subunits and the other ($β_2$) by βγ-dimers derived from dissociation of the heterotrimeric proteins G_o. Although all phospholipase C enzymes are activated by calcium, the δ-isoform is believed to be regulated primarily by changes in the cytosolic calcium concentration.

Inositol 1,4,5-Trisphosphate Receptors

The $Ins(1,4,5)P_3$ formed during activation of phospholipase C binds with high affinity to specific intracellular receptors located in the endoplasmic reticulum, which serves as the internal store of calcium that is released during agonist stimulation. In some cells, $Ins(1,4,5)P_3$ receptors are also present in the plasma membrane. The $Ins(1,4,5)P_3$ receptor is a tetrameric structure composed of four similar subunits, each with several membrane-spanning regions that together form the ion channel through which calcium passes from the endoplasmic reticulum when $Ins(1,4,5)P_3$ binds to the cytoplasmic aspect of the receptor. Three forms of $Ins(1,4,5)P_3$ receptors have been identified, and they differ in their tissue distribution.

In addition to its ligand, the $Ins(1,4,5)P_3$ receptor is also regulated by the Ca^{2+} concentration at regulatory sites close to the mouth of the channel and exhibits a Ca^{2+}-induced Ca^{2+} release process. At low $Ins(1,4,5)P_3$ concentrations, the small amount of Ca^{2+} that is released through the channel exerts a positive feedback that leads to an all-or-none type of Ca^{2+} release. Conversely, high Ca^{2+} concentrations have a negative feedback effect that causes the channel to become inactive, a state from which it only slowly recovers. This biphasic Ca^{2+} regulation of the $Ins(1,4,5)P_3$ receptor channel is the underlying mechanism

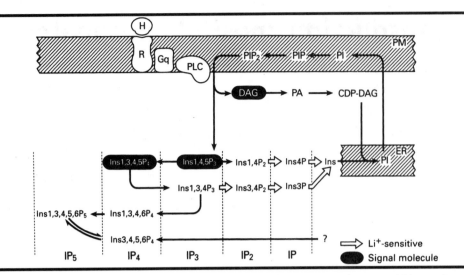

Figure 29.1. Pathways of formation of inositol phosphates and diacylglycerol (DAG) in response to hormones (H) interacting with their receptors (R) in plasma membrane (PM) and metabolic pathways linking various inositol phosphates. Regeneration of phospholipid precursors occurs in endoplasmic reticulum (ER).

for the oscillatory cytosolic Ca^{2+} signals that are observed in many cells during stimulation with low agonist concentrations.

Inositol Polyphosphates

Highly phosphorylated inositols such as $InsP_5$ and $InsP_6$ are present in large amounts in mammalian as well as in avian and plant cells. Their relationship to the second messenger $Ins(1,4,5)P_3$ and its metabolite $Ins(1,3,4,5)P_4$ is not clear, although an enzymatic pathway leading to their formation has been identified. In avian erythrocytes, these molecules serve to regulate the binding of oxygen to hemoglobin, and in the rat brain stem they have been proposed to function as neurotransmitters. A protein that binds $InsP_5$ with high affinity is associated with clathrin, a major component of receptor-mediated endocytosis. These inositides may be synthesized more rapidly in transformed cells and are increased during long-term agonist stimulation and during cell division. These findings may reflect a role for $InsP_5$ and $InsP_6$ in the processes controlling cell growth and proliferation.

Phosphoinositide Kinases

The primary substrate of phospholipase C is a relatively small pool of PIP_2 of the plasma membrane, which is formed from PI by sequential phosphorylations by PI 4-kinases and PIP 5-kinases. Multiple forms of these enzymes have been identified, suggesting that membrane PIP_2 may not be functionally homogeneous. The PI 4-kinase enzymes that synthesize the PIP and PIP_2 pools, which are regulated by agonists, are soluble enzymes and belong to the type III PI 4-kinase family. The function of the more abundant and tightly membrane-bound type II PI 4-kinase is not known at present.

An important group of PI kinases (type I enzymes) phosphorylate PI, as well as PI(4)P and $PI(4,5)P_2$, on the 3 rather than the 4 or 5 position of the inositol ring. These PI 3 kinases are regulated by growth factor receptors and oncogenic tyrosine kinases, and they generate 3-phosphorylated inositol phospholipids. These lipids are not hydrolyzed

by any known phospholipase C, and their regulatory function is probably based on their ability to bind specific protein modules that are present in many signaling proteins. These modules, called pleckstrin homology (PH) domains, are able to recognize and bind various forms of phosphoinositides, which then affect the function of the holoprotein. The interaction of proteins via their PH domains with inositides and the regulation of these inositides by PI kinases and phosphatases represent a novel aspect of inositide-based signaling.

Phosphatidylcholine Signaling

In addition to the lipid second messengers derived from phosphoinositides, agonist stimulation is also associated with the hydrolysis of phosphatidylcholine by a variety of phospholipases (including PLA_2, PLC, and PLD) to form DAG, phosphatidic acid, and arachidonic acid. Both G proteins and PKC have been implicated in the activation of PLD, leading to the release of phosphatidic acid and its subsequent conversion (via phosphatidic acid phosphohydrolase) to DAG. In a given cell type, various agonists can stimulate the activation of PLC and/or PLD, and the proportion of DAG generated from phosphatidylcholine versus phosphoinositide hydrolysis can range from 0% to 100%. During agonist activation of G protein–coupled receptors, the DAG produced from phosphoinositide breakdown can lead to secondary activation of PLD through PKC, causing a further increase in DAG production from the hydrolysis of phosphatidylcholine and metabolism of phosphatidic acid.

SUGGESTED READING

1. Berridge MJ. Inositol trisphosphate and calcium: two interacting second messengers. *Am J Nephrol.* 1997;17:1–11.
2. Divecha N, Irvine RF. Phospholipid signaling. *Cell.* 1995;80:269–278.
3. Exton JH. Cell signalling through guanine-nucleotide-binding regulatory proteins (G proteins) and phospholipases. *Eur J Biochem.* 1997;243:10–20.
4. Exton JH. New developments in phospholipase D. *J Biol Chem.* 1997;272:15579–82.
5. Toker A, Cantley LC. Signalling through the lipid products of phosphoinositide-3-OH kinase. *Nature* .1997;387:673–676.

Chapter 30

Protein Phosphorylation

George W. Booz, PhD; Kenneth M. Baker, MD

KEY POINTS

- Protein phosphorylation plays an important role in the control of many cellular processes, including metabolism, membrane transport, volume regulation, protein synthesis, and gene expression.

- Five principal intracellular signaling systems have been described for eukaryotic cells, which couple to the activation of a particular type of protein kinase (PK): PKA, PKG, Ca^{2+}/calmodulin-dependent kinases, PKC, and protein tyrosine kinases/mitogen-activated protein kinases.

- Transcription factors are important final phosphorylation targets of four of the five principal intracellular signaling systems (the exception being PKG).

See also Chapters 26, 27, 28, 29

For many cellular proteins, phosphorylation by a kinase triggers a conformational change that modifies activity or function. An important feature of this type of covalent modification is that it is reversible through the actions of a phosphatase, thus allowing protein phosphorylation to serve as a molecular switch for turning proteins and cellular systems (eg, channels) on and off. Protein phosphorylation plays an important role in the control of many cellular processes, including metabolism, membrane transport, volume regulation, protein synthesis, and gene expression. The sequential activation of protein kinases in distinct phosphorylation cascades is the principal means by which cells respond to external stimuli. These cascades amplify and prolong an initial signal, allow for the integration of different signals, and often result in a sustained or permanent cellular response to a transient external stimulus. Protein phosphorylation cascades, in particular those involving the mitogen-activated protein kinases (MAPKs), are critically important in development, growth, and programmed cell death or apoptosis (**see Table 30.1 for abbreviations**). The importance of protein phosphorylation to the physiology of the cell is underscored by the fact that protein kinases are the largest known protein family, representing an estimated 1% of all mammalian genes.

Protein Kinases

Protein kinases are structurally related by having a catalytic domain that (1) binds and orients a substrate peptide or protein and a purine nucleotide triphosphate donor (ATP/GTP) as a complex with a divalent cation (Mg^{2+} or Mn^{2+}) and (2) facilitates the transfer of the γ-phosphate of the donor to a hydroxyl residue (serine, threonine, or tyrosine) of the substrate. Based on the amino acid sequence of the catalytic domain, eukaryotic protein kinases can be organized into four groups that have related functions and share substrate preference: the ACG group, which includes the cyclic nucleotide–dependent kinases (PKA and PKG), the PKC family, the RSKs (ribosomal S6 kinases), and β-adrenergic receptor kinases (βARKs), phosphorylate serine/threonine residues near the basic residues arginine and

lysine; Ca^{2+}/calmodulin-regulated kinases (CaMKs) also phosphorylate serine or threonine residues near basic amino acids; CMGC kinases, which include cyclin-dependent kinases, glycogen synthase kinase 3 (GSK3), MAPKs, and Clk (Cdk-like) kinase, phosphorylate serine/threonine residues in proline-rich domains; the protein tyrosine kinase (PTK) group includes both receptor and nonreceptor kinases that phosphorylate tyrosine residues. Several recently described kinases fall outside of these major subgroups, including MAPK-ERK kinases (MEKs) and MEK kinases (MEKKs).

Phosphorylation and Intracellular Signaling

Protein phosphorylation forms the basis of intracellular communication. Five principal intracellular signaling systems have been described for eukaryotic cells that couple to the activation of a particular type of protein kinase: PKA, PKG, Ca^{2+}/calmodulin-dependent kinases, PKC, and PTKs/MAPKs. Each signaling system is activated by a receptor coupled to increased levels of a particular second messenger, or in the case of PTKs/MAPKs, Ras and/or tyrosine phosphorylation events. An important regulatory mechanism for the control of intracellular signaling by phosphorylation is the subcellular location of kinases with targeting proteins and/or the organization of the kinases of a phosphorylation cascade into complexes. However, a single receptor may couple to activation of multiple phosphorylation systems, and cross talk may occur between systems at the level of the signaling components and/or target proteins, resulting in either synergistic or antagonistic effects. The regulation of phosphorylase kinase by both cAMP and Ca^{2+} signals in mammalian skeletal muscle is an example of cross talk that is important in stimulating glycogenolysis during increased muscle activity in vivo. By increasing cAMP, adrenaline activates PKA, which phosphorylates the α- and β-regulatory subunits of phosphorylase kinase, thereby enhancing sensitivity of the catalytic subunit to regulation by the Ca^{2+}-regulated δ calmodulin subunit as well as its maximum kinase activity. Another example of cross talk occurs in cardiac muscle at the level of phospholamban, a small protein that interacts with and sup-

Table 30.1. Selected Abbreviations and Acronyms

CaMK = Ca^{2+}/calmodulin regulated kinase
CBP = CREB-binding protein
CRE = cAMP response element
CREB = CRE-binding protein
eIF = eukaryotic initiation factor
ERK = extracellular signal–regulated kinase
GAP = GTPase activating protein
GEF = guanine nucleotide exchange factor
GPCR = G protein–coupled receptor
JAK = Janus kinase
JNK = c-Jun NH_2 terminal kinase
MAPK = mitogen-activated protein kinase
MAPKAP = MAPK-activated protein
MEK = MAPK-ERK kinase
MEKK = MEK kinase
PI 3-kinase = phosphatidylinositol 3-kinase
PIE = prolactin-inducible element
PKA = protein kinase A
PKC = protein kinase C
PTK = protein tyrosine kinase
RSK = ribosomal S6 kinase
RTK = receptor tyrosine kinase
SAPK = stress-activated protein kinase
SEK = SAPK/ERK kinase
SIE = *sis*-inducible element
SIF = *sis*-inducing factor
SRE = serum response element
STAT = signal transducers and activators of transcription

presses the activity of the Ca^{2+}-ATPase of the sarcoplasmic reticulum. Phosphorylation of phospholamban by either PKA or a calmodulin-dependent protein kinase at different sites relieves this inhibition, increasing the rate at which Ca^{2+} is taken up by the sarcoplasmic reticulum and the rate of relaxation of cardiac muscle.

Regulation of Transcription Factor Activity

Transcription factors can be regulated by changes in their concentration and/or activity. Concentration reflects the activity of multiple steps from transcription to translation, each of which may be regulated by protein phosphorylation. Transcription factors are themselves important final phosphorylation targets of four of the five principal intracellular signaling systems (the exception being PKG). Phosphorylation can regulate transcription factor activity in several ways. First, a phosphorylation event may control the cellular location of a transcription factor. A transcription factor under this type of control is NF-κB, which in the nonstimulated state is found in the cytosol bound to the anchor protein IκB. Phosphorylation of IκB by PKC, PKA, or a ceramide-activated kinase induces its dissociation from NF-κB, permitting the transcription factor to move to the nucleus. Second, phosphorylation may modulate the DNA-binding activity and/or *trans*-activation potential of the transcription factor. For example, stress-activated protein kinase (SAPK) phosphorylates two sites in the N-terminal *trans*-activation domain of c-Jun, thereby enhancing its *trans*-activation potential, and ERK phosphorylates an inhibitor domain in C/EBPβ, disrupting intramolecular binding with the *trans*-activation domain and permitting DNA binding. Last,

phosphorylation of a transcription factor may be required for recruitment of a coactivator. The phosphorylation of cAMP response element (CRE)–binding protein (CREB) in response to the cAMP signal causes it to bind CREB-binding protein, which is required for CREB to function as a transcription factor.

Regulation of Protein Translation

Protein phosphorylation is critically important in regulating protein synthesis. Control occurs primarily at the level of translation initiation, a multistep process whereby the 40S ribosome subunit is positioned at the AUG initiation codon of the mRNA transcript. Attachment of the ribosome to the transcript is facilitated by a cap structure [$m^7G(5')ppp(5')N$, where N is any nucleotide] found at the 5′ terminus of all cytosolic (except organellar) mRNA. Attachment requires the participation of eukaryotic initiation factors (eIFs) and involves ATP hydrolysis. eIF-4F mediates cap function and is composed of three subunits: eIF-4E, a 24-kDa cap-binding polypeptide; eIF-4A, a 50-kDa polypeptide that exhibits RNA-dependent ATPase and bidirectional RNA unwinding activities; and p220, a 220-kDa polypeptide that is required for cap-dependent activity. eIF-4E is present in cells in rate-limiting amounts and has a key role in regulating translation. Phosphorylation of eIF-4E enhances its binding to the cap structure, and a strong correlation occurs between its phosphorylation state and rates of protein synthesis and cell growth. eIF-4E is phosphorylated in vitro and possibly in the cell by PKC. Activity of eIF-4E is repressed by two binding proteins, 4E-BP1 (PHAS-I) and 4E-BP2, that are highly homologous but exhibit different tissue distributions. Binding of 4E-BP1 to eIF-4E has been shown to prevent formation of the eIF-4F complex because of competition with p220 for the same binding site. Phosphorylation of 4E-BP1, which is mediated by the ERKs in vitro and possibly in the cell, decreases its affinity for eIF-4E, thereby allowing translation initiation to occur and resulting in enhanced protein synthesis. Protein phosphorylation may also play a role in the regulation of other aspects of protein synthesis, including the release of mRNA from the nucleus and peptide chain elongation. In addition, phosphorylation of the rDNA transcription factor upstream binding factor (UBF) is one way in which ribosome biogenesis is regulated.

MAPK Phosphorylation Cascades

Three distinct MAPK phosphorylation cascades of similar design have been described in vertebrates. These cascades couple to the selective activation of members of a family of cytosolic serine/threonine kinases, which affect cellular processes and gene expression by phosphorylating structural or functional proteins and transcription factors or activating other kinases. MAPK is a generic term used to classify these kinases, because some are preferentially activated by stress signals rather than mitogens. MAPKs phosphorylate serine or threonine residues that are closely followed by one or more prolines within a motif that is specific for each kinase. Their activation requires phosphorylation on both threonine and tyrosine residues, which is done by the family of cytosolic dual-specificity kinases, activation of which in turn results from phosphorylation by serine/threonine kinases.

The ERK Cascade

The first identified MAPK cascade in vertebrates leads to the activation of the extracellular signal–regulated kinases (ERKs), ERK1

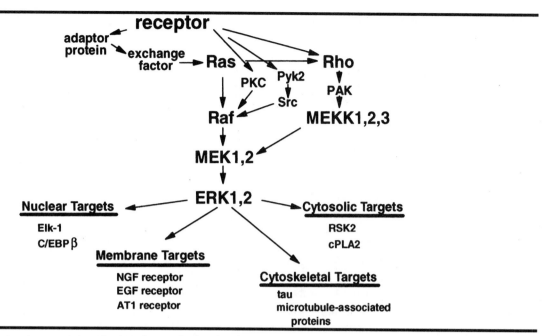

Figure 30.1. Membrane receptors couple to activation of a protein phosphorylation cascade that results in stimulation of cytosolic serine/threonine kinases, ERK1 and 2. Receptor tyrosine kinases couple via GTP-binding protein Ras, with PKC activation contributing synergistically. G protein–coupled receptors may couple via multiple pathways, involving activation of PKC or a nonreceptor tyrosine kinase. The latter can result from either activation by the G protein βγ-subunit or an increase in intracellular calcium (as in the case of Pyk2) and may or may not involve subsequent activation of Ras. Serine/threonine kinase Raf activates dual-specificity kinases MEK1 and 2, which can also be phosphorylated by MEKK1, 2, and 3, upstream components of SAPK/JNK cascade. Activated ERKs phosphorylate numerous membrane, cytosolic, and cytoskeletal proteins. In addition, activated ERKs enhance gene transcription by phosphorylating transcription factors. Other signaling pathways, such as those activated by PKC, Raf, or PI 3-kinase, may be activated as well. One signaling cascade may act synergistically or antagonistically with another.

(p44^{MAPK}) and ERK2 (p42^{MAPK}). This pathway is important in cellular proliferation and differentiation and is activated by polypeptide growth factors or trophic agents binding to cell surface receptors **(Figure 30.1)**. Both receptors that have tyrosine kinase activity, receptor tyrosine kinases (RTKs) and heterotrimeric G protein–coupled receptors (GPCRs), stimulate this cascade. Activation of the ERKs requires phosphorylation on both threonine and tyrosine residues within a Thr-Glu-Tyr motif, which is done by MEK1 and 2, enzymes highly specific for ERK1 and ERK2 (each MEK may have a preference for one ERK). Phosphorylation and activation of MEK1 and MEK2 are mediated in turn by a serine/threonine kinase, Raf. MEK1 and 2 may also be phosphorylated by MEKK1, 2, and 3, although MEKK1 and 2 preferentially stimulate the SAPK/c-Jun NH$_2$ terminal kinase (JNK) pathway.

The Raf proteins (Raf-1, A-Raf, B-Raf) are broadly expressed kinases that phosphorylate and activate MEK1 and 2 but not other MEKs. The prototypical member of this gene family is Raf-1, a protein normally located in the cytosol. Activation of Raf-1 involves its recruitment to the cell membrane by active (GTP-binding) Ras (this does not occur with B-Raf), and the subsequent phosphorylation of certain key serine, threonine, and tyrosine residues. The role of phosphorylation in activating Raf is not fully understood, but it includes autophosphorylation as well as possible tyrosine phosphorylation by membrane-bound Src and serine/threonine phosphorylation by a PKC isoform. Raf-1 may also be phosphorylated by a membrane-bound, proline-directed kinase that is activated by ceramide, the sec-

ond messenger of the sphingomyelin pathway. Raf may also be regulated by a lipid metabolite, because it has a zinc finger–like motif that resembles the lipid-binding domain of PKC. Certain proteins known as 14-3-3 proteins appear to be important in the function of Raf. These are a family of generally acidic, dimeric proteins that comprise at least seven isoforms, some of which (β and ζ) associate with and accompany Raf to the membrane in the presence of activated Ras. 14-3-3 proteins are not required for Raf activation but may prolong stimulated Raf activity by competing with phosphatases for binding to Raf. Their dimer structure may also promote the interaction of Raf with its substrates. 14-3-3 proteins associate with and modify activity of other kinases, including the catalytic p110 subunit of phosphatidylinositol 3-kinase (PI 3-kinase), which is inhibited by 14-3-3, and various PKC isoforms, either enhancing or inhibiting kinase activity depending on the isoform of PKC or 14-3-3.

Ras proteins are small, GTP-binding proteins attached to the inner face of the plasma membrane. In the nonstimulated or relaxed state, Ras binds GDP. Proteins collectively referred to as guanine nucleotide exchange factors (GEFs) catalyze the release of GDP from inactive Ras, thereby allowing GTP (present at a much higher concentration than GDP) to bind to Ras. In binding GTP, Ras undergoes a conformational change that exposes binding sites for other signaling molecules. Hydrolysis of bound GTP by the intrinsic GTPase activity of Ras relaxes its active conformation and terminates the signal. The low intrinsic GTPase activity of Ras is stimulated more than 100-fold by interaction with cytosolic proteins called GTPase activating proteins (GAPs).

Coupling of Cell-Surface Receptors to the ERK Cascade

Upon ligand binding, RTKs undergo dimerization and/or a conformational change, which results in the autophosphorylation of multiple tyrosine residues in the cytoplasmic region of the receptor. These phosphorylated tyrosine residues serve as docking sites for various proteins with one or more Src homology 2 (SH2) domains or phosphotyrosine-binding sequences. One such protein is the nonenzymic adaptor protein Shc, which also has an SH3 domain that recognizes a left-hand polyproline type II helix domain in other proteins. Shc binds to the GEF protein, mSOS, directly by the SH3 domain or via an adaptor protein, GRB2. mSOS binds to and activates Ras by catalyzing the release of GDP. Activated Ras in turn recruits Raf kinase to the membrane, thereby triggering the cascade that results in ERK activation.

GPCRs can couple to ERK activation by different means, depending on which G protein is activated. For G_i-coupled receptors, release of $G\beta\gamma$ may activate a nonreceptor tyrosine kinase that phosphorylates Shc, resulting in formation of the Shc-GRB2-mSOS-Ras complex. For G_q- or G_o-coupled receptors, stimulation of the ERK cascade may occur independently of Ras, via PKC-mediated activation of Raf or an MEKK. G_q/G_i-coupled receptors may also be linked to mSOS and Ras, via activation of the nonreceptor protein tyrosine kinase, Pyk2, which activates Src/leads to Shc phosphorylation. Pky2 can also be activated by increases in intracellular calcium, which often result from activation of GPCRs. Thus, in one cell type, a particular GPCR may couple to ERK activation by multiple means that can be described as independent of or dependent on calcium, PKC, or Ras.

Cytosolic and Nuclear Targets of the ERKs

The ERKs have numerous targets, including membrane, cytoskeletal, and cytosolic proteins and various kinases collectively referred to as MAPK-activated protein (MAPKAP) kinases **(Figure 30.1)**. Phosphorylation of upstream components of the cascade (mSOS, Raf-1, or MEK) by the ERKs may be a way of regulating or shutting off this signaling pathway. The ERKs also phosphorylate 4E-BP1 and eIF4E, although whether the ERK cascade couples to enhanced protein synthesis in the cell is uncertain. Although generally considered functionally interchangeable, ERK1 and 2 probably phosphorylate different substrates.

Activated ERKs, like other MAPKs, may translocate to the nucleus and phosphorylate transcription factors. They stimulate c-*fos* transcription by phosphorylating the protein Elk-1, which together with serum response factor binds to a serum response element located in the c-*fos* promoter. ERKs also stimulate c-*fos* transcription by phosphorylating and activating RSK2, a serine/threonine protein kinase in the p90^rsk family. RSK2 phosphorylates and activates CREB, which binds the CRE in the c-*fos* promoter. Increased c-*fos* expression further activates gene expression by enhancing AP1 activity. AP1 is a heterodimeric transcription complex consisting of members of the c-Fos and c-Jun families of transcription factors.

Cross Talk Between the ERK Cascade and other Signaling Pathways

Raf kinase can function in signaling pathways outside the ERK cascade. In addition to MEK 1 and 2, Raf-1 phosphorylates p53, IκB,

and the dual-specificity phosphatase CDC25A, which dephosphorylates and thereby activates the cyclin CDC2 kinase. Thus, activation of Raf may affect gene expression under control of p53 and NF-κB, as well as progression of the cell cycle. Cross talk between the ERK cascade and other signaling pathways occurs as well. For instance, Ras can activate PI 3-kinase and can indirectly stimulate PKC by activating phospholipases D or C_γ and generating diacylglycerol. Finally, in certain cells, increases in cAMP inhibit the ERK cascade by activating PKA, which by phosphorylating Raf-1 inhibits Ras binding and its kinase activity. The inhibitory effect of PKA activation does not occur in all cells but depends in part on which Raf isoform is expressed predominantly. In some cells, increases in intracellular cAMP stimulate the ERK cascade.

Other MAPK Cascades

Two other MAPK cascades that mediate distinct cellular responses and that may be associated with induction of apoptosis have been identified in vertebrates. One is stimulated by proinflammatory cytokines and stress signals (UV light, heat, hydrogen peroxide, protein synthesis inhibitors) and results in activation of SAPK/JNK. Mitogens can also activate the SAPK/JNK cascade, but less effectively than stress stimuli. In some cells, however, agonists that bind to GPCRs activate the SAPK/JNK cascade more strongly than the pathway leading to ERK activation. SAPKs are phosphorylated on threonine and tyrosine residues within a Thr-Pro-Tyr motif by the dual-specificity kinase SEK, which in turn is activated by MEKK1, 2, or 3. The MEKKs may be activated by the serine/threonine kinase PAK in a cascade that is activated by Rho proteins (Rac 1 and CDC42), GTP-binding proteins closely related to Ras. In some cells, a PKC isoform may activate the MEKKs. Activation of the SAPK/JNK cascade may also be mediated by the nonreceptor tyrosine kinase, c-able, at the level of the nucleus or by the calcium-regulated tyrosine kinase, Pyk2. It is not known what determines the relative extent to which Pyk2 activates the SAPK/JNK or ERK cascade.

SAPK phosphorylates two transcription factors, c-Jun and ATF2, which bind as a heterodimeric complex to the 12-*O*-tetradecanoylphorbol 13-acetate response element on the c-*jun* promoter. This phosphorylation leads to increased c-Jun synthesis, which results in increased AP-1 activity. In addition, SAPK phosphorylates c-Jun in the AP-1 complex, thus enhancing the DNA binding and *trans*-activation potential of AP-1. Activated SAPK may also inhibit PI 3-kinase signaling by forming a complex with the kinase via binding to GRB2.

Physiochemical stress and proinflammatory cytokines, such as interleukin-1 and tumor necrosis factor, can induce another MAPK cascade, which results in the activation of p38 MAP kinase. p38 is activated by MAPK kinase 3 (MKK3) and MKK6 through phosphorylation on tyrosine and threonine residues within a Thr-Gly-Tyr motif. Novel cytokine-suppressive anti-inflammatory drugs (CSAIDs) are potent and selective inhibitors of p38 activity, thus implicating this cascade in cytokine biosynthesis.

PI 3-Kinase–Induced Phosphorylation Cascade

Agonists that stimulate MAPK activity commonly induce a parallel phosphorylation cascade that is linked to PI 3-kinase activation and has been implicated in enhancing protein synthesis. PI 3-kinase represents a family of membrane proteins, composed of an 85-kDa regulatory subunit and a 110-kDa catalytic subunit, that phosphorylate certain lipids in the 3 position and various proteins on serine and threonine, including the insulin receptor substrate 1. Association of SH2 domains in the regulatory subunit with phosphorylated tyrosine residues activates PI 3-kinase. Ras and the $\beta\gamma$-subunit of heterotrimeric G proteins may also activate the catalytic subunit. The phosphorylated lipid products of PI 3-kinase have been implicated in membrane ruffling and the activation of PKC_ζ. Recent studies using the specific PI 3-kinase inhibitor Wortmannin have implicated this kinase in the initiation of a phosphorylation cascade linked to activation of 70-kDa S6 kinase ($p70^{S6K}$) and enhanced protein synthesis. Phosphorylation of the ribosomal S6 subunit is thought to enhance protein translation. In addition, kinases downstream of $p70^{S6K}$ have been implicated in phosphorylation of 4E-BP1 and in causing its dissociation from eIF4E.

JAK-STAT Signaling

This relatively simple signaling cascade linked to gene expression was first shown to be activated by interferon receptors. Subsequently, cytokine receptors, as well as certain RTKs (those for platelet-derived growth factor, epidermal growth factor, and colony-stimulating factor 1) and GPCRs (angiotensin II type 1 and endothelin ETA, and receptors for α-thrombin and serotonin) were shown to couple to this pathway. The Janus kinases, or JAKs, are a family of tyrosine kinases (Tyk2, Jak1, Jak2, Jak3) that phosphorylate members of the signal transducers and activators of transcription (STAT) family of transcription factors. The sequences of six mammalian STAT family members have been reported. Phosphorylated STATs dimerize via reciprocal SH2-phosphotyrosine interactions and translocate to the nucleus, where they bind to DNA elements (c-*sis*–inducible element, SIE, or prolactin-inducable element, PIE, which binds Stat5 dimers) that regulate transcription of downstream genes. Homodimerized or heterodimerized STATs constitute a *sis*-inducing factor (SIF) complex. Different ligands may preferentially induce the formation of a particular SIF complex, eg, SIF-B (Stat1/Stat3 heterodimers).

Activation of JAK-STAT Signaling by Cell Surface Receptors

Coupling of all receptor types to activation of the JAKs appears to involve the noncovalent association of the kinase with the cytoplasmic region of the receptor (or possibly the membrane adaptor protein gp130). Receptor-JAK interactions can be constitutive or ligand-induced. Dimerization of receptors or receptor subunits upon ligand binding brings associated JAKs into juxtaposition, allowing for *trans*-autophosphorylation and activation. Activated JAKs phosphorylate binding motifs on the receptor or gp130 that bind STAT proteins via their SH2 domain. In some cases, activated JAKs may provide docking sites for STAT proteins. The specificity of JAK-STAT signaling is established by which JAK and STAT family members are recruited by a receptor, which is determined by the binding motifs present in the receptor.

Regulation of Transcription

The SIE binding site is present in the promoter region of a number of genes, including those for c-*fos*, serine protease inhibitor 3, and tissue inhibitor of metalloproteinase 1. PIE is also present in the promoter region of a number of genes. Stimulation of gene transcription by growth hormone, prolactin, and various cytokines is mediated mainly by the JAK-STAT pathway. The ability of interferon to induce an antiviral response in cells is dependent on JAK-STAT signaling, and recent evidence indicates that this pathway probably contributes as well to the growth effects induced by RTKs and GPCRs, although less so than the ERK cascade.

Cross Talk With Ras-Mediated Signal Transduction Pathways

Some STAT proteins (Stat1 and Stat3) are also phosphorylated, possibly by the ERKs, on serine residues, which may enhance their *trans*-activating potential. Recent evidence indicates that the JAKs may also mediate ERK activation through a Ras- and Raf-dependent process. Jak2 has been found to associate with the adaptor molecule Shc, which couples to Ras signaling by forming GRB2-mSOS complexes.

SUGGESTED READING

1. Calkhoven CF, Geert AB. Multiple steps in the regulation of transcription-factor level and activity. *Biochem J.* 1996;317:329–342.
2. Denhardt DT. Signal-transducing protein phosphorylation cascades mediated by Ras/Rjo proteins in the mammalian cell: the potential for multiplex signalling. *Biochem J.* 1996;318:729–747.
3. Faux MC, Scott JD. More on target with protein phosphorylation: conferring specificity by location. *Trends Biol Sci.* 1996;21:312–315.
4. Hanks SK, Hunter T. The eukaryotic protein kinase superfamily: kinase (catalytic) domain structure and classification. *FASEB J.* 1995;9:576–596.
5. Leaman DW, Leung S, Li X, Stark GR. Regulation of STAT-dependent pathways by growth factors and cytokines. *FASEB J.* 1996;10:1578–1588.
6. Neary JT. MAPK cascades in cell growth and death. *News Physiol Sci.* 1997;12:286–293.

Chapter 31

Adhesion Molecules

Willa A. Hsueh, MD

KEY POINTS

- Adhesion molecules include intercellular adhesion molecules, integrins, and selectins.

- Adhesion molecules and selectins are regulated by cytokines, growth factors, and shear stress and contribute to the inflammatory process at the vessel wall.

- Integrins regulate remodeling and fibrosis in heart and vascular tissue.

See also Chapters 63, 65

Adhesion molecules allow cells to adhere to each other or to molecules in the extracellular matrix (ECM). The process of adhesion is necessary for a variety of cell functions, including differentiation, growth, migration, and response of the cell to its external milieu. Three types of cell adhesion molecules have been described.

Intercellular Adhesion Molecules

Intercellular adhesion molecules (ICAMS) include ICAM-1, ICAM-2, ICAM-3, neural cell adhesion molecule (NCAM), vascular cell adhesion molecule (VCAM), and platelet/endothelial cell adhesion molecule (PECAM). ICAMs are transmembrane glycoproteins that contain immunoglobulin-like domains. They play an important role in the adhesion of circulating blood cells to vascular tissue, as in the inflammatory response in vascular injury.

Integrins

Integrins are transmembrane receptors composed of α- and β-subunit heterodimers that consist of a large extracellular domain, a transmembrane region, and a relatively short cytoplasmic domain. The extracellular domain binds to proteins in the ECM, such as fibronectin, collagen, vitronectin, osteopontin, and others, whereas the cytoplasmic domains interact with cytoskeletal proteins and intracellular signaling molecules. Integrins transmit information from the external environment of the cell that influences structural changes within the cell and affects cell activity.

Selectins

Selectins occur as P, E, and L forms and are expressed by leukocytes and endothelial cells. These receptors mediate loose contacts between leukocytes and endothelial cells that allow the "rolling" of leukocytes over the endothelium.

Role in Inflammation and Vascular Diseases

The ICAM family and selectins play a key role in immune and inflammatory responses of particular importance in the development of the atherosclerotic plaque. The ICAMS found on endothelial cells, monocytes and macrophages, lymphocytes, and vascular smooth muscle cells contribute to the vascular injury response. They are induced by cytokines such as tumor necrosis factor-α, interleukins,

growth factors such as endothelin and angiotensin II, shear stress, oxidized LDL, and thrombin.

One of the earliest changes in the endothelium in the atherosclerotic process is the attachment of leukocytes. This is mediated by increased expression of ICAM-1 and VCAM-1, which bind in a ligand-receptor fashion to receptors on appropriately activated monocytes or T lymphocytes. PECAM can lead to platelet adhesion if the endothelium is activated appropriately. Increased amounts of ICAM-1, VCAM-1, PECAM, and E-selectin have been found in human atherosclerotic plaques. ICAM-1 can be shed from the vasculature into the circulation in a soluble form. Increased soluble ICAM-1 has been associated with increased risk of myocardial infarction.

Integrins are intimately involved in a variety of cell activities and participate in cell functions that underlie atherosclerosis, cardiac and vascular remodeling, angiogenesis, and other cardiovascular processes. The engagement of integrins by certain ECM proteins initiates the localization of cytoskeletal proteins into focal adhesions, areas of tight association between the plasma membrane and the ECM. Focal adhesions represent the colocalization of cytoskeletal proteins such as talin and α-actin, focal adhesion kinase (FAK), integrins, growth factor receptors, and other signaling molecules. In general, this colocalization is dependent on the integrin β-cytoplasmic domain, which is highly conserved between species and for each of the β-subtypes. Signal-transducing molecules such as c-*src*, phosphatidylinositol 3-kinase, phospholipase C, and various protein kinases are associated with focal adhesions.

Activation of integrins can induce proto-oncogene expression and regulate the production of cell cycle proteins. Integrins may also affect the apoptotic process. The tyrosine kinase FAK is phosphorylated in various cells when the cells are attached to fibronectin, laminin, vitronectin, collagen, and other ECM proteins. FAK appears to be an important regulator of the movement of cells, because cells deficient in FAK have reduced motility in vitro, whereas overexpression of FAK is associated with increased motility. Integrins contribute to vascular smooth muscle cell growth and migration; inhibition of certain integrins on these cells can inhibit intimal hyperplasia and restenosis.

Endothelial cell migration related to angiogenesis is integrin-mediated. Antibodies against integrins inhibit angiogenesis associated with certain cancers and may inhibit cancer growth and metastasis. Because of their effects on cell attachment to the ECM and influence on ECM production, integrins may also play a key role in the fibrotic response of the myocardium and vasculature and contribute to remodeling processes in these tissues.

SUGGESTED READING

1. Ashizawa N, Graf K, Do Y, Nunihiro T, Giachelli CM, Meehan P, Tuan T-L, Hsueh WA. Osteopontin is produced by rat cardiac fibroblasts and mediates AII-induced DNA synthesis and collagen gel contraction. *J Clin Invest.* 1996;98:2218–2227.

2. Giachelli CM, Schwartz SM, Liaw L. Molecular and cellular biology of osteopontin. *Trends Cardiovasc Med.* 1995;5:88–95.

3. Hsueh WA, Law RE, Do YS. Integrins, adhesion and cardiac remodeling. *Hypertension.* 1998;31:176–180.

4. Meredith J, Winitxz S, McArthur LJ, Hoss S, Ren X-D, Rewshaw MW, Schwartz MA. The regulation of growth and intracellular signaling by integrins. *Endocr Rev.* 1996;17:207.

5. Ridker PM, Hennekens CH, Roitman-Johnson B, Stampfer MJ, Allen J. Plasma concentration of soluble intercellular adhesion molecule 1 and risk of future myocardial infarction in apparently healthy men. *Lancet.* 1998;351: 88–92.

6. Ross R. Cell biology of atherosclerosis. *Annu Rev Physiol.* 1995;57:791–804.

Chapter 32

Vascular Smooth Muscle Contraction and Relaxation

Anna F. Dominiczak, MD; David F. Bohr, MD

KEY POINTS

- The contractile state of vascular smooth muscle depends on the state of phosphorylation of myosin light chains.

- Increased vascular smooth muscle cytosolic Ca^{2+} content promotes myosin light chain phosphorylation and vasoconstriction.

- Increased cytosolic cGMP or nitric oxide favors myosin light chain dephosphorylation and vasodilation.

- A subregion of the cell, the plasmERosome, which responds to ouabain, regulates Na,K-ATPase activity, cellular Na^+ content, and Na^+ gradient–dependent Na^+-Ca^{2+} exchange.

See also Chapters 14, 20, 25, 26, 27, 28, 29, 30

The machinery for contraction of vascular smooth muscle (VSM) is composed of its thick and thin filaments, the contractile proteins myosin and actin, respectively. Contraction occurs when the enzyme myosin ATPase releases energy that causes myosin cross-bridges to cycle. This cycling displaces myosin in relation to the actin filament to which the bridges are attached. This displacement is contraction. The regulation of contraction of VSM depends on the extent of phosphorylation of the myosin light chain (MLC). An understanding of this regulation must therefore deal with the processes of both phosphorylation and dephosphorylation of MLC.

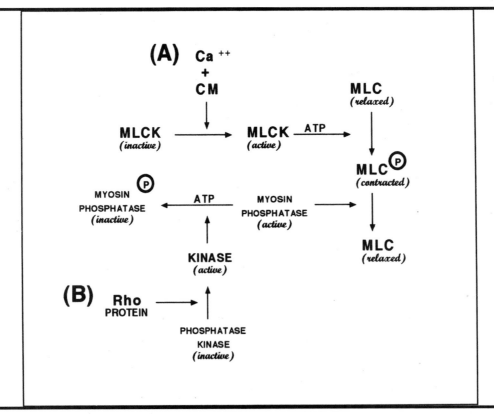

Figure 32.1. Regulation of phosphorylation and contraction of VSM. Contractile process is initiated (A) by an increase in intracellular calcium, which combines with calmodulin (CM) to activate myosin light chain kinase (MLCK). This active kinase phosphorylates myosin light chain (MLC) and causes contraction. Relaxation occurs when MLC is dephosphorylated by myosin phosphatase. However, phosphatase is itself inactivated when it is phosphorylated (B). This phosphorylation occurs physiologically when small G protein RhoA activates a Rho-associated kinase. Resultant inactivation of myosin phosphatase inhibits relaxation and potentiates contraction.

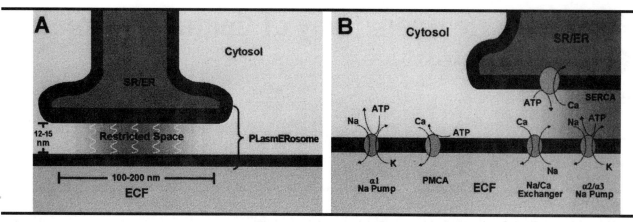

Figure 32.2. Diagram of plasmERosome region. A, Relationship between plasma membrane (unlabeled dark horizontal thick line above extracellular fluid ECF), restricted cytosolic space (12 to 15 nm high × 100 to 200 nm in diameter), and junctional SR/ER. B, Enlarged region of plasmERosome and adjacent plasma membrane (PM), showing key Na^+ and Ca^{2+} transporters present in plasmERosome region of PM and remainder of PM. Reproduced with permission from Blaustein MP, Juhasszova M, Golovina VA. *Clin Exp Hypertens.* 1998;691–703.

Role of Calcium

Contraction is initiated by an increase in intracellular calcium concentration ($[Ca^{2+}]_i$). This cytosolic calcium, either from the extracellular space or from the sarcoplasmic reticulum (SR), combines with calmodulin to activate myosin light chain kinase, which then phosphorylates MLC **(Figure 32.1)**. The SR is not only a source of Ca^{2+} but also an important regulator of Ca^{2+} entry from the extracellular space. Functional regulation of sodium and calcium transport occurs in a cellular subregion that includes the plasma membrane, the subjacent SR, and the narrow cytoplasmic space between the two. This subregion is now called the "plasmERosome" **(Figure 32.2)**. In contrast to the plasma membrane of the remainder of the cell, the plasma membrane of the plasmERosome contains Na,K-ATPase molecules with high ouabain affinities, along with sodium-calcium exchanger molecules. Because calcium extrusion by this exchanger depends on the sodium gradient established by Na,K-ATPase, inhibition of the Na,K-ATPase by ouabain and the resultant increase in sodium in the plasmERosome lead to an increased calcium content of the plasmERosome and the SR.

Role of Phosphatase

The regulation of contraction by the $[Ca^{2+}]_i$/phosphorylation system is balanced by a dephosphorylation process. The myosin phosphatase enzyme responsible for this dephosphorylation is itself inhibited by being phosphorylated **(Figure 32.1)**. This phosphorylation is effected by a G protein RhoA-associated kinase. Inhibition of myosin phosphatase caused by the Rho protein increases calcium sensitivity and VSM contraction. Y-27632, an agent that blocks the action of the Rho protein, lowers blood pressure in hypertensive but not in normotensive rats. This observation suggests that overactivity of the Rho system may contribute to hypertension.

Role of Nitric Oxide and cGMP

A very important stimulus of vasodilation involves the cascade that begins with arginine and includes nitric oxide (NO) and cGMP.

The activity of this cascade depends primarily on the activity of two forms of the enzyme NO synthase. The constitutive enzyme present in endothelial cells and neurons is activated by increases in cytosolic calcium caused by physiological agents such as acetylcholine or bradykinin. The other form of NO synthase is induced by cytokines or endotoxin, a lipopolysaccharide associated with infections, and is calcium-independent. NO produced by inducible NO synthase is responsible for much of the VSM relaxation associated with inflammation and endotoxic shock. Both enzymes are rendered inactive by analogues of arginine, such as N^G-monomethyl-L-arginine (L-NMMA), N^ω-nitro-L-arginine methyl ester (L-NAME), and N^G-nitro-L-arginine (L-NNA). When used in animals in vivo, these blocking analogues cause vasoconstriction and a rise in blood pressure, demonstrating a tonic vasodilator action of NO.

The next step in the cascade leading to VSM relaxation is activation by NO of the enzyme guanylate cyclase to produce cGMP. When cellular concentrations of cGMP are increased, a cGMP-dependent protein kinase is activated. It is not known which protein is phosphorylated by this enzyme, but it results in decreased $[Ca^{2+}]_i$ and relaxation of VSM.

SUGGESTED READING

1. Hai CM, Murphy RA. Ca^{2+} crossbridge phosphorylation and contraction. *Annu Rev Physiol.* 1989;51:285–298.
2. Van Breemen C, Chen Q, Laher I. Superficial buffer barrier function of smooth muscle sarcoplasmic reticulum. *Trends Pharmacol Sci.* 1995;16:98–105.
3. Juhaszova M, Blaustein MP. Na^+ pump low and high ouabain affinity α subunit isoforms are differently distributed in cells. *Proc Natl Acad Sci U S A.* 1997;94:1800–1805.
4. Songu-Mize E, Vassallo DV, Rashed SM, Varner KJ. Ouabain amplifies contractile responses to phenylephrine in rat tail arteries in hypertension. *J Basic Clin Physiol Pharmacol.* 1995;6:309–319.
5. Somlyo AP. Rhomantic interludes raise blood pressure. *Nature.* 1997;389:908–911.
6. Förstermann U, Closs EL, Pollock JS, Nakane M, Schwarz P, Gath I, Kleinert H. Nitric oxide synthase isozymes: characterization, purification, molecular cloning, and functions. *Hypertension.* 1994;23:1121–1131.

Functional Neuroanatomy of Central Vasomotor Control Centers

Donald J. Reis, MD

KEY POINTS

- Neural regulation is the result of actions on the discharge of sympathetic postganglionic neurons, which are excited by preganglionic neurons of the spinal cord.

- Spinal preganglionic sympathetic neurons are spontaneously (tonically) active and normally generate a background of vasoconstriction, cardiac contractility, and adrenal catecholamine secretion.

- The medulla oblongata is the central integrative area of the brain in controlling the circulation.

- The supramedullary networks are closely allied with the elaboration and execution of a range of emotional and consummatory behaviors reflecting the very close linkage between cardiovascular performance and emotional behaviors.

See also Chapters 34, 35, 42, 43, 128

The central nervous system plays a critical role in the short- and long-term regulation of arterial pressure. Short-term regulation is exerted from second to second by modulation of the activity of sympathetic postganglionic and cardiovagal neurons. Long-term arterial pressure regulation is also exerted by hormonal and neural control of blood volume. In this chapter, only short-term control will be considered.

Patterns of Hemodynamic Control

The brain can regulate blood pressure by influencing several physiological relationships: (1) arterial pressure = total peripheral resistance (TPR) $\times$ cardiac output (CO); (2) TPR = R1 + R2 + R3 ... (where R = resistance in a specific vascular bed); (3) CO = stroke volume $\times$ heart rate (HR); and (4) stroke volume = ventricular filling volume $\times$ contractile force. Sympathetic postganglionic neurons (via their innervation of blood vessels, adrenal medulla, and heart) control blood pressure by increasing or decreasing TPR via selective and differentiated actions on specific vascular beds or globally on CO. CO can be modified by changing the volume of large veins (capacitance vessels), thereby influencing cardiac filling; by regulation of the force of cardiac contractility; or by varying HR.

Neural regulation is the result of the discharge of sympathetic postganglionic neurons, driven by preganglionic neurons of spinal cord. The latter represent the principal effectors of cardiovascular centers in brain. Although it was once believed that sympathetic preganglionic neurons discharged en masse, it is now accepted that their discharge is highly differentiated, with vasoconstriction of selective beds occurring in patterns appropriate to different behaviors. For example, during feeding, blood flow may be directed to the gut at the expense of skeletal muscle. During defense behaviors, the reverse is true. Because arterial pressure reflects the sum of the resistances in individual beds, it is possible that wide changes in blood flow to one organ, if counterbalanced by changes in the opposite direction in another organ, may result in no net changes in arterial pressure.

Segmental Mechanisms

Preganglionic sympathetic neurons are localized within the intermediolateral columns of the thoracic and upper lumbar segments of the spinal cord. Their axons emerge through the ventral roots to innervate postganglionic sympathetic neurons in sympathetic ganglia that, in turn, innervate blood vessels and the heart. They also directly innervate chromaffin cells of the adrenal medulla, thereby governing the release of the adrenomedullary hormones epinephrine and norepinephrine. Preganglionic sympathetic neurons are topographically organized within the spinal cord, with upper thoracic segments innervating the head, lumbar segments innervating blood vessel in the legs, and intervening levels innervating the viscera.

Preganglionic neurons are spontaneously (tonically) active and normally generate a background of sympathetic nerve activity (tone), which imposes a corresponding background of vasoconstriction, cardiac contractility, and adrenal catecholamine secretion. This tonic activity is required to maintain resting (normal) levels of blood pressure and HR. Reductions of preganglionic neuronal discharge result in a fall in blood pressure, whereas excitation results in a rise in blood pressure. The tonic activity of spinal preganglionic neurons is itself generated normally by excitatory signals originating in higher centers. Interruption of such inputs after transsection of the cervical spinal cord results in a collapse of blood pressure (also called spinal shock).

Brainstem Control Mechanisms

The medulla oblongata is the central integrative area of the brain in controlling the circulation. Neurons localized to precisely defined regions (1) generate the tonic excitatory background transmitted to spinal preganglionic neurons and are responsible for maintaining normal resting levels of arterial pressure, (2) integrate most reflexes that regulate arterial pressure, (3) couple signals generated in higher brain areas during behavior with appropriate circulatory patterns, (4) sense metabolic and hormonal signals of importance in regulating arterial pressure to elicit specific circulatory responses, and (5) serve as the principal targets of drugs acting in brain to lower arterial pressure.

Rostral Ventrolateral Medullary Control Centers

The major source of tonic excitation of spinal preganglionic sympathetic neurons is a small pool of neurons lying within the rostral ventrolateral medulla, specifically the C1 area of the rostral ventrolateral reticular nucleus (RVL). The critical neurons appear to be a small population of adrenaline-synthesizing neurons of the C1 group and/or neurons in their immediate proximity, all of which directly (monosynaptically) innervate preganglionic neurons. Electrophysiologically, these reticulospinal neurons of the RVL are spontaneously active and discharge with a rhythm locked to the HR. The cardiac rhythmicity is imposed by their phasic inhibition by baroreceptor stimulation. Conversely, baroreceptor withdrawal excites them. RVL neurons excite preganglionic neurons and elevate blood pressure and HR. When they are inhibited or injured, their absence reduces background discharge of spinal preganglionic neurons, resulting in vasodilation and a fall of blood pressure, as well as slowing of the heart. Excitation of preganglionic neurons by RVL neurons is believed to be mediated by release of the excitatory amino acid neurotransmitter L-glutamate.

Vasomotor neurons of the RVL are very few in number, are highly collateralized, and have potent actions on preganglionic neurons. They are embedded in a rich network of neurons lying in a tract running between the nucleus tractus solitarii (NTS) and ventral medulla. The many neurons of this region express a wide range of neurotransmitters and modulators, and form the principal autonomic networks in brain.

Reflex Control Mechanisms

The medulla oblongata is critical for the integration of most reflexes controlling arterial pressure. Most reflex activity is in turn mediated by baroreflex regulation of the rate of discharge of RVL neurons.

Baroreceptor Reflexes

Baroreflexes are initiated in response to stimulation of two types of stretch-sensitive receptors: one in the carotid and aortic regions, which are innervated by branches of the IXth (glossopharyngeal) and Xth (vagus) cranial nerves, the other in the heart. Cardiac mechanoreceptor afferents travel in the Xth cranial nerves to the NTS. Baroreflex stimulation causes inhibition of sympathetic nerve activity, resulting in vasodilation, a fall of blood pressure, and a slowing of HR, the latter of which results from cardiovagal excitation and cardiosympathetic inhibition.

Baroreceptor afferents terminate on neurons within circumscribed regions of the NTS, along with all other visceral afferents. In this manner, the NTS is a homologue of the dorsal horn of the spinal cord. Baroreceptor information received in the NTS is relayed through the network of neurons between the NTS and the vasomotor and cardiomotor nuclei of ventral medulla, but primarily within a tonic vasodepressor region of the caudal ventrolateral medulla.

Neurons of the NTS tonically and phasically inhibit RVL neurons by the release of the inhibitory neurotransmitter GABA. This same pathway presumably also mediates sympathoinhibitory reflexes arising from other cardiac and pulmonary receptors. Stimulation of baroreceptors therefore acts to lower blood pressure by "dis-facilitating" (ie, by withdrawing excitatory) inputs from the RVL onto preganglionic neurons. Similarly, reduction or interruption of baroreceptor inputs elevates blood pressure by "dis-inhibiting" RVL neurons (ie, by withdrawing baroreceptor inhibition) and, in turn, increasing their excitation of preganglionic neurons.

Interruption of baroreceptor activity by denervation of the peripheral baroreceptor nerves or by lesions of the NTS leads to vasoconstriction and transient elevations of blood pressure by a chronic state of increased second-to-second variability of blood pressure (lability), which is also associated with exaggerated reactivity of blood pressure during behavioral stresses.

Chemoreceptor Reflexes

Stimulation of arterial chemoreceptors of the carotid and aortic bodies by hypoxia (or by some agents such as cyanide) excites sympathetic neurons and increases ventilation rate without appreciably altering HR. When ventilation is controlled (eg, in paralyzed subjects or during submersion), the response is modified, with the sympathetic excitation coupled to inspiratory apnea and bradycardia. This latter constellation represents an oxygen-conserving reflex (such as seen in the diving reflex in ducks, seals, and whales) that can be produced by facial immersion in humans.

The increase in sympathetic activity elicited by hypoxic stimulation of carotid chemoreceptors is also mediated by RVL neurons. However, whereas chemoreceptors terminate in the NTS, the pathway over which these metabolic signals reach the RVL is probably direct.

Somatosympathetic Reflexes: Pain and Exercise

The increases in blood pressure and HR stimulated by pain or exercising muscle can activate the sympathoadrenal system. These afferent impulses are transmitted over small myelinated and unmyelinated fibers in somatic sensory nerves. The pathway consists of an initial synapse onto neurons in the ipsilateral dorsal horn, a pathway ascending in the contralateral ventrolateral funiculus, and a termination on dorsal neurons in the contralateral RVL. Impairment of the RVL contralateral, but not ipsilateral, to the site of stimulation abolishes reflex cardiovascular responses to pain or exercise.

Sympathoadrenal excitation and tachycardia in the face of elevated blood pressure during exercise or in response to pain appears paradoxical, because elevated pressure should stimulate baroreceptors and reduce HR. In this setting, tachycardia reflects a profound inhibition of the baroreflex pathway within the central nervous system characteristic of certain patterns of cardiovascular integration during some behaviors. Such central baroreceptor inhibition may represent one mechanism through which central neural imbalances may lead to a hypertensive state.

Direct Excitation of RVL Neurons by Hypoxia or Distortion

Neurons in the RVL are also excited rapidly and reversibly by transient ischemia of the brain stem, by hypoxia, and by brainstem distortion. The response to ischemia is called the cerebral ischemic reflex, and the response to distortion is called the Cushing reflex. These stimuli elicit typical oxygen-conserving responses, including apnea, sympathoexcitation, hypertension, and bradycardia. Clinically, these responses may be triggered by intracranial hypertension resulting from many causes, including trauma, tumors, or vascular compression. They are a serious sign of brainstem dysfunction.

Elevations in blood pressure during the ischemic and Cushing responses are the result of direct excitation of RVL neurons or their axons by hypoxia. Hypercarbia, lactic acid, and H^+ are without effect when locally administered experimentally. Moreover, excitation by hypoxia seems to be specific, because adjacent respiratory neurons are silenced (leading to apnea) or unaffected. The rapid response of RVL neurons to hypoxia suggests that they, like glomus cells of the carotid body, may act as oxygen sensors. Their responses to hypoxia are not a consequence of pathological cellular disruption produced by prolonged oxygen deprivation or energy depletion.

Effects of Angiotensin II and other Circulatory Substances: Chemosensitive Zones

Neurons of the medulla are responsive to circulating agents (drugs and hormones) that may evoke patterned changes in autonomic activity. Many of these agents act at the area postrema, one of the circumventricular organs that does not have a blood-brain barrier. Notable is the role of the area postrema in the integration of autonomic actions associated with emesis. Neurons in the area postrema may also participate in the cardiovascular responses to circulating angiotensin II, which causes sympathoadrenal excitation. Sites along the ventral surface of the brainstem overlying the RVL are also sensitive to chemical stimulation and may represent zones in which agents in the cerebrospinal fluid may act to directly modify blood pressure.

The medulla also is the site of action of a class of drugs typified by clonidine and guanabenz. These drugs, which are centrally acting antihypertensive agents, appear to act by inhibiting the activity of RVL neurons.

Suprasegmental Control

Neuroanatomic and physiological studies have established that control of cardiovascular function in the brain occurs through a network of specific neuronal areas. These nuclei relate to each other by sharing projections from the major afferent nucleus of the cardiovascular system, the NTS, or by projecting neurons directly to the principal autonomic motor outputs such as the intermediolateral columns, the cardiovagal nuclei, the RVL, or its adjacent interneuronal tracks. Electrical or chemical stimulation of these areas elicits powerful actions on the circulation.

The network contains a series of nuclear groups represented at every level of the brain. The principal way stations are the parabrachial nuclei of the pons and adjacent periventricular zones; the periaqueductal gray matter of the midbrain; the lateral, anterior, and paraventricular nuclei of the hypothalamus; the amygdala (notably the central amygdaloid nucleus); and areas of the limbic cortex, including the cingulate, parahippocampal, insular, and orbitofrontal cortices. All of these regions are highly reciprocally interconnected, are closely connected to major neuroendocrine nuclei of the hypothalamus, and are richly innervated by major pathways relating to monoamine and peptide transmitters. In addition, the pathways are in close relationship to circumventricular zones of the forebrain and upper brain stem. The rich interconnection may be a neuroanatomic substrate supporting the often sustained activity of centrally generated sympathetic drive.

Cardiovascular-Behavioral Coupling

The supramedullary networks are closely allied with the elaboration and execution of a range of emotional and consummatory behaviors reflecting the very close linkage between cardiovascular performance and emotional behaviors.

Stimulation of all of these areas in experimental animals under anesthesia will initiate changes in HR, blood pressure, and other autonomic events. In unanesthetized animals, excitation of the same areas will often elicit behaviors to which are linked the appropriate patterned response of blood pressure. Unlike the medulla, these regions do not appear to contribute substantially to tonic blood pressure, nor are they required for integration of most reflexes, although they may modulate reflex reactivity. The suprasegmental regions are also closely linked to other circumventricular zones of the hypothalamus, which may act to process hormonal signals such as those generated by angiotensin II into appropriate behaviors such as drinking, and at the same time couple these with appropriate patterns of sympathetic activation.

SUGGESTED READING

1. Dampney RA. Functional organization of central pathways regulating the cardiovascular system. *Physiological Reviews.* 1994;74:323–364.
2. Golanov EV, Reis DJ. Contribution of oxygen-sensitive neurons of the rostral ventrolateral medulla to hypoxic cerebral vasodilatation in the rat. *J Physiol (Lond).* 1996;495:201–216.
3. Jeske I, Morrison SF, Cravo SL, Reis DJ. Identification of baroreceptor reflex interneurons in the caudal ventrolateral medulla. *Am J Physiol.* 1993;264: R169–R178.
4. Reis DJ, Golanov EV, Ruggiero DA, Sun M-K. Sympatho-excitatory neurons of the rostral medulla are oxygen sensors and essential elements in the tonic and reflex control of the systemic and cerebral circulations. *J Hypertens.* 1994;12(suppl): S159–S180.
5. Sun M-K, Reis DJ. Hypoxia selectively excites vasomotor neurons of rostral ventrolateral medulla in rats. *Am J Physiol.* 1994;266:R245–R256.
6. Sun M-K. Central neural organization and control of sympathetic nervous system in mammals. *Prog Neurobiol.* 1995;47:157–233.

Chapter 34

Arterial Baroreflexes

Mark W. Chapleau, PhD

KEY POINTS

- Arterial baroreceptors in the aortic arch and carotid sinus regions, which are activated by vascular distension, buffer acute fluctuations in blood pressure and reduce pressure lability and its adverse consequences.

- Vascular distensibility, which may be decreased by structural vascular changes in pathological states, is an important determinant of arterial baroreceptor sensitivity.

- Arterial baroreflex resetting during acute and chronic hypertension helps preserve buffering of pressure fluctuations at the prevailing higher pressure level.

- Endothelial dysfunction, oxidative stress, platelet activation, and angiotensin may each contribute, independently of pressure per se, to baroreflex dysfunction in hypertension.

See also Chapters 33, 35, 42, 43, 115, 135, 136

Arterial baroreceptors (ABRs) are sensory nerve endings located in carotid sinuses and the aortic arch that function as blood pressure sensors (**Figure 34.1**). Afferent baroreceptor (BR) activity is transmitted to the nucleus tractus solitarii in the medulla oblongata, where the signals are integrated and relayed through a network of central neurons that determine sympathetic and parasympathetic nerve activity to the heart and vasculature.

Cellular Events

ABRs, which do not respond directly to increased pressure, require acute vascular distension for their activation. The mechanism by which ABR deformation is transduced into electrical activity probably involves mechanosensitive ion channels present on the sensory nerve endings (**Figure 34.2**) that have been identified in numerous cell types, including cultured ABR neurons. Opening of these channels depolarizes ABRs, leading to generation of action potentials at the "spike initiating zone" near the peripheral endings (**Figure 34.2**).

Baroreflex Buffering of Arterial Pressure Fluctuations

The arterial baroreflex is the primary mechanism for rapid buffering of acute fluctuations in arterial pressure that occur during postural changes, behavioral stress, and changes in blood volume. Increases in pressure and ABR activity trigger reflex parasympathetic activation, sympathetic inhibition, and decreases in heart rate (HR) and vascular resistance that oppose the rise in pressure. Conversely, ABR activity decreases during a fall in pressure, producing reflex-mediated increases in HR and vascular resistance. Thus, the baroreflex provides moment-to-moment negative feedback regulation of arterial pressure that minimizes pressure lability. The extreme pressure lability observed in BR-denervated subjects underscores the importance of the baroreflex in buffering fluctuations in pressure.

Baroreflex-mediated changes in circulating hormones contribute to blood pressure regulation, although not as rapidly as efferent autonomic nerves. For example, vasopressin is also released during hypotension.

In addition to responding to changes in pressure, the baroreflex also tonically inhibits resting sympathetic nerve activity and release of vasopressin and renin and thus decreases arterial pressure. The tonic inhibitory influence of ABR activity is appreciated by observation of the profound autonomic changes and increase in blood pressure that occur after acute ABR denervation.

Baroreflexes and Sudden Death After Myocardial Infarction

Ventricular arrhythmias are a common cause of death after myocardial infarction. Parasympathetic and sympathetic nerve activity modulate the electrical properties of the heart. Recent animal and clinical studies have demonstrated that decreased baroreflex sensitivity predicts susceptibility to arrhythmias and sudden death after acute myocardial infarction. Thus, measurements of baroreflex sensitivity may provide a valuable method of screening patients. Furthermore, the results raise the interesting possibility that the baroreflex may protect the heart from arrhythmias by providing appropriate and rapid modulation of autonomic activity to the heart.

Baroreflex During Acute and Chronic Hypertension

During a sustained increase in arterial pressure, ABR activity declines or adapts if the elevated pressure is sustained. The mechanism of ABR adaptation involves mechanical viscoelastic relaxation and activation of 4-aminopyridine–sensitive K^+ channels. Upon return of pressure to lower levels after periods of acute hypertension (5 to 30 minutes), the ABR pressure threshold is increased and ABR activity is suppressed (**Figure 34.3**). The resulting rightward shift of the ABR pressure-activity curve, referred to as "rapid ABR resetting," is caused in part by activation of an electrogenic Na^+ pump, which hyperpolarizes the ABR nerve endings. Rapid resetting does not al-

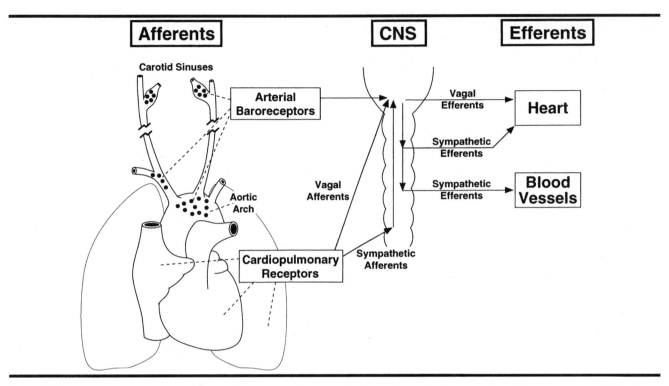

Figure 34.1.   Cardiopulmonary and arterial baroreflex neural pathways involved in cardiovascular homeostasis and blood pressure regulation. Locations of arterial baroreceptors are indicated by filled circles. For discussion of cardiopulmonary baroreflexes, see chapter A35. CNS indicates central nervous system.

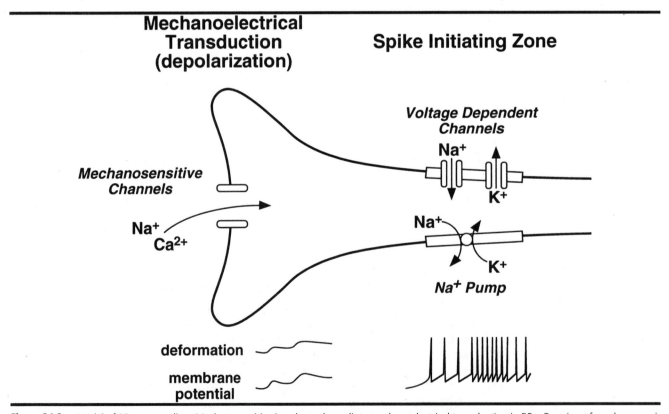

Figure 34.2.   Model of BR nerve ending. Mechanosensitive ion channels mediate mechanoelectrical transduction in BRs. Opening of mechanosensitive channels allows Na^+ and Ca^{2+} influx and depolarization of the endings. Sufficient depolarization opens voltage-dependent Na^+ and K^+ channels at the "spike initiating zone," triggering action potentials at frequencies related to the magnitude of depolarization. An electrogenic Na^+ pump maintains Na^+ and K^+ gradients and influences membrane potential.

ter the slope of the pressure-activity curve or attenuate maximum ABR activity **(Figure 34.3)**. ABR resetting results in a corresponding resetting of the arterial pressure–HR and pressure–sympathetic activity relations and allows effective buffering of pressure fluctuations to persist at the new prevailing pressure level **(Figure 34.3)**.

In chronic hypertension, the ABR is reset to higher pressures **(Figure 34.3)**. The resting level of ABR activity is relatively normal despite the high pressure, but the slope of the curve (ie, change in HR/change in pressure) may be decreased. Several mechanisms contribute to baroreflex resetting and decreased ABR sensitivity in hypertension, including reduced vascular distensibility of the carotid sinuses and aortic arch and altered central mediation of the reflex.

Importantly, the changes in baroreflex function in chronic hypertension can be at least partially reversed by treatment of the hypertension. Rapid baroreflex resetting occurs during decreases as well as increases in pressure and is preserved in treated chronic hypertension. Therefore, the baroreflex function curve may be shifted to lower

pressures soon after therapy is initiated, and this resetting facilitates further lowering of pressure. Reversal of structural vascular changes with longer periods of treatment contributes further to restoration of ABR sensitivity.

Baroreflex-mediated changes in sympathetic activity are decreased in normotensive subjects with a family history of hypertension, suggesting that genetic factors may also influence baroreflex sensitivity independently of blood pressure.

Neurohumoral and Paracrine Modulation of the Baroreflex

Neurohumoral and paracrine factors modulate the baroreflex and contribute to altered reflex control in disease states. For example, circulating angiotensin resets the baroreflex function curve to higher pressures independently of its effect on arterial pressure. In contrast, vasopressin resets the baroreflex curve to lower pressures. These actions are mediated in part through effects of circulating angiotensin

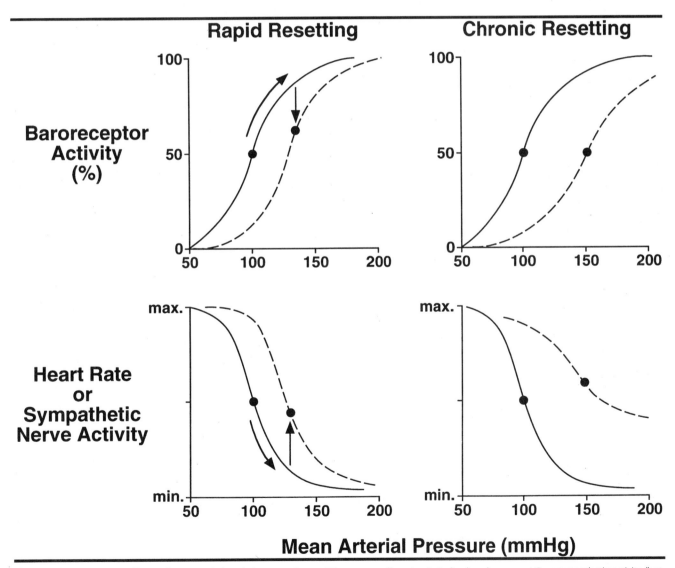

Figure 34.3. Shown are effects of acute and chronic hypertension on BR pressure–afferent activity (top) and pressure-HR or sympathetic activity (bottom) relations. Left, Initial responses to increased pressure are increased BR activity and reflex decreases in HR and sympathetic activity. Sustained acute hypertension results in BR adaptation, a return of HR and sympathetic activity toward control, and a shift in the BR function curves to the right. Right, In chronic hypertension, resting BR activity is relatively normal, function curves are shifted further to right, and slope and range of curves may be decreased.

and vasopressin on the area postrema, a circumventricular region that lacks a blood-brain barrier and has neurons that project to the vasomotor control centers.

Hypertension and heart failure are often associated with neuro-humoral activation, including increases in angiotensin and/or vasopressin. The magnitude and selectivity of the increases in these hormones, which may depend on the underlying cause of the disease, influence the net effect on the baroreflex. For example, renal hypertension associated with high levels of angiotensin is characterized by pronounced baroreflex resetting, decreased slope of the pressure-HR relation, reduced maximum range of HR modulation, and increased sympathetic nerve activity at rest. The altered baroreflex results not only from the elevated pressure but also from the central nervous system actions of angiotensin. In contrast, other types of hypertension may exhibit less baroreflex resetting and lower levels of sympathetic activity.

Paracrine factors produced near ABR endings may alter afferent ABR activity through effects on vascular tone and/or ABR membrane excitability. Factors that increase excitability include norepinephrine and prostacyclin. Factors that decrease excitability include reactive oxygen species, factor(s) released from activated platelets, and nitric oxide.

Baroreflex sensitivity may be favorably influenced by an increase in endogenous prostacyclin production or by use of antioxidants, antiplatelet agents, ACE inhibitors, or angiotensin receptor antagonists.

SUGGESTED READING

1. Chapleau MW, Abboud FM. Mechanisms of adaptation and resetting of the baroreceptor reflex. In: Hainsworth R, Mark AL, eds. *Cardiovascular Reflex Control in Health and Disease.* London, England: WB Saunders; 1993:165–193.

2. Chapleau MW, Cunningham JT, Sullivan MJ, Wachtel RE, Abboud FM. Structural versus functional modulation of the arterial baroreflex. *Hypertension.* 1995;26:341–347.

3. Hamill OP, McBride DW Jr. The cloning of a mechano-gated membrane ion channel. *Trends Neurosci.* 1994;17:439–443.

4. Korner PI. Cardiac baroreflex in hypertension: role of the heart and angiotensin II. *Clin Exp Hypertens.* 1995;17:425–439.

5. Kunze DL, Andresen MC. Arterial baroreceptors: excitation and modulation. In: Zucker IH, Gilmore JP, eds. *Reflex Control of the Circulation.* Boca Raton, Fla: CRC Press; 1991:139–164.

6. Mancia G, Mark AL. Arterial baroreflexes in humans. In: *Handbook of Physiology.* Section 2, vol III, part 2. Bethesda, Md: American Physiological Society; 1983:755–793.

7. Persson PB, Kirchheim HR. *Baroreceptor Reflexes: Integrative Functions and Clinical Aspects.* Berlin, Germany: Springer-Verlag; 1991.

8. Schwartz PJ, LaRovere MT, Vanoli E. Autonomic nervous system and sudden cardiac death: experimental basis and clinical observations for post–myocardial infarction risk stratification. *Circulation.* 1992;85(suppl I):I-77-I-91.

Chapter 35

Cardiopulmonary Baroreflexes

Pramod K. Mohanty, MD

KEY POINTS

- Cardiopulmonary mechanoreceptors, via vagal afferents, tonically inhibit vasomotor centers, strongly influencing sympathetic nervous system, renin-angiotensin system, and arginine vasopressin activity.

- Cardiopulmonary baroreceptors (CPBRs) are intimately involved in volume homeostasis: decreased preload or cardiac stretch deactivates CPBRs, resulting in augmentation of sympathetic activity and vasoconstriction; increased cardiac volume or pressure has the opposite effect.

- CPBR signals modify inputs from arterial baroreceptors in regulating sympathetic output.

- CPBR signals are blunted by left ventricular hypertrophy, thereby contributing to the "volume-vasoconstrictor imbalance" in hypertension.

See also Chapters 33, 34, 42, 43, 115, 135, 136

Cardiopulmonary Baroreceptors

Influences of cardiopulmonary baroreflexes (CPBRs), which are intimately involved with volume homeostasis, are initiated by a group of mechanoreceptors located in the cardiac atria, venoatrial junction, ventricular myocardium, and lungs (see Figure 1 of chapter 34). In normal animals and humans, ventricular and atrial sensory endings play the dominant role in the mediation of cardiopulmonary reflexes. In heart transplant patients, the absence of ventricular innervation causes an attenuated response of sympathetic activity and forearm vasoconstriction when central blood volume is decreased by lower-body negative pressure (LBNP). This finding emphasizes the importance of ventricular mechanoreceptors in systemic neurocirculatory control.

Cardiopulmonary Baroreflex Physiology

Cardiopulmonary baroreflexes constitute one of the two major neural reflex pathways that modulate blood pressure (see Figure 1 of chapter 34). These low-pressure baroreceptors are located predominantly in ventricles but also occur in atria and the venoatrial junction. They fire during systole, and the frequency of firing is directly related to myocardial contraction and cardiac filling pressure ("preload"). Ventricular receptors and their vagal afferents generally function in an inhibitory capacity on the arterial baroreceptors.

The effects of direct stimulation of ventricular mechanoreceptors is inhibitory to cardiac and peripheral sympathetic outflow but excitatory to cardiac vagal outflow. In addition, ventricular mechanoreceptors can inhibit the secretion of angiotensin II, catecholamines, and vasopressin during conditions in which the levels of these hormones are increased. In contrast, arterial or "high-pressure" baroreceptors discharge in response to stretch induced by arterial pressure waves, and their firing rate is directly related to the level of arterial blood pressure.

Feedback from afferent signals from arterial baroreceptors and CPBRs converges on the nucleus tractus solitarii in the brain stem, and their signals are processed there (Figure 1 of chapter 34). Excitation of either of these receptors causes (1) augmentation of efferent parasympathetic outflow, resulting in a decrease in heart rate and atrioventricular conduction, and (2) inhibition of efferent sympathetic outflow to heart and blood vessels, resulting in decreased vascular resistance. Bradycardia and hypotension in the clinical syndrome of vasovagal syncope may occur by this mechanism. In contrast, during reductions in arterial and cardiac filling pressures, the discharge of these receptors decreases, and efferent neural sympathetic outflow increases, with resultant augmentation of vascular resistance. In parallel, efferent parasympathetic outflow decreases, resulting in increased heart rate and enhanced atrioventricular conduction.

Influence of Cardiopulmonary Receptors on Blood Volume

Cardiopulmonary receptors act as "low-pressure" sensors in the afferent limb of the volume homeostasis reflex. The cardiopulmonary volume receptors are sensitive to small changes in cardiac stretch and affect sympathetic discharge during low-grade physiological changes not detected by arterial baroreceptors. Small increases (or decreases) in cardiac filling pressure and volume result in directionally opposite neurohormonal responses (ie, decreased renin-angiotensin system and sympathetic nervous system activity) to preserve volume homeostasis and arterial blood pressure. Studies in humans in which low-level LBNP was used to decrease central blood volume have demonstrated activation of both renin and sympathetic systems despite minimal changes in blood pressure. Investigations of the steady-state vasomotor and humoral responses to prolonged LBNP in normal humans indicate that there is early activation of sympathetic activity (3 to 10 minutes) followed by delayed activation of the renin-angiotensin system (>20 minutes), implying a contribution of angiotensin II to the sustained vasoconstriction. The observation that renin release can be abolished by β-adrenergic receptor blockade with propranolol (without alteration in renal hemodynamics) demonstrates the major influence of renal sympathetic nerves on the renin secretory process. These data, along with other related observations, suggest that low-pressure cardiopulmonary receptors tonically inhibit vasomotor centers and strongly influence sympathetic nerve activity and renin release, thereby controlling volume homeostasis by both neurohumoral and renal functional mechanisms.

Relationship to Atriopeptin Release

Atrial natriuretic peptide (ANP), another cardioregulatory hormone, has also been shown to influence the reflex control of the cardiovascular system. Cardiac stretch–mediated atriopeptin release patterns are the inverse of sympathetic activation. During volume expansion, cardiac ANP release is inhibited, whereas central blood volume reduction inhibits ANP release. ANP has a profound effect on sodium and volume homeostasis and also interferes with the reflexes originating from cardiopulmonary receptors in the control of vasomotor tone. The influence of ANP on the baroreflex control of circulation is probably important in conditions characterized by volume overload (ie, congestive heart failure), and ANP may contribute to impaired baroreflex function.

Human Hypertension

There is augmented cardiopulmonary baroreflex gain in early hypertension, but with progression of hypertension and onset of left ventricular hypertrophy, cardiopulmonary baroreflexes are blunted. Animal and human studies support a significant contribution of reflex neurohumoral activation as a cause of the increased peripheral vascular resistance characteristic of human essential hypertension. In this setting, the restrictive influence of ventricular hypertrophy and fibrosis markedly diminishes the ability of CPBRs to suppress sympathetic vasoconstriction during volume overload.

The neurogenic hypothesis of the control of peripheral vascular resistance predicts that excessive sympathetically mediated venoconstriction results in centralization of blood volume, increased cardiac preload, and inappropriately high cardiac output at any given level of vascular resistance. Thus, a mismatch of flow (cardiac output) and vasomotor tone (peripheral resistance) can be viewed as an ongoing dynamic mechanism underlying human hypertension. The time course from borderline to established hypertension suggests that cardiac output returns to normal as long-term structural changes in peripheral arterioles develop, resulting in augmented resistance and decrease in arterial compliance. This peripheral vascular remodeling is associated with β-receptor downregulation of angiotensin and AT_1 receptor expression, allowing α-adrenergic and AT_1receptor–mediated vasoconstriction to be maintained.

SUGGESTED READING

1. Bishop V, Haser EM. Arterial and cardiopulmonary reflexes in the regulation of neurohumoral drive to the circulation. *Fed Proc.* 1985;44:2377–2385.
2. Mancia G, Shepherd JT, Donald DE. Role of cardiac, pulmonary and carotid mechanoreceptor in the control of hind limb and renal circulation in dogs. *Circ Res.* 1975;37:200–208.
3. Mark AL. The Bezold-Jarisch reflex revisited: clinical implications of inhibition reflexes originating in the heart. *J Am Coll Cardiol.* 1983;1:90–102.
4. Mohanty PK, Sowers JR, McNamara C, Thames MD. Reflex effects of prolonged cardiopulmonary baroreceptor unloading in humans. *Am J Physiol.* 1988;23: R320–R324.
5. Rea RF, Hadman M. Baroreflex control of muscle sympathetic nerve activity in borderline hypertension. *Circulation.* 1990;82:856–862.
6. Mohanty PK, Thames MD, Arrowood J, Sowers JR, McNamara C, Szentpetry S. Impairment of cardiopulmonary baroreflex following cardiac transplantation in humans. *Circulation.* 1987;75:914–921.
7. Egan BM, Julius S, Cottier C, Osterziel KJ, Ihsen H. Role of cardiovascular receptors on the neural regulation of renin release in normal man. *Hypertension.* 1983;5: 779–786.
8. DiBona GF. Neural control of the kidney in hypertension. *Hypertension.* 1992; 19(suppl I):I-28-I-35.
9. Wang SY, Manyari DE, Tyberg JV. Cardiac vagal reflex modulates intestinal vascular capacitance and ventricular preload in anesthetized dogs with acute myocardial infarction. *Circulation.* 1996;94:529–533.
10. Massimo V. Atrial natriuretic peptide and baroreflex control of circulation. *Am J Hypertens.* 1992;5:488–493.

Chapter 36

Renal Nerves and Extracellular Fluid Volume Regulation

Jeffrey L. Osborn, PhD; Suzanne G. Greenberg, PhD

KEY POINTS

- Renal nerves modulate urinary sodium chloride excretion by directly altering renin release and tubular sodium reabsorption.

- Cardiac extracellular fluid volume receptors modulate renal sympathetic nerve activity by sympathoexcitation and inhibition via central neural structures.

- Acute and rapid adjustments in sodium excretion during step changes in extracellular fluid volume are mediated by inverse changes in renal sympathetic outflow.

- Renal sympathetic nerve activity accounts for ≈35% of the short-term adjustment in sodium excretion after step changes in sodium intake.

See also Chapters 35, 45

In addition to the regulation of renal blood flow, renal nerves play a critical role in the regulation of renal tubular function, including stimulation of sodium transport in the proximal convoluted tubules and medullary thick ascending limbs. The cellular mechanism(s) responsible for neural regulation of sodium excretion include α-adrenergic stimulation of sodium-hydrogen (Na^+-H^+) exchange (with accompanying bicarbonate reabsorption) in the proximal convoluted tubule, activation of sodium potassium adenosine triphosphatase (Na^+-K^+ ATPase) (proximal convoluted tubules), and stimulation of the sodium, potassium-2 chloride ($2\ Cl^- > Na^+$-K) cotransporter of the thick ascending limb. In addition to direct effects of renal nerves on tubular transport, neurogenic sodium balance may be critically influenced by activation of the renin-angiotensin-aldosterone axis via direct neural stimulation of renin release (β_1-adrenergic stimulation) and indirectly by α_1-adrenergic stimulation of tubular sodium reabsorption, which also promotes renin release. These critical effects of renal neuroadrenergic stimulation on kidney function have led to the notion that elevation of renal sympathetic nerve activity vitally influences the regulation of sodium balance and extracellular fluid volume (ECFV).

Afferent Mechanisms Controlling Renal Sympathetic Nerve Activity

Neurogenic influences on the control of ECFV involve both sodium intake and urinary sodium excretion. Behavioral factors and hypothalamic control of sodium intake are critical to the overall level of ingested sodium and consequently ECFV. Changes in ECFV, however, are controlled predominantly via urinary sodium excretion **(Figure 36.1)**.

Basal efferent renal nerve activity is mediated predominantly by high-pressure aortocarotid baroreflexes and exhibit a bursting sympathetic pattern coincident with the cardiac cycle. Thus, renal nerve activity is low or silent during systole, with peaks during diastole. Changes in efferent renal sympathetic tone occur inversely in response to both low-pressure baroreflex afferent input (cardiopulmonary stretch receptors) and high-pressure baroreflex mechanisms of the carotid sinus and aortic arch. Recent experiments have also confirmed significant input from numerous somatosensory afferent inputs as well as potential sodium receptors located in the hepatic and portal regions of the systemic circulation. These efferent renal sympathetic responses are closely and inversely associated with increases and decreases in cardiac filling pressure after dietary changes in sodium intake, suggesting that low-pressure cardiac vagal afferent nerve fibers leading to the central nervous system are significant in the "sensing" of ECFV status and total body sodium content. The summation of these afferent inputs by the vasomotor control centers of the medulla oblongata allows specific and selective control of urinary sodium excretion via control of renal sympathetic outflow.

Efferent Renal Sympathetic Nerve Activity and Control of Sodium Balance

The renal efferent responses to increased or decreased sodium intake are associated with inverse changes in urinary sodium excretion. After a decrease in sodium intake in dogs, renal efferent nerve activity increases within 8 hours, and this neurogenic activation is associated with a simultaneous decrease in urinary sodium excretion **(Figure 36.2)**. The renal neurogenic response to a step decrease in sodium intake becomes maximal within 10 hours, approximately the same time period in which the antinatriuretic response is also maximal. These rapid changes in urinary sodium excretion are abolished by bilateral renal denervation. In the absence of renal nerve traffic, regulation of urinary sodium excretion is mediated solely by long-term controllers of ECFV, including humoral factors,

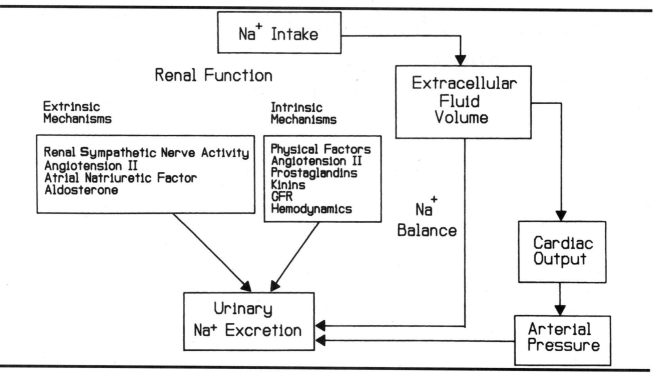

Figure 36.1.   Major factors modulating urinary sodium excretion as a function of regulation of extracellular fluid volume. GFR indicates glomerular filtration rate.

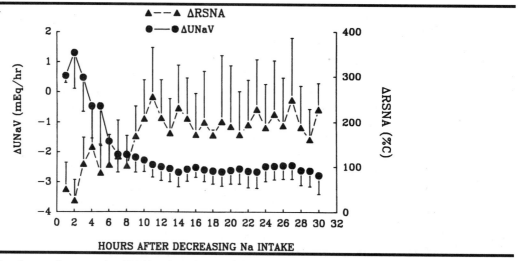

HOURS AFTER DECREASING Na INTAKE

Figure 36.2.   Hourly changes in urinary sodium excretion (UNaV) and renal sympathetic nerve activity (RSNA) during the first 30 hours after a step decrease in Na intake. Changes in RSNA are depicted by triangles and those in UNaV by circles.

renal blood flow, glomerular filtration rate, and physical forces (ie, oncotic pressure) present in the plasma.

In similar studies using step increases in sodium intake, the contributions of neural and nonneural factors to sodium balance and regulation of ECFV have been partially quantified by comparison of sodium balance in conscious animals with that in innervated and denervated kidneys during the first 72 hours after a step increase in sodium intake. In the absence of renal nerves, the rate of achieving sodium balance is significantly delayed **(Figure 36.3)**. The neural

component of the summed controllers of sodium balance (and consequently ECFV) has been estimated at ≈35% of the total sodium intake.

Although the central-neural regulation of ECFV is critical to the overall rate of achieving sodium balance, numerous other intrinsic and extrinsic renal factors mediate changes in urinary sodium excretion and contribute substantially to the overall sodium balance. These other controllers provide important redundancy to the volume-regulatory system **(Figure 36.1)**. Thus, renal efferent nerve traffic is critical primarily to the control of the rate at which sodium

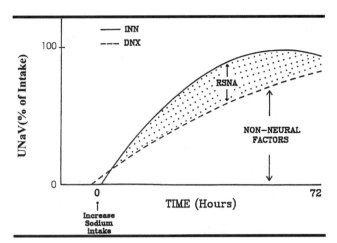

Figure 36.3. Hourly changes in urinary sodium excretion (UNaV) in rats with innervated (INN) and denervated (DNX) kidneys for 72 consecutive hours after a step increase in sodium intake. Stippled area represents sodium excretion response that can be attributed to inhibition of renal sympathetic outflow.

balance is achieved during increases and decreases in sodium intake, whereas other regulators of sodium excretion maintain appropriate long-term sodium excretion.

Pathophysiological Conditions of Altered Neural Control of ECFV

There are several pathophysiological conditions in which altered control of renal efferent sympathetic nerve activity con-tributes significantly to an imbalance in the regulation of sodium excretion and consequently leads to excess fluid and water retention. These diseases, which represent major edema-forming states, include congestive heart failure, cardiac tamponade, nephrotic syndrome, and cirrhosis of the liver. In each of these conditions, one or a combination of the regulators of urinary sodium excretion identified in Figure 1 may contribute to the overall ECFV status. Activation of renal sympathetic outflow is of crucial importance in promoting sodium and water retention, edema formation, and further pathogenesis of these edema-forming conditions. Activation of renal sympathetic outflow functions occurs as a consequence of afferent sensory signals that are responding to overall cardiovascular dysfunction, and this activation may prevent complete cardiovascular collapse. Thus, even in those conditions in which overall cardiovascular function is declining, activation of renal sympathetic nerve activity may importantly circumvent more rapid dysfunction and loss of blood pressure and/or cardiac output (ie, cardiovascular collapse).

SUGGESTED READING

1. Awazu M, Ichikawa I. Alterations in renal function in experimental congestive heart failure. *Semin Nephrol.* 1994;14:401–411.
2. Greenberg SG, Tershner S, Osborn JL. Neurogenic regulation of rate of achieving sodium balance after increasing sodium intake. *Am J Physiol.* 1991;261: F300–F307.
3. Kopp UC, DiBona GF. The neural control of renal function. In: Seldin DW, Giebisch G, eds. *The Kidney: Physiology and Pathophysiology.* 2nd ed. New York, NY: Raven Press Ltd; 1992:1157–1204.
4. Osborn JL. Relation between sodium intake, renal function, and the regulation of arterial pressure. *Hypertension.* 1991;17(suppl I):I-91–I-96.

Chapter 37

Systemic Hemodynamics and Regional Blood Flow Regulation

Thomas G. Coleman, PhD; John E. Hall, PhD

KEY POINTS

- Regional blood flows are precisely and powerfully regulated to satisfy the metabolic needs of the tissues; these needs can be relatively constant (eg, brain) or highly variable (eg, skeletal muscle). In other instances, regulation satisfies a special homeostatic need (eg, skin blood flow and temperature regulation).

- Regional blood flow regulation is, for the most part, normal in essential hypertension, with most organs showing a normal flow and an elevated vascular resistance that is proportional to the increase in arterial pressure.

- Exercise-induced vasodilation is impaired in essential hypertension.

- The kidney often shows decreased blood flow in long-standing hypertension; this could be a sign of a renal defect that is contributing to the hypertension.

See also Chapters 44, 45

The whole-body hemodynamic pattern seen most often in essential hypertension, at least in supine humans, is one of increased total peripheral resistance and normal cardiac output. This flow and resistance pattern is determined by regional blood flow regulation, because cardiac output is equal to the mathematical sum of all regional blood flows, and total peripheral resistance is equal to the parallel sum of all regional vascular resistances **(Figure 37.1)**.

Principles of Blood Flow Regulation

The metabolic state of a tissue is maintained by a stable relationship between metabolism and blood flow **(Figure 37.2)**.

The following discussion travels counterclockwise around Figure 37.2, beginning at top center. Blood flow through a tissue is equal to the pressure gradient across the tissue divided by the vascular resistance of the tissue. The pressure gradient is arterial pressure minus venous pressure; because this latter pressure is relatively small, it is often omitted. Thus,

(1) blood flow = arterial pressure/vascular resistance.

According to the theory of Poiseuille, vascular resistance is proportional to the viscosity of the blood and the length of the vessels, whereas resistance is inversely proportional to the radius of the vessels raised to the 4th power. Under normal conditions, the radius is the most important of these three factors.

(2) Resistance $\propto$ (viscositylength)/radius^4.

The radius of small, high-resistance blood vessels is determined by the tension generated by the smooth muscle in the vessel wall. Tension is influenced by local metabolic factors that are determined by the balance between metabolic need and nutrient transport. Nutrient transport is a function of blood flow, completing the circular and stable relationship. In addition to local metabolic factors, smooth muscle tension can be modified by overriding neural and humoral factors. This is particularly important in the control of skin blood flow and in preserving blood flow to vital organs in cardiovascular crises, such as severe hemorrhage.

Normal Regional Blood Flow Regulation

Regional blood flow is highly varied and in some cases highly variable. Many tissues have a blood flow of 3 to 5 mL·min^{-1}·100 g^{-1}, a value that just meets basal metabolic demands. The brain and heart have flows of 50 to 100 mL·min^{-1}·100 g^{-1} because of their relatively high rates of metabolism. The kidney has a blood flow of 350 mL·min^{-1}·100 g^{-1}, a value that greatly exceeds its metabolic needs.

Cerebral blood flow is relatively constant because of autoregulation, yet it is very sensitive to CO_2 tension in the brain. CO_2 tension, in turn, is a function of blood flow, with increased flow washing out excess cerebral CO_2. This interrelationship provides a stable environment for cerebral neural function. The stimulatory effect of cerebral CO_2 on ventilation and the ability of ventilation to remove excess CO_2 provides an additional stabilizing factor for the cerebral environment as well as for all of the body's other tissues.

Myocardial blood flow is proportional to myocardial oxygen use, which, in turn, is proportional to myocardial workload. Under normal conditions, the heart extracts ≈50% of the oxygen delivered to it; this percentage is close to the practical maximum and is about twice the whole-body oxygen extraction. Thus, it is not the increases in extraction but rather increases in coronary blood flow that satisfy myocardial oxygen demands during increased myocardial workload.

Skeletal muscle blood flow is proportional to skeletal muscle workload and generally to cardiac output, ranging from a low of 4 mL·min^{-1}·100 g^{-1} at rest to nearly 100 mL·min^{-1}·100 g^{-1} during strenuous exercise. Because a trained athlete's body typically

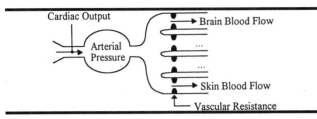

Figure 37.1. Flow and resistance patterns.

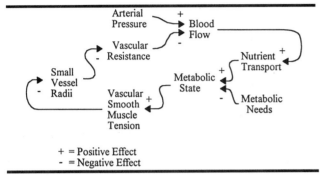

+ = Positive Effect
- = Negative Effect

Figure 37.2. Interrelationships between pressure, resistance, blood flow, and metabolic state.

contains >20 kg of skeletal muscle, total muscle blood flow can approach 20 L/min in these individuals during strenuous exercise.

Skin blood flow regulates heat loss from the body by metering the flow of heat from the core to the surface of the body, where heat is lost to the environment. Skin blood flow is controlled by the central nervous system via sympathetic nerves. Normal skin blood flow is ≈250 mL·min^{-1}·m^{-2} of surface area, but marked increases and decreases from that value occur as needed. Even with severe vasoconstriction, skin blood flow is great enough to meet the basic metabolic demands of the skin.

Renal blood flow is relatively constant and very large, averaging ≈20% of cardiac output. On a unit weight basis, the kidney has twice the oxygen consumption of the brain but 7 times the blood flow **(Table 37.1)**. A high renal blood flow makes possible a high rate of glomerular filtration. The kidney generally filters 125 mL/min from a renal plasma flow of 660 mL/min. The total plasma volume is processed (ie, filtered and reabsorbed) more than 60 times each day.

Control of Natriuresis

Renal sodium excretion rises or falls in a very precise way to match dietary sodium intake; the half-time of the response is <2 days. Renal blood flow, in partnership with the renin-angiotensin system, helps to implement control of sodium excretion while keeping glomerular filtration relatively steady. When dietary sodium intake is decreased, renal blood flow decreases; this is associated with decreased sodium filtration and excretion and increased sodium reabsorption, renin secretion, angiotensin formation, and renal vascular resistance **(Figure 37.3)**.

As mentioned above, the very high and relatively fixed kidney blood flow supports the basic functions of the kidney: filtering unwanted metabolites and controlling sodium balance. High, fixed flow may also be related in some way to erythropoiesis, by which the kidney is able to detect with great precision not only hypoxemia but also anemia.

Importance of Arterial Pressure in Regional Blood Flow Regulation

Regional blood flow regulation requires an adequate arterial pressure, as illustrated by the response to physical exercise in patients with autonomic dysfunction. As the normal person begins to exercise, skeletal muscle resistance decreases markedly, while skeletal muscle blood flow and cardiac output increase markedly and arterial pressure remains relatively constant. As persons with autonomic dysfunction begin to exercise, skeletal muscle resistance decreases markedly, but skeletal muscle blood flow and cardiac output increase only modestly. Consequently, arterial pressure plummets, exercise is not well tolerated, and syncope is likely.

Arterial pressure is determined by the balance between the filling effect of cardiac output and the draining effect of regional blood flow **(Figure 37.1)**. Tissue dilation drains additional blood from the arterial tree. If arterial pressure is to be held constant, this blood must be replaced by an increase in cardiac output. Several mechanisms make important contributions. The vasodilation itself increases venous return and, therefore, cardiac output. Repetitive contractions of skeletal muscle pump blood back to the heart. Venous valves prevent backflow. The autonomic nervous system increases venous pressure, heart rate, and myocardial contractility. These factors combine to provide the cardiac output and arterial pressure needed for proper regional flow regulation.

When cardiac outflow is inadequate, as in heart failure or hypovolemia, neural and humoral factors produce a vasoconstriction that overrides normal flow control in many organs. This keeps arterial pressure from falling too low; adequate blood flow is maintained in the vital organs, especially the brain and heart.

Essential Hypertension

The hemodynamic pattern seen most often in essential hypertension is normal blood flow with elevated vascular resistance. This pattern suggests that regulation of regional blood flow is generally not impaired. Oxygen consumption is normal.

Cerebral blood flow shows a normal value of ≈ 50 mL·min^{-1}·100 g tissue^{-1} in essential hypertension **(Table 37.2)**.

Table 37.1. Kidney Versus Brain Blood Flow and Oxygen Use

	ORGAN WEIGHT, g	OXYGEN USE, mL/min	BLOOD FLOW, mL/min
Kidney	300	22	1200
Brain	1400	50	720

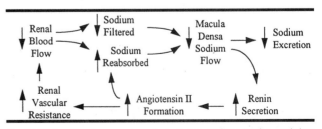

Figure 37.3. Events occurring when dietary sodium intake, and thus renal blood flow, is decreased.

Table 37.2. Cerebral Hemodynamics in Essential Hypertension

	MEAN ARTERIAL PRESSURE, mm Hg	CEREBRAL BLOOD FLOW, mL·min^{-1}·100 g^{-1}	VASCULAR RESISTANCE, mm Hg·mL^{-1}·min^{-1}·100 g^{-1}
Normal subjects	86	54	1.6
Essential hypertension	159	54	3.0

Coronary blood flow is elevated in essential hypertension in proportion to the prevailing amount of myocardial hypertrophy. Blood flow per unit weight of heart muscle is normal, with a value of ≈80 mL·min^{-1}·100 g^{-1}.

Splanchnic blood flow is slightly reduced in essential hypertension, having a typical value of 750 mL·min^{-1}m^{-2} of surface area compared with 800 mL·min^{-1}·m^{-2} in normotensive subjects. Skin blood flow is normal.

Control of *skeletal muscle blood flow* is for the most part normal in essential hypertension, but several peculiarities have been identified. The ability of skeletal muscle to dilate is less than normal in essential hypertension, as characterized by the minimum attainable vascular resistance. This impairment is probably due to structural limitations imposed by vessel wall hypertrophy. In addition, skeletal muscle blood flow per gram of tissue at rest is somewhat elevated.

The *hemodynamic response to exercise* is altered. The maximum level of exercise, quantified by oxygen uptake, is depressed in proportion to the severity of hypertension. Arterial pressure is high before exercise and goes even higher during exercise. In the presence of the dilation defect noted above, elevated blood pressure boosts blood flow through the skeletal muscle (**see Equation 1**), but it also creates an increased, detrimental cardiac afterload that limits both cardiac output and exercise performance. At each level of exercise below maximum, cardiac output and skeletal muscle blood flow are identical to flows seen in normotensive subjects. These flows are achieved at a higher vascular resistance (**Figure 37.4**) and higher arterial pressure; the resistance and pressure influences cancel each other (**Equation 1**) to yield a normal flow.

Renal blood flow has been observed to be increased, normal, or decreased in essential hypertension. These flow data must be interpreted with regard to the special functional needs of the kidney. For instance, dietary protein, dietary sodium, and weight gain all require increases in renal blood flow, whereas nephron damage and nephron loss lead to decreases. The common observations that renal blood flow tends to be normal or increased early in hypertension, particularly in obese subjects, whereas flow is generally reduced in longer-standing hypertension and nonobese subjects, parallel data obtained for cardiac output in these different conditions.

Although there is no proof, inadequate renal blood flow may be related to the etiology of essential hypertension in several ways.

Renovascular Hypertension

In experimental renal artery stenosis, increased renal preglomerular resistance produces a predictable rise in arterial pressure that is proportional to the severity of the constriction. The immediate response to preglomerular vasoconstriction is a decrease in renal blood flow (**Equation 1**). A secondary increase in arterial pressure then follows, which is a combination of increased renin secretion and renal sodium retention, with hyperreninemia having an important

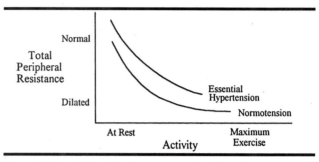

Figure 37.4. Relationship between total peripheral resistance and physical activity in normotensive and hypertensive individuals.

early role and sodium retention having an important chronic role. The eventual hemodynamic picture is elevated total peripheral resistance, normal cardiac output and plasma renin activity, and decreased renal blood flow.

Although many factors have been postulated to be the cause of essential hypertension, the similarities between the hemodynamics of essential hypertension and experimental renovascular hypertension indirectly support the idea that renal blood flow control is abnormal in both. The abnormality may raise preglomerular resistance, decrease renal blood flow, and, in fact, be a cause of the hypertension.

ACKNOWLEDGMENT

This study was supported in part by National Institutes of Health grant HL-51971.

SUGGESTED READING

1. Amery A, Julius S, Whitlock LS, Conway J. Influence of hypertension on the hemodynamic response to exercise. Circulation. 1967;36:231–237.
2. Bevegård S, Jonsson B, Karlöf I. Circulatory responses to recumbent exercise and head-up tilting in patients with disturbed sympathetic cardiovascular control (postural hypotension). Acta Med Scand. 1962;172:623–636.
3. Coleman TG, Guyton AC, Young DB, DeClue JW, Norman RA, Manning RD Jr. The role of the kidney in essential hypertension. Clin Exp Pharmacol Physiol. 1975;2:571–581.
4. Goldblatt H, Lynch J, Hanzal RF, Summerville WW. Studies on experimental hypertension, I: the production of persistent elevation of systolic blood pressure by means of renal ischemia. J Exp Med. 1934;59:347–379.
5. Hollenberg NK, Merrill JP. Intrarenal perfusion in the young "essential" hypertensive: a subpopulation resistant to sodium restriction. Trans Assoc Am Physicians. 1970;83:93–101.
6. Kety SS, Hafkenschiel JH, Jeffers WA, Leopold IH, Shenkin HA. The blood flow, vascular resistance, and oxygen consumption of the brain in essential hypertension. J Clin Invest. 1948;27:511–514.
7. Ljungman S, Aurell M, Hartford M, Wikstrand J, Wilhelmsen L, Berglund G. Blood pressure and renal function. Acta Med Scand. 1980;208:17–25.
8. Rowe GG, Castillo CA, Maxwell GM, Crumpton CW. A hemodynamic study of hypertension including observations on coronary blood flow. Ann Intern Med. 1961;54:405–412.
9. Wilkins RW, Culbertson JW, Rymut AA. The hepatic blood flow in resting hypertensive patients before and after splanchnicectomy. J Clin Invest. 1952;31:529–531.

Chapter 38

Autoregulation of Blood Flow

Richard J. Roman, PhD

KEY POINTS

- Blood flow, especially in the renal and cerebral circulations, remains relatively constant despite fluctuations in arterial pressure; this phenomenon is known as autoregulation.

- Two major mechanisms contribute to autoregulation: myogenic activation of vascular smooth muscle cells in arteries and metabolic release of mediators from the vascular endothelium and surrounding tissues.

- Shear stress also modulates vascular tone and autoregulation by stimulating the release of nitric oxide, prostacyclin, epoxyeicosatrienoic acids and other endothelium-derived relaxing factors from the vascular endothelium.

- Vascular resistances are elevated in hypertension and the range of blood flow autoregulation is shifted toward higher pressures.

See also Chapter 71

Blood flow in most vascular beds is highly regulated and remains relatively constant despite fluctuations in arterial pressure from 70 to 130 mm Hg. This is especially true in the renal and cerebral circulations. This phenomenon is known as autoregulation, and the range of constant perfusion is referred to as the autoregulation plateau (**Figure 38.1**).

Mechanisms of Autoregulation of Blood Flow

Two major mechanisms are responsible for the autoregulation of blood flow. The first is myogenic activation of precapillary arterioles. Elevations in transmural pressure induce contraction of these arterioles. This myogenic response is associated with depolarization of vascular smooth muscle and a rise in intracellular calcium that is dependent on calcium influx through voltage-sensitive calcium channels. Recent studies have suggested that activation of stretch-activated cation channels, protein kinase C, and vasoconstrictor P450 metabolites of arachidonic acid may all participate in this response.

The second mechanism involves the metabolic regulation of blood flow. When perfusion pressure and blood flow are reduced in a vascular bed, the tissue becomes hypoxic and triggers the release of vasodilator mediators such as nitric oxide, prostacyclin, prostaglandins, epoxyeicosatrienoic acids and adenosine from the vascular endothelium and surrounding parenchymal tissues. Changes in intracellular pH and Po_2 also exert direct effects on ion channels in vascular smooth muscle cells that act to diminish tone. Conversely, increases in blood flow diminish the accumulation of vasodilator mediators and promote vasoconstriction. In addition, there is recent evidence that the production of vasoconstrictor P450 metabolites of arachidonic acid in vascular smooth muscle cells is stimulated by elevations in tissue Po_2 and that they also contribute to the vasoconstrictor response to elevations in tissue oxygen delivery.

Renal Circulation

Autoregulatory mechanisms are especially well developed in the kidney to allow for the maintenance of constant glomerular capillary pressure, glomerular filtration rate, and a uniform rate of clearance of metabolic wastes despite physiological variation in arterial pressure. Two major mechanisms are responsible for the autoregulation of blood flow in the kidney. The first is the myogenic activation of preglomerular arterioles. Elevations in transmural pressure induce contraction of preglomerular arteries, predominantly at the level of afferent arterioles (vessel diameters of 20 μm).

The other mechanism, tubuloglomerular feedback, acts in concert with the myogenic response. It senses changes in chloride concentration of the fluid reaching the macula densa cells in the distal tubule and adjusts the diameter of the afferent arteriole accordingly. Tubuloglomerular feedback is an effective autoregulatory mechanism, because the chloride concentration of the fluid reaching the macula densa is dependent on flow rate, which, in turn, is directly related to the rate of filtration and glomerular capillary pressure. Elevations in renal arterial pressure and flow initially increase glomerular capillary pressure and glomerular filtration rate, which in turn increase tubular flow rate and the concentration of chloride reaching the macula densa. The rise in chloride concentration, which is sensed by an unknown mechanism, causes contraction of the portion of the afferent arteriole adjacent to the juxtaglomerular apparatus, completing the feedback loop. The nature of the substances involved in mediating this response remains to be determined but may include adenosine or metabolites of arachidonic acid.

Cerebral Circulation

In the brain, autoregulatory mechanisms are also well developed to maintain adequate perfusion, oxygenation, and substrate delivery as blood pressure varies. Two major mechanisms contribute to the autoregulation of cerebral blood flow: the myogenic behavior of larger cerebral arteries and metabolic autoregulatory adjustments of small arterioles in the cerebral cortex. The large cerebral arteries originating from the circle of Willis and the smaller pial arteries on the surface of the brain are highly myogenically active. They constrict

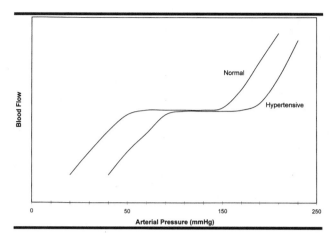

Figure 38.1. Autoregulation of renal and cerebral blood flow in normal and hypertensive individuals. Blood flow in these circulations in normal subjects is maintained nearly constant over a range of arterial pressures from 70 to 120 mm Hg. The autoregulatory range is shifted to higher pressures in hypertensive individuals due to elevations in vascular tone and structural changes in the microcirculation.

in response to elevations in transmural pressure. Since these vessels account for a major fraction of total cerebral vascular resistance, myogenic responses of these arteries increase cerebral vascular resistance sufficiently to minimize changes in blood flow and pressure in downstream elements of the cerebral circulation.

The remainder of the autoregulatory adjustments in cerebral vascular resistance occur at the level of small arterioles supplying the capillary networks in the cerebral cortex. These changes in vascular resistance are mediated by the release of vasoactive metabolites from metabolically active neural tissue and the vascular endothelium. These responses are highly sensitive to changes in pH, P_{CO_2}, and P_{O_2}. Elevations in blood or tissue pH or P_{CO_2} or hypoxia increase cerebral blood flow and impair autoregulation. The nature of the metabolites that mediate the changes in cerebral vascular resistance remain to be identified but evidence supports a role for nitric oxide, prostacyclin, prostaglandins, epoxyeicosatrienoic acids and adenosine. In addition, changes in intracellular pH and P_{O_2} have direct effects on tone in cerebral vascular smooth muscle cells.

Shear Stress and Blood Flow Regulation

Shear stress represents the frictional forces acting upon the intimal surface of vessels in response to blood flow. Shear stress can be calculated by the following equation:

$$\text{Shear Stress} = 8\eta V/R$$

where; η is the viscosity of blood, V is the flow velocity, and R is the inner diameter of the vessel. Shear stress is directly dependent on the velocity of flow in a vessel and is inversely proportional to vascular diameter. Increases in shear stress stimulate the release of vasodilator mediators from the endothelium as summarized in **Figure 38.2.** These products include nitric oxide, prostacyclin, epoxyeicosatrienoic acids and perhaps other endothelium-derived relaxing factors, which dilate vessels by hyperpolarizing vascular smooth muscle cells and lowering intracellular calcium. Each uses a different signal transduc-

tion pathway. Nitric oxide stimulates the formation of cGMP, which opens potassium channels to hyperpolarize the cell and diminish calcium entry through voltage sensitive channels. Prostacyclin acts on a receptor to promote vasodilation via a cAMP-dependent pathway. Epoxyeicosatrienoic acids are potent vasodilators that also open potassium channels in vascular smooth muscle cells.

In general, shear stress stimulates the release of these endothelially derived relaxing factors that act as negative modulators of autoregulatory responses. For example, acute elevations in perfusion pressure promote myogenic responses in vessels to autoregulate blood flow. The reduction in vascular diameter, however, increases shear stress, which promotes the release of nitric oxide and other endothelially derived relaxing factors, thus opposing further vasoconstriction.

Besides acting as a negative modulator of myogenic responses, shear-related changes in vascular tone also play an important role in dilating large vessels and augmenting blood flow to skeletal muscle during exercise or in response to increases in metabolic demand. The accumulation of metabolic products during exercise lowers vascular resistance in the skeletal muscle microcirculation to increase blood flow. The increase in blood flow and flow velocity in the larger upstream feed vessels then stimulates the release of nitric oxide and other mediators to dilate these vessels.

Shear Stress and Autoregulation in Hypertension

Elevations in vascular resistance, especially in the renal and cerebral vascular beds, are characteristic of hypertension. In addition, there is generalized dysfunction of the vascular endothelium associated with diminished vasodilatory responses to shear stress and other stimuli. In mild to moderate hypertension, the elevation in vascular resistances is appropriate for the degree of hypertension, so cerebral and renal blood flow remain relatively normal. In more severe hypertension, however, renal blood flow is reduced, while cerebral blood flow remains relatively normal until pressure exceeds the upper limit of autoregulation and hypertensive encephalopathy occurs.

The autoregulatory plateau in renal and cerebral blood flow is shifted to higher pressure ranges in hypertensive patients, and the

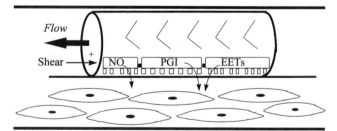

Figure 38.2. Effects of shear stress on the release of vasoactive mediators from the vascular endothelium. Increases in flow within a vessel increase shear stress, which promotes the release of nitric oxide (NO), prostacyclin (PGI), and epoxyeicosatrienoic acids (EETs) from the vascular endothelium. Each of these factors are potent vasodilators that open potassium channels in vascular smooth muscle cells through different signal transduction pathways.

magnitude of the shift is dependent on the severity and duration of the hypertension **(Figure 38.1).** This shift is due to hypertrophy and thickening of the wall of arterioles, endothelial dysfunction and potentiation of myogenic responses. Generally, the shift in autoregulatory relationships in moderate hypertension is not severe, so that arterial pressure can be lowered into the normotensive range without compromising renal or cerebral perfusion. However, in patients with severe or long standing hypertension, the structural changes in the cerebral and renal circulations may be so severe that it may not be possible to lower blood pressure to the normotensive range without compromising blood flow. Under these conditions, gradual reduction in blood pressure is accompanied by regression of vascular

hypertrophy and a shift in the autoregulatory curve back toward the normal range.

SUGGESTED READING

1. Cohen RA, Vanhoutte PM. Endothelium-dependent hyperpolarization: beyond nitric oxide and cGMP. *Circulation.* 1995;92:3337–3349.

2. Heistad DD, Kontos JP. Cerebral circulation. In: Berne RM, Sperelakis N, eds. *Handbook of Physiology: The Cardiovascular System.* Bethesda, Md: American Physiological Society; 1979.

3. Navar LG, Inscho EW, Majid SA, Imig JD, Harrison-Bernard LM, Mitchell KD. Paracrine regulation of the renal microcirculation. *Physiol Rev.* 1996;76:425–536.

4. Strandgaard S, Paulson OB. Cerebral blood flow and its pathophysiology in hypertension. *Am J Hypertens.* 1989;2:486–492.

Chapter 39

Monogenic Determinants of Blood Pressure

Disorders in the Renin-Angiotensin-Aldosterone System

Robert G. Dluhy, MD

KEY POINTS

- Monogenic, or single-gene, forms of human hypertension involve gain-of-function mutations that can be divided into overproduction of mineralocorticoids versus increased mineralocorticoid action.

- The clinical phenotype usually includes severe hypertension from birth, volume expansion, suppression of plasma renin activity, and variable hypokalemia.

See also Chapters 40, 41, 80, 81, 107

Progress has recently been made in identifying the genetic mutations of mendelian, or single-gene, forms of human hypertension **(Table 39.1)**. These syndromes are usually characterized by severe hypertension occurring from birth onward. In several of these syndromes (glucocorticoid-remediable aldosteronism and Liddle's syndrome), there appears to be high morbidity and mortality from early hemorrhagic stroke, underscoring the importance of identifying and treating affected persons. These monogenic hypertensive syndromes are confined to mutated genes involving gain of function of various components of the renin-angiotensin-aldosterone system, resulting in excessive renal sodium retention. In a broad sense, these syndromes divide into overproduction of mineralocorticoids versus increased mineralocorticoid action. Identification of these mutated genes has also permitted targeted antihypertensive therapies.

Overproduction of Mineralocorticoids
Glucocorticoid-Remediable Aldosteronism

Glucocorticoid-remediable aldosteronism (GRA), an autosomal dominant disorder that is characterized by moderate to severe hypertension in affected patients from birth onward, is the most common form of monogenic human hypertension. Because the majority of patients with GRA are not hypokalemic, a potassium level lacks sensitivity as a screening test for this disorder. Early hemorrhagic stroke (mean age, 32 years) is characteristic of GRA pedigrees. In a recent study, 48% of all GRA pedigrees and 18% of all GRA patients had cerebrovascular complications.

In GRA, aldosterone secretion is positively and solely regulated by adrenocorticotropic hormone (ACTH), and not by angiotensin II and potassium. As a consequence, exogenous glucocorticoid administration profoundly suppresses aldosterone secretion in affected subjects and reverses the syndrome. As in other causes of primary aldosteronism, plasma renin levels are suppressed.

Genetic analysis of GRA kindreds has revealed linkage of GRA to a mutation in the aldosterone synthase gene, which is closely related to steroid 11β-hydroxylase, a second gene involved in adrenal steroidogenesis. Both genes are 95% identical in DNA sequence, have identical intron-exon structures, and are located in close proximity on chromosome 8. In all GRA kindreds, affected subjects have two normal copies of genes encoding aldosterone synthase and 11β-hydroxylase, but in addition, they have a novel gene duplication: a hybrid, or chimeric, gene. This gene duplication, containing the 5' regulatory sequences confirming ACTH responsiveness of 11β-hydroxylase fused to more distal coding sequences of aldosterone synthase, results from an unequal crossing-over between these two homologous genes **(Figure 39.1, left)**. In GRA kindreds, the sites of crossing-over are variable, indicating that in different pedigrees, these gene duplications arise independently and do not descend from a single ancestral mutation. In addition, the sites of crossing-over are upstream of exon 5 of aldosterone synthase, suggesting that encoded amino acids in exon 5 are essential for aldosterone synthase enzymatic functions **(Figure 39.1, right)**.

This gene duplication appears to explain all of the known physiology and biochemistry previously reported in GRA. First, the promoter region of this chimeric gene contains regulatory sequences of 11β-hydroxylase and would be expected to be regulated by ACTH. In addition, this chimeric gene would allow ectopic expression of aldosterone synthase enzymatic activity in the ACTH-regulated zona fasciculata, which normally secretes only cortisol. Finally, the sole regulation of aldosterone secretion by ACTH and the suppression of aldosterone secretion by glucocorticoids in GRA is explained by the fact that aldosterone synthase gene is abnormally regulated by ACTH promoter sequences. Direct genetic screening for the presence of the gene duplication in GRA is 100% sensitive and specific for diagnosing GRA and is recommended for patients with primary aldosteronism without radiographic evidence of tumors, for young hypertensive individuals with suppressed levels of plasma renin activity (especially children), and for at-risk individuals in affected families. Treatments with low-dose glucocorticoids, amiloride, and spironolactone are effective.

Disorders of Steroid Hormone Biosynthesis (Congenital Adrenal Hyperplasia)

Various abnormalities of hydroxylase enzymes of the P450 class have been identified. These include C21, C17, and C11 hydroxylases, which are important steps in steroidogenesis. Disordered volume regulation and hypertension are usually not the presenting

Table 39.1. Monogenic Forms of Human Hypertension

DISORDER	SITE OF ALTERATION IN RAAS	GENES MUTATED
Glucocorticoid-remediable aldosteronism (GRA)	Adrenal (aldosterone)	Aldosterone synthase
11β-Hydroxylase, 17α-hydroxylase deficiencies	Adrenal (mineralocorticoids)	*CYP11B1; CYP17*
Liddle's syndrome	Renal epithelial Na+ channel (ENa C)	β- or α-subunit of ENa C genes
Syndrome of apparent mineralocorticoid excess (AME)	Renal mineralocorticoid receptor	*11βHSD2* (renal isoform) gene

RAAS indicates renin-angiotensin-aldosterone system; ENa C, amiloride sensitive epithelial sodium channel; and 11βHSD, 11β-hydroxysteroid dehydrogenase.

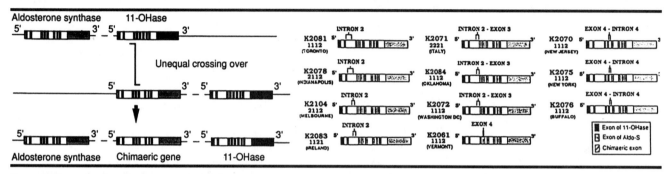

Figure 39.1. Left, The chimeric gene duplication in GRA, a result of unequal crossing-over between the homologous 11β-hydroxylase and aldosterone synthase genes. The chimera fuses the 5′-regulatory sequences of the 11β-hydroxylase gene and the 3′-coding sequences of the aldosterone synthase gene. Reproduced from Lifton et al (4) with permission. Right, Cross-over break points in 11 GRA pedigrees. The sites of crossing-over are all upstream of exon 5 of aldosterone synthase. Reproduced by permission from Lifton et al. Hereditary hypertension caused by chimaeric gene duplications and ectopic expression of aldosterone synthase. *Nat Genet.* 1992;2:66–74.

symptoms in the majority of patients with congenital adrenal hyperplasia (CAH). Rather, excessive androgenic effects in female patients or hypogonadism in male patients are more characteristic of the clinical phenotypes. 21-Hydroxylase deficiency, resulting from a mutated gene encoding P450C21 and accounting for >90% of the CAH genetic disorders, is not associated with hypertension but rather with sodium wasting in the severe clinical variant presenting in childhood.

P450C11β Deficiency

P450C11β deficiency causes a hypertensive variant of CAH, in which hypertension and hypokalemia variably occur because impaired conversion of 11-deoxycorticosterone to corticosterone results in the accumulation of 11-deoxycorticosterone, a potent mineralocorticoid. Increased shunting into the androgen pathway leads to ambiguous external genitalia at birth in girls (female pseudohermaphroditism) or hirsutism/virilization in girls in the postnatal period. P450C11β deficiency is an uncommon cause of CAH in individuals of European ancestry but accounts for 15% of cases in Moslem and Jewish Middle Eastern populations. Mutations causing P450C11β deficiency cluster in exons 6 to 8 of the CYP11B1 gene.

P450C17α Deficiency

P450C17α deficiency is characterized by hypogonadism, hypokalemia, and hypertension. This rare disorder causes decreased production of cortisol and shunting of precursors into the mineralocorticoid pathway; usually, 11-deoxycorticosterone production is elevated. Because P450C17α hydroxylation is required for biosynthesis of adrenal and gonadal testosterone and estrogen, this defect is

associated with sexual immaturity, high urinary gonadotropin levels, and low urinary 17-ketosteroid excretion. Female patients have primary amenorrhea and lack of development of secondary sexual characteristics. Because of deficient androgen production, male patients have either ambiguous external genitalia or a female phenotype (male pseudohermaphroditism). Exogenous glucocorticoids can correct the hypertensive syndrome, and treatment with appropriate gonadal steroids results in sexual maturation. A large number of random mutations can cause 17α-hydroxylase deficiency, making genetic diagnosis difficult.

Increased Mineralocorticoid Action
Syndrome of Apparent Mineralocorticoid Excess

In vitro, both cortisol and aldosterone are potent activators of renal mineralocorticoid receptors. Yet aldosterone is the primary regulator of renal mineralocorticoid activity in vivo, because cortisol is normally excluded from occupying renal mineralocorticoid receptors by the enzyme 11β-hydroxysteroid dehydrogenase (11β-HSD). There are two isoforms of the 11β-HSD enzyme: 11β-HSD1, which is NADP-preferring and active primarily as a reductase (cortisone to cortisol) in the liver; and 11β-HSD2, which is NAD-requiring and is active as a dehydrogenase in the kidney (**Figure 39.2**). Normally, cortisol is metabolized to the biologically inactive cortisone by 11β-HSD2 in the kidney, thus serving to "protect" the receptor from activation by cortisol. 11β-HSD–deficiency states allow cortisol to act as a mineralocorticoid and activate the type I renal mineralocorticoid receptor. As a result, sodium is retained and the renin-angiotensin-aldosterone system is suppressed. The syndrome of apparent mineralocorticoid excess (AME) occurs as an autosomal

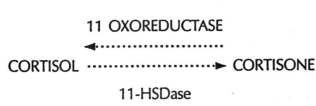

GLUCOCORTICOID SHUTTLE

Figure 39.2.   The "glucocorticoid shuttle" whereby the two isoforms of the 11β-HSD enzyme act either as a reductase in the liver (cortisone to cortisol, 11β-HSD1) or a dehydrogenase in the kidney (11β-HSD2).

recessive disorder and is the result of mutations in the gene coding for the kidney-specific isoform 11β-HSD2. Patients with either the congenital or acquired (licorice ingestion) AME syndrome characteristically exhibit an increased ratio of cortisol to cortisone metabolites in the urine. The plasma half-life of cortisol is also prolonged in patients with AME.

Liddle's Syndrome

Liddle's syndrome, a rare autosomal dominant disorder with variable penetrance, is characterized by hypertension, excessive sodium retention, hypokalemia (usually), and low plasma renin activity. Aldosterone levels are undetectable, and antagonism of the mineralocorticoid receptor with spironolactone has no effect on blood pressure or serum potassium. The syndrome is ameliorated by amiloride, which blocks sodium reabsorption and potassium excretion by mineralocorticoid receptor–independent mechanisms. The defect in Liddle's syndrome results from constitutive activation of amiloride-sensitive epithelial sodium channels on distal renal tubules, which causes excess sodium reabsorption. This channel is composed of at least three subunits and is normally regulated by aldosterone. The mutations causing Liddle's syndrome have been localized to genes on chromosome 16 that encode the β- and α-subunits of the epithelial sodium channels. These β- and α-subunit mutations result in a gain of function, probably secondary to slower disappearance of activated sodium channels from the renal distal tubule apical cell surfaces.

SUGGESTED READING

1. Curnow KM, Slutsker L, Vitek J, Cole T, Speiser PW, New MI, White PC, Pascoe L. Mutations in the CYP11β 1 gene causing congenital adrenal hyperplasia and hypertension cluster in exons 6, 7, and 8. *Proc Natl Acad Sci U S A.* 1993;90: 4552–4556.
2. Funder JW, Pearce PT, Smith R, Smith AI. Mineralocorticoid action: target tissue specificity is enzyme, not receptor, mediated. *Science.* 1988;242:583–585.
3. Liddle GW, Bledsoe T, Coppage WS Jr. A familial renal disorder simulating primary aldosterone but with negligible aldosterone secretion. *Trans Assoc Am Physicians.* 1963;76:199–213.
4. Lifton RP, Dluhy RG, Powers M, Rich GM, Cook S, Ulick S, Lalouel J-M. A chimaeric 11β-hydroxylase/aldosterone synthase gene causes glucocorticoid-remediable aldosteronism and human hypertension. *Nature.* 1992;355:262–265.
5. Lifton RP, Dluhy RG, Powers M, Rich GM, Gutkin M, Fallo F, Gill JR Jr, Feld L, Ganguly A, Laidlaw JC, Murnaghan DJ, Kaufman C, Stockigt JR, Ulick S, Lalouel J-M. Hereditary hypertension caused by chimaeric gene duplications and ectopic expression of aldosterone synthase. *Nat Genet.* 1992;2:66–74.
6. Lifton RP. Molecular genetics of human blood pressure variation. *Science.* 1996;272:676–680.
7. Litchfield WR, Anderson BF, Weiss RJ, Lifton RP, Dluhy RG. Intracranial aneurysm and hemorrhagic stroke in glucocorticoid-remediable aldosteronism. *Hypertension.* 1998;31(pt 2):445–450.
8. Mune F, Rogerson FM, Nikkila H, Agarwal AK, White PC. Human hypertension is caused by mutations in the kidney isozyme of 11β-hydroxysteroid dehydrogenase. *Nat Genet.* 1995;10:394–399.
9. Shimkets RA, Warnock DG, Bositis CM, Nelson-Williams C, Hansson JH, Schambelan M, Gill JR Jr, Ulick S, Milora RV, Findling JW. Liddle's syndrome: heritable human hypertension caused by mutations in the β subunit of the epithelial sodium channel. *Cell.* 1994;79:407–414.
10. Yanase T, Simpson ER, Waterman MR. 17α-Hydroxylase/17,20 lyase deficiency: from clinical investigation to molecular definition. *Endocrinol Rev.* 1991;12: 91–108.

Chapter 40

Polygenic Determinants of Blood Pressure

George T. Cicila, PhD

KEY POINTS

- Blood pressure is a continuously variable quantitative trait that is determined by many genes (ie, is polygenic) and is normally distributed in both human and animal populations.

- Affected sib-pair analysis and association studies have been used to identify regions of human chromosomes that may contain genes that influence blood pressure, called blood pressure quantitative trait loci (QTLs).

- Blood pressure QTLs have also been identified on several rat chromosomes.

- Congenic strains confirm the presence and location of many blood pressure QTLs and may facilitate the identification and positional cloning of the genes that cause blood pressure QTLs in the future.

See also Chapters 39, 41, 80, 81, 107

Blood Pressure as a Quantitative Trait

Blood pressure is a quantitative trait with continuous variation from low to high values in outbred populations of humans or animals. As with most quantitative traits, differences in blood pressure result from the contributions of many genes (ie, blood pressure is a polygenic trait) interacting with each other and the environment. In outbred human populations, blood pressure values show a skewed normal distribution, with values over a certain threshold defined as hypertensive. The influence of genes on hypertension was initially studied by comparing adopted with biological children, identical and nonidentical twins, and other family studies. Such studies indicate that ≈30% to 50% of the blood pressure variation observed in the general population can be explained by genetic factors.

Recently, mutations that cause a number of human diseases have been identified by first detecting chromosomal regions in which genetic markers cosegregate with the disease trait in families and then using positional cloning to identify the single defective gene responsible for the disease. This approach has been useful in identifying a number of mutant genes that cause rare, monogenic, forms of heritable hypertension. However, the situation is much more complex for the 90% to 95% of patients designated as having primary or essential hypertension in whom the cause is not due to obvious lesions in a single gene. Here, the many genetic alterations responsible for high blood pressure would be expected to be subtle, such as upregulated or downregulated expression of an active gene or point mutations that alter but do not abolish the activity of a protein.

Human Essential Hypertension

Human essential hypertension is a polygenic disorder and as such is genetically heterogeneous in nature, with different patients carrying different subsets of genes that lead to elevated blood pressure. These genes that affect blood pressure can be described as having alternate (or allelic) variant forms associated with either increased or decreased blood pressure, ie, "low" or "high" blood pressure alleles.

The genetic component of essential hypertension is thought to be largely additive in nature, such that the blood pressure observed in a particular patient is dependent, in part, on the balance between the number and relative strength of the low and high blood pressure alleles present. Epistasis, or the interaction between two or more nonallelic genes (ie, those located at different positions in the genome), can lead to nonadditive effects, which complicates identification of disease-related genes by linkage analysis. Understanding of the molecular basis of blood pressure regulation is further complicated by the existence of genes that have no direct effect on blood pressure but that influence blood pressure in a specific environmental context, such as a high dietary salt intake.

Studying the Genetics of Human Essential Hypertension

Linkage analysis of extended families and positional cloning approaches are unlikely to identify genes that cause essential hypertension, because they require the presence of a single major disease gene having a specific mode of inheritance. Headway can be made in the understanding of a polygenic trait by simplifying the analysis or the system or both. One way to identify genes involved in heritable forms of hypertension is to ignore quantitative differences in blood pressure and substitute a dichotomous, qualitative threshold criterion to define which individuals are affected (hypertensive) and which are not.

Affected Sib-Pair Analysis

Affected sib-pair analysis searches for increased levels of similarity in polymorphic genetic markers (ie, markers that differ greatly in size or sequence, allowing the identification of different alleles) in pairs of affected siblings. In this analysis, chromosomal regions showing higher degrees of marker similarity in hypertensive siblings (presumably from inheritance of the same alleles) are more likely to contain alleles that affect blood pressure.

Polymorphic genetic markers, initially examined for candidate genes, can also be examined at regular distances along each chromosome. Thus, the whole genome can be examined (scanned) for chromosomal regions with elevated levels of genetic marker similarity. Genome scanning approaches now dominate the study of polygenic determinants of traits like blood pressure, particularly in animal models of genetic hypertension. Computer programs are used to identify chromosomal regions most likely to contain genes (or loci) associated with variation in blood pressure. Genes that control quantitative traits like blood pressure, ie, traits with values having a continuous distribution, are known as quantitative trait loci (QTLs).

Association Studies

Association studies are another approach, complementary to linkage analysis, for identifying the genetic determinants of hypertension. Association studies are particularly useful in identifying a particular gene as a strong candidate after a chromosomal region has been linked to the disease. Frequencies of the different alleles for this locus are examined in hypertensive patients and normotensive control subjects carefully matched for confounding factors such as age, sex, or race. Linkage disequilibrium occurs when combinations of alleles at different loci (haplotypes) are observed at frequencies significantly higher than expected from chance association alone. When alleles have strikingly different frequencies in patients compared with unaffected control subjects, such differences could arise either from causal involvement of the gene in disease susceptibility or from linkage disequilibrium with a different locus that is actually responsible for the disease susceptibility.

Although linkage disequilibrium can arise from several sources, including recent admixtures of groups within a population, selection for a specific allele, or random genetic drift, disequilibrium occurring between tightly linked loci is expected to persist longer. In this way, linkage disequilibrium between a genetic marker and a disease or trait locus could lead to identifying one of the genes responsible for susceptibility to high blood pressure.

Animal Models of Genetic Hypertension

Identification of QTLs in animal models is a powerful method for simplifying and dissecting the genetic basis of human polygenic traits, such as blood pressure. Indeed, in some crossbred animal populations, ≥60% of the variation in blood pressure can be explained by genetic factors.

Selectively bred rat strains have been developed that are divergent for a polygenic, quantitative trait, such as blood pressure. After blood pressure measurement of a large, heterogeneous population, several pairs of rats with the highest blood pressures are selected for mating to produce a high blood pressure strain, such as the spontaneously hypertensive rat. Blood pressures of progeny from these matings are also measured, and again, several pairs of rats with the highest blood pressures are selected for mating. Repetition of this procedure further concentrates alleles associated with high blood pressure.

At some point, usually after further selection does not result in progeny with higher blood pressures compared with the parents, the selectively bred strain is inbred to fix the genes responsible for the trait. After such brother-sister mating of rats from the selectively bred strain for at least 20 additional generations, >99% of its loci become homozygous (ie, having two copies of the same allele), and the inbred strain can be considered genetically identical. Creation of inbred strains results in homozygous alleles at virtually all loci, including genes that are not involved in the genetic determination of blood pressure. Similar procedures can also be used to select and breed contrasting, low blood pressure strains.

Different selectively bred strains do not carry identical sets of genes that affect blood pressure because (1) different populations of rats were used for selective breeding, (2) strains were subjected to different selective pressures because of different breeding or selection schemes, and (3) alleles were fixed randomly while the strains were being inbred. The spontaneously hypertensive rat was developed to concentrate high blood pressure alleles, but other strains have been developed that will not become hypertensive without alteration of an environmental factor. The Sabra hypertension-sensitive strain develops hypertension only when fed an excessive intake of dietary NaCl. Other strains, such as the inbred Dahl salt-sensitive rat, are both spontaneously hypertensive and sensitive to excessive intake of dietary NaCl. Conversely, the inbred Dahl salt-resistant rat will not develop high blood pressure, even when fed a high-NaCl diet.

Identifying Blood Pressure QTLs in Animal Models

Studying inbred rats rather than human populations has several advantages. (1) In such a population, a single set of genetic factors is segregating (ie, the alleles carried by each of the inbred strains that were crossbred), making all polymorphic genetic markers fully informative for the genotype at all chromosomal loci. (2) The environment in which a segregating population is maintained can be manipulated by nutritional, pharmacological, or other interventions. Unlike studies with humans, environmental conditions can be controlled for artificially bred animal populations, ensuring that each rat is maintained under the same conditions. (3) Most important, if variation in environmental factors is minimized, much of the observed phenotypic variation in blood pressure can be attributed to genetic components.

Segregating populations are bred by mating of inbred rats with contrasting phenotypes to produce first filial generation (F_1) animals that are genetically identical but heterozygous for every locus (ie, carrying an allele from each parent at every locus). Hence, phenotypic variation observed in F_1 animals is due to environmental factors. Populations in which all alleles are segregating can be produced either by intercrossing male and female F_1 rats or by backcrossing F_1 rats with one of the parental strains.

Genome scanning approaches have been used to identify blood pressure QTLs in segregating populations bred by crossing hypertensive rats from a number of different genetic models with contrasting normotensive strains. To date, blood pressure QTLs have been identified on many rat chromosomes, confirming the complex, polygenic nature of blood pressure regulation in this species. One blood pressure QTL in the Dahl rat model contains a gene, steroid 11β-hydroxylase (*Cyp11b1*), with allelic variants encoding proteins with amino acid sequence differences that cosegregate with both enzymatic activity and blood pressure differences.

As with human patients, blood pressure QTLs identified in crossbred rodent populations can be only crudely localized to regions of 10 to 30 cM (≈10 million to 60 million bp) that contain many genes. Studies showing blood pressure QTLs have often been difficult to replicate in both animal and human populations.

Using Congenic Strains to Study Blood Pressure

Chromosomal regions containing a blood pressure QTL allele can be genetically transferred from one strain (donor) to another inbred (recipient) strain by selective breeding. F_1 (donor × recipient) rats are backcrossed to the appropriate parental strain, and the resulting progeny are examined for polymorphic genetic markers present in a selected chromosomal region. Progeny heterozygous for markers in this region are backcrossed to the recipient strain, with the process repeated until rats are identified that carry only the selected region of donor chromosome on a background of alleles from the recipient strain. The chosen rats are then brother-sister mated to become homozygous for the selected donor strain alleles and maintained as inbred strains. Such inbred strains, carrying a small portion of donor chromosomal material on an otherwise uniform background of recipient strain alleles, are known as congenic strains.

Blood pressures can be compared between such congenic strains and the inbred recipient, parental, strain. Findings of significant blood pressure differences between the congenic and recipient strains confirm the presence of a blood pressure QTL allele in the introgressed chromosomal region and define physical limits for the location of the QTLs. In the Dahl rat model alone, 8 blood pressure QTLs have been confirmed by use of congenic strains, including the rat chromosome 7 region containing *Cyp11b1*.

Further selective breeding can be used to develop congenic substrains carrying a blood pressure QTL allele in a reduced portion of introgressed donor chromosome, further narrowing the region in which the allele responsible for this blood pressure QTL can be located. These congenic substrains should facilitate the subsequent identification and positional cloning of genes responsible for the development of hypertension.

Future Studies

Homologous genes, found both in human essential hypertension and in animal genetic models, are likely to explain at least some of the observed blood pressure variation. Fine mapping of human chromosomal regions carrying blood pressure QTLs, in conjunction with positional cloning of blood pressure QTL alleles present in congenic strains carrying the equivalent rat chromosomal regions, should facilitate the eventual identification of genes that cause hypertension in humans.

SUGGESTED READING

1. Cicila GT, Dukhanina OI, Kurtz TW, Walder R, Garrett MR, Dene H, Rapp JP. Blood pressure and survival of a chromosome 7 congenic strain derived from Dahl rats. *Mamm Genome.* 1997;8:896–902.

2. Cicila GT, Rapp JP, Wang J-M, St Lezin E, Ng SC, Kurtz TW. Linkage of 11β-hydroxylase mutations with altered steroid biosynthesis and blood pressure in the Dahl rat. *Nat Genet.* 1993;3:346–353.

3. Falconer, DS, Mackay TFC. *Introduction to Quantitative Genetics.* 4th ed. New York, NY: Longman; 1996.

4. Julier C, Delépine MBK, Terwilliger J, Davis S, Weeks DE, Bui T, Jeunemaître X, Velho G, Froguel P, Ratcliffe P, Corvol P, Soubrier F, Lathrop GM. Genetic susceptibility for human familial essential hypertension in a region of homology with blood pressure linkage on rat chromosome 10. *Hum Mol Genet.* 1997;6:2077–2085.

5. Rapp JP, Deng AY. Detection and positional cloning of blood pressure quantitative trait loci: is it possible? Identifying the genes for genetic hypertension. *Hypertension.* 1995;25:1121–1128.

6. Rapp JP. The search for the genetic basis of blood pressure variation in rats. In: Laragh JH, Brenner BM, eds. *Hypertension: Pathophysiology, Diagnosis, and Management.* New York, NY: Raven Press Ltd; 1995;1289–1300.

7. Schork NJ, Nath SP, Lindpaintner K, Jacob HJ. Extensions to quantitative trait locus mapping in experimental organisms. *Hypertension.* 1996;28:1104–1111.

8. Siffert W, Rosskopf D, Siffert G, Busch S, Moritz A, Erbel R, Sharma AM, Ritz E, Wichman H-E, Jakobs KH, Horsthemke B. Association of human G-protein β3 subunit variant with hypertension. *Nat Genet.* 1998;18:45–48.

9. Weeks DE, Lathrop GM. Polygenic disease: methods for mapping complex disease traits. *Trends Genet.* 1995;11:513–519.

Chapter 41

Renin-Angiotensin Genetics

James R. Sowers, MD

KEY POINTS

- Angiotensinogen gene mutations may contribute to the development of hypertension before the age of 60 years in whites.

- ACE gene polymorphisms have stronger associations with atherosclerosis than hypertension; the DD allele is a marker of vascular diseases, including coronary artery and cerebrovascular diseases.

See also Chapters 3, 4, 5, 6, 7, 8, 39, 40, 51, 80, 81, 107, 129, 130

Mounting evidence demonstrates a genetic contribution of the components of the renin-angiotensin system to cardiovascular disease.

Angiotensinogen

The possibility that inherited variability in the renin gene might contribute to genetic hypertension was originally raised by linkage analysis of blood pressure in F2 and backcross populations derived from inbred Dahl salt-sensitive and Dahl salt-resistant rats. Subsequent sib-pair linkage analysis and case-control studies in humans suggested that the angiotensinogen gene on chromosome 1 was potentially important in the pathogenesis of essential hypertension.

In a study conducted in Utah, a 33% excess of shared angiotensinogen alleles was observed among male sibling pairs with diastolic hypertension, and it was estimated that mutations in the angiotensinogen gene might be responsible for up to 6% of hypertension in whites whose hypertension was present before the age of 60 years. These same investigators reported that the T235 variant of the angiotensinogen gene was associated with increased plasma concentrations of angiotensinogen, giving a plausible biochemical basis for the hypertension.

Renin

Studies in other white populations have not yielded a relationship between the renin and ACE gene and essential hypertension. In contrast, a modest association between essential hypertension and a 5.0-kb *Bgl* II restriction fragment length polymorphism in the renin gene has been reported in an Afro-Caribbean population. These preliminary studies suggest the need for larger population studies exploring a genetic linkage between the renin-angiotensin system and hypertension in different ethnic groups.

Nonmodulator Trait

There is a group of salt-sensitive hypertensives with normal or elevated plasma renin activity who are unable to mount normal aldosterone responses to volume manipulation. These nonmodulators are candidates for studies of linkage between the renin-angiotensin system and salt-sensitive hypertension. First, there is a strong positive family history of hypertension in nonmodulators: 85% of nonmodulators were reported by the Brigham group to have a positive family history of hypertension. When a Utah population was tested for concordance between nonmodulation and hypertension, a high degree of concordance was seen.

Angiotensin-Converting Enzyme

In contrast to equivocal results in hypertension, there is more definitive evidence that ACE gene polymorphism is associated with atherosclerotic vascular disease. Two basic alleles have been identified for the ACE gene, called insertion (I) and deletion (D). In Ireland and France, a highly significant relationship has been observed between the DD ACE genotype and coronary heart disease. Furthermore, the frequency of the DD allele was increased in persons with a parental history of coronary heart disease. A recent autopsy study showed an association of aortic atherosclerosis and the DD and ID genotypes in diabetic persons. Two studies in Europe in older subjects from a general population showed associations of increased carotid artery intimal-medial thickness, plasma ACE levels, and the DD genotype. Similarly, a study on older Japanese type II diabetic subjects showed an association between the D allele of the ACE gene and carotid artery intimal-medial thickness, a surrogate for carotid atherosclerosis. Finally, when a population of patients with cerebrovascular disease was compared with an age-matched control group without stroke or myocardial infarction, the DD genotype was more prevalent in persons with lacunar stroke or hypertension. Thus, the association between polymorphism of ACE and cardiovascular disease is striking and consistent, regardless of the presence or absence of such a relationship between hypertension and ACE polymorphism.

SUGGESTED READING

1. Cambien F, Costerousse O, Tiret L, Poirier O, Lecerf L, Gonzalez MF, Evans A, Arveiler D, Cambou JP, Luc G, Rakotovao R, Ducimetiere P, Soubrier F, Alhenc-Gelas F. Plasma level and gene polymorphism of angiotensin-converting enzyme in relation to myocardial infarction. *Circulation.* 1994;90:669–676.

2. Gardemann A, Weib T, Schwartz O, Eberbach A, Katz N, Hehrlein FW, Tillmans H, Waas W, Waberbosch W. Gene polymorphism but not catalytic activity of angiotensin I–converting enzyme activity is associated with coronary artery disease and myocardial infarction in low-risk patients. *Circulation.* 1995;92: 2796–2799.

3. Kauma H, Paivansalo M, Savolainen MJ, Rantala AO, Kiema TR, Lilja M, Renanen A, Kesaniemi YA. Association between angiotensin converting enzyme gene polymorphism and carotid atherosclerosis. *J Hypertens.* 1996;14:1183–1187.

4. Lindpaintner K, Pfeffer MA, Kreutz R, Stampfer MJ, Grodstein F, LaMotte F, Buring

J, Hennekens CH. A prospective evaluation of an angiotensin-converting-enzyme gene polymorphism and the risk of ischemic heart disease. *N Engl J Med.* 1995;332:706–711.

5. Ludwig E, Corneli PS, Anderson JL, Marshall HW, Lalouel JM, Ward RH. Angiotensin-converting enzyme gene polymorphism is associated with myocardial infarction but not with development of coronary stenosis. *Circulation.* 1995;91:2120–2124.

6. Markus HS, Barley J, Lunt R, Bland JM, Jeffery S, Carter ND, Brown MM. Angiotensin-converting enzyme gene deletion polymorphism: a new risk factor for lacunar stroke but not carotid atheroma. *Stroke.* 1995;26: 1329–1333.

7. Tarnow L, Cambien F, Rossing P, Nielsen FS, Hansen BV, Lecerf L, Poirier O, Danilov S, Boelskifte S, Borch-Johnsen K, Parving HH. Insertion/deletion polymorphism in the angiotensin-I-converting enzyme gene is associated with coronary heart disease in IDDM patients with diabetic nephropathy. *Diabetologia.* 1995;38: 798–803.

8. Zee RY, Lou YK, Griffiths LR, Morris BJ. Association of the polymorphism of the angiotensin I-converting enzyme gene with essential hypertension. *Biochem Biophys Res Commun.* 1992;184:9–15.

Chapter 42

Sympathetic Nervous System Abnormalities in Hypertension

J. Michael Wyss, PhD

KEY POINTS

- There are increased numbers of adrenergic neurons and increased activity of the rostral ventrolateral medulla (RVLM) in several animal models of hypertension.

- Lesions in the anteroventral hypothalamus or nucleus tractus solitarius raise blood pressure, demonstrating the depressor effect of these regions, whereas lesions in the RVLM, anteroventral third ventricle, posterolateral hypothalamus, and area postrema increase blood pressure, demonstrating the pressor effect of these regions.

- Angiotensins, neuropeptide Y_1 calcitonin gene–related peptide, and atriopeptins modulate sympathetic nervous function and may play a role in chronic blood pressure elevation.

- Increased sympathetic activity is an early feature of renovascular, steroid-induced, and genetic hypertension in rats and is necessary for full expression of hypertension.

See also Chapters 33, 34, 35, 43, 128

Those physiologists who have held that the kidney plays the dominant role in setting long-term arterial pressure have viewed the nervous system as only a short-term regulator of arterial pressure, adjusting arterial pressure to acute challenges (standing, running, stress stimuli, etc). In several animal models, however, inappropriate regulation of the cardiovascular system by the sympathetic nervous system contributes directly to chronic hypertension.

Peripheral Autonomic Neuroanatomy

The autonomic nervous system and the neuroendocrine system are the major final output pathways by which the brain regulates arterial pressure in health and disease. The autonomic nervous system comprises separate sympathetic and parasympathetic effector mechanisms and the afferent (sensory) feedback associated with each of these divisions **(see Table 42.1)**. The peripheral sympathetic nervous system contains motor neurons located in ganglia that lie either immediately lateral to the spinal cord (paravertebral) or anterior to the vertebral column (prevertebral). The prevertebral neurons appear to innervate primarily visceral organs, including the heart and kidney, whereas the paravertebral neurons project more to blood vessels throughout the body and mediate "fight-or-flight" responses.

The parasympathetic motor axons that innervate tissue above the transverse colon are innervated by preganglionic neurons that reside in the brain stem, whereas those associated with organs below the transverse colon are innervated by preganglionic neurons in the sacral spinal cord segments 2 through 4. The cell bodies of the postganglionic neurons are located near the target organ and regulate digestive and regenerative functions.

Sensory afferent feedback from the innervated tissue is projected back through the ganglia to the central nervous system. Sympathetic afferents are directed into the spinal cord and terminate at the level of the spinal cord that correlates with the ganglia through which they course. The kidney is innervated by the lower thoracic sympathetic ganglia, and the sensory feedback terminates in the lower thoracic spinal cord. Parasympathetic sensory innervation follows the projection pattern of the motor fibers.

Sympathetic Neuromodulation

Synaptic transmission may be modulated by hormones and peripheral interplay between neurons. Kopp and associates demonstrated that neurotransmitters released from efferent nerve terminals can affect conduction of information in other afferent nerves. Similarly, Kruelen and associates have shown that some peripheral afferent nerves appear to directly innervate neurons in the sympathetic ganglia. Neuroactive agents synthesized in peripheral sensory axons can also function locally as coneurotransmitters or neuromodulators. Perhaps the best example is calcitonin gene–related peptide (CGRP), which is released by peripheral afferent neurons onto blood vessels, causing profound vasodilation. Release of CGRP is inhibited by α_2-adrenergic receptor activation. Thus, an overabundance of norepinephrine in a target tissue could increase vasoconstriction directly by stimulation of α_1-adrenergic receptors and indirectly via inhibition of CGRP release. New studies in the rat suggest that a decrease in peripheral CGRP release may contribute to pregnancy-related hypertension.

Of the several neuropeptides that interact with the sympathetic nervous system, angiotensin II and atrial natriuretic peptide (ANP) have been most extensively studied. Angiotensin II directly enhances release of norepinephrine centrally and in the periphery and blunts baroreflexes. Both of these actions are considered to be important contributors to hypertension in the spontaneously hypertensive rat (SHR) and other models. Other angiotensin metabolites may mimic

Table 42.1. Autonomic Effects on Cardiovascular Tissue

ORGAN	SYMPATHETIC	PARASYMPATHETIC
HEART MUSCLE	**INCREASED RATE AND INCREASED CONTRACTION**	**SLOWED RATE AND DECREASED FORCE OF CONTRACTION**
Coronary arteries	α_1 = receptor constricted β_2 = receptor dilated	Dilated
Peripheral arteries	α_1 = receptor vasoconstriction β = receptor vasodilation Muscarinic vasodilation	Not applicable
Kidney	Decreased output and renin secretion	Not applicable

Areas that increase blood pressure: anteroventral third ventricle (especially median preoptic nucleus); rostroventrolateral medulla; posterolateral hypothalamus; area postrema.

Areas that decrease blood pressure: anterior hypothalamus; nucleus tractus solitarius.

(eg, angiotensin III) or oppose (angiotensin 1–7) the effects of angiotensin II on arterial pressure regulation. ANP and type C natriuretic peptide cause sympathoinhibition and decrease the release of norepinephrine from nerve terminals. In some models of hypertension, eg, the SHR, decreased circulating ANP appears to contribute to hypertension, and this may be via a direct effect on the sympathetic nervous system.

Neuropeptide Y is another cotransmitter released along with norepinephrine by sympathetic nerve terminals. By itself, neuropeptide Y does not exert potent vasoconstriction or activation of other sympathetic nervous system target tissues, but it does enhance the responses of target cells to catecholamine stimulation. In both deoxycorticosterone acetate (DOCA)-NaCl–induced hypertension and pulmonary hypertension induced by veratrine stimulation of the sympathetic nervous system, increases in plasma concentrations of neuropeptide Y parallel the increases in plasma norepinephrine concentrations. In contrast to neuropeptide Y, adenosine and galanin inhibit norepinephrine release, and recent studies have suggested that a deficit in inhibition by either or both of these neuromodulators may contribute to hypertension.

Hypertension in Animal Models

Abnormalities in peripheral sympathetic innervation may contribute to essential hypertension. Several groups have shown that in genetic forms of hypertension in the rat, there is an increase in the number of sympathetic postganglionic neurons. This is suggestive of an increased sympathetic drive to the organs and appears to be related to a failure of the nervous system to appropriately prune down the number of postganglionic neurons during development. Increased sensory feedback from vital organs or diminished baroreflex control may also contribute to hypertension.

Many studies have examined the relationship between sympathetic nerve activity and hypertension. In several animal models of hypertension, sympathetic nerves appear to be overly active, and this is presumed to lead to greater vasoconstriction and hypertension. The relationship between the sympathetic nervous system and hypertension in animal models has been studied extensively in relation to renal innervation. Using renal denervation as a primary tool, many studies indicate that the renal nerves contribute to the development of hypertension but are much less influential in the maintenance phase of the disease. In SHRs of the Okomoto strain, in rodent mod-

els with renovascular hypertension, and in DOCA-NaCl–treated rats, renal sympathetic innervation is necessary for the full development of hypertension. Recent studies suggest that renal nerves also mediate enhanced afferent arteriolar responsiveness to chronic angiotensin II infusion in rats. In contrast, one-kidney, one-clip renovascular hypertension in rats and aortic coarctation hypertension in dogs are mediated, at least in part, by the renal sensory (but not motor) nerves. In these latter cases, there is no associated sodium retention, in contrast to the models in which the renal sympathetic efferent nerves are important. Rather surprisingly, the renal nerves do not appear to contribute to NaCl-sensitive hypertension in the SHRs or Dahl NaCl-sensitive rats or to the nephrotoxic effects of cyclosporin A therapy in rats, despite the observation that sympathetic nervous system overactivity plays a prominent role in all three forms of hypertension. Similarly, although the hypertension induced by inhibition of NO synthase is associated with enhanced renal nerve activity, this increased renal sympathetic nerve activity does not appear to contribute to the hypertension in this model.

The principal neurotransmitter that is released by the sympathetic nerves is norepinephrine, and the adrenergic receptors most likely involved in the development of sympathetic nervous system–related hypertension would seem to be α_1-adrenergic receptors. However, recent studies suggest that this view should be somewhat modified. In SHRs, the sympathetic nervous system contributes importantly to the development of hypertension, but blockade of the α_1-adrenergic receptor from 4 to 12 weeks of age does not eliminate the development of hypertension. Furthermore, in the reduced renal mass model of hypertension, a failure of the presynaptic α_2-adrenergic receptor to adequately inhibit norepinephrine release appears to accelerate the development of hypertension. Very recent studies in transgenic mouse models demonstrate that stimulation of peripheral α_{2c}-adrenergic receptors is prohypertensive.

Participation of Brainstem, Hypothalamic, Periventricular, and Cortical Centers in Hypertension

Several brainstem regions can modify blood pressure. Lesions of the nucleus tractus solitarius, for example, produce increased sympathetic activity and cause fulminant hypertension. A closely related region of the rostral ventrolateral medulla also seems to play a role in almost any form of central nervous system–driven hypertension, and several studies suggest that the contribution may be more primary. For instance, inhibitory input to these neurons is blunted in SHRs, and microinjections of angiotensin into this region elicit greater responses in SHRs than in normotensive control rats. In the area postrema, which is dorsal to the nucleus tractus solitarius, the lack of a blood-brain barrier allows its neurons to monitor concentrations of hormones (including angiotensin II) and peptides in the general circulation. Lesions of this area decrease arterial pressure in SHRs, normotensive dogs, and DOCA-NaCl–induced hypertension in the rat, suggesting that the area postrema participates in the pathogenesis of several forms of hypertension.

The role of the hypothalamus in hypertension has been demonstrated by lesion, stimulation, and neuronal transplantation studies in the rat. Transplantation of a hypothalamus from a genetically hypertensive rat induces hypertension in a genetically normotensive recipient. Transplantation of tissue from a normotensive donor has no significant effect on arterial pressure in the recipient. The lateral and posterior hypothalamic areas are sympathoexcitatory regions that increase arterial pressure and heart rate. Lesions of the posterior hypothalamic area reduce arterial pressure in DOCA-NaCl rats. In the posterior hypothalamus of SHRs, imbalances in norepinephrine, acetylcholine, and γ-aminobutyric acid may contribute to hypertension.

The paraventricular nucleus has a well-known role in arterial pressure regulation because the magnocellular division of this nucleus and the associated supraoptic nucleus produce vasopressin and release it into the general circulation. Studies over the past decade demonstrate that the parvicellular portion of the paraventricular nucleus projects to the brainstem. SHRs display abnormal regulation of neurons in the paraventricular nucleus, and the interaction between angiotensin II and the paraventricular nucleus appears to be altered in several forms of hypertension.

The anterior hypothalamus contains several cardiovascular control regions that may contribute to hypertension. The anteroventral third ventricle is perhaps the leading hypertension-inducing candidate in this group. Lesions of the median preoptic nucleus of the anteroventral third ventricle region, which receives input from circumventricular organs and brainstem nuclei, prevent hypertension or decrease blood pressure in hypertensive animal models. Other preoptic nuclei regulate thirst and water balance. The anterior hypothalamic area, along with the preoptic area, provides important sympathoinhibitory influences, most of which are mediated by projections to sympathoexcitatory nuclei in the diencephalon and brainstem. Stimulation of these nuclei elicits a decrease in arterial pressure and heart rate, whereas lesions in the anterior hypothalamic area increase arterial pressure in SHRs. Furthermore, in SHRs, diets high in NaCl exacerbate hypertension, at least in part by reducing sympathoinhibitory drive from the anterior hypothalamic area.

Several regions of the forebrain have received considerable attention in relation to hypertension. Subcortical nuclei that have been described as playing a role in arterial pressure changes include the basal ganglia, the septal nuclei, and the amygdala. Of these areas, the amygdala, which regulates defense responses, has the closest linkage to hypertension. Cortical areas that appear to be involved in hypertension include the insular and cingulate cortices. These telencephalic areas are also involved in emotional responses and are most likely involved in forms of hypertension related to environmental stress.

SUGGESTED READING

1. Brooks VL, Osborn JW. Hormonal-sympathetic interactions in long-term regulation of arterial pressure: an hypothesis. *Am J Physiol.* 1995;268:R1343–R1358.

2. Ichihara A, Inscho EW, Imig JD, Michel RE, Navar LG. Role of renal nerves in afferent arteriolar reactivity in angiotensin-induced hypertension. *Hypertension.* 1997;29:442–449.

3. Loewy AD. Anatomy of the autonomic nervous system. In: Loewy AD, Speyer KM, eds. *Central Regulation of Autonomic Functions.* New York, NY: Oxford University Press; 1990:3–16.

4. McCarty R, Gold PE. Catecholamines, stress, and disease: a psychobiological perspective. *Psychosom Med.* 1996;58:590–597.

5. Oparil S, Chen YF, Berecek KH, Calhoun DA, Wyss JM. The role of the central nervous system in hypertension. In: Laragh JH, Brenner BM, eds. *Hypertension: Pathophysiology, Diagnosis and Management.* 2nd ed. New York, NY: Raven Press; 1995:713–740.

6. Reinhart GA, Lohmeier TE, Mizelle HL. Temporal influence of the renal nerves on renal excretory function during chronic inhibition of nitric oxide synthesis. *Hypertension.* 1997;29:199–204.

7. Wyss JM, Oparil S, Sripairojthikoon W. Neuronal control of the kidney: contribution to hypertension. *Can J Physiol Pharmacol.* 1992;70:759–770.

Chapter 43

The Sympathetic Nervous System in Human Hypertension

Joseph L. Izzo, Jr, MD

KEY POINTS

- In humans there is evidence of inappropriately high sympathetic nervous system (SNS) activity early and late in essential hypertension and in all forms of secondary hypertension.

- Increased SNS activity causes a spectrum of responses of cardiac output or vascular resistance depending on the type of CNS stimulation and the relative proportion of α- and β-receptors in a given individual.

- Age-related increases in SNS activity directly and indirectly promote vasoconstriction and hypertrophy of cardiac and vascular smooth muscle, which are at least partially reversible.

See also Chapters 33, 34, 35, 42, 128

Speculation that the autonomic nervous system is involved in the pathogenesis of chronic arterial hypertension can be found in the writings of Claude Bernard. Yet 150 years later there remains significant controversy about the precise role of the sympathetic nervous system (SNS) in long-term BP control in humans. There is little debate that acute stimulation of SNS control centers in animals or humans activates the heart and causes arteriolar and venous constriction, with a resulting increase in systemic BP. Where opinion has diverged, however, is whether or not the SNS can play an ongoing role in sustained BP elevation.

The SNS as Initiator of Early Hypertension

The prevalent current view suggests that the SNS is a critical initiating factor in human hypertension but plays little if any role in maintaining elevated BP chronically. In this analysis, hypertension begins as a syndrome of high cardiac output initiated by overactivity of cardiac sympathetic nerves. This hyperdynamic phase eventually gives way to a long-term phase of vascular adaptation that includes the "hallmark abnormality" of chronic hypertension: increased systemic vascular resistance. During the chronic phase, structural changes such as vascular hypertrophy are thought to be the sustaining forces for maintenance of high vascular resistance. With aging, cardiac function declines and vascular changes continue to progress, leading to further vasoconstriction.

It is noteworthy that this sympathetic-hemodynamic model, which was developed largely from animal studies, has little data to support it in humans. Julius and others have defined a group of younger hypertensive individuals with relatively high cardiac outputs, whose BPs were easily normalized by β-blockade. Yet the vast majority of hypertensives experience BP elevations in later life, usually beyond the age of 60. There is no evidence that these older hypertensives begin with a high cardiac output phase and for that matter, they do not respond as well as younger individuals to β-blockade.

The Alternate Model: the SNS as Facilitator of Chronic Hypertension

A less popular view, yet one much more consistent with clinical observations, is that the SNS not only plays an initiating role in hypertension but also contributes directly to the maintenance of the true hallmark abnormality in hypertension: a dynamic blend of inappropriately high cardiac output *and* inappropriately high systemic vascular resistance. The SNS is the only physiological system capable of instantaneous (eg, during postural change) and long-term BP control and is therefore the prime candidate to be an obligatory facilitator of chronic hypertension. The central position of SNS activation in BP regulation is shown in **Figure 43.1.** In this model, inappropriate SNS output causes both cardiac output and vascular resistance to be inappropriately high. Whether flow or resistance is predominantly elevated at any given moment is dependent on the type of CNS stimulation (mental stress, posture, cold, etc) and on the relative proportion of β-receptors (principally cardiac) and α-receptors (principally systemic vascular) in that individual. Variable patterns of hemodynamic stress responses can occur within and across individuals; these patterns are the subject of several new studies. For example, supranormal systemic resistance is the prevalent abnormality in hypertensives when they are studied resting in the supine position. However, supranormal cardiac output maintains elevated BP values in hypertensives when they are studied during upright posture.

A further adaptation of this integrated model is necessary to explain the effect of age on BP and systemic hemodynamics. Inappropriately high SNS output early in hypertension causes a relatively balanced increase in cardiac output and systemic resistance through roughly equal α- and β-receptor stimulation. The well-documented age-related decline in β-receptors is one mechanism underlying the age-related decrease in cardiac output. At the same time, age-related increases in SNS activity cause increased systemic resistance and cardiac impedance **(Figure 43.2)**. Age-related decrease in plasma renin activity may also be triggered by age-related loss of renal β-receptors.

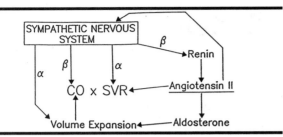

Figure 43.1. Central position of the sympathetic nervous system (SNS) in the control of blood pressure. Cardiac output (CO) and total systemic vascular resistance (SVR) are controlled by interacting adrenergic receptor influences. Renal α-adrenergic mechanisms, through vasoconstriction and tubular sodium retention, directly favor volume expansion. β_1-mediated increases in heart rate and renin release further enhance the "prohypertensive" effects of the SNS. Angiotensin II facilitates ongoing sympathoadrenal activity by central and peripheral mechanisms.

Evidence for SNS Overactivity in Chronic Hypertension

For the integrated model to be true, there must be abnormal or inappropriate SNS activity during all phases of essential hypertension. Attempts to study early and late hypertension in humans are confounded by genetic heterogeneity, the coincidence of aging, increased SNS activity, and BP elevation, and by different rates of "biological aging" in the population. Cost has been a barrier as well because studies of SNS function are very expensive.

Yet there are clear, well-conducted studies corroborating inappropriate SNS activity in all phases and forms of human hypertension. In early hypertension, there is general agreement that SNS overactivity exists as evidenced by elevated plasma norepinephrine (NE) concentrations, increased total-body NE spillover (as detected by radiotracer infusions), and increased muscle sympathetic nerve traffic (as demonstrated by direct peripheral nerve recordings).

In established hypertension, the relatively "normal" plasma NE values that are often present have been responsible in large measure for the conjecture that the SNS overactivity seen in earlier phases of the condition disappears chronically. Yet this interpretation requires further analysis. A strong argument can be made that "normal" values for plasma NE in the setting of increased systemic BP are actually *inappropriate* because plasma NE should be physiologically suppressed when BP is increased acutely or chronically. This implies, of course, that there are negative feedback mechanisms that control SNS outflow.

In studies using arteriolar dilators such as α-blockers or K-channel activators to normalize BP chronically (6 to 8 weeks) in essential hypertension, plasma NE doubled, suggesting that the SNS overactivity present in established hypertension had been suppressed by the chronic BP elevation itself and was unmasked when BP was lowered to normal levels (**Figure 43.3**). Note that ACE inhibition was not associated with the same patterns of SNS response to BP normalization, suggesting that renin-angiotensin blockade removes part of the stimulus to ongoing inappropriate SNS activation. The increases in plasma NE during vasodilator therapy also are consistent with the theory advanced by Chalmers and associates of "disinhibition failure," in which the primary abnormality in hyperten-

sion, SNS overactivity, is caused by the failure of inhibitory neurons to limit activity of SNS stimulatory cells in the rostral ventrolateral medulla.

Critics of this "inhibitory failure" argument believe that the SNS does not respond to negative feedback control by systemic BP and point to the fact that arterial baroreceptors "reset" rather quickly at any BP level. Resetting of arterial baroreflexes is part of the reason why "disinhibition failure" occurs. In addition, there is cardiopulmonary baroreflex dysfunction in hypertension. Cardiopulmonary baroreflexes are at least as important in chronic control of SNS out-

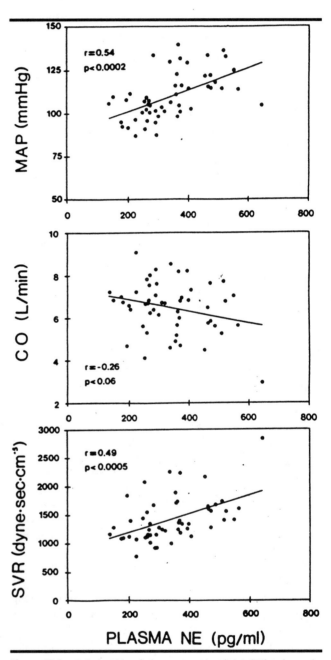

Figure 43.2. Relationship of plasma norepinephrine (NE) to hemodynamic variables. CO indicates cardiac output; SVR, systemic vascular resistance. Age and plasma NE are also related but plasma NE correlates better with hemodynamics than does age.

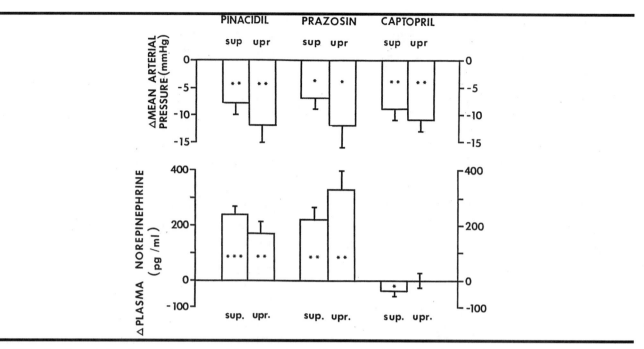

Figure 43.3. Despite equivalent decreases in mean arterial pressure, the arterial dilator pinacidil and the α-blocker prazosin increased plasma NE in both supine (sup.) and upright (upr.) positions. Captopril lowered supine plasma NE but did not change upright plasma NE. *$P < .05$, **$P < .005$, ***$P < .0005$ compared with placebo baseline values for each drug, probably due to the dependency of sympathetic nervous system outflow on angiotensin II.

flow. In a survey study of established hypertensives, a stronger inverse relationship was found between stroke volume and plasma NE than between arterial pressure and plasma NE, suggesting that cardiac stretch mechanisms have an important influence on chronic SNS outflow **(Figure 43.4)**. These data suggest that those with lower stretch volumes will have the greatest degree of inappropriate SNS outflow. Age-related decreases in cardiac function (and cardiac stretch) would also be expected to perpetuate inappropriate SNS outflow, which tends to increase in parallel with age and BP.

Further evidence of excessive specific SNS overactivity to specific organs in chronic hypertension has also been provided by organ-specific radiotracer spillover studies by Esler and colleagues, who have found markedly elevated cardiac and renal sympathetic activity in essential hypertension. Both of these influences would be expected to sustain the inappropriate level of cardiac output seen through increased preload, heart rate, and contractility. Studies demonstrating increased peripheral sympathetic nerve firing rates to the leg muscles in humans, though conducted in few subjects, corroborate the ongoing role of inappropriate SNS-mediated peripheral vasoconstriction in chronic hypertension.

Role of Mutual Reinforcement of the SNS and Renin-Angiotensin Systems on Vasoconstriction and Cardiovascular Hypertrophy

An important feature that underlies the maintenance of inappropriate SNS activity found in chronic hypertension is the mutually reinforcing effect of the SNS and renin-angiotensin systems (Figure 43.1). Renal sympathetic nerve traffic, as mediated by β_1-adrenergic receptors, is the major controller of J-G cell renin release. Subsequent increased generation of angiotensin II then acts centrally and pe-

ripherally to increase SNS outflow and catecholamine release. Teleologically, these mutually reinforcing pressor systems probably evolved to sustain humans during times of dehydration or hemorrhage. In modern times, however, and especially with longer life spans, they cause a disadvantage. These interactions must necessarily exist at a low level or there would be a runaway increase in systemic BP any time the organism was physiologically stimulated.

Structural changes induced by catecholamines and angiotensin II are additional factors perpetuating chronic hypertension. Recent investigations have demonstrated parallel growth-promoting or "trophic" influences of NE and angiotensin II on the heart and vascular smooth muscle. These two hormones thus contribute to long-term cardiac and vascular degenerative changes by causing acute and chronic increases in contractile forces and by promoting cardiac and vascular hypertrophy, which accentuate and maintain the elevated BP. It is increasingly recognized that these structural changes are at least partially reversible by pharmacological blockade of the ongoing influence of catecholamines and angiotensin II.

Pharmacological Evidence of Sustained SNS Overactivity in Hypertension

Among the strongest evidence for an ongoing role of the SNS in chronic hypertension is the body of pharmacological studies indicating that anti-adrenergic drugs consistently lower BP. In young hypertensives, β-blockade alone is often extremely effective. In early hypertension, increased vascular α-adrenergic tone has also been demonstrated by virtue of the supranormal responses of forearm blood flow to phentolamine (α_1-blockade). Perhaps most revealing is that central sympatholytic drugs or combined α,β-blockade lower BP (though not always to normal) in all forms of early and late

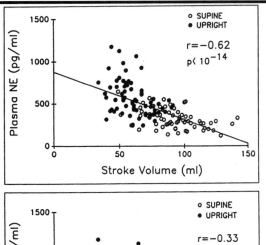

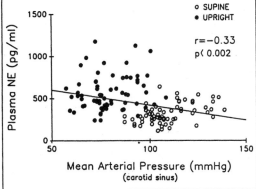

Figure 43.4. Top, Correlation between supine and upright plasma nor-epinephrine (NE) and corresponding values of stroke volume (used an in-dicator of cardiac stretch and cardiopulmonary baroreflex input). The high correlation coefficient (r=−.62) has extraordinary statistical significance (P< 10⁻¹⁴). When supine values alone are used (n=68), the negative cor-relation persists (r=−.43, P< .001), as it does for the corresponding up-right values of plasma NE and stroke volume (n=68, r=−.40, P<.001). Bottom, Correlation between plasma NE and estimated carotid sinus pressure (used as a measure of aortocarotid baroreflex input). This weaker relation than the one in Figure 43.4, top, reflects the lesser input of the carotid sinus on sympathetic nervous system activity.

essential hypertension. These observations attest to an ongoing functional contribution of the SNS in chronic hypertension.

SNS Overactivity in Secondary Forms of Hypertension

The universal permissive role of the SNS in chronic hyperten-sion is perhaps most dramatically illustrated by studies in animals and human demonstrating SNS overactivity in all forms of sec-ondary hypertension. In steroid-induced hypertension, alterations in central nervous BP control mechanisms and increased CNS sympathetic outflow are thought to maintain the elevated BP. In re-nal parenchymal hypertension, there is increased whole-body sympathetic outflow and abnormal peripheral catecholamine re-lease. In renovascular hypertension (Goldblatt model), early treat-ment with anti-sympathetic drugs prevents the development of sustained hypertension. Finally, in pheochromocytoma, the quint-essential catecholamine-dependent model of hypertension, re-moval of the tumor usually normalizes the BP. With the exception of pheochromocytoma, elevated BP levels in all hypertensive con-ditions are improved or fully controlled by the use of central sym-patholytic drugs. In pheochromocytoma and all forms of primary and secondary hypertension, combined α,β-blockade lowers or normalizes BP.

SUGGESTED READING

1. Esler M, Jennings G, Lambert G, Meredith I, Horne M, Eisenhofer G. Overflow of catecholamine neurotransmitters to the circulation: source, fate, and functions. *Physiol Rev.* 1990;70:963–985.
2. Goldstein DS, Kopin IJ. The autonomic nervous system and catecholamines in nor-mal blood pressure control and in hypertension. In: Laragh JH, Brenner BM, eds. *Hypertension: Pathophysiology, Diagnosis, and Management.* New York, NY: Raven Press Ltd;1990:711–747.
3. Izzo JL Jr, Smith RJ, Larrabee PS, Kallay MC. Plasma norepinephrine and age as de-terminants of systemic hemodynamics in men with established essential hyper-tension. *Hypertension.* 1987;9:415–419.
4. Izzo JL Jr, Licht MR, Smith RJ, Larrabee PS, Radke KJ, Kallay MC. Chronic effects of direct vasodilation (pinacidil), alpha-adrenergic blockade (prazosin) and angiotensin-converting enzyme inhibition (captopril) in essential hypertension. *Am J Cardiol.* 1987;60:303–308.
5. Izzo JL Jr. Sympathoadrenal activity, catecholamines, and the pathogenesis of vasculopathic hypertensive target-organ damage. *Am J Hypertens.* 1989; 2: 305S-312S.
6. Izzo JL Jr, Sander E, Larrabee PS. Effect of postural stimulation on systemic he-modynamics and sympathetic nervous activity in systemic hypertension. *Am J Cardiol.* 1990;65:339–342.
7. Mark AL. The sympathetic nervous system in hypertension: a potential long-term regulator of arterial pressure. *J Hypertens Suppl.* 1996;14:S159-S165.
8. Anderson EA, Sinkey CA, Lawton WJ, Mark AL. Elevated sympathetic nerve activ-ity in borderline hypertensive humans: evidence from direct intraneural record-ings. *Hypertension.* 1989;14:177–183.
9. Egan B, Panis R, Hinderliter A, Schork N, Julius S. Mechanism of increased alpha adrenergic vasoconstriction in human essential hypertension. *J Clin Invest.* 1987; 80:812–817.
10. Julius S, Mejia A, Jones K, Krause L, Schork N, van de Ven C, Johnson E, Petrin J, Sekkarie MA, Kjeldsen SE, et al. "White coat" versus "sustained" borderline hyper-tension in Tecumseh, Michigan. *Hypertension.* 1990;16:617–623.

Chapter 44

Hyperkinetic Hypertension and Vascular Hyperresponsiveness

Mark A. Creager, MD, Marie D. Gerhard, MD

KEY POINTS

- Many young borderline hypertensive patients have features consistent with increased sympathetic nervous system activity at rest, including rapid heart rate, high cardiac output, and increased stroke volume, and normal vascular resistance.

- Exaggerated increases in cardiac output during stress ultimately may result in structural vascular changes and contribute to the development of sustained hypertension.

- Structural changes in the blood vessel wall not only increase basal vascular resistance but further augment vascular responsiveness to vasoconstrictive stimuli.

- Angiotensin II and endothelin-1 act independently and together with the sympathetic nervous system to increase vascular resistance in patients with hypertension.

- Counterregulatory vasodilator functions may be reduced in patients with hypertension. In particular, endothelium-dependent vasodilation, mediated by nitric oxide, is impaired.

See also Chapters 37, 43, 45, 125

Blood pressure is determined by cardiac output and total peripheral resistance. Both cardiac hyperreactivity resulting in increased cardiac output and vascular hyperreactivity resulting in increased total resistance are found in hypertension. Although increased total resistance is a hallmark of established hypertension, it is less frequent in patients with borderline hypertension. In contrast, increased resting cardiac output is uncommon in established hypertension but common in borderline hypertension.

Hyperkinetic (Hyperdynamic) Hypertension

A hyperkinetic circulation has been well characterized in certain young borderline hypertensive patients. The hyperkinetic or hyperdynamic features in this group that suggest increased sympathetic nervous system activity include rapid heart rate, high cardiac output, and increased stroke volume with normal systemic vascular resistance. Type A behavior pattern, another state characterized by increased sympathetic drive, is often present in borderline patients. Also, plasma renin activity is elevated in this hyperkinetic subgroup, in keeping with the idea that the pathogenesis of the condition involves excessive β_1 adrenergic receptor stimulation.

Experiments with specific sympathetic antagonists and agonists provide additional evidence that a hyperkinetic circulation results from increased sympathetic drive. In borderline hypertensive subjects with high cardiac indices, sympathetic blockade with propranolol decreases cardiac output and reduces blood pressure. Furthermore, cardiogenic hypertension (as is found in persons with a hyperkinetic circulation) can be produced experimentally by interventions that chronically increase sympathetic activity and enhance myocardial contractility. In dogs, chronic sympathetic activation induced by either left stellate ganglion stimulation or intracoronary dobutamine infusion increases cardiac output and causes hypertension. Cardiac output and blood pressure return to normal with cessation of these stimuli.

Increased Vascular Adrenergic Tone

Peripheral adrenergic receptor responsiveness is increased in hypertensive subjects in comparison with age- and weight-matched control subjects. Phentolamine, an α-adrenergic receptor antagonist, decreases forearm vascular resistance to a greater extent in established hypertensive patients than in normotensive subjects. At high doses, intra-arterial norepinephrine, an α-adrenergic receptor agonist, causes greater vasoconstriction in hypertensive than in normotensive subjects. The vasoconstrictive response to increased doses of angiotensin II is also greater in hypertensive subjects, indicating that these responses may reflect generalized hyperreactivity of the resistance vessels.

Neurohumoral Interactions

The renin-angiotensin system may interact with or act independently of the sympathetic nervous system to increase vascular resistance in patients with borderline hypertension. Sympathetic efferent stimuli increase renal release of renin; conversely, angiotensin II facilitates neural release of norepinephrine. ACE inhibitors and angiotensin II antagonists reduce blood pressure in these persons, particularly when plasma renin activity is elevated.

Plasma levels of endothelin-1 are normal or slightly elevated in patients with hypertension. The vasoconstrictive response to endothelin-1 is depressed in subcutaneous resistance vessels of hypertensive patients studied in vitro, but the vasoconstrictive response to endothelin-1 is enhanced in hand veins of hypertensive patients in vivo. Moreover, endothelin-1 potentiates sympathetically mediated vasoconstriction in hypertensive but not normotensive subjects.

Endothelial dysfunction and vascular hyperreactivity

Increased vascular resistance in hypertension may occur when counterregulatory vasodilator functions are impaired. In particular, endothelium-dependent vasodilation, mediated by endothelium-derived nitric oxide, is abnormal in forearm and coronary resistance vessels of patients with hypertension. Vasodilator responses to acetylcholine, a drug that stimulates endothelial release of nitric oxide, are reduced in patients with hypertension and in their normotensive offspring. Also, the vasoconstrictive response to N^G-monomethyl-L-arginine, a nitric oxide synthase antagonist, is attenuated in hypertensive patients, implicating reduced contribution of nitric oxide to basal vascular resistance.

Linked Vascular Structural Changes

Structural changes in the blood vessel not only increase basal vascular resistance but also augment vascular responsiveness to vasoconstrictive stimuli. Increased systemic flow that results from excess cardiac responses to environmental stimuli ultimately may result in structural vascular changes and development of sustained hypertension. Arterioles undergo morphological modification in response to increased flow and pressure. As the media/lumen ratio increases, there is enhanced resistance to flow and an increase in blood pressure. Morphologic abnormalities may precede and potentially contribute to the development of hypertension. Capillary rarefaction and impaired dermal vasodilation to ischemia and heating have been observed in young adults with a family predisposition to high blood pressure.

SUGGESTED READING

1. Egan B, Panis R, Hinderliter A, Schork N, Julius S. Mechanisms of increased alpha adrenergic vasoconstriction in human essential hypertension. *J Clin Invest.* 1987;80:812–817.

2. Haynes WG, Hand MF, Johnstone HA, Padfield PL, Webb DJ. Direct and sympathetically mediated venoconstriction in essential hypertension: enhanced responses to endothelin-1. *J Clin Invest.* 1994;94:1359–1364.

3. Heagerty AM, Aalkjaer C, Bund SJ, Korsgaard N, Mulvany MJ. Small artery structure in hypertension: dual processes of remodeling and growth. *Hypertension.* 1993;21:391–397.

4. Julius S. Transition from high cardiac output to elevated vascular resistance in hypertension. *Am Heart J.* 1988;116:600–606.

5. Matsukawa T, Mano T, Gotoh E, Ishii M. Elevated sympathetic nerve activity in patients with accelerated essential hypertension. *J Clin Invest.* 1993;92:25–28.

6. Noll G, Wenzel RR, Schneider M, Oesch V, Binggeli C, Shaw S, Weidmann P, Luscher TF. Increased activation of sympathetic nervous and endothelin by mental stress in normotensive offspring of hypertensive parents. *Circulation.* 1996;93:866–869.

7. Noon, JP, Walker BR, Webb DJ, Shore AC, Holton DW, Edwards HV, Watt GC. Impaired microvascular dilatation and capillary rarefaction in young adults with a predisposition to high blood pressure. *J Clin Invest.* 1997;99:1873–1879.

8. Panza JA, Garcia CE, Kilcoyne CM, Quyyumi AA, Cannon RO III. Impaired endothelium-dependent vasodilation in patients with essential hypertension: evidence that nitric oxide abnormality is not localized to a single signal transduction pathway. *Circulation.* 1995;91:1732–1738.

9. Schiffrin EL. Endothelin: potential role in hypertension and vascular hypertrophy. *Hypertension.* 1995;25:1135–1143.

10. Taddei S, Virdis A, Mattei P, Ghiadoni L, Sudano I, Salvetti A. Defective L-arginine–nitric oxide pathway in offspring of essential hypertensive patients. *Circulation.* 1996;94:1298–1303.

Chapter 45

Hemodynamic Profiles and Responses

Fetnat Fouad-Tarazi, MD; Joseph L. Izzo, Jr, MD

KEY POINTS

- There is a wide spectrum of cardiac output and systemic vascular resistance in essential and secondary hypertension.

- Conditions with disproportionately high cardiac output include hyperdynamic hypertension, hemodialysis, and early diabetes.

- Conditions with disproportionately high vascular resistance include accelerated or malignant hypertension, advanced age, heart failure, hypovolemia, and steroid-induced hypertension

- Variable stress-induced hemodynamic responses depend on physiological factors (gender, etc) and on perceived state of well-being.

See also Chapters 37, 43, 44, 96, 125, 151

Arterial BP is always determined by the product of cardiac output (CO) and systemic vascular resistance (SVR). In both normotensive and hypertensive subjects, however, there is a wide spectrum of CO (about "Three-to-four fold range") with reciprocal changes in vascular resistance for any given level of BP. This hemodynamic heterogeneity exists both in the resting condition and in response to stimulation by physiological and psychological stressors.

General Considerations

Many factors can influence CO, including myocardial contractility and relaxation, circulating blood volume, venous return, and heart rate, which are in turn controlled by systemic neuroendocrine systems and modified by local factors. Although these factors are interdependent, there also may be predominant abnormalities in subtypes of persons with hypertension. Similarly, systemic and regional changes in resistance are determined by a variety of vasoconstrictor and vasodilator mechanisms including the sympathetic nervous system, the renin-angiotensin system, and local endothelial and vasomotor modulation. Arterial resistance is also dependent on the thickness of arterial walls because increased wall thickness magnifies the effects of normal vasoconstrictor stimuli. The interdependence of each of the parameters that determine flow and resistance is demonstrated by the effect of systemic sympathoadrenal stimulation, which simultaneously increases myocardial contractility, facilitates ventricular relaxation, increases heart rate, and increases peripheral vascular constriction while promoting renal sodium retention. The net result is a balanced increase in CO and SVR.

Resting Hemodynamic Profiles in Hypertensive Subtypes

Certain forms of hypertension are associated with: (1) high CO and low SVR, (2) mixed hemodynamic abnormalities with inappropriate CO and inappropriate vascular resistance, or (3) low CO and high SVR.

High-CO Hypertension

Hyperdynamic (hyperadrenergic") hypertension. A fraction of hypertensives, usually younger in age, manifest a syndrome of high CO and low SVR. They have an increased prevalence of essential hypertension in later life. Many of these individuals present with resting tachycardia while others present with increased systolic blood pressure and high stroke volume. There are no good estimates of prevalence of this condition, but given the age dependence of hypertension, the hyperdynamic subgroup probably comprises <5% of persons with essential hypertension. The cause of this condition is not fully known but is believed to result from excessive cardiac sympathetic nerve stimulation. These individuals respond well clinically to β-blockers and in unpublished data to ACE inhibitors.

Dialysis patients. Most persons with chronic renal failure exhibit a degree of volume expansion and sodium overload, particularly on interdialytic days. Both high heart rate and increased stroke volume are seen in this condition. Monotherapy with β-blockade is occasionally successful, but the improved efficacy of combined α- and β-blockade in these individuals also suggests that their hypertension is dependent in part on inappropriate increases in vascular resistance as well.

Diabetes mellitus (early phase). The early phases of diabetes are marked by a syndrome of increased CO with relatively normal SVR. The renal hyperperfusion and glomerular hyperfiltration that are so prevalent in diabetes may therefore be manifestations of a broader systemic problem of overperfusion. Increased renal perfusion pressure in these individuals is particularly responsive to therapy with ACE inhibitors, which have been shown to favorably affect the natural history of diabetic renal disease. β-blockers can also be used in diabetics as long as precautions are taken to instruct the individuals in alterations in signs of hypoglycemia (less tachycardia or sweating, etc).

Mixed Hemodynamic Abnormalities

Essential hypertension. The hallmark of essential hypertension is a combined abnormality of increased CO and increased SVR under different physiological conditions, as discussed elsewhere in this volume. Generally speaking, there is age dependency of the hemodynamics of essential hypertension, with higher CO values present in younger subjects and lower CO values present in the large number of older subjects who comprise the bulk of the population of hypertensives. Broad overlaps exist within these groups, however.

Pheochromocytoma. The balanced influence of circulating norepinephrine on CO and SVR is best demonstrated in pheochromocytoma, where neither increased CO nor increased SVR predominates hemodynamically. Appropriate BP lowering in pheochromocytoma requires combined α- and β-adrenergic blockade. In those rare cases of epinephrine-secreting pheochromocytoma, cardiac arrhythmias and hypotension are more common. This subgroup is more appropriately treated with isolated β-blockade.

Renovascular hypertension. The balanced effect of increased renin-angiotensin activity on systemic hemodynamics is demonstrated by the fact that angiotensin II–dependent hypertension in renal artery stenosis is associated with proportional increases in both CO and SVR. Appropriate blockade of the renin-angiotensin system causes a return of these proportional hemodynamic abnormalities toward normal.

High Vascular Resistance Hypertension

Accelerated and malignant hypertension. The most extreme example in human hypertension of severe vasoconstriction with normal or low CO occurs in the syndrome of accelerated or malignant phase hypertension. In these individuals, blood volume can be diminished by 30% to 40%. Although unproven, it seems likely that this volume contraction is in part due to long-term pressure diuresis with concomitant contraction of the circulating erythron mass. Further volume depletion in these cases, often caused by the introduction of diuretic therapy, can destabilize the precarious hemodynamic balance, leading to extraordinary degrees of additional vasoconstriction and further BP increases. This severe reflex vasoconstriction is mediated by increased activity of the sympathetic nervous and renin-angiotensin systems and may depend in part on failure of endothelial and other buffer mechanisms.

Treatment of accelerated and malignant hypertension requires that the clinician understand that severe hypovolemia and vasoconstriction coexist and that vasodilator therapies are first-line agents in this condition. After appropriate vasodilation, it is not uncommon to see a dramatic fall in hematocrit/hemoglobin as the erythron mass is diluted in the newly increased vascular space. Diuretics should be given with great caution to individuals with accelerated or malignant hypertension and in general should be reserved for those with pulmonary edema. After euvolemic status has been restored, however, diuretics may be useful adjunctive agents in the maintenance of normal BP.

Elderly hypertensives. Most older individuals with long-standing hypertension have low or normal CO and high SVR. Because most elderly individuals also have significant arteriosclerosis, the high SVR is manifested predominantly by an increase in systolic BP (isolated systolic hypertension). In this case, decreases in aortic compliance and the corresponding increases in reflected pulse waves cause increased systolic pressure and contribute substantially to left ventricular hypertrophy. Of note, these individuals tend to have low-renin status in conjunction with high vascular resistance, demonstrating

that low plasma renin activity is not necessarily associated with "volume overload." Appropriate vasodilator therapy such as thiazide diuretics and low doses of calcium antagonists tend to restore the hemodynamic profile toward normal.

Hypertension in Blacks. In contrast to the mixed hemodynamic patterns seen in whites, there is a tendency toward exaggerated increases in SVR in blacks. The mechanism for this difference is not known but may involve abnormalities in cellular transport mechanisms at the level of vascular smooth muscle. Appropriate vasodilator agents such as thiazides, calcium antagonists, and in some cases ACE inhibitors are effective in lowering BP. Monotherapy with β-blockers is less effective, presumably because CO is not abnormally high. These individuals also manifest low renin essential hypertension associated with systemic vasoconstriction that is independent of volume states.

Steroid-induced hypertension. It has been widely taught that hypertension due to steroid excess is associated with volume overload and increased CO. In the DOCA-hypertensive swine model, however, sympathetic overactivity causes a predominant increase in SVR rather than CO. Similar profiling in humans has not been done. Of note, blockade of the sympathetic nervous system centrally or peripherally returns the hemodynamic and BP abnormalities toward normal, while β-blockade is relatively ineffective as monotherapy in this condition.

Vasoconstrictive syndromes without hypertension. Other syndromes of intense vasoconstriction without hypertension are worth mentioning because their existence demonstrates that the coexistence of inappropriately high CO and systemic resistance is necessary for sustained BP elevations. The most obvious example of "normotensive vasoconstriction" is systolic dysfunction (heart failure), where cardiac contractility is insufficient to maintain an elevated BP despite marked increase in sympathetic activity, renin-angiotensin activity, and systemic resistance. Syndromes of hypovolemia are other circumstances in which decreased ventricular filling and the associated low CO prevents systemic BP from rising despite marked vasoconstriction induced by sympathoadrenal and renin-angiotensin activation. In the uncommon syndrome of idiopathic hypovolemia, unknown mechanisms promote chronic renal salt loss. The associated orthostatic hypotension, which occurs despite intense vasoconstriction, may require the use of fludrocortisone and central sympatholytic agents.

Hemodynamic Responses to Acute Stressors

One of the most important areas in which further investigation is required is the area of hemodynamic stress responses of the cardiovascular system, particularly in hypertension. Emerging work in the field indicates that the pattern of hemodynamic response to a given stimulus is a function of genes, other physiological states, the diseases present in the individual, and other psychological and environmental influences. Dynamic exercise, the most common stimulus used to date, either in the form of treadmill or bicycle exercise, uniformly increases CO. Essential hypertensives or those with a parental history of hypertension, however, exhibit significantly less exercise-induced vasodilation than their normotensive counterparts and also exhibit a trend toward a supranormal CO response as well.

Different experimental stressors used in the laboratory tend to produce predominant patterns of response but with significant heterogeneity. For example, premenopausal women respond to mental arithmetic predominantly with increases in CO, whereas their male counterparts respond generally with increases in vascular resistance. Postmenopausal women tend to respond similarly to men, supporting a role of estrogen in modifying the hemodynamic impact of stress. Acute stress responses are also dependent on endothelial function, as discussed in the chapter on Endothelial Dysfunction. Thus, cigarette smoking, dyslipidemia, insulin resistance, and other factors can influence the hemodynamic response to stress. Finally, caffeine and other agents can accentuate stress responses.

Recent work indicates that the "state of well-being" of the individual is an important determinant of hemodynamic responses. For example, perception of a task as a threat causes a systemic vasoconstrictive response, whereas perception of a task as a challenge causes a vasodilation-CO response. Of interest, either pattern may occur within the same individual depending on whether the stimulus was perceived as a threat or challenge. Another aspect of perception or "state of well-being" that affects hemodynamics is the available social support level. Those individuals who have effective social support systems tend to perceive stimuli as challenges and respond with increases in CO. Individuals with low levels of social support, on the other hand, tend to perceive stimuli as threats and respond with increased vascular resistance. Logistic regression techniques showed that social support and perceptive mechanisms were more predictive of response patterns than family history of hypertension. The role of

additional personality factors in hemodynamic responses remains unclear at this time.

SUGGESTED READING

1. Lund-Johansen P, Omvik P. Hemodynamic patterns of untreated hypertensive disease. In: Laragh JH, Brenner BM. *Hypertension: Pathophysiology, Diagnosis, and Management.* New York, NY: Raven Press Ltd; 1990:305–327.
2. Zambraski EJ, Ciccone CD, Izzo JL Jr. The role of the sympathetic nervous system in 2-kidney DOCA-hypertensive Yucatan miniature swine. *Clin Exp Hypertens [A].* 1986;8:411–424.
3. Safar ME, Weiss YA, Levenson JA, London GM, Milliez PL. Hemodynamic study of 85 patients with borderline hypertension. *Am J Cardiol.*1973;31:315–319.
4. Julius S, Randall OS, Esler MD, Kashima T, Ellis C, Bennett J. Altered cardiac responsiveness and regulation in the normal cardiac output type of borderline hypertension. *Circ Res.* 1975;37(suppl 1):199–207.
5. Sung BH, Wilson MF, Izzo JL Jr, Ramirez L, Dandona P. Moderately obese, insulin-resistant women exhibit abnormal vascular reactivity to stress. *Hypertension.* 1997; 30:848–853.
6. Allen K, Shykoff BE, Izzo JL Jr. Cognitive appraisal of threat or challenge predicts hemodynamic responses to mental arithmetic and speech tasks. *Am J Hypertens.* 1998;11:134A. Abstract.
7. Shykoff BE, Allen K, Izzo JL Jr. Interactions of social support and family history in blood pressure reactivity to psychological stressors. *Am J Hypertens.* 1998;11:135A. Abstract.
8. Frohlich ED, Tarazi RC, Dustan HP. Hyperdynamic beta-adrenergic circulatory state: increased beta-receptor responsiveness. *Arch Intern Med.* 1969;123:1–7.
9. Fouad FM, Tadena-Thome T, Bravo EL, Tarazi RC. Idiopathic hypovolemia. *Ann Intern Med.* 1986:104:298–303.
10. Tarazi RC, Dustan HP, Frohlich ED, Gifford RW Jr, Hoffman GC. Plasma volume and chronic hypertension: relationship to arterial pressure levels in different hypertensive disease. *Arch Intern Med.* 1970;125:835–842.

Chapter 46

Obesity

Lewis Landsberg, MD

KEY POINTS

- Hypertension and obesity are closely linked: blood pressure increases with increasing body weight, and the incidence of hypertension among the obese approaches 50%.

- Obesity and hypertension frequently occur in a risk factor constellation that includes insulin resistance and a characteristic dyslipidemia (low HDL cholesterol, high triglycerides).

- The pathophysiology of obesity-related hypertension is complex and involves insulin resistance, salt sensitivity, and the sympathetic nervous system.

- Treatment should be directed at decreasing overall cardiovascular risk by use of weight loss and other lifestyle modifications as important components of therapy.

See also Chapters 47, 93, 94, 144

Epidemiology and Importance

The relationship between hypertension and obesity is well documented. As shown in **Figure 46.1,** from the Framingham study, the prevalence of hypertension in men and women as a function of age increases substantially with increases in relative weight, so that the prevalence of hypertension is almost 50% in the most obese groups. It is well established, moreover, that this association does not reflect "cuff artifact" imposed by increased arm circumference, nor does the relationship depend on increased salt intake in the obese. Recent weight gain, however, is a very important factor in the development of hypertension. In the Framingham study, obesity or recent weight gain accounted for 70% of new-onset hypertension. It is abundantly clear, therefore, that obesity is a major factor in the development of hypertension.

Body fat distribution also plays a critical role as a risk factor for hypertension. Observations made >50 years ago by Vague that the cardiovascular and metabolic consequences of obesity were most marked in individuals with the abdominal or upper-body form of obesity were confirmed in the mid-1980s by large-scale epidemiological studies from Scandinavia. An increase in waist-to-hip ratio or abdominal circumference **(Figure 46.2)**, surrogate markers for the upper-body fat pattern, is an independent risk factor for the development of high blood pressure and is independently associated with other cardiovascular risk factors.

Risk Factor Constellation (Metabolic Syndrome, Insulin Resistance Syndrome, Syndrome X)

Both obesity and hypertension independently increase cardiovascular risk. Hypertension and upper body obesity, moreover, are part of a larger risk factor constellation that includes, as additional major manifestations, insulin resistance and a characteristic dyslipidemia (low HDL cholesterol and high triglycerides), type II diabetes

mellitus, salt sensitivity, microalbuminuria, small dense (atherogenic) LDL, and prothrombotic coagulation abnormalities. These additional factors increase the likelihood of adverse cardiovascular events, thereby accentuating the danger imposed by both obesity and hypertension.

Pathophysiology of Obesity-Related Hypertension

The relationship between obesity and blood pressure is not explained adequately by hemodynamics. Although it is true that the obese have an increased blood volume and increased cardiac output compared with lean individuals, these variables normalize when corrected for the increased body mass. Peripheral resistance, moreover, is elevated in obese hypertensives compared with obese normotensives. Intake of sodium in the obese is frequently greater than in lean individuals, but increased sodium intake is not a sufficient explanation for the hypertension, because weight loss in obese hypertensive individuals decreases blood pressure even when salt intake is undiminished.

The shift in the pressure-natriuresis curve in the obese, implied by salt sensitivity, may be secondary to the effects of increased insulin and sympathetic nervous system activity on sodium reabsorption. Insulin levels track with hypertension in the obese, and insulin has been demonstrated to be antinatriuretic. Obese persons have increased sympathetic nervous system activity, and sympathetic activation at the level of the kidneys and the vasculature exerts a hypertensive effect. The origin of sympathetic hyperactivity in obesity may be related to hyperinsulinemia, because insulin stimulates the sympathetic nervous system, but other factors may contribute as well.

Treatment

The goal of therapy is global cardiovascular risk reduction, which includes lowering blood pressure and addressing other risk factors. The threshold for treatment and the goal blood pressure should follow standard Joint National Committee VI guidelines, which take into

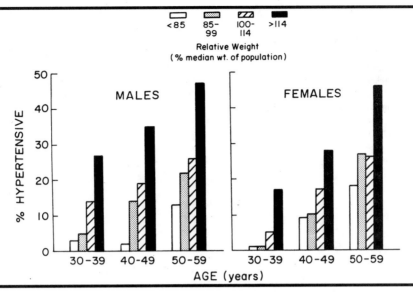

Figure 46.1.   Prevalence of hypertension (systolic >160 mm Hg or diastolic >95 mm Hg) by age and sex in four relative weight groups at the first Framingham Heart Study examination. All trends are significant at *P*=.05. Reprinted from Kannel et al. The relation of adiposity to blood pressure and development of hypertension: the Framingham study. *Ann Intern Med.* 1967;67:48–59 with permission.

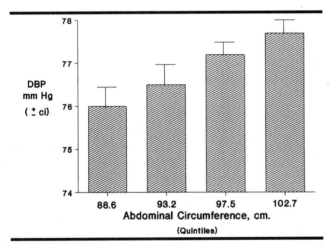

Figure 46.2.   Diastolic blood pressures ±95% CIs are shown for 1972 subjects from the Normative Aging Study as a function of abdominal circumference. Note that blood pressure and abdominal girth increased together. Data from Cassano PA, Segal MR, Vokonas PS, Weiss ST. Body fat distribution, blood pressure, and hypertension: a prospective cohort study of men in the normative aging study. *Ann Epidemiol.* 1990;1:33–48. Figure reprinted from Landsberg L. Obesity and hypertension: experimental data. *J Hypertens.* 1992;10:S195-S201 with permission.

Table 46.1.   Relative Effectiveness of Nonpharmacological Measures in Hypertension

	BLOOD PRESSURE REDUCTION	CORONARY PROTECTION
Weight control	+++	++
Alcohol reduction*	+++	+
Salt restriction	++	?
Moderate exercise	++	++
Vegetarian-like diets†	+	++
Dietary fish	+	+++
Stopping smoking	−	++

*Reducing from 4 or 5 to 1 or 2 drinks a day.
†Low-fat, fruit and vegetables.
From Beilin L. "Non-pharmacological management of hypertension optimal strategies for reducing cardiovascular risk." *J Hypertens.* 1994;12(suppl 10):S71-S81.

account the presence of target organ damage and concurrent disease as well as the risk factor profile. In general, obese hypertensive patients are at high risk because of their associated risk factors.

Lifestyle modification, particularly weight loss, plays a central role in blood pressure lowering and risk reduction **(Table 46.1)**. Caloric restriction, a sensible exercise regimen, and salt and alcohol reduction have the greatest impact on blood pressure, whereas smok-

ing cessation and restriction in dietary fat have the greatest impact on coronary artery disease. Caloric restriction and exercise, moreover, will diminish insulin resistance and associated sympathetic nervous system hyperactivity, thereby modifying the underlying pathophysiology in a favorable manner. In many obese hypertensives, pharmacological agents will be required for adequate blood pressure control, although lifestyle modification continues to play an important adjunctive role in these patients.

Most of the currently used drugs have demonstrated efficacy in obesity-related hypertension. Treatment should be individualized depending on target organ damage, concomitant disease, and the risk factor profile. Calcium channel blockers, ACE inhibitors, and α-blockers do not worsen and may actually improve the metabolic abnormalities common in obese hypertensive patients.

SUGGESTED READING

1. Grassi G, Seravalle G, Cattaneo BM, Bolla GB, Lanfranchi A, Colombo M, Giannattasio C, Brunani A, Cavagnini F, Mancia G. Sympathetic activation in obese normotensive subjects. *Hypertension.* 1995;25:560–563.

2. Kannel WB, Brand N, Skinner JJ Jr, Dawber TR, McNamara PM. The relation of adiposity to blood pressure and development of hypertension: the Framingham study. *Ann Intern Med.* 1967;67:48–59.

3. Krieger DR, Landsberg L. Obesity and hypertension. In: Laragh JH, Brenner BM, eds. *Hypertension: Pathophysiology, Diagnosis, and Management.* 2nd ed. New York, NY: Raven Press Ltd; 1995:2367–2388.

4. Reaven GM, Lithell H, Landsberg L. Hypertension and associated metabolic abnormalities: the role of insulin resistance and the sympathoadrenal system. *N Engl J Med.* 1996;334:374–381.

5. Reisin E, Abel R, Modan M, Silverberg DS, Eliahou HE, Modan B. Effect of weight loss without salt restriction on the reduction of blood pressure in overweight hypertensive patients. *N Engl J Med.* 1978;298:1–6.

6. Tuck ML, Sowers J, Dornfeld L, Kledzik G, Maxwell M. The effect of weight reduction on blood pressure, plasma renin activity, and plasma aldosterone levels in obese patients. *N Engl J Med.* 1981;304:930–933.

Chapter 47

Insulin Resistance and Hypertension

Helmut O. Steinberg

KEY POINTS

- Insulin resistance (IR) is a risk factor for the development of hypertension and cardiovascular disease.

- The prevalence of IR is $\approx$ 20% in the United States.

- IR is almost always associated with a cluster of cardiovascular risk factors, including obesity, dyslipidemia, dysfibrinolysis, endothelial dysfunction, salt sensitivity, and hypertension.

- IR is associated with increased vascular reactivity.

See also Chapters 46, 93, 94, 144

Insulin resistance (IR) is a potent risk factor for the development of cardiovascular diseases. IR is defined as the inability of the body to achieve normal rates of glucose uptake in response to insulin. IR occurs at multiple organ sites, including the liver, fat, and skeletal muscle cells, this last organ being the most important on a quantitative basis. The "gold standard" for the quantification of IR is the euglycemic hyperinsulinemic clamp technique, which under steady-state conditions measures the glucose uptake into skeletal muscle. With IR progression, there is increasing fasting hyperinsulinemia, another hallmark of IR.

Prevalence

IR often occurs in association with a cluster of other metabolic abnormalities, such as impaired glucose tolerance, type II diabetes mellitus, obesity, low HDL cholesterol, elevated triglyceride and free fatty acid levels, and hypertension. This clustering of cardiovascular risk factors has been named "insulin resistance syndrome" or "syndrome X" and is associated with a 2- to 3-fold increase in rates of cardiovascular morbidity and mortality.

IR and essential hypertension are common in the American population. More than 45 million subjects exhibit IR, which is seen mostly in obese and type II diabetic subjects, and hypertension is found in nearly 60 million Americans. Whether IR is one cause of hypertension or whether both conditions result from a more basic defect remains unanswered.

IR and essential hypertension are polygenic conditions (ie, one or several sets of genes contribute to their expression). To add even more complexity, the expression of both hypertension and IR is modified by environmental factors, such as diet and degree of activity. If IR and hypertension genes were independent, one would expect the incidence of the combination of IR and hypertension in patients to exceed that predicted by chance.

Prospective studies have demonstrated that hypertension develops more often in subjects with hyperinsulinemia than in subjects with normal insulin levels. This finding indicates that IR is a risk factor for hypertension. Furthermore, cross-sectional studies also have shown that IR is accompanied by hypertension more often than expected by chance alone. IR is found in up to 50% of hypertensive subjects, and nearly 50% of obese subjects exhibit hypertension. Taken together, these findings provide evidence that IR and hypertension are strongly linked.

The link between IR and hypertension is further supported by the observation that worsening of IR through weight gain or sedentary life style is associated with higher incidence of hypertension. Conversely, maneuvers that decrease IR, such as weight loss or exercise, diminish blood pressure levels. Furthermore, drugs that improve insulin sensitivity (such as troglitazone) have also been reported to lower blood pressure. Importantly, the lowering of blood pressure in response to these drugs was independent of weight loss or increased levels of exercise.

The mechanism by which IR predisposes to hypertension is unknown. It has been suggested that elevated insulin levels per se cause blood pressure elevation. At the cellular level, insulin stimulates a number of ion channels/pumps regulating intracellular sodium and calcium. Intracellular Ca^{2+} is one determinant of vascular smooth muscle cell tension and contractility in response to vasopressor substances. Increased ion fluxes due to elevated insulin levels were initially thought to play a role in the development of hypertension in IR.

However, insulin is a vasodilator substance in vivo. Recent data indicate that Ca^{2+} flux into vascular smooth muscle cells and into platelets is actually decreased by insulin. Importantly, this insulin action to reduce Ca^{2+} influx is impaired in IR and thus could contribute to the development of hypertension.

At the level of the whole organism, both insulin and leptin (a hormone produced by fat cells in proportion to fat mass) increase sympathetic nervous system activity, and it has been shown that obese IR (hyperinsulinemic and hyperleptinemic) subjects exhibit higher sympathetic nervous system activity. Increased activity of the sympathetic nervous system can lead to elevation of cardiac output and peripheral vasoconstriction, which could cause a rise in blood pressure. Another possible mechanism thought to be responsible for the development of hypertension is the acute ability of insulin to cause sodium and volume retention. However, more recent studies have suggested that elevated insulin levels per se are most likely not the cause of hypertension.

Insulin administered to normal subjects even in high pharmacological doses does not cause blood pressure elevation but often results in a small but significant decrease in blood pressure. Furthermore, insulin attenuates the pressor effects of the pressor hormones norepinephrine and angiotensin II in normal insulin-sensitive but not in IR subjects. These findings demonstrate that in insulin-sensitive subjects, insulin modulates vascular reactivity and acts as a vasodepressor agent. In fact, insulin is a potent vasodilator of skeletal muscle vasculature in insulin-sensitive but not in IR subjects. The vasodilator action of insulin is mediated, in part, through the release of nitric oxide, a potent endogenous vasodilator. Nitric oxide also displays a host of antiatherogenic properties, suggesting that decreased production or release of endothelial nitric oxide in IR could explain, at least in part, the higher rates of hypertension and macrovascular diseases in IR.

IR could cause hypertension via the following hypothetical steps. Early in the course of IR, the production/release of nitric oxide decreases, and responses to pressor hormones become exaggerated. Later, with progressive obesity and IR, hyperinsulinemia and hyperleptinemia increase, causing higher sympathetic nervous system activity and perhaps sodium and water retention. It is also possible that increased catecholamine levels in hypertensives exacerbate IR. In either case, the vasodepressor system is impaired in IR, and the unopposed higher sympathetic nervous system activity, the heightened reactivity to pressors, and the retention of sodium and water could lead to hypertension. However, this hypothetical scenario has not yet been fully experimentally confirmed.

SUGGESTED READING

1. Baron AD. Hemodynamic actions of insulin. *Am J Physiol.* 1994;267:E187-E202.
2. Ferrannini E, Buzzigoli G, Bonadonna R, Giorico MA, Oleggini M, Graciadei L, Pedrinelli R, Brandi L, Bevilacqua S. Insulin resistance in essential hypertension. *N Engl J Med.* 1987;317:350–357.
3. Haffner SM, Valdez RA, Hazuda HP, Mitchell BD, Morales PA, Stern MP. Prospective analysis of the insulin-resistance syndrome (syndrome X). *Diabetes.* 1992;41: 715–722.
4. Reaven GM. Banting lecture 1988: role of insulin resistance in human disease. *Diabetes.* 1988;37:1595–1607.
5. Steinberg HO, Chaker H, Leaming R, Johnson A, Brechtel G, Baron AD. Obesity/insulin resistance is associated with endothelial dysfunction: implications for the syndrome of insulin resistance. *J Clin Invest.* 1996;97:2601–2610.

Chapter 48

Salt Sensitivity

Myron H. Weinberger, MD

KEY POINTS

- Increased salt intake does not raise blood pressure in all hypertensive persons.

- Sensitivity to dietary salt intake is greatest in hypertensive persons with obesity, low renin status, increased sympathetic nervous activity, or renal insufficiency.

- Older, black, and diabetic hypertensive persons are often salt sensitive.

- Salt sensitivity can be demonstrated in some normotensive persons.

See also Chapters 47, 90, 123, 118, 124

Alterations in sodium balance and extracellular fluid volume have heterogeneous effects in normotensive and hypertensive humans. Studies in relatively large groups of subjects have yielded inconsistent evidence for a relationship between salt and blood pressure (BP), yet when individual responses are examined, most studies demonstrate that BP in some individuals is responsive (or "sensitive") to manipulation of sodium, whereas others are resistant.

Several different approaches to the identification of salt responsivity have been reported. These studies have revealed characteristics associated with salt sensitivity and resistance of BP as well as some evidence regarding the mechanisms that may be involved. Recently, genetic factors have been identified that may simplify the recognition of salt sensitivity.

Clinical Investigation

Clinical Studies

Anecdotal observations relating excessive salt intake to raised BP were followed by population studies confirming this relationship. Social groups that typically ingest <50 to 100 mEq/d of sodium (or chloride) have a substantially lower incidence of both hypertension and its cardiovascular consequences than groups in whom habitual sodium chloride intake is higher. Other characteristics that may differentiate these groups are physical activity, body mass, genetic factors, calcium and potassium intake, and other lifestyle components.

Interventional efforts have not consistently demonstrated a decrease in BP when dietary sodium intake is reduced. This has led some to conclude that sodium is not an important factor in the pathogenesis of essential hypertension but has stimulated others to examine for individual differences in BP responses to salt.

Techniques for the Evaluation of Salt Responsivity

Kawasaki and colleagues studied 19 hypertensives during 1 week of low sodium intake (9 mEq/d) followed by 1 week of high sodium intake (249 mEq/d). Nine subjects who had a mean arterial BP on the last day of the high-sodium period >10% greater than that on the last day of the low-sodium intake were defined as salt sensitive, and the remainder were called salt insensitive. The BP at the end of the high-salt period was not significantly different from that observed during a normal-sodium (109-mEq/d) diet in either group. The difference between the salt-sensitive and the salt-insensitive populations was primarily the degree of BP reduction during the low-salt diet compared with baseline measures.

Our group examined the BP responses of 375 normotensives and 192 essential hypertensives using a reproducible protocol of rapid sodium and extracellular volume expansion. Intravenous infusion of 2 L of normal (0.9%) saline over a 4-hour period was followed on the next day by sodium and volume depletion induced by a low-sodium (10-mEq/d) diet and enhanced by three doses of 40 mg furosemide. The mean arterial BP on the morning after sodium and volume depletion was compared with that after the saline infusion. A decrease in mean arterial pressure of ≥10 mm Hg was designated as salt sensitive, and a decrease of ≤5 mm Hg (or an increase in mean arterial pressure) after sodium and volume depletion was designated as a salt-resistant response. Decreases in mean arterial pressure of 6 to 9 mm Hg were deemed indeterminate. The responses to this protocol were congruent with those of longer periods of dietary sodium manipulation and are reproducible.

Characteristics of Salt Responsivity

Clinical groups with salt sensitivity are shown in the **Table 48.1.** It has been suggested that impaired renal sodium handling may be responsible for salt sensitivity of BP, but this possibility has not been convincingly demonstrated.

In addition to the greater prevalence of salt sensitivity in older individuals, a recent study has demonstrated that salt sensitivity in normotensive subjects is associated with a significantly greater age-related increase in BP than in salt-resistant subjects, implying that the age-related rise in BP may be a reflection of salt sensitivity. Some studies suggest that salt-sensitive subjects have enhanced sympathetic nervous system activity. A more consistent abnormality, relative renin suppression, also called low-renin hypertension, may play a permissive role in the BP response to sodium depletion by reducing the degree of counterregulatory vasoconstrictive response to this challenge.

Table 48.1. Clinical Groups with Enhanced Salt Sensitivity

Older persons
Low-renin hypertensives (including blacks)
Diabetics
Persons with renal failure
Persons with increased sympathetic activity

A blunting of the renin response to volume depletion may explain the enhanced fall in BP with a low-salt diet, but it does not account for the rise in BP with salt loading. The influence of sodium balance on pressor responses to vasoactive substances provides a potential explanation for the enhanced rise in BP during a high-salt diet in persons with increased catecholamine or renin levels. It has been proposed that the renal dopaminergic system may have a role in modulating renal sodium excretion and the BP response to sodium loading. It has also been suggested that it is the chloride rather than sodium that is responsible for the rise in BP; of the dietary sources of sodium, >95% is in the form of sodium chloride.

Finally, correlation of different degrees of BP sensitivity to salt in subjects with differing haptoglobin, α-adducin, or β-adrenergic receptor phenotypes suggests that salt sensitivity may have a genetic basis. A better understanding of the genetic basis for this finding may help prevent hypertension in predisposed persons.

SUGGESTED READING

1. Campese VM, Romoff MS, Levitan D, Saglikes Y, Friedler RM, Massry SG. Abnormal relationship between sodium intake and sympathetic nervous system activity in salt-sensitive patients with essential hypertension. *Kidney Int.* 1982;21:371–378.
2. Gill JR Jr, Grossman E, Goldstein DS. High urinary dopa and low urinary dopamine-to-dopa ratio in salt-sensitive hypertension. *Hypertension.* 1991;18:614–621.
3. Kawasaki T, Delea CS, Bartter FC, Smith H. The effect of high-sodium and low-sodium intakes on blood pressure and other related variables in human subjects with idiopathic hypertension. *Am J Med.* 1978;64:193–198.
4. Kurtz TW, AL-Bander HA, Morris RC Jr. "Salt-sensitive" essential hypertension in men: is the sodium ion alone important? *N Engl J Med.* 1987;317:1043–1048.
5. MacGregor GA. Sodium is more important than calcium in essential hypertension. *Hypertension.* 1985;7:628–640.
6. Rankin LI, Luft FC, Henry DP, Gibbs PS, Weinberger MH. Sodium intake alters the effects of norepinephrine on blood pressure. Hypertension 1981;3:650–656.
7. Weinberger MH, Fineberg NS. Sodium and volume sensitivity of blood pressure: age and pressure change over time. *Hypertension.* 1991;18:67–71.
8. Weinberger MH, Miller JZ, Fineberg NS, Luft FC, Grim CE, Christian JC. Association of haptoglobin with sodium sensitivity and resistance of blood pressure. *Hypertension.* 1987;10:443–446.
9. Weinberger MH, Miller JZ, Luft FC, Grim CE, Fineberg NS. Definitions and characteristics of sodium sensitivity and blood pressure resistance. *Hypertension.* 1986;8(suppl II):II-127-II-134.
10. Weinberger MH. Salt sensitivity of blood pressure in humans. *Hypertension.* 1996;27:481–490.

Chapter 49

Divalent Cations in Essential Hypertension

Lawrence M. Resnick, MD

KEY POINTS

- Hypertension, cardiac hypertrophy, insulin resistance, obesity, and type II diabetes are all characterized by similar alterations of intracellular free calcium and magnesium content.

- An ionic model can be used to describe all forms of hypertension, which is the net combination, present to a variable extent in different subjects, of extracellular calcium-dependent (salt-sensitive, high α-adrenergic activity, low-renin) and intracellular calcium release–dependent (salt-insensitive, high-renin) pressor mechanisms.

- Dietary salt and calcium have opposite effects on blood pressure due to their reciprocal, hormone-mediated promotion/suppression, respectively, of cellular calcium uptake, from the extra cellular space.

- Identifying the predominant operative calcium (hormone) mechanism predicts blood pressure responsiveness to dietary and antihypertensive drug therapies.

See also Chapters 25, 92, 131, 132

Hypertension is one sign of heterogeneous pathophysiological events that only appear clinically as a uniform entity. Focussing on steady-state cellular ion activity as a final common pathway mediating blood pressure (BP) homeostasis and tissue responsiveness, hypertension is best understood as one manifestation of a generalized cellular ionic defect, which is expressed in other tissues as insulin resistance, hyperinsulinemia, left ventricular hypertrophy, increased platelet aggregation, enhanced sympathetic nerve activity, and accelerated atherosclerotic disease, all components of what has been called syndrome X. Furthermore, the activity of ion-active hormone systems appears to underlie the heterogeneous responses to dietary minerals, nutrients, and antihypertensive drugs observed in different subjects.

Intracellular Calcium and Magnesium as Determinants of Blood-Pressure, Vascular, and Metabolic Disturbances

In vascular smooth muscle, plasma membrane depolarization-induced T- and L-channel Ca^{2+} current and subsequent Ca^{2+} release from the sarcoplasmic reticulum elevates cytosolic free Ca^{2+} levels ($[Ca^{2+}]_i$) and trigger a cascade of molecular rearrangements of calmodulin and myosin light-chain kinase, ultimately leading to myofilament shortening and vasoconstriction. Conversely, vasorelaxation involves cellular Ca^{2+} egress and Ca^{2+} reuptake into sarcoplasmic reticulum stores. Similar Ca-related events also regulate a wide spectrum of cellular responses, including cardiac function, hormone secretion, renal ion excretion, and neural excitation. Levels of $[Ca^{2+}]_i$ and intracellular free Mg ($[Mg^{2+}]_i$) are reciprocally related. Mg buffers the constrictor and other effects of $[Ca^{2+}]_i$, and cellular Mg deficiency leads to enhanced Ca-induced cell stimulation and vasoconstriction.

Clinically, elevated $[Ca^{2+}]_i$ levels and/or suppressed $[Mg^{2+}]_i$ levels have been found in essential hypertension, obesity, and type II diabetes. Quantitatively, the higher the $[Ca^{2+}]_i$ and the lower the $[Mg^{2+}]_i$, the more elevated the BP, cardiac hypertrophy, vascular stiffness, hyperinsulinemia, insulin resistance, and abdominal visceral fat mass. Hence, each of the above aspects of hypertensive disease appears to reflect a shared cellular ionic lesion defined at least in part by excess steady-state $[Ca^{2+}]_i$ and reciprocally suppressed $[Mg^{2+}]_i$ levels. According to this ionic hypothesis, for example, rather than hypertension "causing" insulin resistance, or conversely, insulin resistance and hyperinsulinemia causing hypertension, it is more likely that each represents altered responses of different tissues to the same altered intracellular ionic environment (**Figure 49.1**).

Extracellular Regulation of Intracellular Divalent Ions

The intracellular ionic environment common to hypertension and the other conditions mentioned above is influenced extracellularly by environmental factors that affect ion-active hormone systems (**Table 49.1**).

Circulating Divalent Cations and the Renin-Angiotensin System

Low-renin hypertensive subjects exhibit significantly lower serum ionized Ca^{2+} and calcitonin levels and reciprocally higher serum Mg, parathyroid hormone (PTH), and 1,25-dihydroxyvitamin D (1,25D) levels compared with normotensive or other hypertensive subjects. High-renin subjects exhibit oppositely skewed values. These deviations in divalent cation metabolism in both directions away from normotensive values suggest an extracellular Ca^{2+} deficiency in low-renin subjects, and in high-renin subjects, a Ca^{2+} surfeit.

How can the uniform elevations of $[Ca^{2+}]_i$ levels in all hypertension be reconciled with the heterogeneous deviations, both higher and lower than normotensive values, of extracellular Ca^{2+} and Mg^{2+} ion and hormone levels among different subjects?

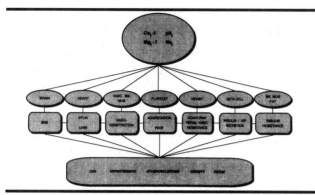

Figure 49.1. Ionic hypothesis of cardiovascular and metabolic disease, in which multiple disease entities (bottom) are clinical manifestations of underlying cellular ion abnormalities shared in common (top) but expressed differently in different organ systems (middle) (see text).

Dietary Salt, Dietary Ca, and Intracellular Divalent Cations. Since $[Ca^{2+}]_i$ levels reflect the steady-state equilibrium between exchange of systolic Ca with extracellular Ca, and with intracellular Ca stores, elevated $[Ca^{2+}]$ in hypertension implies, by definition, an altered participation of at least one of these two calcium equilibria, present in varying degrees in different subjects and under different circumstances in the same subject **(Figure 49.2).** Thus, volume excess or high-salt diets may transiently lower extracellular Ca^{2+}, increasing levels of Ca hormones such as 1,25D and other factors such as digitalis-like molecules and parathyroid hypertensive factor. These Ca-active hormones stimulate extracellular Ca uptake intracellulary, promoting vasoconstriction and suppressing renal renin release. BP remains unchanged as long as steady-state $[Ca^{2+}]_i$ levels also remain unchanged, the increased salt-induced extracellular Ca component of $[Ca^{2+}]_i$ offset by an equal and opposite suppression of renin-stimulated angiotensin II–dependent, intracellular Ca^{2+} release. Conversely, a low dietary salt intake, associated with a more positive Ca^{2+} balance, a transient rise of extracellular Ca, and a fall in Ca-regulating hormones, digitalis-like factors, etc, result in opposite responses. Here, the fall in extracellular Ca^{2+}-dependent Ca^{2+} entry is precisely offset by reciprocal increases in the intracellular Ca^{2+}-release component of $[Ca^{2+}]_i$, mediated by appropriate stimulation of the renin-angiotensin system. Again, BP is maintained, constant.

Thus, BP and cellular Ca homeostasis are coordinately regulated in a seesaw fashion. BP homeostasis remains intact unless an increase in the activity of one $[Ca^{2+}]_i$-regulating mechanism, extracellular Ca^{2+} entry or intracellular Ca^{2+} release, either exceeds the limits of physiological compensation (eg, primary aldosteronism, low-renin essential hypertension, unilateral renal artery stenosis, renin-secreting tumors) or fails to cause a sufficient reciprocal suppression of its companion Ca_i mechanism (eg, Nl-high renin or nonmodulating hypertension, bilateral renal artery stenosis, preeclampsia, and malignant hypertension). For example, in salt-sensitive subjects, salt loading reproduces the cellular ionic-hormonal profile of the low-renin subject, with extracellular Ca^{2+}-dependent, high-1,25D, digitalis-like factor, α-adrenergic activity–mediated increased $[Ca^{2+}]_i$ and BP and reciprocally decreased serum $[Ca^{2+}]_i$ and $[Mg^{2+}]_i$ levels.

The importance of extracellular Ca^{2+} and Ca^{2+} hormones in hypertension is demonstrated by the effects of (1) oral Ca^{2+} supplementation, which physiologically suppresses Ca^{2+} ionophoric hor-

Table 49.1 Evidence of Altered Divalent Cation Metabolism in Hypertension

Epidemiology
  Increased incidence/prevalence of hypertension with decreased dietary Ca and/or Mg intake
  Relation of salt to BP selectively in subjects with low calcium intakes
  Increased urinary Ca relative to Na
Pathophysiology
  Intracellular
    Elevated steady-state fasting $[Ca^{2+}]_i$/suppressed $[Mg^{2+}]_i$
    BP $\propto [Ca^{2+}]_i, \propto (-)[Mg^{2+}]_i$
  Extracellular
    Opposite deviations in different renin forms of hypertension
    Low-renin hypertension
      Decreased Ca-io, calcitonin
      Increased Mg-o, PTH, 1, 25D
    High-renin hypertension
      Increased Ca-io, calcitonin
      Decreased Mg-o, PTH, 1, 25D
  Salt-sensitive hypertension
    $\Delta BP \propto$ salt-induced $\Delta 1,25D, \Delta[Ca^{2+}]_i, (-)\Delta [Mg^{2+}]_i, (-) \Delta Ca$-io
  Other risk factors in hypertension are $\propto$ fasting
  $[Ca^{2+}]_i, \propto (-) [Mg^{2+}]_i$
    LV mass
    Arterial stiffness
    Abdominal visceral fat
    Insulin resistance
    $HbA_{I}c$ and fasting blood sugar in normal and Type II diabetic subjects
Therapy
  PO calcium can lower BP
    Preferentially effective in low-renin, salt-sensitive, elderly subjects
    Lowers 1,25D, $[Ca^{2+}]_i$
    $\Delta BP \propto$ Ca-io, PRA, $\propto (-)$ 1, 25D, $(-)$ UNaV
  All antihypertensive drugs reverse the elevated $[Ca^{2+}]_i$ and/or decreased $[Mg^{2+}]_i$ of hypertension
    $\Delta BP \propto \Delta[Ca^{2+}]_i, (-) \Delta[Mg^{2+}]_i$

mones such as 1,25D and parathyroid hypertensive factor; (2) Ca^{2+} antagonists, which directly block extracellular Ca^{2+} uptake; and (3) α-adrenergic antagonists to reverse the ionic and BP effects of salt. Indeed, these three maneuvers are effective clinically in lowering pressure among elderly, low-renin, salt-sensitive subjects.

Role of Glucose and Insulin in Regulating Intracellular Ions

Hyperglycemia, after oral ingestion or in vitro, raises $[Ca^{2+}]_i$ and lowers $[Mg^{2+}]_i$ levels, thus reproducing the abnormal intracellular ionic "profile" found in both diabetes and hypertension. Indeed, because fasting glucose and HbA_{Ic} levels in nondiabetic and diabetic subjects closely predict fasting $[Ca^{2+}]_i, [Mg^{2+}]_i$, and BP levels, glucose levels even within the normal range may be one physiological determinant of basal $[Ca^{2+}]_i$ and $[Mg^{2+}]_i$ content and thus of basal vascular tone. Insulin, independent of glucose, also has primary ionic effects, raising $[Mg^{2+}]_i$ and under some circumstances, $[Ca^{2+}]_i$ in vascular and other tissues. In hypertension, these ionic actions are blunted in direct proportion to the deviation of basal $[Ca^{2+}]_i$ and $[Mg^{2+}]_i$ values from normal, demonstrating not only that insulin resistance is an ionic phenomenon but that it is only one example of ion-dependent alterations of cell responsiveness.

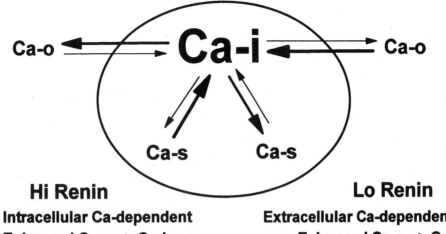

Dual Calcium Mechanisms in Hypertension

Ca-o ← **Ca-i** ← → **Ca-o**

Ca-s   **Ca-s**

Hi Renin
Intracellular Ca-dependent
Enhanced Ca-s --> Ca-i
BP ∝ Ca-i ∝ Ca-o
Salt insensitive

Lo Renin
Extracellular Ca-dependent
Enhanced Ca-o --> Cai
BP ∝ Ca-i ∝ (-)Ca-o
Salt sensitive

$$BP \propto (Ca\text{-}i) = f\,(Ca\text{-}o) + g\,(Ca\text{-}s)$$

Figure 49.2. Dual Ca mechanisms in hypertension, in which an inappropriate excess cytosolic free Ca (Ca-i) can result alternatively from either enhanced, eg, salt-dependent, extracellular Ca (Ca-o, right) transport intracellularly or from enhanced, eg, angiotensin II–mediated intracellular Ca release from intracellular Ca stores (Ca-s, left). Primary increases in Ca-i from either source may be at least partially offset by a secondary increase in Ca extrusion from cytosol into Ca stores (right) or into extracellular space (left). Altogether, net blood pressure (BP) is proportional to ambient steady-state $[Ca^{2+}]_i$ level, which is, in turn, determined by reciprocating contributions of each Ca source, defined here as f(Ca-o) and g(Ca-s) (bottom) (see text).

Table 49.2 Equivalent Descriptions of Blood Pressure Homeostasis

Clinical/physiological level:
BP = volume × vasoconstriction
(salt) × (renin)

Tissue/organ level:
BP = cardiac output × peripheral resistance
(C.O.) × (T.P.R.)

Cellular/ionic level:
BP = k$[Ca^{2+}]_i$ = k {f (Ca-o) × g (Ca-s)}
(extracellular Ca) × (cellular ca stores)

$[Ca^{2+}]_i$ cytosolic free intracellular calcium; Ca-o, extracellular ionized calcium; Ca-s, intracellular Ca stores; k, proportionality factor (either a constant or a function of other non-calcium, eg, magnesium-reltated variables) describing blood pressure as a function of $[Ca^{2+}]_i$ (and thus BP) level.
At each level of description above, the two terms on the right, defining blood pressure (salt, elevations of one calling forth a reduction in the other, the resulting blood pressure remaining constant (see text).

In summary, it is now possible to describe blood pressure at the cellular level in a manner equivalent to older formulations (**Table 49.2**), as a reciprocating homeostatic balance between intracellular Ca^{2+} stores and extracellular Ca^{2+} entry– dependent, Mg^{2+}-buffered processes. Hypertension is then best understood as a multisystem disease manifested clinically by elevated BP and other tissue consequences of an inappropriate, unbalanced ionic state, defined at least in part by excess $[Ca^{2+}]_i$ and deficient $[Mg^{2+}]_i$ values.

SUGGESTED READING

1. Altura BM, Altura BT, Gebrewold A, Ising H, Günther T. Magnesium deficiency and hypertension: correlation between magnesium-deficient diets and microcirculatory changes in situ. *Science.* 1984;223:1315–1317.
2. Barbagallo M, Gupta RK, Bardicef O, Bardicef M, Resnick LM. Altered ionic effects of insulin in hypertension: role of basal ion levels in determining cellular responsiveness. *J Clin Endocrinol Metab.* 1997;82:1761–1765.
3. Erne P, Bolli P, Bürgissen E, Bühler FR. Correlation of platelet calcium with blood pressure: effect of antihypertensive therapy. *N Engl J Med.* 1984;310:1084–1088.
4. Hunt SC, Williams RR, Kuida H. Different plasma ionized calcium correlations with blood pressure in high and low renin normotensive adults in Utah. *Am J Hypertens.* 1991;4:1–8.
5. Laragh JH, Resnick LM. Recognizing and treating two types of long-term vasoconstriction in hypertension. *Kidney Int Suppl.* 1988;25:S162-S174.
6. Resnick LM, Gupta RK, DiFabio B, Barbagallo M, Mann S, Marion RM, Laragh JH. Intracellular ionic consequences of dietary salt loading in essential hypertension: relation to blood pressure and effects of calcium channel blockade. *J Clin Invest.* 1994;94,1269–1276.
7. Resnick LM, Gupta RK, Laragh JH. Intracellular free magnesium in erythrocytes of essential hypertension: relation to blood pressure and serum divalent cations. *Proc Natl Acad Sci USA.* 1984;81 6511–6515.
8. Resnick LM, Laragh JH, Sealey JE, Alderman MH. Divalent cations in essential hypertension: relations between serum ionized calcium, magnesium, and plasma renin activity. *N Engl J Med.* 1983;309:888–891.
9. Resnick LM, Müller FB, Laragh JH. Calcium-regulating hormones in essential hypertension: relation to plasma renin activity and sodium metabolism. *Ann Intern Med.* 1986;105:649–654.
10. Resnick LM. Ionic disturbances of calcium and magnesium metabolism in essential hypertension. In: Laragh JH, Brenner BM, eds. *Hypertension: Pathophysiology, Diagnosis, and Management.* 2nd ed. New York, NY: Raven Press; 1995:1169–1193.

Chapter 50

Experimental Models of Hypertension

Donald J. DiPette, MD

KEY POINTS

- Because human hypertension is heterogeneous, several animal models have been developed to mimic its many facets.

- Hypertension can be produced by various vascular, renal, adrenal, brain, and genetic manipulations.

- Newer molecular techniques have become increasingly important in the development of animal models to determine the involvement of a particular gene or genetic locus in hypertension.

The difficulty in studying a disease process such as hypertension begins with the fact that the etiology of hypertension is heterogeneous. Hypertension can be primary ("essential") or secondary to a defined process, such as renal artery stenosis. The pathophysiology of essential hypertension is also heterogeneous and varies by renin status, sodium dependency, etc. Therefore, a spectrum of experimental animal models of hypertension has been developed to aid in our investigation of both essential hypertension and secondary forms of hypertension.

Genetic Animal Models of Experimental Hypertension

Genetic models of experimental hypertension developed to approximate the pathogenesis of human essential hypertension include the spontaneously hypertensive rat (SHR), the SHR-stroke-prone strain, Dahl salt-sensitive and salt-resistant rat strains, Milan hypertensive and normotensive rat strains, and Lyon hypertensive and normotensive rat strains. Although these models may differ in genetics, cellular alterations, or neurohumoral mechanisms, under appropriate conditions they all share one thing: the spontaneous development of an elevation of blood pressure. The two most commonly studied are the SHR and the Dahl salt-sensitive and -resistant strains.

The SHR was developed in 1959 by Okamoto and Aoki through selective inbreeding of Wistar-Kyoto normotensive rats. In 1970, Okamoto and Aoki developed the SHR-stroke-prone rat strain from the SHR. Both these strains develop hypertension spontaneously, without additional modalities such as salt loading, and also develop target organ complications such as cerebrovascular (especially the stroke-prone strain), cardiovascular, and renal complications. As in human essential hypertension, the pathogenesis of the SHR appears to be heterogeneous; cellular, central nervous system, neurohumoral, and renal abnormalities have been proposed. The SHR is a "normal-renin" model, and its blood pressure is relatively sodium independent (ie, only a modest blood pressure rise is seen after an excess sodium diet). More recently, a substrain SHR that is salt sensitive has been developed in which a central nervous system mechanism may be involved in the sodium dependency.

As with any experimental model, there has been intense debate over the applicability of the SHR to human essential hypertension. Part of this debate revolves around the appropriate normotensive control for the SHR. Most investigators use the normotensive Wistar-Kyoto rat, which can vary genetically among differing colonies and suppliers. The model remains useful in studies of the target organ complications of hypertension and in screening of potential pharmacological antihypertensive agents. More recently, the genetic basis for the SHR has been under intense investigation. At least three, and possibly more, gene loci are thought to be involved, one of which may be in close association with the angiotensinogen gene. It has been speculated that a similar multiple gene interaction is involved in human essential hypertension.

The Dahl salt-sensitive and corresponding salt-resistant strains were developed in 1961 from the normotensive Sprague-Dawley strain. In contrast to the SHR, genetic and environmental factors are involved in the development of hypertension in the Dahl salt-sensitive strain. In this regard, increased dietary sodium is required for the rapid and full development of the blood pressure elevation. Typically, when a low-salt diet ($\approx$0.4% NaCl) is consumed, both the salt-sensitive and salt-resistant Dahl rats will remain normotensive. However, when both strains are placed on a high-salt diet (8% NaCl), only the Dahl salt-sensitive rats exhibit a blood pressure rise within 4 to 6 weeks of salt administration. Because salt is necessary to induce the full expression of the hypertension, most attention to the mechanism responsible for the blood pressure elevation has centered on the role of the kidney. As would be expected in view of the sodium dependency, the Dahl salt-sensitive strain is a "low-renin" experimental model.

Renal Artery Stenosis

Two classic animal models of renovascular disease have been developed in multiple species by constriction of one or both of the renal arteries, and they are named after the pioneering work of Goldblatt and colleagues. The two models are the "two-kidney, one-clip" and the "one-kidney, one-clip" Goldblatt hypertension models. Importantly, both animal models have human hypertensive counterparts.

In the two-kidney, one-clip model, both native kidneys are intact, but a constricting clip (to resemble a clinical stenosis) is placed on one renal artery (usually the left in the rat model). Depending on the degree of constriction, the blood pressure may reach levels >200 mm Hg systolic. In the absence of damage to the contralateral nonclipped kidney, this model is a classic renin-dependent model, at least in its early phases. During this initial period, administration of an ACE inhibitor or an angiotensin II receptor antagonist or removal of the renal artery clip will result in abrupt lowering of the blood pressure. However, if the hypertension is allowed to persist, the contralateral kidney (and probably other organs) undergoes significant damage, and removing the clip on the clipped kidney may have little effect on the hypertension. It is important to note that this same scenario is seen clinically in patients with prolonged unilateral renal artery stenosis with renovascular hypertension and an intact nonstenosed kidney.

In the one-kidney, one-clip model, complete unilateral nephrectomy is followed by a constricting renal artery clip on the remaining kidney. This model resembles patients who have only a solitary kidney and a significant renal artery stenosis in that remaining kidney (ie, a congenital solitary kidney, previous surgical nephrectomy, a renal transplant with stenosis, or a thrombosed kidney with subsequent kidney loss). This model may also approximate the pathophysiology of bilateral renal artery stenosis. In contrast to the two-kidney, one-clip model, in which plasma renin activity is significantly elevated and the hypertension is clearly renin-dependent, in the one-kidney, one-clip model, the plasma renin activity is increased only in the first few days after renal artery constriction. After this initial phase, the plasma renin activity decreases into the normal range. Furthermore, in this chronic phase, blockade of the renin-angiotensin system does not significantly decrease the blood pressure. Conversely, if aggressive diuresis with accompanying sodium depletion is achieved, the model becomes renin dependent again. Thus, in this model there is interplay between early activation of the renin-angiotensin system and sodium retention in that both are required for the full development and maintenance of the hypertension. It is important to note that a similar pathophysiology is seen in the clinical counterparts of this model.

Renal Parenchymal Hypertension

Clinically, the most common secondary cause of hypertension is a loss of renal function from any cause (diabetes mellitus, glomerular diseases, etc). As many as 90% to 95% of patients entering dialysis have hypertension. The animal model that most closely approximates this clinical condition is the renal mass reduction-salt-induced model, most commonly studied in the rat and dog. In this model, a renal mass reduction of ≈85% is required. To accomplish this, a unilateral nephrectomy is followed by surgical removal of ≈66% of renal mass from the remaining kidney. This degree of mass reduction is usually accompanied by biochemical evidence of renal insufficiency (ie, an increased blood urea nitrogen or serum creatinine). By itself, this degree of renal mass reduction results in only a slight blood pressure increase over sham-operated, normotensive control animals. To further exacerbate the increase in blood pressure to hypertensive levels, excess salt is usually administered in the drinking water or in the diet. Thus, the renal mass reduction-salt-induced hypertensive model is another example of a sodium-dependent, low-renin model. Interestingly, blockade of the renin-angiotensin system with ACE or AT-1 receptor antagonist results in a lowering of blood pressure. Explanations for this apparent paradox include effects of anti-renin-angiotensin drugs on the local tissue renin-angiotensin systems, the sympathetic nervous system, the vasopressin system, and/or an increase in vasodilators, such as calcitonin gene-related peptide, and substance P.

Although not as commonly used for experimental purposes, there are many other renal animal models of experimental hypertension, such as renal ischemic models, perinephric ("renal wrap") hypertension, and the chronic administration of angiotensin II ("angiotensin-induced hypertension").

Adrenal Models of Experimental Hypertension

The most common adrenal model studied is the mineralocorticoid-salt or deoxycorticosterone-salt model. This model resembles the clinical situation of aldosterone excess (Conn's syndrome) from an adrenal adenoma or bilateral zona glomerulosa hyperplasia. Typically, this model is produced in differing animal strains by a surgical uninephrectomy followed by excess mineralocorticoid (usually deoxycorticosterone) and salt (usually 0.9% NaCl drinking water) administration. After these manipulations, the blood pressure rises (within a few weeks) into the hypertensive range. If left untreated, the hypertension will transform to a progressive phase accompanied by weight loss and target-organ damage. If a more gradual blood pressure rise is wanted, the kidneys can be left intact. This model is a sodium-dependent, low-renin experimental model. As in other models, nonsodium mechanisms have been suggested to play a role in the full development of the hypertension, including sympathetic nervous system activation, renin-angiotensin and vasopressin activation, disturbances of cation transport and homeostasis (such as calcium), and enhanced vascular reactivity. This model, in conjunction with the renin-dependent two-kidney, one-clip Goldblatt model, is useful to study dependency on the renin-angiotensin system of a given therapeutic agent.

In addition to excess aldosterone production, excess production of glucocorticoids, such as cortisol (Cushing's syndrome or disease), clinically leads to secondary hypertension. Glucocorticoid-induced hypertension, the animal model that approximates this clinical situation, is produced by the administration of excess glucocorticoid to the normotensive animal. The rat has been the most commonly used species. Unlike some of the other models, no other manipulation, such as surgery and/or salt administration, is necessary. Although the blood pressure rises to hypertensive levels, it usually does not reach as high a level as that seen in other experimental models. As with other models, the mechanism of the blood pressure elevation is most likely multifactorial. The blood pressure is extremely difficult to treat pharmacologically, often requiring blockade of multiple pressor systems. The adrenal cortex produces other steroid hormones, such as the sex steroids, which may also participate in blood pressure regulation. As with glucocorticoids, these hormones can be manipulated experimentally with adrenalectomy and/or can be given in excess by exogenous administration.

The adrenal medulla produces the catecholamines epinephrine and norepinephrine. Excess catecholamine production accompanied by hypertension is seen in the clinical syndrome of pheochromocytoma. Models of pheochromocytoma include the chronic exogenous administration of catecholamines and the New England Deaconess pheochromocytoma tumor-bearing rat. There are other models of adrenal experimental hypertension, such as adrenal regeneration.

Neural Models of Experimental Hypertension

The brain is a major target organ of the hypertensive process, and it also plays a major role in blood pressure regulation and the pathophysiology of hypertension. There are many neural models of experimental hypertension. The stroke-prone SHR is often used to investigate the pathophysiology of cerebrovascular disease. For example, dietary potassium supplementation has recently been shown to decrease the frequency of stroke, independently of blood pressure, in this experimental model. Other neurally induced models of experimental hypertension include the surgical manipulation of specific brain areas, such as the periventricular (AV3V) region, and peripheral sinoatrial deafferentation. Recently, borderline hypertension has been modeled as well.

Other Models of Experimental Hypertension

A great deal of recent investigation of hypertension has revolved around the molecular basis of hypertension and the use of molecular biology techniques. Some studies have used antisense oligonucleotides targeted to knock out a specific mRNA and thus delete a given protein. Others use whole-animal transgenic technology to either knock out or overexpress a particular gene. This technology has led to the recent development of a knockout model of the angiotensin ATII receptor as well as mice that overexpress the renin gene. Currently, a great deal of ongoing investigation is targeted at identifying the gene or genes that contribute to an increase in blood pressure. Experimental animal models are integral to these efforts. Newer animal models may arise from studies that attempt to segregate genetic hypertensive markers by use of "congenic methodology," which uses repetitive inbreeding, resulting in a generation of animals that is almost entirely devoid of or entirely contains a certain genetic locus. Thus, the blood pressure phenotype can be correlated with the presence or absence of a certain locus. It is interesting to note that even

with these newer molecular techniques, the elucidation of the genes that may contribute to hypertension is far from complete. Multiple other models using these techniques will be developed and will aid the investigation of the hypertension. For example, manipulation of nitric oxide, particularly its inhibition with N^{ω}-nitro-L-arginine methyl ester, has led to newer models of experimental hypertension, including pregnancy-induced hypertension.

SUGGESTED READING

1. Bohr DF, Dominiczak AF. Experimental hypertension. *Hypertension.* 1991;17 (suppl I):I-39-I-44.
2. DiPette DJ, Simpson K, Rogers A, Holland OB. Haemodynamic response to magnesium administration in mineralocorticoid-salt and two-kidney, one-clip renovascular hypertension. *J Hypertens.* 1988;6:413–417.
3. Gavras H, Brunner HR, Thurston H, Laragh JH. Reciprocation of renin dependency with sodium volume dependency in renal hypertension. *Science.* 1975;188: 1316–1317.
4. Kreutz R, Higuchi M, Ganten D. Molecular genetics of hypertension. *Clin Exp Hypertens.* 1992;14:15–34.
5. Laragh JH, Brenner BM. *Hypertension: Pathophysiology, Diagnosis, and Management.* New York, NY: Raven Press; 1990.
6. Mockrin SC, Dzau VJ, Gross KW, Horan MJ. Transgenic animals: new approaches to hypertension research. *Hypertension.* 1991;17:394–399.
7. Phillips MI. Antisense inhibition and adeno-associated viral vector delivery for reducing hypertension. *Hypertension.* 1997;29(pt 2):177–187.
8. Smithies O. Theodore Cooper Memorial Lecture: a mouse view of hypertension. *Hypertension.* 1997;30:1318–1324.
9. Tobian L. Salt and hypertension: lessons from animal models that relate to human hypertension. *Hypertension.* 1991;17(suppl I):I-52-I-58.
10. Yamori Y. Overview: studies from spontaneous hypertension: development from animal models toward man. *Clin Exp Hypertens.* 1991;13:631–644.

Chapter 51

Pathophysiology of Renovascular Hypertension

Luis Gabriel Navar, PhD; David W. Ploth, MD

KEY POINTS

- Reduced renal perfusion pressure resulting from stenosis of the arterial vasculature in one or both kidneys causes unilateral or bilateral renovascular hypertension.

- Activation of the renin-angiotensin system contributes to the pathophysiology of both bilateral and unilateral renovascular hypertension through systemic and renal effects.

- Increased angiotensin II blunts the kidney's ability to excrete a salt load, sustaining the elevation of blood pressure.

See also Chapters 5, 41, 129, 130, 141, 153

Sustained elevations in arterial pressure caused by stenosis, constrictions, or lesions of the arterial supply to one or both kidneys are categorized as renovascular hypertension. The derangements may be quite variable, ranging from overt renal arterial stenosis of one or both renal arteries to subtle microvascular alterations that are not easily detectable clinically. When the degree of stenosis results in marked impairment of renal perfusion and glomerular filtration rate (GFR), the resulting hypertension is characterized by failure to maintain adequate renal excretion of water and electrolytes, sodium retention, and expansion of extracellular fluid volume similar to chronic renal insufficiency. Subtle alterations in the renal vasculature that may be present in only one kidney can result in sustained hypertension even though overall renal perfusion and GFR are only slightly reduced or even unchanged. In unilateral renal vascular impairment, it is quite intriguing that hypertension is not prevented by the presence of one normal kidney. Thus, there are pathophysiologically significant interactions between the kidneys that permit sustained hypertension.

There are two main types of renovascular hypertension: unilateral renovascular involvement and symmetrical, or bilateral, renovascular involvement, which also includes conditions in which there is only one remaining kidney, as in renal transplant patients with stenosis of the transplanted kidney. In large part, the resultant hypertension is due to inappropriate increases in the activity of the renin-angiotensin system, which can exert powerful and long-lasting intrarenal and systemic actions. Although other hormonal and neural mechanisms are also involved, the renin-angiotensin system appears to be of critical importance in the mediation of both unilateral and bilateral renovascular hypertension, but the mechanisms are different.

Bilateral Renal Vascular Hypertension

Bilateral renal hypertension involves a stenosis or lesion in the vasculature of both kidneys or of a single remaining kidney that reduces glomerular perfusion pressure and compromises renal blood flow. The stenosis can be caused by arteriosclerotic vascular disease of the renal artery, fibromuscular dysplasia, external compression by a tumor, or stenosis at the anastomosis in transplanted kidneys. This condition can also be caused by microvascular lesions due to diffuse arteriosclerosis or arteritis of the intrarenal vasculature. Experimentally, this condition is elicited by placing constrictive clips on both renal arteries or on the aorta proximal to the origin of the renal arteries.

The critical initiating event is the decrease in renal perfusion pressure with or without marked or sustained reductions in renal blood flow and GFR. Reductions in renal arterial pressure down to the range of 70 to 80 mm Hg will not cause sustained decreases in renal blood flow and GFR because the kidneys are able to maintain renal hemodynamic function by autoregulatory adjustments of preglomerular vascular tone. Nevertheless, the reduced intrarenal perfusion pressure markedly compromises sodium excretory capability.

The initial phase in bilateral renal hypertension involves an increased release of renin, resulting in increased systemic and intrarenal generation of angiotensin I. Angiotensin I is rapidly converted to angiotensin II by angiotensin-converting enzyme present on endothelial cells of many tissues and particularly abundant in the lungs. Angiotensin II causes generalized systemic vasoconstriction, increases aldosterone release, and elicits other actions that attempt to restore elevated renal perfusion pressure distal to the stenosis. Subsequent intrarenal pressure increases and then diminishes the stimulus for renin release.

With time, the angiotensin dependency of the systemic hypertension is also markedly attenuated because of progressive retention of salt and water, leading to expansion of extracellular fluid volume and blood volume. Salt and water retention occurs for at least two reasons. Because all of the functional renal mass is subjected to reduced perfusion pressure, there is a direct pressure-dependent effect causing reduced sodium excretion related to the pressure-natriuresis phenomenon (**Figure 51.1**). This phenomenon serves as the critical link between arterial pressure and sodium excretion. For any given hormonal and neural setting, there is a direct relationship between arterial pressure and the rate of sodium excretion. In the presence of bilateral renal arterial stenosis, the reduced intrarenal pressure directly lowers sodium excretion and minimizes sodium excretory responsiveness to natriuretic stimuli activated by volume expansion. Furthermore, the reduced renal perfusion pressure increases renal renin activity and local generation of angiotensin II.

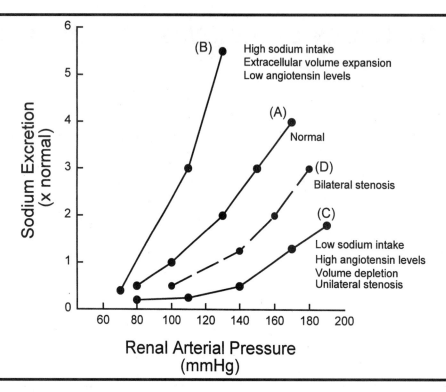

Figure 1. Relationship between renal arterial pressure and sodium excretion for normal conditions, high angiotensin states, and reduced angiotensin states. The increase in sodium excretion in response to an increase in renal arterial pressure is referred to as pressure natriuresis and serves as the critical link between the regulation of arterial pressure and the renal regulation of sodium balance and extracellular volume. In bilateral renal vascular hypertension, the curve is shifted to the right (curve D) because of the reduced intrarenal perfusion pressure. In unilateral renovascular hypertension, the curve for the stenotic kidney is shifted to the right (curve D), and the relationship in the nonstenotic kidney remains inappropriately suppressed because of elevated intrarenal angiotensin II levels (curve C).

The increased intrarenal angiotensin II activity elicits vasoconstrictor effects on the kidney, directly stimulates net tubular sodium reabsorption, and increases sodium retention via increased aldosterone levels. These changes are synergistic with the direct effects of reduced perfusion pressure to cause sodium and water retention, leading to expansion of the extracellular and intravascular compartments. The progressive salt and water retention and resultant volume expansion slowly transform this condition into a second phase in which the hypertension becomes primarily volume dependent, with progressive diminution in renin release and circulating and intrarenal angiotensin II levels. Chronically, salt and water balance is restored, at the expense of systemic hypertension. Even if the pressure-natriuresis relationship is restored to the normal profile, as shown for curve A in Figure 1, the entire relationship is shifted to a higher systemic pressure because of the pressure gradient caused by the stenotic lesions. This situation is represented by curve D, showing that the extent of the shift is dependent on the degree of stenosis.

The precarious balance between volume-dependent and angiotensin II–dependent components of the hypertension has direct clinical relevance. Vasodilator therapy to reduce arterial pressure lowers renal perfusion pressure and causes further volume retention. Diuretic therapy to enhance sodium excretion will lead to volume depletion and augmentation of the activity of the renin-angiotensin system. In both cases, there is "pseudoresistance" to drug therapy. In the extreme case, volume-depleted subjects can become extremely

sensitive to reductions in arterial pressure and may respond to antihypertensive medication by exhibiting reduction in creatinine clearance or even by developing acute renal failure. Treatment with angiotensin-converting enzyme inhibitors or angiotensin receptor antagonists may also exert deleterious effects on renal function, depending on the severity of the bilateral stenosis. Because of the stenosis, renal perfusion pressure is either at or below the lower limit of the autoregulatory range. The effects of the increased intrarenal angiotensin II levels on the afferent arterioles are counteracted by autoregulatory afferent arteriolar dilatation, whereas the vasoconstrictive effects of angiotensin II on efferent arterioles are maintained. When angiotensin blockade is imposed in this setting, the resulting decreased glomerular capillary pressure falls below the autoregulation range and decreases GFR. Secondary vasodilation of the efferent arterioles further contributes to precipitous decreases in glomerular pressure and renal function.

Unilateral Renovascular Hypertension

One normal kidney is sufficient to maintain fluid and electrolyte balance, yet does not prevent hypertension in unilateral renal arterial stenosis. The pathophysiology of hypertension in this model depends on progressive changes in the hormonal, neural, and hemodynamic influences caused by the stenotic kidney (**Figure 51.2**). This mechanism may also be relevant to understanding basic pathophysiological mechanisms in other forms of hypertension, including es-

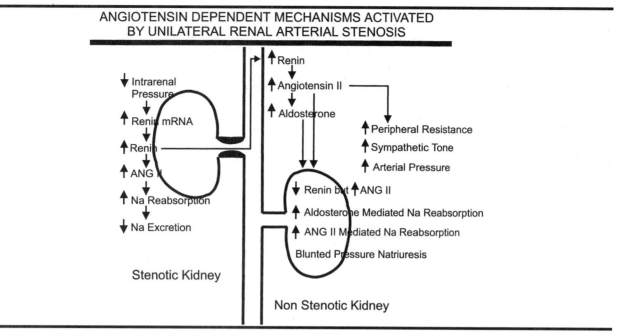

ANGIOTENSIN DEPENDENT MECHANISMS ACTIVATED
BY UNILATERAL RENAL ARTERIAL STENOSIS

Figure 2. Effects of the changes occurring in the stenotic kidney on the systemic circulation and on the contralateral non-stenotic kidney.

sential hypertension. While the nonstenotic kidney is not an initial causative factor, it develops inappropriately enhanced sodium reabsorption, resulting in an expanded extracellular fluid volume that can be counteracted only by the elevated arterial pressure.

In response to a reduction in perfusion pressure of a single kidney or even a segment of the renal vasculature, the hypoperfused tissue increases renin production and releases renin, resulting in elevated circulating levels of angiotensin I and II. Unlike the situation in bilateral stenosis, however, the resulting hypertension can influence the nonstenotic kidney to increase sodium excretion. However, increased angiotensin II levels blunt the expected pressure-natriuresis effect. In the presence of sustained elevations in angiotensin II and aldosterone levels, the pressure-natriuresis relationship of the nonstenotic kidney remains suppressed, as shown in curve C of Figure 1.

The elevated circulating angiotensin II levels influence the nonstenotic kidney through multiple other mechanisms as well. Angiotensin II exerts renal vasoconstrictor effects to reduce renal plasma flow and GFR and also directly enhances proximal and distal tubule sodium reabsorption. Through its adrenal actions to stimulate aldosterone secretion, angiotensin II further augments distal tubular sodium reabsorption. Thus, there is a marked diminution in the ability of the nonstenotic kidney to respond to the elevated arterial pressure with an appropriate pressure-natriuresis response; subsequent restoration of salt and water balance depends on the maintenance of the hypertension. The combined effects of angiotensin II and aldosterone are so powerful that they cannot be compensated by various other physiological responses such as increased natriuretic peptides. The unique difference between hypertension caused by unilateral renal stenosis and that caused by bilateral renal arterial stenosis is persistent angiotensin dependency of the unilateral condition, especially of the nonstenotic kidney, which remains during the more chronic phases of hypertension. The pressure distal to the

stenosis is apparently never completely restored, so that there is continuous stimulation of renin release from the stenotic kidney. Thus, as shown in Figure 2, the nonstenotic kidney remains influenced by the inappropriately elevated angiotensin II levels.

Recent studies have suggested the presence of an additional amplification mechanism that leads to progressive increases in intrarenal angiotensin II levels of the nonstenotic kidney. In response to relatively subtle but sustained increases in circulating angiotensin II concentrations, there is accumulation of circulating angiotensin II by a receptor-mediated internalization mechanism. In addition, the nonstenotic kidney maintains its local production of angiotensin II even though the renin activity is markedly diminished.

Nonrenal (ie, systemic) pressor effects of angiotensin II also contribute to chronic blood pressure elevation. In experimental renovascular hypertension, an early neurogenic phase occurs, during which the administration of antibody to nerve growth factor blunts subsequent blood pressure elevations. This phenomenon is probably due to the actions of angiotensin II to increase or sustain sympathoadrenal discharge. Angiotensin II also exerts a direct constrictive effect on systemic arterioles, leading to increased vascular resistance.

Renal Damage and Treatment Effects

Sustained elevations of arterial pressure to the nonstenotic kidney eventually cause hypertension-induced glomerular injury, which can lead to progressive decreases in renal function. Persistent hypertension leads to permanent damage, which further compromises renal function and elevates arterial pressure. Once this occurs, repair of the vascular stenosis or even nephrectomy of the stenotic kidney will not restore arterial pressure to normal, probably because of progressive damage in the nonstenotic kidney. Thus, it is essential to detect and treat or surgically correct the hypertension due to renal vascular lesions at the earliest possible time.

Treatment of unilateral renovascular hypertension with ACE inhibitors or angiotensin receptor antagonists results in variable decreases in renal blood flow and GFR in the stenotic kidney but increased renal blood flow and GFR in the nonstenotic kidney unless it has already developed hypertension-induced injury. Blockade or inhibition of angiotensin II and aldosterone effects on the nonstenotic kidney allows it to markedly increase its sodium excretion by shifting the pressure-natriuresis relationship from curve C to curve A or B. This phenomenon leads to a restoration of extracellular fluid volume and intravascular volume and reduction of the elevated arterial pressure. The differences in vascular responses are the basis of the captopril renal scintigram scan, a useful screening test for renovascular hypertension.

SUGGESTED READING

1. Guan S, Fox J, Mitchell KD, Navar LG. Angiotensin and angiotensin-converting enzyme tissue levels in two-kidney, one clip hypertensive rats. *Hypertension*. 1992; 20:763–767.

2. Imamura A, Mackenzie HS, Hutchison FN, Fitzgibbon WR, Ploth DW. Effects of chronic treatment with angiotensin converting enzyme inhibitor or an an-giotensin receptor antagonist in two-kidney, one-clip hypertensive rats. *Kidney Int*. 1995;47:1394–1402.

3. Laragh JH. The modern evaluation and treatment of hypertension:the causal role of the kidneys. *J Urol*. 1992;147:1469–1477.

4. Martinez-Maldonado M. Pathophysiology of renovascular hypertension. *Hypertension*. 1991;17:707–719.

5. Mitchell KD, Navar LG. Intrarenal actions of angiotensin II in pathogenesis of experimental hypertension. In: Laragh JH, Brenner BM, eds. *Hypertension: Pathophysiology, Diagnosis, and Management*. New York. NY:Raven Press Ltd; 1995: 1437–1450.

6. Navar LG. The kidney in blood pressure regulation and development of hypertension. *Med Clin North Am*. 1997;8:1165–1198.

7. Ploth DW. Renovascular hypertension. In: Jacobson HR, Striker GE, Klahr S, eds. *The Principles and Practice of Nephrology*. 2nd ed. St Louis, Mo: Mosby-Year Book; 1995:379–386.

8. Pohl MA. Renal artery stenosis, renal vascular hypertension and ischemic nephropathy. In: Schrier RW, Gottschalk CW, eds. *Diseases of the Kidney*. 6th ed. Boston, Mass: Little Brown & Co; 1997:1367–1423.

9. Vari RC, Navar LG. Normal regulation of arterial pressure. In: Jacobson HR< Striker GE, Klahr S, eds. *The Principles and Practice of Nephrology*. 2nd ed. St. Louis, Mo: Mosby-Year Book; 1995:354–361.

10. Ram CVS. Renovascular Hypertension. *Curr Opin Nephrol Hypertens*. 1997;6: 575–579.

Chapter 52

Pathophysiology of Renal Parenchymal Hypertension

Vito M. Campese

KEY POINTS

- Excessive intravascular volume is a major pathogenetic factor, and dietary sodium restriction, administration of diuretics, or removal of excessive fluids with dialysis are important adjuncts in the management of hypertension in these patients.

- Excessive renin secretion in relation to the state of sodium/volume balance has long been recognized as an important factor in the pathogenesis of hypertension in patients with renal parenchymal diseases.

- Mechanisms potentially responsible for the increase in sympathetic nerve activity in uremic patients include reduced central dopaminergic tone, reduced baroreceptor sensitivity, abnormal vagal function, increase $[Ca^{2+}]_1$ concentration, and increased plasma β-endorphin and β-lipotropin.

- Endothelial dysfunction, perhaps due to inhibition of NO synthesis, may contribute to hypertension in renal failure.

See also Chapters 73, 78, 112, 141

The association between hypertension and chronic renal disease has been recognized since the pioneering work of Richard Bright at Guy's Hospital in 1836. Renal disease is by far the commonest cause of secondary hypertension, which occurs in approximately 80% of patients with chronic renal failure, and it contributes to the progression of renal disease.

Cardiovascular disease is the leading cause of death in patients with end-stage renal disease (ESRD), especially in the first year of treatment. Hypertension is the single most important predictor of coronary artery disease in uremic patients, even more predictive than cigarette smoking or hypertriglyceridemia. The nocturnal dipping of blood pressure is significantly blunted in these patients, probably because of autonomic dysfunction or alteration of sleeping patterns, and this factor also has been associated with increased cardiovascular morbidity. Because blood pressure is usually measured during the day, this may lead to the erroneous impression of good anti-hypertensive control.

Pathogenesis

Role of Sodium and Volume Status

Several factors have been implicated in the pathophysiology of hypertension in renal patients (**Table 52.1**). Excessive intravascular volume is a major pathogenetic factor, and dietary sodium restriction, administration of diuretics, or removal of excessive fluids with dialysis are important adjuncts in the management of hypertension in these patients.

The mechanisms by which sodium excess may lead to arterial hypertension in the uremic patient are complex. In early phases, sodium excess leads to volume expansion and to increased cardiac output. Later, hypertension is sustained by an increase in peripheral vascular resistance. Restriction of dietary sodium intake to 1 g/d helps to control the volume status in these patients.

Role of the Renin-Angiotensin System

The role of excessive renin secretion in relation to the state of sodium/volume balance has long been recognized as an important factor in the pathogenesis of hypertension in patients with renal parenchymal diseases. Several factors support this notion. First, one can frequently find in these patients an abnormal relationship between exchangeable sodium or blood volume and plasma renin activity or plasma levels of angiotensin II. This finding suggests that even "normal" plasma concentrations of renin are inappropriately high in relation to the state of sodium and volume balance. Second, a direct relationship between plasma renin activity and blood pressure frequently can be found. Third, blood pressure can be effectively reduced in most of these patients by the administration of angiotensin-converting enzyme inhibitors or angiotensin II blockers. Finally, bilateral nephrectomy results in normalization of blood pressure in most of these patients.

Role of the Autonomic Nervous System

The kidney is not only an elaborate filtering device but also a sensory organ richly innervated with afferent nerves. There are two main functional types of renal sensory receptors and afferent nerves: renal baroreceptors, which increase their firing in response to changes in renal perfusion and intra-renal pressure, and renal chemoreceptors, which are stimulated by ischemic metabolites or uremic toxins. Activation of renal chemoreceptors or baroreceptors and renal afferent nerves that disinhibit integrative nuclei of the central nervous system can activate efferent sympathetic pathways and raise blood pressure. We have also shown that an acute renal injury caused by an intrarenal injection of phenol in the rat raises blood pressure and increases the secretion of norepinephrine from the posterior hypothalamic nuclei. These effects are permanent and occur in the absence of any change in renal function. Thus, an injury to a lim-

Table 52.1. Factors Implicated in the Pathogenesis of Hypertension in End-Stage Renal Disease

Sodium and volume excess
The renin-angiotensin-aldosterone system
The adrenergic system and baroreceptor activity
Endothelium-derived vasodepressor substances
Endothelium-derived vasoconstrictor substances
Erythropoietin
Divalent ions and parathyroid hormone
Atrial natriuretic peptide
Structural changes in the arteries
Preexistent essential hypertension
Miscellaneous:
    Anemia
    Arteriovenous fistula
    Vasopressin
    Serotonin
    Thyroid function
    Calcitonin gene-related peptide

ited portion of one kidney may cause a permanent elevation of no-radrenergic activity and blood pressure.

In patients with chronic renal failure, plasma norepinephrine levels are frequently but not always increased. This variability is probably related to the complex effects of uremia on prejunctional modulation of norepinephrine release and on plasma catecholamines clearance, as well as on the methods used to measure plasma catecholamines. More recently, Converse and others performed direct microelectrode recordings of postganglionic sympathetic action potentials in peroneal nerves of chronic hemodialysis patients with and without bilateral nephrectomy. They found that the rate of sympathetic nerve discharge was much higher in dialysis patients with their native kidneys than in those who had undergone bilateral nephrectomy or in control subjects. In both groups of uremic patients, plasma norepinephrine levels varied widely and no correlation was found between those levels and sympathetic nerve discharge in the peroneal nerves. In patients with bilateral nephrectomy, the decrease in sympathetic nerve firing was associated with lower regional vascular resistance and mean arterial pressure.

These findings support the notion that increased afferent nervous input from the injured kidney to the central nervous system may play a role in the pathogenesis of hypertension in uremic patients.

Other mechanisms potentially responsible for the increase in sympathetic nerve activity in uremic patients include reduced central dopaminergic tone, reduced baroreceptors sensitivity, abnormal vagal function, increased $[Ca^{2+}]_i$ concentration, and increased plasma β-endorphin and β-lipotropin.

Role of the Vascular Endothelium

In rats, chronic inhibition of nitric oxide (NO) synthesis by N^{ω}-nitro-l-arginine methyl ester causes systemic hypertension, marked renal vasoconstriction and hypoperfusion, a fall in glomerular filtration rate, an increase in filtration fraction, a rise in plasma renin levels, focal arteriolar obliteration, and segmental fibrinoid necrosis of the glomeruli. Administration of N^g-methyl-l-arginine (an NO synthase inhibitor) increased renal sympathetic nerve activity and systemic blood pressure in male Wistar rats. In vitro and in vivo NO

synthesis can be inhibited by an endogenous compound, N^G,N^G-dimethylarginine (asymmetrical dimethylarginine, ADMA). Significantly higher plasma levels of ADMA and significantly lower plasma arginine:dimethylarginine ratios have been observed in some uremic patients on chronic hemodialysis. This raises the possibility that hypertension in the uremic patient might be due to NO synthesis inhibition caused by increased levels of this circulating endogenous inhibitor.

Compelling evidence that endothelin (ET)-1 might play a role in the pathophysiology of hypertension was reported in two cases of hemangioendothelioma, a rare malignant vascular neoplasm. In these cases, plasma levels of ET were 10-fold to 15-fold greater than those of normal or essential hypertensive subjects. Surgical removal of the tumor led to resolution of hypertension in both cases. In one patient, recurrence of the tumor was accompanied by a rise in plasma ET levels and in blood pressure. Hypertensive patients with chronic renal failure have higher plasma ET-1 levels than normotensive subjects. Elevated plasma ET-1 and ET-3 levels have also been observed in hemodialysis patients, along with a positive correlation between blood pressure and ET-1 serum levels.

Role of Erythropoietin

Recombinant human erythropoietin (rHu-EPO), which is currently widely used to treat anemia in patients with chronic renal failure, can worsen hypertension and increase the requirement for antihypertensive drugs. The rise in blood pressure during treatment with rHu-EPO has not been observed in patients receiving rHu-EPO for other reasons, suggesting that renal disease may confer a particular susceptibility to the hypertensive action of rHu-EPO. The rise in blood pressure during rHu-EPO administration usually occurs within 2 to 16 weeks, although some patients may experience a rise in blood pressure several months after the initiation of therapy. Patients who are at greater risk for developing hypertension during rHu-EPO therapy are those with severe anemia, those whose anemia is corrected too rapidly, or those with preexisting hypertension.

Clinical and experimental studies have confirmed the importance of hematocrit in the regulation of both systemic and renal hemodynamics. Anemia causes a hyperdynamic state characterized by increased cardiac output and decreased total peripheral vascular resistance (TPR). Correction of the anemia with rHu-EPO leads to a decrease in cardiac output and a rise in TPR. Patients who become hypertensive or experience an exacerbation of hypertension during rHu-EPO therapy either have an exaggerated rise of TPR in response to the increase in hematocrit or do not suppress cardiac output to the same extent as patients who remain normotensive. The increase in blood viscosity during rHu-EPO therapy correlates with the increase in TPR but not with blood pressure changes. Hypertension induced by rHu-EPO therapy could also be a result of enhanced pressor responsiveness to norepinephrine and angiotensin II. Other potential mechanisms responsible for the rise in blood pressure during therapy with rHu-EPO are an increase in cytosolic free calcium, or an increase in ET-1 secretion.

Role of Divalent Ions and Parathyroid Hormone

Chronic renal failure is associated with secondary hyperparathyroidism and increased $[Ca^{2+}]_i$ in many organs, including the myocardium and circulating platelets. A relationship between platelet or lymphocyte $[Ca^{2+}]_i$ and blood pressure has been demonstrated in essential hypertension.

A study in 36 patients with chronic renal failure found that 10 had normal serum parathyroid hormone (PTH) levels, 17 had elevated serum PTH, and 9 had elevated PTH but were treated with nifedipine. A significant relation was present between serum PTH and platelet $[Ca^{2+}]_i$ or between platelet $[Ca^{2+}]_i$ or PTH and mean blood pressure. In patients with high serum PTH receiving nifedipine, platelet $[Ca^{2+}]_i$ was not increased. Nine patients with hyperparathyroidism were restudied during treatment with alfacalcidisl, a Vitamin D metabolite. In these patients, serum PTH, platelet $[Ca^{2+}]_i$, and mean blood pressure all decreased significantly. The changes in blood pressure during treatment with alfacalcidisl were linearly related with the changes in serum PTH and $[Ca^{2+}]_i$. These studies suggest that increased serum levels of PTH may be responsible for both the rise in $[Ca^{2+}]_i$ and the increase in blood pressure in these patients.

SUGGESTED READING

1. Baumgart P, Walger P, Gemen S, von Eiff M. Raidt H, Rahn KH. Blood pressure elevation during the night in chronic renal failure, hemodialysis, and renal transplantation. *Nephron.*. 1991;57:293–298.

2. Baylis C, Mitruka B, Deng A. Chronic blockade of nitric oxide synthesis in the rat produces systemic hypertension and glomerular damage. *J Clin Invest.* 1992;90: 278–281.

3. Campese VM, Chervu I. Hypertension in dialysis subjects. In: Henrich WL, ed. *Principles and Practice of Dialysis.* Baltimore, Md: Williams & Wilkins;1994: 148–169.

4. Converse RL Jr, Jacobsen TN, Toto RD, Jost CMT, Cosentino F, Fouad-Tarazi F, Victor RG. Sympathetic overactivity in patients with chronic renal failure. *N Engl J Med.*. 1992;327:1912–1918.

5. Katholi RE. Renal nerves and hypertension: an update. *Fed Proc.*. 1985;44: 2846–2850.

6. Raine AEG, Bedford L, Simpson AW, Ashley CC, Brown R, Woohead JS, Ledingham JG. Hyperparathyroidism, platelet intracellular free calcium and hypertension in chronic renal failure. *Kidney Int.* 1993;43:700–705.

7. Shichiri M, Hirata Y, Ando K, Emori T, Ohta K, Kimoto S, Ogura M, Inoue A, Marumo F. Plasma endothelin levels in hypertension and chronic renal failure. *Hypertension.* 1990;15:493–496.

8. Steffen HM, Brunner R, Müller R, Degenhardt S, Pollock M, Lang R, Baldamus CA. Peripheral hemodynamics, blood viscosity, and the renin-angiotensin system in hemodialysis patients under therapy with recombinant human erythropoietin. *Contrib Nephrol.* 1989;76:292–298.

9. Weidmann P, Maxwell MH, Lupu AN, Lewin AJ, Massry SG. Plasma renin activity and blood pressure in terminal renal failure. *N Engl J Med.* 1971;285:757-.762.

10. Ye S, Ozgur B, Campese VM. Renal afferent impulses, the posterior hypothalamus, and hypertension in rats with chronic renal failure. *Kidney Int.* 1997;51:722–727.

Chapter 53

Pathophysiology of Adrenal Cortical Hypertension

Burl R. Don, MD; Morris Schambelan, MD

KEY POINTS

- Mineralocorticoid hypertension follows a sequence of initial volume expansion and high cardiac output; as the volume excess subsides ("mineralocorticoid escape"), hypertension is maintained by systemic vasoconstriction that may be due in part to augmented sympathoadrenal activity.

- Glucocorticoid hypertension is more complex than mineralocorticoid hypertension; it involves potentiation of sympathoadrenal and renin-angiotensin activity and may involve inhibition of vasodilator systems.

- Monogenic forms of mineralocorticoid-induced hypertension include Liddle's syndrome, 11-steroid hydroxygenase deficiency, and glucocorticoid-remediable hyperaldosteronism.

See also Chapters 9, 10, 11, 155

Aldosterone, the principal mineralocorticoid hormone, is synthesized in the outer zone of the adrenal cortex (zona glomerulosa) because of the unique presence in this zone of aldosterone synthase, the enzyme that converts corticosterone to aldosterone. Aldosterone secretion by the zona glomerulosa is regulated primarily by the renin-angiotensin system and the concentration of potassium but is also affected by the circadian secretion of adrenocorticotropic hormone (ACTH). By virtue of its effects on transepithelial ion transport, aldosterone modulates sodium, potassium, and acid-base balance and is therefore a major participant in the physiological regulation of extracellular fluid volume. Deoxycorticosterone, another steroid with mineralocorticoid activity, is synthesized in the inner zone of the adrenal cortex (zona fasciculata) under the control of ACTH. At normal plasma concentrations, deoxycorticosterone has only weak mineralocorticoid activity, but when produced in large quantities, it can cause hypertension and other features typical of a hypermineralocorticoid state.

The principal glucocorticoid in humans, cortisol, is synthesized in the zona fasciculata under the control of ACTH. Although cortisol normally has minimal mineralocorticoid activity in vivo, it has an affinity equivalent to that of aldosterone for the mineralocorticoid receptor in vitro. The presence of the enzyme 11β-hydroxysteroid dehydrogenase, which converts cortisol to cortisone (a steroid with little affinity for the mineralocorticoid receptor) in specific tissues (kidney, parotid, colon), gives rise to their selectivity as mineralocorticoid targets. When activity of this enzyme is reduced or absent, as occurs in several clinical settings described here, cortisol can produce robust mineralocorticoid effects, including severe hypertension.

Mineralocorticoids
Pathogenesis of Mineralocorticoid Hypertension

Although primary aldosteronism is a relatively rare cause of hypertension, it is important to recognize patients with this disorder because affected individuals, particularly those with aldosterone-producing adenomas (APAs), can be cured or their hypertension ameliorated by unilateral adrenalectomy. The cardinal clinical features of primary aldosteronism are hypertension, hypokalemia, renal potassium wasting, hyporeninemia, and elevated plasma and/or urine levels of aldosterone.

Aldosterone binds to mineralocorticoid receptors in the collecting tubule of the nephron, thereby initiating a series of cellular processes that result in increased reabsorption of sodium and chloride and secretion of potassium and hydrogen ion. Chronic administration of supraphysiological doses of mineralocorticoids (aldosterone or deoxycorticosterone) to normal subjects ingesting an adequate salt intake causes salt and water retention, extracellular fluid volume expansion, and a rise in blood pressure. After an initial retention of 1 to 3 L, a spontaneous diuresis occurs that returns the plasma volume to normal, yet hypertension persists. This natriuretic response is referred to as "mineralocorticoid escape" and is due to decreased sodium reabsorption in other segments of the nephron. From a hemodynamic perspective, persistence of hypertension in these subjects is due to an increase in total peripheral vascular resistance.

In clinical states of mineralocorticoid excess, hypertension is presumed to result from a similar pathogenetic sequence. This is best illustrated in studies performed in patients with primary aldosteronism whose blood pressure has been maintained normal with the aldosterone antagonist spironolactone. When spironolactone treatment is discontinued, mean arterial blood pressure increases within 2 weeks in association with an increase in cardiac output, stroke volume, plasma volume, and total exchangeable sodium. In some individuals, cardiac output remains elevated, but in most, cardiac output and plasma volume return to their initial levels and peripheral vascular resistance increases. Thus, as in normal subjects given deoxycorticosterone, increased peripheral vascular resistance is the predominant cause of hypertension in patients with chronic mineralocorticoid excess. However, the increased total body sodium that is characteristic in such patients, particularly when it occurs in the presence of an increase in peripheral vascular resistance, may contribute to the hypertension.

Increased peripheral vascular resistance in patients with chronic mineralocorticoid excess may be due in part to augmented vascular sensitivity to catecholamines. Aldosterone may also affect blood pressure by binding to mineralocorticoid receptors in the central nervous system: in the rat, infusion of aldosterone into the cerebral ventricular system induces hypertension that can be attenuated by infusion of an aldosterone antagonist.

Aldosterone-Producing Adenoma and Idiopathic Hyperaldosteronism

A benign APA, as originally described by Conn, accounts for ≈75% of the cases of primary aldosteronism. Idiopathic hyperaldosteronism (IHA), a disorder with many similar clinical features, accounts for most of the remaining cases. In IHA, the adrenal glands either are normal in appearance or, more commonly, reveal bilateral (or rarely unilateral) micronodular or macronodular adrenal hyperplasia.

Patients with IHA tend to have a milder form of hyperaldosteronism than those with APA, although there can be overlap in the severity of the biochemical features of the two groups. Patients with APA typically exhibit a diurnal pattern of aldosterone secretion, with peak values in the early morning (4 am to 8 am) and a nadir in the late afternoon or evening (4 pm to midnight), suggesting that aldosterone production is under the control of ACTH. In such patients, aldosterone secretion does not increase normally in response to assumption of an upright posture because of marked suppression of the renin-angiotensin system and insensitivity of the adenoma to angiotensin II. While recumbent, patients with IHA demonstrate a diurnal variation in aldosterone secretion similar to that seen in patients with adenomas. However, in contrast to patients with adenoma, those with IHA have a 2-fold to 3-fold increase in aldosterone concentration during upright posture, suggesting that adrenal sensitivity to angiotensin II persists. The observation that aldosterone secretion is responsive to changes in the renin-angiotensin axis in IHA has been used to discriminate IHA from APA. Increased aldosterone secretion in IHA may be due to increased adrenal sensitivity to angiotensin II or to a pituitary factor other than ACTH.

Glucocorticoids
Pathogenesis of Glucocorticoid Hypertension

Glucocorticoids modulate a wide variety of cellular processes by altering the rate of gene transcription. Owing to the wide distribution of glucocorticoid receptors and the recently appreciated importance of the nature of the interaction with other transcription factors, it is not surprising that the mechanisms by which glucocorticoids cause hypertension are more complex than those attributed to mineralocorticoids.

One possible mechanism for "glucocorticoid-induced hypertension" is a direct mineralocorticoid effect of excess cortisol. Although cortisol is a relatively weak mineralocorticoid in vivo, the circulating levels are normally a thousand times greater than those of aldosterone and may be further augmented in states of cortisol excess. However, since most patients with Cushing's syndrome do not have findings consistent with hypermineralocorticoidism (eg, hypokalemia and hyporeninemia), the mineralocorticoid effects of cortisol excess are probably not the major factors in the pathogenesis of hypertension.

There are several mechanisms by which glucocorticoids raise blood pressure. Production of the potent vasoconstrictor angiotensin II is increased because of glucocorticoid-induced increased hepatic synthesis of the angiotensin precursor angiotensinogen. Enhanced glucocorticoid-mediated vascular reactivity to vasoconstrictor hormones and inhibition of extraneuronal uptake and degradation of norepinephrine results in vasoconstriction. Inhibition of vasodilatory systems such as prostaglandins and kinins occurs as well. A shift of sodium from the intracellular to the extracellular compartment results in an increase in plasma volume, with further augmentation of cardiac output from increased epinephrine production due to enhanced phenylethanolamine-N-methyltransferase activity in the adrenal medulla.

Hypercortisolism

Hypercortisolism is characterized clinically by truncal obesity, moon face, purple striae, muscle atrophy, neuropsychiatric disturbances, diabetes mellitus, easy bruisability, and menstrual abnormalities. Hypertension occurs in ≈80% of patients. This constellation of findings is commonly referred to as Cushing's syndrome, in honor of the neurosurgeon who first recognized this disorder. Cortisol excess may be caused by increased ACTH secretion by the pituitary gland (70%), ectopic secretion of ACTH by extrapituitary neoplasms (15%), and primary neoplasms (benign and malignant) of the adrenal zona fasciculata (15%). Increased ACTH secretion by the pituitary is usually due to microadenomas or macroadenomas of the ACTH-secreting cells (corticotrophs). Ectopic sources of ACTH include bronchial carcinoid and malignancies of the lung, thymus, pancreas, and thyroid. Increased ACTH secretion from either a pituitary or ectopic source causes bilateral adrenal hyperplasia. Cortisol-producing adrenal adenomas are usually encapsulated tumors of zona fasciculata–like cells that typically secrete cortisol alone. Cortisol-producing adrenal carcinomas may resemble adenomas histologically, but their invasiveness and evidence of metastatic spread betrays their apparent innocence.

Increased ACTH production of either pituitary or ectopic origin may result in increased secretion of ACTH-dependent mineralocorticoids such as deoxycorticosterone. Cortisol-producing adrenal carcinomas may also secrete excessive amounts of deoxycorticosterone. Thus, hypertension in some patients with Cushing's syndrome may be due to excess secretion of mineralocorticoids as well as cortisol. This may explain why hypertension is not common in patients receiving exogenous glucocorticoids, inasmuch as these steroids have minimal mineralocorticoid activity.

Other Clinical Syndromes
Glucocorticoid-Remediable Hyperaldosteronism

Glucocorticoid-remediable hyperaldosteronism (GRA) is a rare autosomal dominant disorder in which the typical features of primary aldosteronism can be ameliorated by small doses of glucocorticoids such as dexamethasone. Affected individuals appear to have an increased adrenal sensitivity to the aldosterone-stimulating effects of ACTH. These patients also excrete large quantities of 18-hydroxycortisol and

18-oxocortisol, steroids that are normally present in small or undetectable amounts. Recently, the abnormal gene that causes GRA has been shown to result from unequal crossing over on chromosome 8q, leading to the formation of a chimeric gene consisting of the 5′ regulatory region of 11β-hydroxylase and the coding sequence of aldosterone synthase. As a result, aldosterone synthase, normally found only in the zona glomerulosa, is expressed in the zona fasciculata under the control of the ACTH-sensitive 11β-hydroxylase regulatory sequence, accounting for the increased production of aldosterone as well as increased conversion of cortisol to 18-hydroxycortisol and 18-oxocortisol. With the advent of molecular genetic techniques, recognition of patients with this disorder has been greatly simplified and should be undertaken in all patients with evidence for familial primary aldosteronism.

Enzymatic Deficiencies

Two enzyme-deficiency states can result in hypermineralocorticoidism: 11β- and 17α-hydroxylase deficiency. 11β-Hydroxylase converts 11-deoxycortisol to cortisol; deficiency of this enzyme leads to reduced cortisol levels, increased secretion of ACTH, and increased production of deoxycorticosterone as a consequence of increased activity of the 17-deoxy pathway in the zona fasciculata. The elevated levels of deoxycorticosterone induce volume expansion, hypertension, and suppression of aldosterone secretion. Affected individuals tend to be virilized as a consequence of increased androgen production. 17α-Hydroxylase converts progesterone to 17-hydroxyprogesterone; a deficiency of 17α-hydroxylase leads to reduced cortisol levels, augmented ACTH secretion, and increased production of deoxycorticosterone from the zona fasciculata. In contrast to 11β-hydroxylase deficiency, virilization does not occur, inasmuch as 17α-hydroxylation is required for androgen production in the adrenal gland.

Syndrome of Apparent Mineralocorticoid Excess

A rare disorder, initially designated as the syndrome of apparent mineralocorticoid excess, is characterized by typical features of a hypermineralocorticoid state (hypertension, sodium and water retention, hyporeninemia, hypokalemia, and amelioration with spironolactone) despite low mineralocorticoid levels. The syndrome was first described in children with severe, and often lethal, hypertension and has been reported in at least one young adult. An abnormally high ratio of cortisol to cortisone metabolites in the urine was the clue that eventually led to the hypothesis that apparent mineralocorticoid excess is caused by a deficiency of 11β-hydroxysteroid dehydrogenase. Deficiency of this enzyme in the kidney would be expected to result in high renal levels of cortisol, which would bind to

and activate mineralocorticoid receptors. An acquired form of this syndrome has been described in persons ingesting large quantities of licorice and chewing tobacco. Originally, it was thought that the active alkaloid in licorice, glycyrrhetinic acid, caused a hypermineralocorticoid state by binding to mineralocorticoid receptors. Recently, it has been appreciated that glycyrrhetinic acid inhibits 11β-hydroxysteroid dehydrogenase, producing high renal levels of cortisol and therefore increased mineralocorticoid activity in the kidney.

Pseudohyperaldosteronism: Liddle's Syndrome

In 1963, Liddle et al described a familial disorder in which the affected individuals had features of a mineralocorticoid-excess state, despite subnormal levels of aldosterone. None of the known mineralocorticoids were found to be present in increased amounts and, more important, neither treatment with the mineralocorticoid antagonist spironolactone nor inhibitors of adrenal biosynthesis ameliorated this disorder. The inheritance pattern in this large family was that of an autosomal dominant disorder. The observation that hypertension and hypokalemia can be ameliorated in such patients with the use of drugs that inhibit sodium reabsorption in the distal nephron (amiloride, triamterene) suggests that the primary abnormality in Liddle's syndrome is due to enhanced distal sodium reabsorption caused by a defect in the cytoplasmic domain of either the β- or γ-subunit of the epithelial sodium channel that results in constitutive activation of the channel. This results in augmented sodium reabsorption (hypertension) and impaired potassium excretion (hyperkalemia).

SUGGESTED READING

1. Biglieri EG, Irony I, Kater CE. Adrenocortical forms of human hypertension. In: Laragh JH, Brenner BJ, eds. *Hypertension: Pathophysiology, Diagnosis, and Management.* New York, NY: Raven Press Publishers; 1990:1609–1623.

2. Farese RV Jr, Biglieri EG, Shackleton CH, Irony I, Gomez-Fontes R. Licorice-induced hypermineralocorticoidism. *N Engl J Med.* 1991;325:1223–1227.

3. Greminger P, Tenschert W, Vetter W, Luscher T, Vetter H. Hypertension in Cushing's syndrome. In: Mantero F, Biglieri EG, Edwards CRW, eds. *Proceedings, Serono Symposia No. 50, Endocrinology of Hypertension.* London, UK/New York, NY: Academic Press Inc; 1982:103–110.

4. Lifton RP, Dluhy RG, Powers M, Rich GM, Cook S, Ulick S, Lalouel J-M. A chimaeric 11β-hydroxylase/aldosterone synthase gene causes glucocorticoid-remediable aldosteronism and human hypertension. *Nature.* 1992;355:262–265.

5. Shimkets RA, Warnock DG, Bositis CM, Nelson-Williams C, Hansson JH, Schambelan M, Gill JR Jr, Ulick S, Milora RV, Findling JW, et al. Liddle's syndrome: heritable human hypertension caused by mutations in the beta subunit of the epithelial sodium channel. *Cell.* 1994;79:407–414.

6. Stewart PM, Corrie JE, Shackleton CH, Edwards CR. Syndrome of apparent mineralocorticoid excess: a defect in the cortisol-cortisone shuttle. *J Clin Invest.* 1988;82:340–349.

7. Wenting GH, Man in 'T Veld AJ, Verhoeven RP, Derkx FH, Schalekamp DH. Volume-pressure relationships during development of mineralocorticoid hypertension in man. *Circ Res.* 1977;40(suppl I):I-163–I-170.

Chapter 54

Pathophysiology of Pheochromocytoma

William M. Manger, MD, PhD

KEY POINTS

- Pheochromocytoma, a rare neuroendocrine tumor occurring in the abdomen, pelvis, chest, or neck, may be multiple; 10% are familial and may be associated with hyperplasia or tumors of thyroid and parathyroid glands and other neuroectoderm tumors.

- Clinical and laboratory manifestations are caused mainly by secretion of catecholamines, but various secreted peptides and amines may also participate. Pheochromocytomas can mimic many diseases, some of which also secrete catecholamines.

- Chromosome abnormalities are important in detecting familial disease; abnormal DNA patterns occur in up to 39% of malignant pheochromocytomas.

See also Chapter 1, 2, 154

Pheochromocytoma is a treacherous neuroendocrine tumor that causes manifestations, often paroxysmal and dramatic, mainly via excess catecholamines. If unrecognized, it will almost invariably cause lethal cardiovascular complications from excess circulating catecholamines and hypertension.

Origin, Pathophysiology, and Pathology

Pheochromocytomas occur in perhaps 0.05% of hypertensives. They occur at any age and arise from neuroectodermal chromaffin cells, which are part of the adrenergic (sympathoadrenal) system; 98% occur in the abdomen or pelvis, major sites being the adrenal medullae (85%; 15% are extra-adrenal), organ of Zuckerkandl, and paraganglia chromaffin cells, which are found in association with sympathetic nerves and plexuses; <1% occur in the urinary bladder. Tumors rarely arise in the chest (<2%) in a paraspinal location or intrapericardially, in the neck (<1%) from the base of the skull and extending intracranially through the jugular foramen, or from ectopic chromaffin tissue (eg, spermatic cord). Multiple pheochromocytomas are more common in children (35%) than adults (8%).

Genetics of Pheochromocytoma

Ten percent of pheochromocytomas are familial with a dominant autosomal mode of inheritance. Mutations of the *RET* proto-oncogene on chromosome 10 appear to be involved in the pathogenesis of familial pheochromocytomas, which usually arise in both adrenals and coexist with other tumors, ie, multiple endocrine neoplasia (MEN) type 2 or 2a and type 3 or 2b. In MEN 2 pheochromocytoma, medullary thyroid carcinoma (MTC), parathyroid adenoma or hyperplasia often coexist, whereas in MEN 3, parathyroid disease is extremely rare, and a characteristic phenotype (neuromas of lips and tongue, thickened corneal nerves, intestinal ganglioneuromatosis, marfanoid habitus) exists. Deletions on chromosomes 1p, 3p, 11, 17p, and 22q have also been reported. It is noteworthy that pheochromocytomas occur in 14% of patients with familial Von Hippel-Lindau disease (which has a deletion on chromosome 3p) and in 1% of pa-

tients with peripheral neurofibromatosis (which has a deletion on 17q). Rarely, pheochromocytomas coexist with pancreatic neoplasms or occur in families without other tumors, but chromosome mutations are unclear.

Pathophysiology

Hypertension and excess circulating catecholamines cause morbidity or lethal cerebrovascular or cardiac complications. Pheochromocytomas average 5 cm in diameter but may be microscopic or weigh up to 4 kg. Tumors are usually encapsulated and vascular but sometimes are avascular or cystic and, rarely, may contain calcium. Tumor cells, usually pleomorphic and polygonal or spheroidal, harbor multiple storage vesicles containing norepinephrine or epinephrine. Ten percent of adrenal and up to 40% of extra-adrenal tumors metastasize or invade adjacent structures. Although malignancy cannot be determined histologically, a normal flow cytometric DNA pattern of pheochromocytoma cells predicts benignancy, whereas an abnormal pattern (polyploidy) portends malignancy in up to 39%. Malignancy is more frequent in extra-adrenal tumors and those secreting dopamine or its precursor (dopa). Rarely, benign tumors are multicentric. Pheochromocytomas usually secrete norepinephrine and epinephrine but predominantly norepinephrine; rarely only norepinephrine or epinephrine is secreted, and very rarely only dopamine.

Embryologically related diseases arising from neural crest maldevelopment (eg, pheochromocytoma, neuroblastoma, neurofibromatosis, MTC, carcinoid, and MEN) have been designated neurocrestopathies. Some of these tumors are capable of *a*mine and amine *p*recursor *u*ptake and *d*ecarboxylation (the APUD system) and they may secrete catecholamines and a variety of peptides.

Many substances have been identified in some pheochromocytomas eg, chromogranins, vasoactive intestinal peptide, enkephalins, β-endorphin, dynorphin, α-melanocyte–stimulating hormone, adrenocorticotropic hormone, neuropeptide Y, neuron-specific enolase, atrial natriuretic factor, corticotropin-releasing factor, growth hormone–releasing factor, somatostatin, parathyroid hormone, calcitonin, substance P, synaptophysin, gastrin-releasing peptide, neurotensin, insulin-like growth factor, gastrin, cholecystokinin, serotonin, motilin, interleukin-6, erythropoietin-like substance, adrenomedullin, angiotensin II, and ACE. Some may be released into the circulation and cause physiological and/or pharmacological effects with diverse manifestations.

Clinical Presentation

Pheochromocytomas often present with sudden and dramatic manifestations that may mimic many diseases. Absence of sustained or paroxysmal hypertension during "attacks" suggesting excess circulating catecholamines is very atypical; however, familial pheochromocytoma sometimes presents without manifestations or hypertension. Attacks are abrupt in onset and subside more slowly.

Episodic increases in systolic and diastolic pressures occur in ≈45% of patients, whereas 50% have sustained hypertension that often fluctuates. Rarely, patients with predominantly epinephrine-secreting tumors have hypertension alternating with hypotension. Approximately 5% remain normotensive. Orthostatic hypotension may result from desensitized adrenergic receptors. Resistance to certain antihypertensive agents or pressor responses to some (eg, β-blockers) may occur. Attacks usually occur ≥1 time weekly and last <1 hour in ≈75%; however, they may occur at any frequency. Sometimes attacks are precipitated by pressure on a tumor, postural changes, exertion, anxiety, trauma, pain, ingestion of food or beverages containing tyramine (certain cheeses, beer, wine); by administration of certain drugs (eg, histamine, glucagon, tyramine, phenothiazines, metoclopramide, adrenocorticotropic hormone, chemotherapy); or by micturition or urinary bladder distension (with bladder pheochromocytomas), intubation, anesthesia, and operative manipulation.

Manifestations result mainly from excess circulating catecholamines or hypertensive complications but may be influenced by secreted peptides. Signs of tumor encroachment on adjacent structures or metastases may occur. Severe headaches, generalized sweating, and palpitations with tachycardia (rarely reflex bradycardia) are frequently experienced; ≥1 of these manifestations occur in 95% of patients. Acute anxiety, fear of death, and pallor (rarely flushing) are frequent during paroxysmal attacks. Weight loss and severe constipation are not uncommon, but secretion of vasoactive intestinal peptide or serotonin by a pheochromocytoma or secretion of calcitonin, serotonin, or prostaglandin from a coexisting medullary thyroid carcinoma can cause diarrhea. Severe retinopathy (similar to that of essential hypertension) can occur with sustained but not paroxysmal hypertension. Fine tremors and slight fever (rarely hyperpyrexia) may occur. Polydypsia, polyuria, and convulsions are not uncommon in children.

Hypercatecholaminemia can cause hyperglycemia, increased free fatty acids, hypermetabolism, and hyperreninemia. Rarely, intense vasoconstriction can cause lactic acidosis and increase pancreatic, liver, and cardiac enzymes. Some pheochromocytomas or coexisting hemangioblastomas secrete erythropoietin and cause polycythemia.

Transient arrhythmias or ECG changes suggesting ischemia or strain during hypertensive episodes or sudden heart failure may oc-cur, but catecholamine cardiomyopathy, hypertension, and atherosclerosis can cause permanent damage.

Approximately 2% of patients harboring pheochromocytomas present with unexplained shock, abdominal pain, pulmonary edema, and intense mydriasis unresponsive to light; 1% develop pheochromocytoma multisystem crisis, ie, multiple organ system failure, hyperpyrexia, encephalopathy, and severe hypertension and/or hypotension, sometimes associated with lactic acidosis and, rarely, disseminated intravascular coagulation.

Diagnostic Implications

Establishing the diagnosis of pheochromocytoma depends most critically on clinical suspicion. The presence of headache, tachycardia, palpitations, diaphoresis, orthostatic BP decreases, and to a lesser extent paroxysmal hypertension, are cardinal signs and symptoms. Diagnostic testing is then directed at screening tests, principally 24-hour urinary metaephrines (diagnostically superior to VMA) or plasma catecholamines, which are elevated in at least 95% of patients with pheochromocytoma but which may be normal during normotensive periods. Some patients with familial pheochromocytoma are asymptomatic and present with normotension and normal plasma and urinary catecholamines and metabolites.

Symptomatic patients with neurogenic hypertension and modest elevations of plasma catecholamines (eg, 600 to 2000 pg/mL) may be differentiated from pheochromocytoma by the clonidine suppression test, which decreases plasma catecholamines to normal levels in neurogenic hypertension but does not change levels in patients with pheochromocytoma. With few exceptions (eg, neuroblastoma, baroreflex failure, severe physiological or pathological stress), plasma catecholamines >2000 pg/mL are diagnostic of pheochromocytoma. Evaluation of patients with pheochromocytoma should include consideration of hyperparathyroidism, and medullary thyroid carcinomas.

Preoperative localization is mandatory. Computerized axial tomography (CT) identifies 95% of pheochromocytomas (adrenal tumors 1 cm or greater and extraadrenal abdominal tumors >2 cm). Magnetic resonance imaging (MRI) appears superior to CT in locating extraadrenal, recurrent, and metastatic pheochromocytomas and in detecting some familial adrenal pheochromocytomas. Since 85% of the pheochromocytomas take up [131] I-metaiodobenzylguanidine (MIBG), scintigraphy with this radiopharmaceutical agent is highly specific. PET scanning with [11] C-hydroxyephedrine does not appear to be as reliable.

SUGGESTED READING

1. Bravo EL. Evolving concepts in the pathophysiology, diagnosis, and treatment of pheochromocytoma. *Endocr Rev.* 1994;15:356–368.
2. Manger WM, Gifford RW Jr. *Clinical and Experimental Pheochromocytoma.* 2nd ed. Cambridge, Mass: Blackwell Science; 1996.
3. Manger WM, Gifford RW Jr. Pheochromocytoma: a clinical overview. In: Laragh JH, Brenner BM, eds. *Hypertension: Pathophysiology, Diagnosis, and Management.* 2nd ed. New York, NY: Raven Press Ltd; 1995:2225–2244.
4. Sheps SG, Jiang NS, Klee GG, van Heerden JA: Recent developments in the diagnosis and treatment of pheochromocytoma. *Mayo Clin Proc.* 1990; 65: 88–95.
5. Stein PP, Black HR. A simplified diagnostic approach to pheochromocytoma: a review of the literature and report of one institution's experience. *Medicine* (Baltimore). 1990;70: 46–66.

Chapter 55

Hypertension Caused by Thyroid and Parathyroid Abnormalities and Acromegaly

Yoram Shenker, MD

KEY POINTS

- Hypothyroidism is often associated with diastolic hypertension, increased catecholamine levels, and increased vascular resistance. Replacement of thyroid hormone frequently leads to normalization of all these parameters.

- Thyrotoxicosis is often associated with systolic hypertension due to increased cardiac output and decreased peripheral resistance. Treatment of thyrotoxicosis usually leads to normalization of blood pressure.

- Hypertension in hyperparathyroidism is multifactorial and may be related to a direct effect of calcium, effects of parathyroid hormone, renal insufficiency, or changes in the renin-aldosterone system.

- Approximately 50% of acromegalic patients are hypertensive. Hypertension seems to be related to increased left ventricular mass and increased stroke volume induced by a direct effect of growth hormone on heart tissue.

See also Chapter 156

The Thyroid and Hypertension

Most of the effects of thyroid hormones are mediated through activation of specific nuclear receptors, which increase transcription of the specific messenger RNA and increase production of proteins that mediate the function of the thyroid hormones in different organ systems. Some of the effects of thyroid hormones, including cardiovascular effects, occur very rapidly and appear to be directly related to the interaction of the hormone with cell membranes (**Table 55.1**).

Hemodynamic Variations

Thyrotoxicosis, or excess administration of thyroid hormones, is associated with increased cardiac output, stroke volume, heart rate, and mean ejection rate It also leads to increased blood volume, decreased peripheral vascular resistance, and a widened pulse pressure (decreased diastolic pressure and increased systolic blood pressure). Conversely, hypothyroidism is associated with low cardiac output and increased total peripheral resistance, which may be partially related to acceleration of structural changes in vascular tissue caused by thyroid hormone deficiency. Total blood volume is decreased in hypothyroidism.

Autonomic Interactions

The cardiovascular manifestations of thyrotoxicosis closely resemble those caused by epinephrine, and many of the symptoms of thyrotoxicosis are controlled by β-blockers. Yet catecholamine levels in thyrotoxicosis are either low or normal. One possible explanation is increased sensitivity to catecholamines in thyrotoxicosis, which may be related to increased density of β-adrenergic receptors, as was reported to occur in heart tissue and in leukocytes. The absence of increased response to adrenergic agonists in thyrotoxicosis, however, casts some doubt on the receptor sensitivity hypothesis.

Several investigators have shown that hypothyroid patients have higher norepinephrine levels, particularly when they are hypertensive. Sympathetic nerve activity in the muscles in hypothyroid patients also seems to be increased. The number of β-adrenergic receptors in hypothyroid patients is decreased, leading to increased α-adrenergic responses, which may explain the increase in peripheral vascular resistance and hypertension of hypothyroidism.

The Renin-Angiotensin System

Plasma renin activity (PRA) is low in hypothyroidism; it increases when thyroxine is replaced. Aldosterone secretion rate and the response of aldosterone to other secretagogues are also diminished. This suggests that the renin-aldosterone system does not play a role in hypertension of hypothyroidism. PRA is increased in thyrotoxicosis, which may be related to thyroid hormone–induced hepatic synthesis of renin substrate (angiotensinogen), which is similar to the effects of estrogen and cortisol and which leads to stimulation of the entire renin-aldosterone system. Conversely, administration of angiotensin II antagonist in thyrotoxic patients does not necessarily reduce blood pressure, which casts doubt on the role of the renin-aldosterone system in thyrotoxic hypertension.

Clinical Features

The reported prevalence of hypertension in hypothyroidism varies between 0% and 50%. Hypothyroidism has been identified as a cause of hypertension in 3% of hypertensive patients. Many of the hypertensive hypothyroid patients have predominantly diastolic hypertension, and the degree of severity of hypothyroidism seems to be correlated with diastolic blood pressure. Thyroid hormone replacement in hypertensive hypothyroid patients decreases both systolic and diastolic blood pressure. Complete normalization of blood

Table 55.1 Endocrine and Cardiovascular Changes in Thyroid Disorders

ENDOCRINE/ CARDIOVASCULAR FUNCTIONS	HYPOTHYROIDISM	THYROTOXICOSIS
Catecholamine levels	Increased	Normal/decreased
Density of β-adrenergic receptors	Decreased	Increased
Plasma renin activity levels	Decreased	Increased
Aldosterone levels	Decreased	Increased
Blood volume	Decreased	Increased
Cardiac output	Decreased	Increased
Stroke volume	Decreased	Increased
Heart rate	Decreased	Increased
Peripheral vascular resistance	Increased	Decreased

pressure is less likely in older patients and in those with more long-standing hypertension.

The prevalence of hypertension in thyrotoxicosis is probably in the range of 20% to 30%. Systolic hypertension dominates because of the increased cardiac indices and decreased peripheral resistance. High diastolic blood pressure is uncommon in thyrotoxicosis. The prevalence of hypertension in thyrotoxic patients is particularly increased (compared with the euthyroid population) in patients <49 years old. Treatment of thyrotoxicosis and restoration of the euthyroid state usually leads to normalization of systolic blood pressure, particularly in younger patients.

Hyperparathyroidism and Hypertension

Hypertension is frequently associated with primary hyperparathyroidism (due to adenoma or hyperplasia of the parathyroid gland), pseudohypoparathyroidism (due to resistance to the parathyroid hormone, PTH), or secondary hyperparathyroidism, most often caused by advanced renal failure. The prevalence of hypertension in primary hyperparathyroidism varies in different studies from 10% to >70%. Patients with pseudohypoparathyroidism have a 40% to 50% prevalence of hypertension.

Mechanisms of Hypertension in Hyperparathyroidism

Hypertension in different forms of hyperparathyroidism is probably multifactorial. The possibility of coexisting essential hypertension and hyperparathyroidism cannot be ignored, considering the high prevalence of both conditions in the elderly population.

Serum calcium and blood pressure. Acute infusion of calcium in normotensive patients leads to increased peripheral vascular resistance. Conditions of non–PTH-dependent hypercalcemia are also quite frequently associated with hypertension. These observations lead to the hypothesis that hypercalcemia causes increased free intracellular calcium, which is known to increase vascular smooth muscle contractility and hypertension. Conversely, some studies do not support the idea of hypertensive effects of hypercalcemia. Hypocalcemia has also been associated with hypertension, and multiple studies have shown the beneficial effects of calcium supplementation on systolic blood pressure in essential hypertension.

PTH and hypertension. Patients with pseudohypoparathyroidism who are hypocalcemic with high PTH levels have as much hypertension as patients with primary hyperparathyroidism, suggesting that increased PTH itself may be responsible for hypertension. Moreover, patients with pseudohypoparathyroidism and hypertension remain hypertensive after correction of hypocalcemia. In a long-term study, PTH infusion in normotensive subjects led to hypertension, possibly related to ACTH-stimulated cortisol and aldosterone secretion. Conversely, other acute studies have shown vasodilatory and hypotensive effects of high PTH levels.

PTH-induced renal disease and hypertension. Most, but not all, studies have shown that the prevalence of hypertension is much higher in patients with hyperparathyroidism who have renal insufficiency than in hyperparathyroid patients without renal dysfunction.

The renin-aldosterone system in hyperparathyroidism. Many studies have shown increased PRA and aldosterone levels in hyperparathyroidism. In a recent study, hypertensive hyperparathyroid patients were compared with normotensive hyperparathyroid patients and normal control subjects. PRA and plasma aldosterone levels were higher in the hypertensive hyperparathyroid patients, who also had a greater pressor response to infused norepinephrine. Parathyroidectomy normalized blood pressure, PRA, plasma aldosterone, and pressor responsiveness to norepinephrine in 8 of 10 subjects.

Response of Hypertension to Parathyroidectomy

According to different reports, 20% to 100% of patients with hypertension and hyperparathyroidism normalize or improve their blood pressure after undergoing parathyroidectomy. No known factor can predict which patient with hypertension will respond favorably to parathyroidectomy. Some studies suggest that the effect of decreased blood pressure after such surgery will usually not last more than 3 years. At present, the consensus is that hypertension alone is not a reason to perform a parathyroidectomy in hyperparathyroid patients.

Acromegaly and Hypertension

Acromegaly is a disease of adults caused by chronic excess of growth hormone (GH). Gigantism is a similar condition associated with increased height that develops before puberty and closure of the epiphyses.

The vast majority of cases of acromegaly are due to GH-producing pituitary adenomas (usually macroadenomas, which by definition are larger than 1 cm). Another cause of acromegaly is an excess of GH-releasing hormone secreted either eutopically by a hypothalamic tumor or ectopically from carcinoid or islet cell tumors. Ectopic GH secretion is extremely rare, with only one well-documented case of a GH-producing pancreatic islet cell tumor.

Hypertension is very common in acromegaly. In the largest series ever published, 51% of 500 acromegalic patients were hypertensive, with 51% of these having borderline hypertension and 49% having frank hypertension.

An increase in left ventricular mass is a very frequent finding in acromegaly. Cardiac stroke volume is increased in active acromegaly before the onset of high blood pressure. Hypertensive acromegalics also have a reduction in end-systolic stress, which is an index of afterload. These changes result in increased cardiac output, which may be involved in the development of hypertension. All of these abnormalities also suggest the existence of a specific acromegalic cardiomyopathy, which leads to hypertension. An alternative hypothesis is that acromegalic cardiomyopathy and acromegalic hypertension are independent of each other and that their pathophysiologies are different and unknown.

The structural and functional cardiovascular abnormalities of acromegaly respond to treatment when GH levels are successfully controlled. In many cases, such treatment also leads to cure or at least amelioration of hypertension, particularly if patients are diagnosed and treated relatively early in the course of the disease.

SUGGESTED READING

1. Akpunonu BE, Mulrow PJ, Hoffman EA. Secondary hypertension: evaluation and treatment: thyrotoxicosis and hypertension [published correction appears in *Dis Mon.* 1997;43:62]. *Dis Mon.* 1996;42:689–696 and 696–703.

2. Ezzat S, Forster MJ, Berchtold P, Redelmeier DA, Boerlin V, Harris AG. Acromegaly: clinical and biochemical features in 500 patients. *Medicine.* 1994;73:233–240.

3. Gennari C, Nami R, Gonnelli S. Hypertension and primary hyperparathyroidism: the role of adrenergic and renin-angiotensin-aldosterone systems. *Miner Electrolyte Metab.* 1995;21:77–81.

4. López-Velasco R, Escobar-Morreale HF, Vega B, Villa E, Sancho JM, Moya-Mur JL, García-Robles R. Cardiac involvement in acromegaly: specific myocardiopathy or consequence of systemic hypertension? *J Clin Endocrinol Metab.* 1997;82: 1047–1053.

5. Saito I, Saruta T. Hypertension in thyroid disorders. *Endocrinol Metab Clin North Am.* 1994;23:379–386.

Chapter 56

Coarctation of the Aorta

Albert P. Rocchini, MD

KEY POINTS

- Coarctation of the aorta is the most common cardiovascular cause of hypertension.

- Coarctation is diagnosed by the presence of higher blood pressures in the arms than in the legs.

- Coarctation can be corrected with either surgery or balloon angioplasty.

- Despite successful repair of coarctation, individuals may have persistent cardiovascular problems, including hypertension, coronary artery disease, aneurysms of the aorta, and stroke.

See also Chapter 147

Coarctation of the aorta is the most common cardiovascular cause of hypertension. Coarctation is the fourth most frequent (7.5%) form of congenital heart disease. It requires either cardiac catheterization or surgery during the first year of life, and it affects boys more often than girls (1.74:1). Coarctation of the aorta usually occurs sporadically but has been reported in monozygotic twins, in one family in which coarctation occurred in an autosomal dominant pattern, and in 35% of children with Turner's syndrome.

Diagnosis

The physical findings diagnostic of coarctation are diminished femoral pulses and a systolic pressure gradient between right arm and leg blood pressures. A grade 2 or 3 over 6 systolic murmur, heard best in the posterior left interscapular area, is frequently present and is important in localizing the coarctation to the thoracic aorta. Among patients with well-developed collateral blood flow, systolic or continuous murmurs may be heard over the left and right sides of the chest. Noninvasive conformation of the diagnosis can be made by chest radiograph and echocardiogram. On the frontal projection of the chest radiograph, a discrete thoracic coarctation may show a "3 sign," consisting of the proximal aorta, the coarcted segment, and poststenotic dilatation. Barium swallow may reveal indentations from the same structures on the esophagus in a "reverse 3" configuration. Echocardiogram and Doppler determinations are useful not only in localizing the site of the coarcted segment but also in assessing the anatomy of the aortic arch and in estimating the pressure gradient across the coarctation. Cardiac catheterization is now reserved for those infants and children in whom the echocardiogram or physical examination suggests either abnormal location of the coarctation (ie, abdominal aorta), the presence of other associated cardiac lesions, or abnormal aortic arch anatomy or to enable nonsurgical treatment with balloon angioplasty (**Figure 56.1**).

Management

The poor prognosis of untreated patients with coarctation of the aorta is well established. Twenty percent of patients die between the first and second decades of life, and 80% die before 50 years of age. Coarctation of the aorta should be treated as early in childhood as possible. The two current approaches used for treating coarctation of the aorta are surgery and balloon angioplasty. Surgical treatment can consist of either resection and extended end-to-end anastomosis, left subclavian flap angioplasty, synthetic patch angioplasty, or, rarely, the use of a tube interposition graft. The incidence of restenosis depends more on the age at the time of repair than the type of surgical repair (occurring in up to 20% of children operated on at <1 year of age and in only 3% of children operated on at >3 years of age). In selected cases, balloon angioplasty can be used for the initial treatment of coarctation of the aorta. Balloon angioplasty is the treatment of choice in patients who develop restenosis after surgical repair.

Prognosis

Many individuals with repaired coarctation of the aorta do not have a normal life expectancy. They can suffer from significant cardiovascular problems, including ischemic heart disease, cerebral hemorrhage, aortic aneurysms, and persistent hypertension. Recently, we evaluated the long-term results of 254 survivors of coarctation repair performed between 1948 and 1976. After we excluded 20 individuals who died during the initial repair, use of estimated survival analysis showed that 95% of patients were alive at 10 years, 89% at 20 years, 82% at 30 years, and 79% at 40 years after operation. The mean age at death among those 45 individuals who died late after repair was 34.4 ± 22.1 years. Age at the time of initial surgical repair and preoperative blood pressure significantly affected long-term survival. The 30-year survival rate after successful correction of coarctation is $93.2 \pm 2.7\%$ in individuals operated on at <5 years of age, $91.2 \pm 2.4\%$ in individuals operated on between 5 and 10 years of age, and $75.6 \pm 3.6\%$ in individuals operated on at >10 years of age ($P<.001$ for <5 versus between 5 and 10 years and <5 versus >10 years of age). Coronary artery disease was the most common cause of late death, along with unexplained sudden death, ruptured thoracic aortic aneurysm, and perioperative death in those who underwent repeat surgery.

Mechanisms of Hypertension

There are three different types of hypertension associated with coarctation of the aorta: prerepair hypertension, postrepair paradoxical hypertension, and late postrepair hypertension.

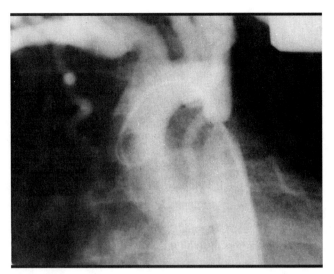

Figure 56.1. Left anterior oblique angiogram of a 15-year-old boy with a discrete thoracic coarctation.

Prerepair Hypertension

Three main theories are used to explain prerepair hypertension: the mechanical theory, the neural theory, and the Goldblatt-type phenomenon. The basis for the mechanical theory is that hypertension proximal to the coarcted segment is simply a function of the high resistance to left ventricular output imposed by the narrowing. The observations that many patients with coarctation have hypertension below as well as above the narrowing and that hypertension persists despite the presence of large collateral channels have cast doubt on this theory. The neural theory proposes that hypertension is the result of readjustment of the baroreceptors in the aortic arch such that the increased proximal pressure is necessary to ensure an adequate blood supply to the organs distal to the obstruction. There are no objective data to support or refute this theory. The third and most likely explanation for the hypertension observed in patients with coarctation of the aorta is the Goldblatt-type phenomenon, with renal underperfusion and stimulation of the renin-angiotensin-aldosterone system. Studies creating coarctation in dogs showed that hypertension could be prevented if one kidney was transplanted above the coarctation and the other kidney removed. Until recently, the major criticism of the renal underperfusion theory was that hypertensive children with coarctation did not have elevated plasma renin activity and did not have a decrease in renal blood flow. However, when coarctation patients are volume depleted, plasma renin activity is dramatically increased and their blood pressures become very responsive to antagonists of the renin-angiotensin system. A similar situation has been documented in experimental models of one-kidney, one-clip Goldblatt hypertension, and thus the analogy.

Paradoxical Hypertension

During the first week after surgical repair of coarctation of the aorta, activation of the sympathetic nervous system and the renin-angiotensin system causes paradoxical hypertension. Because balloon angioplasty is not associated with paradoxical hypertension, it appears that during the surgical repair of the coarctation, disruption of some of the afferent thoracic sympathetic fibers occurs, leading to a loss of the normal balance of excitatory and depressor sympathetic mechanoreceptors. Increased sympathetic activity in turn stimulates renin release and leads to the development of paradoxical hypertension. Paradoxical hypertension can be prevented by propranolol pretreatment, blockade of the renin-angiotensin system, or balloon angioplasty.

Late Postrepair Hypertension

Many individuals with good hemodynamic repairs and no resting gradients develop significant upper-extremity hypertension with treadmill but not arm exercise. These patients have increased vascular reactivity to exogenous norepinephrine in the right arm, normal reactivity in the legs, abnormal baroreceptor activity, and abnormal compliance and responsiveness of the vessels in the vascular bed proximal to the original coarctation. Hypertension in children or adults with absent or minimal resting arm-leg gradient and resting or exercise hypertension can be treated with standard antihypertensive medications, including ACE inhibitors and calcium channel blockers.

SUGGESTED READING

1. Campbell M. Natural history of coarctation of the aorta. *Br Heart J.* 1970;32:633–640.
2. Clarkson PM, Nicholson MR, Barratt-Boyes BG, Neutze JM, Whitlock RM. Results after repair of coarctation of the aorta beyond infancy. a 10 to 28 year follow-up with particular reference to late systemic hypertension. *Am J Cardiol.* 1983;51:1481–1488.
3. Cohen M, Fuster V, Steele PM, Driscoll D, McGoon DC. Coarctation of the aorta: long-term follow-up and prediction of outcome after surgical correction. *Circulation.* 1989;80:840–845.
4. Gidding SS, Rocchini AP, Beekman R, Szpunar CA, Moorehead C, Behrendt D, Rosenthal A. Therapeutic effect of propranolol on paradoxical hypertension after repair of coarctation of the aorta. *N Engl J Med.* 1985;312:1224–1228.
5. Markel H, Rocchini AP, Beekman RH, Martin J, Palmisano J, Moorehead C, Rosenthal A. Exercise-induced hypertension after repair of coarctation of the aorta: arm versus leg exercise. *J Am Coll Cardiol.* 1986;81:165–171.
6. Salazar O, Steinberger J, Carpenter B, et al. Predictors of hypertension in long-term survivors of repaired coarctation of the aorta. *J Am Coll Cardiol.* 1996;27(suppl A):35A. Abstract.
7. Scott HW, Bahnson HT. Evidence for a renal factor on the hypertension of coarctation of the aorta. *Surgery.* 1951;30:206–217.
8. Stewart AB, Ahmed R, Travill CM, Newman CG. Coarctation of the aorta: life and health 20–44 years after surgical repair. *Br Heart J.* 1993;69:65–70.

Chapter 57

Pathophysiology of Sleep Apnea

Barbara J. Morgan, PhD

KEY POINTS

- In a large proportion of middle-aged adults, apneas and hypopneas during sleep result in intermittent asphyxia, marked transient blood pressure elevations, and sleep fragmentation.

- A dose-response relationship exists between sleep-disordered breathing and daytime blood pressure.

- Abnormalities of sympathetic nervous function and vascular reactivity occur in sleep apnea.

- A causal link between sleep-disordered breathing and hypertension has been demonstrated in animal models; thus, sleep-disordered breathing may be an underlying pathophysiological factor in some persons with "essential" hypertension.

See also Chapter 157

Epidemiology

The estimated prevalence of clinically significant sleep-disordered breathing (≥ 5 apneas or hypopneas per hour of sleep plus complaints of daytime sleepiness) in middle-aged adults is 2% for women and 4% for men. Although daytime hypersomnolence is the predominant symptom reported by those affected by this disorder, declines in cognitive function and increased incidence of psychiatric disorders have also been reported. Sleep apnea syndrome is also associated with long-term cardiovascular morbidity from systemic and pulmonary hypertension, myocardial infarction, and stroke.

Pathophysiology

The onset of sleep is associated with a decrease in neural drive to the muscles of the respiratory pump and also to those that stiffen and maintain patency of the upper airway. This loss of muscle tone reduces airway caliber, thereby increasing transpulmonary resistance, and renders the airway more collapsible. In individuals with anatomic compromise, eg, pharyngeal fat deposition, enlargement of the soft palate or tongue, or craniofacial abnormalities, sleep-induced loss of muscle tone predisposes them to complete collapse of the upper airway, or apnea. Both apneas and hypopneas (episodes of partial airway collapse) produce transient hypoxemia, hypercapnia, acidosis, and in most cases, arousal from sleep. Each event triggers marked increases in sympathetic nervous system activity and blood pressure (**Figure 57.1**). Individuals with obstructive sleep apnea syndrome may experience hundreds of these events throughout the course of a single night's sleep.

Sleep Apnea and Hypertension

Hypertension is highly prevalent (50% to 90%) in individuals with sleep apnea syndrome. Although some of the blood pressure elevation may be attributed to comorbid obesity, several lines of evidence suggest that the relationship between sleep apnea and hypertension is causal. First, blood pressure decreases in some but not all individuals when sleep apnea is successfully treated. Second, a dose-response relationship between sleep-disordered breathing and daytime blood pressure has been observed in a large, population-based study; however, more than half of this effect can be attributed to confounding factors such as obesity, age, and male sex. Finally, evidence obtained using two distinct animal models strongly supports the notion of a cause-and-effect relationship.

Recently, persistent daytime hypertension has been produced by frequent tracheal occlusions during nocturnal sleep in a canine model (**Figure 57.2**). In parallel experiments, sleep fragmentation produced by acoustic stimuli failed to affect daytime blood pressure, suggesting that the chemical and/or mechanical consequences of the occlusions contributed more importantly to the hypertensive effect of this intervention.

The sympathetic nervous system appears to be involved in the hypertension associated with sleep apnea. A rat model that uses intermittent hypoxia during sleep has produced persistent daytime hypertension with as few as 5 weeks of exposure, but only in animals with intact sympathetic nervous systems. Sleep-disordered breathing events are known to trigger episodes of sympathetic activation and marked transient blood pressure elevations in humans; however, the mechanisms responsible for conversion of these acute pressor responses to persistent daytime hypertension have not been elucidated. Augmented sympathetic activity during wakefulness (when breathing is stable) has been observed in individuals with sleep apnea syndrome.

There is a growing body of evidence that sleep apnea, probably via the resultant hypoxia, interferes with function of the vascular endothelium. Nitric oxide–induced vasodilatation, an important mechanism in regulation of vascular tone, is impaired in patients with sleep apnea. In contrast, the search for a hormonal mediator of sleep apnea hypertension has thus far been fruitless. The renin-angiotensin-aldosterone system is suppressed in individuals with sleep apnea. Atrial natriuretic peptide, the one hormone that is consistently found to be elevated in patients with obstructive sleep apnea, would be expected to have a blood pressure–lowering effect.

Amelioration of some types of sleep-disordered breathing has been observed after treatment of high blood pressure. This finding raises the possibility that the acute and chronic hypertension caused by sleep-

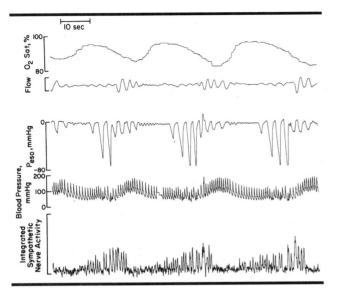

Figure 57.1. Mixed (central and obstructive) sleep apneas produce marked sympathoexcitation and transient blood pressure elevations in a patient with sleep apnea syndrome. From: Skatrud JB, Badr MS, Morgan BJ. Control of breathing during sleep and sleep disordered breathing. In: Altose M, Kawakami Y, eds. *Control of Breathing in Health and Disease.* New York, NY: Marcel Dekker Inc. (in press). Reproduced with permission.

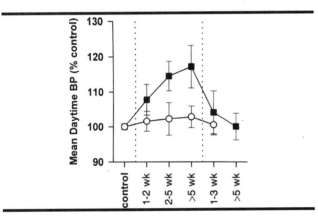

Figure 57.2. Mean daytime blood pressure in four dogs exposed to intermittent tracheal occlusions during sleep (filled squares) and sleep fragmentation (open circles) (mean±SE). The vertical dashed lines represent the durations of the exposures. From: Brooks D, Horner RL, Kozar LF, Render-Teixeira CL, Phillipson EA. Obstructive sleep apnea as a cause of systemic hypertension. *J Clin Invest.* 1997;99:106–109 by copyright permission of The American Society for Clinical Investigation.

disordered breathing can, in turn, exacerbate sleep-disordered breathing. The question of whether the two conditions could be linked by a positive feedback mechanism awaits further exploration.

Mild Sleep-Disordered Breathing and Hypertension

Most clinical investigations linking sleep-disordered breathing and hypertension have focused on individuals with obstructive sleep apnea syndrome, ie, those who represent the severe end of the sleep-disordered breathing spectrum. It has recently been appreciated that marked fluctuations in systolic and diastolic pressure accompany mild to moderate as well as severe sleep-disordered breathing. These less severe events (hypopneas and infrequent apneas) are very common in the undiagnosed population, and they contribute to small but statistically significant elevations in daytime blood pressure. The health risks associated with mild to moderate sleep-disordered breathing and the effects of early intervention in this group of individuals remain to be elucidated.

SUGGESTED READING

1. Brooks D, Horner RL, Kozar LF, Render-Teixeira CL, Phillipson EA. Obstructive sleep apnea as a cause of systemic hypertension: evidence from a canine model. *J Clin Invest.* 1997;99:106–109.
2. Carlson JT, Hedner J, Elam M, Ejnell H, Sellgren J, Wallin BG. Augmented resting sympathetic activity in awake patients with obstructive sleep apnea. *Chest.* 1993;103:1763–1768.
3. Fletcher EC, Lesske J, Culman J, Miller CC, Unger T. Sympathetic denervation blocks blood pressure elevation in episodic hypoxia. *Hypertension.* 1992;20:612–619.
4. Hedner J. Vascular function in OSA. *Sleep.* 1996;19(Suppl.10):S213-S217.
5. Leuenberger U, Jacob E, Sweer L, Waravdekar N, Zwillich C, Sinoway L. Surges of muscle sympathetic nerve activity during obstructive apnea are linked to hypoxemia. *J Appl Physiol.* 1995;79:581–588.
6. Mayer J, Weichler U, Herres-Mayer B, Schneider H, Marx U, Peter JH. Influence of metoprolol and cilazapril on blood pressure and on sleep apnea activity. *J Cardiovasc Pharmacol.*1990;16:952–961.
7. Mayer J, Becker H, Brandenburg U, Penzel T, Peter JH, von Wichert P. Blood pressure and sleep apnea: results of long-term nasal continuous positive airway pressure therapy. *Cardiology.* 1991;79:84–92.
8. Wilcox I, Grunstein RR, Hedner JA, Doyle J, Collins FL, Fletcher PJ, Kelly DT, Sullivan CE. Effect of nasal continuous positive airway pressure during sleep on 24-hour blood pressure in obstructive sleep apnea. *Sleep.* 1993;16:539–544.
9. Young T, Palta M, Dempsey J, Skatrud J, Weber S, Badr S. The occurrence of sleep-disordered breathing among middle-aged adults. *N Engl J Med.* 1993;328:1230–1235.
10. Young T, Peppard P, Palta M, Hla KM, Finn L, Morgan B, Skatrud J. Population-based study of sleep-disordered breathing as a risk factor for hypertension. *Arch Intern Med.* 1997;157:1746–1752.

Chapter 58

Affective Illness and Hypertension

Wayne L. Creelman, MD, MMM, FAPA

KEY POINTS

- The prevalence of depression and anxiety disorders is greater in persons with hypertension.

- The lowering of blood pressure does not cause depression.

See also Chapter 101

General Aspects

Case reports, cohort studies, and other medical literature suggest an association between affective illness (depression) and hypertension. Unfortunately, in most of the clinical literature, differing methods of case findings and differing operational definitions of depression and hypertension are used, but the prevalence of depression among hypertensive individuals may exceed 30%. A causal basis for this association was suggested by B.F. Fuller, who outlined several possibilities, including (1) a common physiological factor that underlies both disorders; (2) depression resulting from side effects of antihypertensive medications; (3) depression secondary to chronic medical illness, including hypertension; (4) depression resulting from medically lowered blood pressure and decreased cerebral perfusion; and (5) coincidence.

Epidemiological Studies

Some investigators have reported that depressive illness occurs in >62% of hypertensive psychiatric outpatients. However, Fuller's own retrospective study using a convenience sample of 175 adult clients of three community mental health centers in a western US state did not support any unusually high prevalence of depressive disorders among psychiatric outpatients. He found no difference in the prevalence of *Diagnostic and Statistical Manual of Diagnostic Disorders* (DSM-III)-diagnosed depressive disorders between hypertensive and normotensive psychiatric outpatient subjects, even when age and drug therapy were considered.

Rabkin et al studied 452 psychiatric outpatients with a DSM-III diagnosis of major depression and found that they were three times as likely to suffer from comorbid hypertensive disease as those without hypertension. It appears from the study that age, sex, chronic medical illness, or current antihypertensive medication did not account for these diagnostic differences. The data in Rabkin's study support a clinically and statistically significant association between hypertension and depression among psychiatric patients. However, the authors also indicate the need for longitudinal cohort studies that would disentangle a variety of causal factors in the relationship and etiologies of the two disorders.

Simonsick et al found an association between depressive symptomatology and blood pressure control as well as the longitudinal association between depressive symptomatology and blood pressure control, stroke, and cardiovascular system-related mortality. Their data indicate that among persons with diagnosed hypertension, 9.4% to 13.5% of men and 20.6% to 27.1% of women had high depressive symptomatology. Such studies open the door to the potential for improved outcomes with appropriate antidepressant medications.

Neuroanatomic Linkages

Neuroanatomic evidence also exists regarding the relationship between depression and hypertension. Krishnan et al found a greater number of subcortical white matter hyperintensities and smaller basal ganglia in late-onset depressive individuals that may also have a common origin in atherosclerotic changes that occur with both aging and hypertensive vascular disease. Because depression is a frequent finding in hypertension and is also associated with an impairment of cognitive function, depression could be the primary determinant of the attentional impairment, related memory defects, and slower psychomotor reaction time found in hypertensive patients. Palombo et al identified the functional nature of cognitive impairment in hypertension and suggested that improvement can be achieved with adequate control of blood pressure using antihypertensive drugs that do not themselves interfere with psychomotor performance. This particular study also underscores that the cognitive impairment associated with depression in hypertensive participants is independent of the presence of cerebral lesions.

Relationship to Anxiety and Personality Disorders

Up to 60% of patients with depressive symptoms also have diagnosable anxiety disorders. Clinicians in primary care and mental health sectors should be prepared to screen and treat individuals with multiple comorbid psychiatric conditions, because anxiety symptomatology may be a precursor to the comorbid association of depression and hypertension. Individuals with a positive family history of hypertension often report greater levels of anxiety and depression compared with those with a negative family history of hypertension. Although the literature suggests a possible genetic link to impaired cognitive abilities and depression among patients with hypertension, further research is necessary to identify specific mechanisms that may be responsible for the deficits observed in individuals with a positive family history of hypertension who exhibit a high prevalence of depressive symptoms.

Wells et al found that depressed adult outpatients with a history of myocardial infarction have a particularly poor clinical prognosis. Persistence of depressive symptoms in outpatients with myocardial infarction is also associated with a poorer clinical prognosis for cardiac improvement. Individuals who report high levels of anxiety or depressive symptoms are at elevated risk for developing cardiovascular disease years later.

There is also an association between alexithymia and essential hypertension. In a sample of 114 hypertensive patients studied with the well-validated 20-item Toronto Alexithymia Scale, Todarello et al found that individuals who suppress their feelings, especially chronic anger, are at an increased risk for developing essential hypertension. It has been hypothesized that a deficit in the cognitive processing and modulation of emotions may leave alexithymic individuals prone to states of heightened sympathetic arousal that may be responsible for the development of essential hypertension.

Stress, Depression, and Hypertension

Many clinical studies indicate that psychosocial stress may indeed be associated with eventual depressive states with or without hypertension. Feelings of exhaustion and emotional distress clearly may lead to clinical states of depression, with the comorbid stress exerting its influence toward an increased risk for hypertension. Anxiety, depression, and stress have all been shown to result in direct acute autonomic arousal and transient increases in blood pressure.

Much evidence exists that the regulatory failure of noradrenergic and serotonergic systems results in a loss of selectivity of responsiveness to environmental stimuli and a delayed return to baseline activity after stressful or depressive stimuli diminish. It is therefore possible that the persistence of any type of dysphoric mood may contribute to the development of chronic hypertension. Recent work by Konopka et al suggests that there may be a relationship of depression to hypertension based on an abnormality of calcium flux. They suggest that increased intracellular calcium levels in platelets from depressed patients are similar to those reported in chronic hypertension. Thus, as a consequence, a defect in calcium regulation may predispose an individual to both hypertension and depression.

Psychopharmacological Issues
Effects of Lowered Blood Pressure on Mood

Much confusion exists regarding the benefit of medication treatment of comorbid depression and hypertension. Treatment of isolated systolic hypertension did not cause deterioration in cognition, emotional state, physical function, or leisure activities in the Systolic Hypertension in the Elderly Program (SHEP) study in 4736 persons. Thus, active treatment of hypertension had no perceptible negative effect on any measures that would constitute either a worsening or an initiation of depression.

Effects of Specific Antihypertensive Drugs

Cardiovascular drugs may contribute to mood disorders. Patten et al found an association between ACE inhibitors and depressive disorders, but their study design was not capable of determining whether the depressive disorder preceded or followed exposure to ACE inhibitors, although the effects may be most evident in women and elderly subjects.

The side-effect profile for propranolol and other lipophilic β-blockers is well known for the induction of hypotension and depression. Similarly, central sympatholytics such as methyldopa, clonidine, guanabenz, and guanfacine frequently cause depression and sedation. Finally, the peripheral noradrenergic antagonists such as reserpine are well known in the literature for their adverse effects of severe psychic depression.

Drug Interactions That Can Raise Blood Pressure

Blood pressure may increase in some depressed patients treated with antidepressants, but cause and effect have not been clearly established. Modest increases in blood pressure may occur with tricyclic antidepressants but are unlikely to be of clinical significance in most patients. Hypertensive crisis can occur with potent serotonergic compounds such as clomipramine, fluoxetine, paroxetine, and sertraline. Lethal reactions have been extremely rare, except when monoamine oxidase inhibitors were given either concomitantly with or shortly after an SSRI. Although the antidepressant venlafaxine may increase blood pressure in a small proportion of normotensive patients at doses >200 mg daily, blood pressure does not tend to increase further in depressed patients with hypertension. Adverse cardiovascular outcomes have not been reported for venlafaxine or other tricyclic antidepressants.

The interaction of tricyclic antidepressants antagonizing guanethidine is well established. Because guanethidine and related antihypertensives are taken up into noradrenergic neurons by the same pump that is responsible for the reuptake of norepinephrine, when tricyclic antidepressants block this pump, they prevent guanethidine from reaching its site of action. Lower doses of cyclic antidepressants may be required when diltiazem or verapamil is coprescribed, because these calcium channel blockers inhibit the metabolism of drugs oxidized by the cytochrome P450–3A4 isoenzyme. The hypotensive effects of clonidine may also be antagonized by cyclic antidepressants, which alter the sensitivity of presynaptic α-adrenergic receptors.

SUGGESTED READING
1. Applegate WB, Pressel S, Wittes J, Luhr J, Shekelle RB, Camel GH, Greenlick MR, Hadley E, Moye L, Perry HM Jr, Schron E, Wegener V. Impact of the treatment of isolated systolic hypertension on behavioral variables. *Arch Intern Med.* 1994;154:2154–2160.
2. Ciraulo DA, Shader RI, Greenblatt DJ, Creelman W. *Drug Interactions in Psychiatry.* 2nd ed. Baltimore, Md: Williams & Wilkins; 1995.
3. Feighner JP. Cardiovascular safety in depressed patients: focus on venlafaxine. *J Clin Psychiatry.* 1995;56:574–579.
4. Fuller BF. DMS-III depression and hypertension in two psychiatric outpatient populations. *Psychosomatics.* 1988;29:417–423.
5. Konopka LM, Cooper R, Crayton JW. Serotonin-induced increases in platelet cytosolic calcium concentration in depressed, schizophrenic, and substance abuse patients. *Biol Psychiatry.* 1996;39:708–713.
6. Krishnan KR, McDonald WM, Doraiswamy PM, Tupler LA, Husain M, Boyko OB, Figiel GS, Ellinwood EH Jr. Neuroanatomical substrates of depression in the elderly. *Eur Arch Psychiatry Clin Neurosci.* 1993;243:41–46.
7. Palombo V, Scurti R, Muscari A, Puddu GM, Di Ioria A, Zito M, Abate G. Blood pressure and intellectual function in elderly subjects. *Age Aging.* 1997;26:91–98.
8. Patten SB, Williams JV, Love EJ. Case-control studies of cardiovascular medications as risk factors for clinically diagnosed depressive disorders in a hospitalized population. *Can J Psychiatry.* 1996;41:469–476.
9. Rabkin JG, Charles E, Kass F. Hypertension and DMS-III depression in psychiatric outpatients. *Am J Psychiatry.* 1983;140:1072–1074.
10. Simonsick EM, Wallace RB, Blazer DG, Berkman LF. Depressive symptomatology and hypertension-associated morbidity and mortality in older adults. *Psychosom Med.* 1995;57:427–435.
11. Todarello O, Taylor GJ, Parker JD, Fanelli M. Alexithymia in essential hypertensive and psychiatric outpatients: a comparative study. *J Psychosom Res.* 1995;39:987–994.
12. Wells KB, Rogers W, Burnam MA, Camp P. Course of depression in patients with hypertension, myocardial infarction, or insulin-dependent diabetes. *Am J Psychiatry.* 1993;150:632–638.

Chapter 59

Pathophysiology of Preeclampsia

Ellen W. Seely, MD; Marshall D. Lindheimer, MD

KEY POINTS

- Preeclampsia is a multisystem disorder of pregnancy characterized by hypertension, proteinuria, often edema, and variable manifestations of liver function and coagulation system abnormalities.

- Preeclampsia is a vasoconstrictive form of hypertension with decreased intravascular volume and increased vascular resistance.

- The pathogenesis of preeclampsia is unknown and is likely to be multifactorial.

See also Chapter 148

Preeclampsia is a hypertensive condition peculiar to pregnancy. Its convulsive phase, eclampsia, remains a leading cause of maternal and fetal morbidity and death. The disorder has been recognized and feared for centuries, but its genesis remains unknown, and there are still no definitive means of prevention or treatment. Preeclampsia complicates >3% of all pregnancies and ≈7% of nulliparous gestations in the United States. The disorder is more apt to occur in several "high-risk" populations, including women with diabetes, twins, chronic hypertension, underlying renal disease, or previous preeclampsia, for whom the incidence is between 20% and 25%. Incidence of the disorder may also be high in patients with dyslipidemias and thrombotic disorders, including women with factor V Leyden, protein C or S deficiency, increased antiphospholipid antibody titers, certain angiotensinogen gene variants, and hyperhomocysteinemia.

Clinical Syndrome

Preeclampsia typically presents in the third trimester of a first pregnancy and resolves in the immediate puerperium. Rarely, "early" (<20 weeks' gestation) forms of the disorder occur. It is a multisystem disease affecting primarily the vasculature, kidneys, liver, and brain. Preeclampsia is diagnosed in a woman with new onset of hypertension (≥140/90 mm Hg), usually after gestational week 20, accompanied by proteinuria ≥300 mg/d. Other common clinical and laboratory manifestations include facial and extremity edema, hemoconcentration, thrombocytopenia, hypoalbuminemia, elevated uric acid levels, liver enzyme abnormalities, and hypocalciuria. The diagnosis is more difficult in women with preexisting chronic hypertension, but it is prudent to consider "superimposed preeclampsia" when systolic or diastolic blood pressure levels increase ≥30 or ≥15 mm Hg, respectively, proteinuria ≥300 mg/d appears, protein excretion increases dramatically, or there is evidence of the "HELLP" syndrome (hemolysis, elevated liver function tests, and low platelets).

The greatest concern is that preeclampsia may progress to a life-threatening convulsive phase called eclampsia, or to a HELLP-like syndrome. Eclampsia is frequently preceded by premonitory symptoms and signs, including hyperreflexia, visual disturbances, severe headaches, right upper quadrant or epigastric pain, and several laboratory changes. The sudden appearance of the HELLP constellation, with microangiopathic hemolytic anemia, a rapidly falling platelet count, and increments in bilirubin and liver enzymes (often marked), is an emergency requiring interruption of the pregnancy to avoid progression to renal failure, sepsis, eclampsia with cerebral hemorrhage, and maternal death. Decreased placental perfusion is another characteristic of preeclampsia and underlies the increase in the incidence of intrauterine growth retardation and fetal loss in these patients. In addition, the frequent need for preterm delivery makes preeclampsia a leading cause of premature birth in the United States.

Pathology and Pathophysiology

Preeclampsia is a complex disorder that affects many organ systems.

Kidney

In contrast to normal pregnancy, both glomerular filtration rate and renal plasma flow decrease in preeclampsia. These changes are accompanied by a microscopic renal lesion characterized by hypertrophy of glomerular capillary endothelial and mesangial cells, called "glomerular endotheliosis." The severity of these lesions correlates with the magnitude of proteinuria and hyperuricemia.

Brain

Fatal cases demonstrate various degrees of cerebral bleeding, from microscopic petechiae to gross hemorrhage. Cerebral edema, usually diagnosed by computerized tomography, was not recognized in the older literature and may reflect improved diagnostic sensitivity, iatrogenic volume loading, or vasogenic edema in cases in which blood pressure exceeds cerebral autoregulatory capacity. In this latter respect, vasoconstriction out of proportion to peripheral blood pressure measurements has been described by use of Doppler ultrasound technology.

Liver

The "HELLP" syndrome was described above. Its pathological counterparts are periportal hepatic lesions characterized by cell necrosis, associated at times with infarction and fibrin deposition. Periportal hemorrhages may become confluent and develop into hematomas. Subcapsular bleeding leading to rupture is a serious complication of preeclampsia.

Placenta

Abnormal placentation is a feature of preeclampsia. Major lesions occur in the placental arteries ("acute atherosis"), and the uterine spiral arteries do not undergo normal dilation and remodeling. The compromised placenta may be the source of the disease, with the hypoxemic environment leading to abnormal metabolism and the release of hormones and cytokines that may enter the maternal circulation. In preeclampsia, cytotrophoblastic cells express adhesion molecules believed to be crucial to the process of vascular remodeling. Other data suggest that women with the angiotensin gene variant T235 have abnormalities of the local renin-angiotensin system in placental vessels, leading to inappropriate angiogenesis and perhaps clotting.

Cardiovascular System and Volume Homeostasis

Hypertension in preeclampsia is primarily due to a reversal of the pattern of vasodilation and blood volume expansion characteristic of normal gestation. Instead, preeclampsia is characterized by striking increments in peripheral vascular resistance and low blood volume. Even when peripheral edema is marked, intravascular volume, cardiac filling pressures, and cardiac output are decreased or normal. A rise in hematocrit is evidence of hemoconcentration. Another feature of the disease is persistence of pressor effects of infused angiotensin, and perhaps catecholamines as well; in normal pregnancies, there is decreased pressor sensitivity. The increased vascular reactivity to endogenous pressor substances may contribute to the blood pressure lability seen in some of these patients and the marked increments in peripheral resistance.

Endothelial Dysfunction

In preeclampsia, there is decreased activity of the constitutive nitric oxide synthase in maternal and fetal vessels and in the placenta. Evidence for NO deficiency is more consistent in animal models than in human disease. Aberrations in the NO-independent endothelium-derived relaxing factor systems, mainly potassium channels, have also been implicated in preeclampsia. Whether this is a primary abnormality or a phenomenon secondary to vascular damage is not yet known.

Hypocalciuria and Low Vitamin D

Hypocalciuria is a characteristic finding in women with preeclampsia. Low urinary calcium is associated with lower $1,25(OH)_2$ vitamin D levels and higher parathyroid hormone levels than in normal pregnancy. The higher parathyroid hormone levels may result in an increase in intracellular calcium, which in vascular smooth muscle would result in vasoconstriction.

Insulin Resistance and Sympathetic Activity

Insulin resistance is a hallmark of pregnancy, and some studies have shown greater insulin resistance in preeclampsia than in normal pregnancy. Increased sympathetic nervous activity, which has also been described in preeclampsia, could explain the exaggerated vasoconstriction seen in this disorder.

Renin-Angiotensin-Aldosterone System and Volume Homeostasis

Disordered regulation of the renin-angiotensin-aldosterone system (RAAS) appears to play a role in the pathophysiology of preeclampsia. Unlike the activation of this system seen in normotensive pregnancy, women with preeclampsia have lower levels of all circulating RAAS components despite activation of local cellular systems, such as in the developing placental vasculature. Coexistent suppression of the systemic RAAS in the setting of decreased plasma volume and increased sensitivity to the vasoconstrictive effects of angiotensin II define a profile of abnormal relationships between volume regulatory and vasoconstrictive systems. Excessive angiotensin II responsiveness in preeclampsia may be due to upregulation of angiotensin II receptors.

Prostaglandin Imbalance

An excess of vasoconstrictor over vasodilatory prostaglandins has been proposed as another mechanism for the vasoconstriction seen in preeclampsia. Relative overproduction of thromboxane A_2 (TXA_2) compared with prostacyclin (PGI_2) could cause vasoconstriction and increased platelet aggregation. Investigations in this field have been limited by the technical difficulties in accurate measurement of prostaglandins. Of interest, clinical trials aimed at decreasing thromboxane production, such as the prophylactic administration of low-dose aspirin, have failed to prevent preeclampsia.

Endothelins

Higher endothelin levels have been reported in women with preeclampsia, but it is unclear whether this is a primary event or secondary to vascular damage during the disease process.

Cytokines

Elevated plasma levels of several cytokines, including tumor necrosis factor-α, interleukin-1, and interleukin-6, have been demonstrated in preeclamptic women. The site of genesis of these cytokines is not known but has been postulated to be a hypoxic placenta. These cytokines may cause endothelial damage.

Oxidants and Antioxidants

There is evidence that the balance between circulating oxidant and antioxidant activity is challenged by the gravid state. In preeclampsia, the dominance of the former leads to endothelial damage. Areas of interest relate to a host of substances that stimulate, temporize, or counterbalance the production of free radicals (eg, serum iron, xanthine oxidase, LDLs, isoprostanes, and vitamin C).

Etiology

Limitation of understanding of the pathophysiology of preeclampsia is in part a result of the unknown etiology of the disorder. However, renewed interest in this disorder has produced a plethora of research activity, including the application of modern technology pertinent to molecular and cell biology. The mystique surrounding the cause of preeclampsia, which has fascinated us for centuries, may not survive the first decade of this millenium. There are three schools of thought in current investigation: (1) that preeclampsia is of placental origin (discussed above); (2) that the pathogenesis resides in factors initiated in the maternal environment; and, of course, (3) that pathology related to the placenta and to the mother must interact to cause the disease. Those investigating the maternal environment focus primarily on known cardiovascular risks found in nonpregnant populations. Although some still seek a single unifying hypothesis, others maintain that there will be multiple causes of the disorder.

Genetic

Inheritance of a gene or genes that predispose to the development of preeclampsia is suggested by the familial nature of this disorder. The familial nature was first described by Chesley in the 1960s. Recently, there has been a report of several specific allelic substitutions that have been associated in different reports with preeclampsia. The increased incidence of preeclampsia associated with a number of inherited genes (eg, variants of the angiotensinogen gene) and clotting and lipid disorders have already been discussed.

Immunology

An immune response to paternal antigen in the fetoplacental unit is proposed as a cause of preeclampsia. This may explain the occasional reports of "inflammatory" responses associated with preeclampsia, including activation of circulating leukocytes. The propensity of preeclampsia to occur in the first pregnancy supports the immune hypothesis. Preeclampsia usually decreases in frequency with subsequent pregnancies, but if the father is different, the incidence is similar to the first pregnancy. Women who had formerly used barrier methods of contraception have a greater chance of being preeclamptic than those with a prior history of oral contraceptive use. Finally, the incidence of preeclampsia decreases with length of cohabitation, suggesting that long-term exposure causes accommodation to paternal antigens.

SUGGESTED READING

1. August P, Lindheimer MD. Pathophysiology of preeclampsia. In: Laragh JH, Brenner BM, eds. *Hypertension: Pathophysiology, Diagnosis, and Management.* 2nd ed. New York, NY: Raven Press; 1995:2407–2426.
2. Brown MA, Wang J, Whitworth JA. The renin-angiotensin-aldosterone system in pre-eclampsia. *Clin Exp Hypertens.* 1997;19:713–726.
3. Conrad KP, Benyo DF. Placental cytokines and the pathogenesis of preeclampsia. *Am J Reprod Immunol.* 1997;37:240–249.
4. Decker GA, Sibai BM. Early detection of preeclampsia. *Am J Obstet Gynecol.* 1998;165:160–172.
5. Ness RB, Roberts JM. Heterogeneous causes constituting the single syndrome of preeclampsia: a hypothesis and its implications. *Am J Obstet Gynecol.* 1996;175:1365–1370.
6. Schobel HP, Fischer T, Heuszer K, Geiger H, Schmieder RE. Preeclampsia: a state of sympathetic overactivity. *N Engl J Med.* 1996;335:1480–1485.
7. Witlin AG, Sibai BM. Hypertension in pregnancy: current concepts of preeclampsia. *Annu Rev Med.* 1997;48:115–127.

Chapter 60

Hypertension and Transplantation

Stephen C. Textor, MD

KEY POINTS

- Hypertension is relatively common after solid organ transplantation.

- The hallmark of transplantation-associated hypertension is increased vasoconstriction.

- Cyclosporine and other drugs used in suppressing rejection contribute directly to the pathogenesis of this hypertension.

See also Chapter 158

Hypertension, either de novo or aggravated from pretransplantation levels, has been a regular feature of solid organ transplantation since the introduction of immunosuppression based on cyclosporin A (CSA) in the early 1980s. This has been particularly common in patients receiving liver, heart, and renal allografts. Disturbances of renal function and vasomotor tone leading to elevated systemic vascular resistance are nearly universal (**Table 60.1**). Newer agents and formulations, such as tacrolimus (FK506) and neoral, share these features, with minor modifications. In most instances, these agents are administered in combination with glucocorticoids, which may themselves raise arterial pressure (**see Figure 60.1**). This section will summarize current views regarding the pathophysiology and management of this disorder.

Incidence of Hypertension After Transplantation

Serial studies in patients treated with CSA demonstrate a rise in systemic vascular resistance within days or weeks of the beginning of immunosuppression. The prevalence of hypertension ranges from 42% in patients treated with CSA alone to 100% in some allograft settings with both CSA and steroids. Particularly in the case of renal transplant recipients, pretransplantation hypertension may be worsened. In conditions such as liver transplantation, pretransplantation blood pressures are normal or low and may rise 40 to 50 mm Hg over the course of a few weeks. Within 6 to 12 months, blood pressure in between 75% and 100% of allograft recipients reaches hypertensive levels (**Figure 60.2**).

Clinical Features

The rate of blood pressure rise after transplantation differs among the various organ settings and may reflect other posttransplantation changes, including volume expansion, preexisting hypertension, graft rejection, and infections.

A loss of the normal nocturnal fall in blood pressure is nearly universal in the first months after transplantation. In some cases, there is a nocturnal rise in blood pressure, associated with increased sodium excretion, nocturnal headache, and sleep disturbances. This may be partly a result of high steroid doses early after transplantation. Over time, diurnal blood pressure variation returns in some but not all patients, regardless of steroid dose.

Hypertensive target organ effects can appear rapidly after transplantation. If untreated, posttransplantation hypertension can progress to an accelerated phase with encephalopathy, seizures, and vascular injury, including microangiopathic hemolysis. Intracranial hemorrhage has occurred. The most severe clinical manifestations seem to occur in previously normotensive subjects and children.

Within days of administration, CSA immunosuppression produces a fall in glomerular filtration caused by renal vasoconstriction and impaired sodium excretion. Although changes in kidney function do not entirely explain increased blood pressure in these patients, hypertension after transplantation is considered "sodium sensitive" and may worsen during volume expansion.

The natural history of posttransplantation hypertension is not well understood. Despite reduction in CSA and steroid doses in later periods, most patients require continued antihypertensive therapy. Antihypertensive drug doses may be lowered, however, and occasionally may be discontinued, despite long-term alterations in kidney function.

Pathophysiology

Several mechanisms appear to participate in the development of hypertension after transplantation (**Table 60.2**). The dominant hemodynamic feature is widespread vasoconstriction, leading to a rise in regional and total peripheral vascular resistance. CSA and tacrolimus are highly lipophilic materials and freely permeate cell membranes, including vascular endothelial cells. CSA produces a generalized distur-

---

Table 60.1. Clinical Manifestations of Hypertension After Transplantation

Rapid rise in arterial pressure after introduction of cyclosporine/steroid immunosuppression
Vasoconstriction in most vascular beds
Accelerated hypertension if untreated
    Encephalopathy
    Microangiopathic hemolysis
    Intravascular thrombosis
        Intracranial hemorrhage
        Reversal of circadian blood pressure patterns
        Acceleration of atherosclerosis

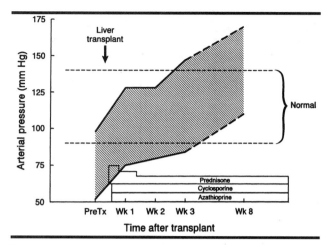

Figure 60.1. Arterial pressures during the first weeks after liver transplantation. Doses of immunosuppressive drugs, including glucocorticoids (prednisone) and cyclosporine, are highest immediately after transplantation. The progressive rise of arterial pressure over several weeks was accompanied by a reduction in cardiac output and increased system vascular resistance.

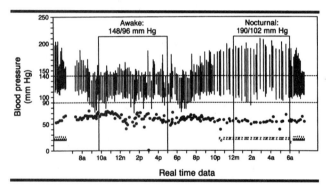

Figure 60.2. Ambulatory blood pressure monitoring in a young woman 4 months after transplantation. Pressures when the patient is awake underestimate the average 24-hour pressure because of a paradoxical nocturnal rise in pressure. This is sometimes associated with a distinctive syndrome of nocturia, headache, and disturbed sleep. Reprinted with permission from Textor SC, Taler SJ, Canzanello VJ, Schwartz L. Cyclosporine, blood pressure and atherosclerosis. *Cardiol Rev.* 1997;5:141–151.

Table 60.2. Proposed Mechanisms of Hypertension After Clinical Transplantation

Endothelial dysfunction with disturbed vasomotor systems
   Reduced nitric oxide production
   Reduced prostacyclin excretion
   Increased endothelin release
   ?Increased thromboxane
Renal dysfunction with impaired sodium excretion
Increased adrenergic sympathetic neural activity

---

bance of endothelial control, both stimulating vasoconstrictor mechanisms (including release of the potent vasoconstrictor endothelin) and inhibiting vasodilating systems (including prostacyclin and nitric oxide). Some studies indicate increased adrenergic activation and modification of intracellular calcineurin. The renin-angiotensin system is suppressed early after transplantation, although it appears to become more active during late phases (>1 year) after transplantation.

Management of Hypertension After Transplantation

Primary principles affecting the choice of antihypertensive agents in transplant recipients include (1) recognition of a high incidence of diminished glomerular filtration rate associated with relatively impaired potassium excretion and hyperuricemia and (2) thorough knowledge of interactions between antihypertensive drugs and cyclosporine/tacrolimus levels. For the most part, the same considerations regarding any other hypertensive state apply to patients with solid organ transplants. Dihydropyridine calcium channel blocking agents, such as nifedipine, felodipine, amlodipine, and isradipine, are effective vasodilators and have negligible effects on cyclosporine disposition. Diltiazem, verapamil, and nicardipine have substantial effects on CSA and warrant close follow-up of drug levels during administration. When combined with diuretics, ACE inhibitors have been used successfully, although caution must be exercised and the patient must be observed for hyperkalemia and hyporeninemic hypoaldosteronism (type IV renal tubular acidosis). In animals, nephrotoxicity related to cyclosporine is blunted by blockade of the renin-angiotensin system, although the applicability of this observation to human subjects is not known.

It should be emphasized that long-term immunosuppression commonly leads to increased lipid levels and adverse changes in overall cardiovascular risk. Morbidity and mortality after the early years are common and are related to accelerated manifestations of atherosclerotic disease in allograft recipients, particularly coronary artery disease. Hence, management of transplant recipients requires careful attention to both posttransplantation hypertension and lipid changes for optimal long-term success.

SUGGESTED READING

1. Canzanello VJ, Schwartz L, Taler SJ, Textor SC, Wiesner RH, Porayko MK, Krom RA. Evolution of cardiovascular risk after liver transplantation: a comparison of cyclosporine A and tacrolimus (FK506). *Liver Transpl Surg.* 1997;3:1–9.
2. Roullet JB, Xue H, McCarron DA, Holcomb S, Bennett WM. Vascular mechanisms of cyclosporine-induced hypertension in the rat. *J Clin Invest.* 1994;93:2244–2250.
3. Sander M, Victor RG. Hypertension after cardiac transplantation: pathophysiology and management. *Curr Opin Nephrol Hypertens.* 1995;4:443–451.
4. Taler SJ, Textor SC, Canzanello VJ, Schwartz L, Porayko M, Wiesner RH, Krom RA. Role of steroid dose in hypertension early after liver transplantation with tacrolimus (FK506) and cyclosporine. *Transplantation.* 1996;62:1588–1592.
5. Taler SJ, Textor SC, Canzanello VJ, Wilson DJ, Wiesner RH, Krom RA. Loss of nocturnal blood pressure fall after liver transplantation during immunosuppressive therapy. *Am J Hypertens.* 1995;8:598–605.
6. Textor SC, Taler SJ, Canzanello VJ, Schwartz L. Cyclosporine, blood pressure and atherosclerosis. *Cardiol Rev.* 1997;5:141–151.
7. Van den Dorpel MA, van den Meiracker AH, Lameris TW, Boomsma F, Levi M, Man in 't Veld AJ, Weimar W, Schalekamp MA. Cyclosporin A impairs the nocturnal blood pressure fall in renal transplant recipients. *Hypertension.* 1996;28:304–307.

Chapter 61

Mechanisms of Vascular Hypertrophy

Paul R. Standley, PhD

KEY POINTS

- A variety of endocrine and autocrine/paracrine factors work in concert to regulate vascular smooth muscle cell growth.

- The hallmark of vascular hypertrophy is an increase in vascular smooth muscle cell size and DNA content.

See also Chapters 62, 114

Hypertrophy can be strictly defined as growth brought about by an increase in cell size rather than number. In contrast, hyperplastic growth results from an abnormal increase in cell number rather than cell size. Arterial media (or muscularis) is composed of phenotypically heterogeneous vascular smooth muscle cell (VSMC) populations with unique developmental lineage. In adulthood, VSMCs normally reside in the vascular wall in a relatively quiescent state characterized by an extremely low (<5%) mitotic index. However, in pathological states such as hypertension and atherosclerosis, VSMCs display phenotypic modulation characterized by enhanced hypertrophic and/or hyperplastic growth, altered lipid metabolism, altered expression of receptors, and enhanced extracellular matrix deposition.

Role of the Endothelium

Although vascular hypertrophy/hyperplasia occurs primarily as a result of VSMC growth and increased extracellular matrix protein deposition, the vascular endothelium plays a vital modulating role in such growth. Vascular endothelial cells transduce myriad chemical and hemodynamic signals that ultimately enhance or diminish the overall growth status of VSMCs. For example, adhesion of T cells and monocytes to endothelial immune elements fosters monocytic infiltration, altered lipid metabolism, formation of foam cells, and platelet aggregation at sites of vascular injury (eg, in atherosclerosis and after balloon angioplasty). This ultimately leads to vascular hypertrophy/hyperplasia, as is seen in restenosis and in hypertensive states after angioplasty.

Autocrine Regulation by VSMCs and Platelets

VSMCs themselves express a variety of growth factors that, in an autocrine manner, regulate their own growth. These include insulin-like growth factor 1 (IGF-1), fibroblast growth factor (FGF), and platelet-derived growth factor (PDGF). VSMCs also express specific receptors for these growth factors that transduce mitogenic and antimitogenic signals. Various other stimuli enhance or attenuate expression of such autocrine growth factors and their receptors, including endothelium-derived growth factors, hemodynamic factors such as circumferential and axial stretch, shear stress, platelet-derived mitogens, VSMC redox state, and extracellular matrix proteins and their molecular fragments.

At sites of injury, platelet aggregation enhances VSMC growth promoting/inhibiting signals. For example, PDGF stimulates VSMC hypertrophy and hyperplasia both indirectly via modulation of endothelial cell function and directly by binding to VSMC receptors. In addition, nitric oxide (NO) secreted by activated platelets decreases proliferation and contributes to programmed cell death (apoptosis; see below).

Hemodynamic Factors and Mechanotransduction

The pulsatile flow of blood in arteries and veins is a major stimulus to VSMC structure and function. Changes in flow velocity or shear stress on the endothelium combine with changes in axial and circumferential stress of VSMCs on the vessel wall to produce powerful cell signals that affect vascular structure and function. During a single cardiac cycle at normal blood pressure, VSMCs are stretched by ≈10% of their initial resting length. Increased pulse pressures can double the stretch stimulus and activate a subset of stretch-activated calcium and sodium channels that alter vascular tone, sodium pump activity, intracellular pH, and gene expression. Mechanical deformation of the extracellular matrix by pressure waveforms stimulates VSMC growth via activation of integrin-associated tyrosine kinases and subsequent activation of gene promoter elements (see below).

Experimental cyclic stretch of VSMCs cultured on extracellular matrix protein elastomeres also enhances expression and secretion of IGF-1 and FGF, which promote cellular hypertrophy and hyperplasia. Blockade of these receptors or their key intermediate cellular signaling molecules eliminates stretch-induced growth.

Diversity of Mitogenic Stimuli

Most circulating vasoconstrictors (eg, catecholamines, angiotensin II, vasopressin, and endothelins) identified to date are mitogenic. These vasoconstrictors decrease vascular lumen diameter and, given equivalent blood flow, increase blood pressure. With chronic blood pressure elevation, enhanced muscle cell mass or extracellular matrix protein density would increase contractile force, vascular wall thickening, and wall tension (as would be predicted by the law of Laplace).

VSMCs can synthesize several vasoconstrictor/growth-promoting substances, such as angiotensin II, endothelins, and growth factors (such as PDGF, FGF, IGF-1, and transforming growth factor-β [TGF-β]), which act in autocrine fashion to stimulate VSMC growth (**Figure 61.1**). Several of these growth factors serve the role of

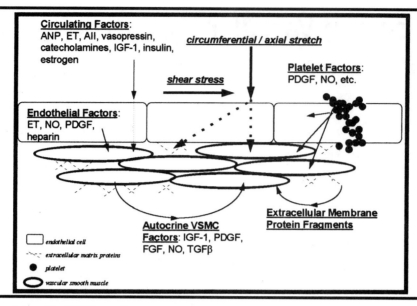

Figure 61.1.   Multiple stimuli that affect VSMC growth. ANP indicates atrial natriuretic peptide; ET, endothelin; and AII, angiotensin II. Other abbreviations as in text.

competence factors (eg, PDGF is sufficient to allow VSMCs to transit from the quiescent G_0 phase). Other molecules (eg, IGF-1) serve as progression factors that stimulate cells to proceed through the remainder of the cell cycle. VSMCs are capable of expressing both types of factors, because cultured VSMCs proliferate in the absence of exogenously added serum or associated growth factors.

Antimitogenic Stimuli and Apoptosis

Many vasodilators inhibit VSMC growth, including vasodilatory prostaglandins (PGI_1, PGI_2), prostacyclin, NO, endothelium-derived heparin, estrogen, atrial natriuretic peptide, and TGF-β. Consequently, NO and other vasodilators/growth inhibitors provide counterregulation not only of blood pressure but also of vascular growth status compared with the actions of vasoconstrictors/growth promoters.

Apoptosis, a ubiquitous and highly regulated form of programmed cell death, is another important mechanism to delete nonfunctional or aging cells. In normal growth and development, apoptosis of specific VSMC lineages is required to provide space for new, differentiated cell types to establish themselves. In a similar fashion, vascular remodeling, as seen in hypertension and other pathological states, seems to involve VSMC apoptotic events coupled to VSMC proliferative sequelae. A steady state requires equal rates of entry and exit of cells. The presence of growth can be viewed as an equilibrium shift in favor of proliferation or hypertrophy over apoptosis or atrophy. In this regard, NO not only slows VSMC hyperproliferation in pathological states but also is probably required for physiological remodeling of the vasculature by deletion of certain VSMCs of distinct lineages.

Cellular Signaling Abnormalities

In some hypertensive states, overproduction of vasoconstrictor mitogens, such as angiotensin II, has been implicated in pressure-induced vascular growth. However, derangements in cellular signaling of such hormones also probably underlie such remodeling, be-

cause VSMCs obtained from hypertensive humans and animals display hyperproliferation in the face of normal binding kinetics of some mitogens. For example, enhanced intracellular calcium as brought about by mutant receptor-operated calcium channels, alterations in membrane Ca-ATPase expression/activity, enhanced phospholipase C action (leading to greater than normal intracellular release of calcium from sarcoplasmic reticulum), and alterations in voltage sensitivity of L-type calcium channels have long been implicated in hypercontractile VSMCs. This enhanced contractile nature is often viewed as a key mechanism involved in enhanced vascular tone and consequent hypertension. Similarly, such changes in cytoplasmic calcium homeostasis may be pivotal in the overexpression of many VSMC genes involved in enhanced VSMC growth responses.

Enhanced sensitivity of tyrosine kinases coupled to vasoconstrictor and growth factor receptors has also been assigned a key role in abnormal mitogenic signaling, which is enhanced at the postreceptor level rather than by the presence of excess mitogen. Alterations in receptor binding kinetics thus may be sufficient but not necessary for the observed VSMC hyperproliferation seen in pathological states. The growing list of signaling cascade derangements in hypertensive vessels now includes protein kinase C, cAMP, cGMP, phospholipases C and D, and mitogen-activated protein kinases. Because this list represents signaling modalities shared by vasoconstrictors and mitogens alike, it is clear that molecules that use such signaling pathways have dual roles in their regulation of vascular tone as well as vascular growth. Additional genetic and hormonally and hemodynamically induced alterations in a variety of such signaling cascades will most likely be implicated in the near future.

DNA Synthesis and Hypertrophy

Wall thickening in blood vessels is usually hypertrophic, ie, numbers of cell nuclei remain constant while protein synthesis increases. The process by which cells hypertrophy rather than proliferate remains incompletely understood. In hypertrophy, cells may synthesize more DNA but do not divide, whereas in hyperplasia, the nuclei divide. The ploidy of VSMCs (ie, the number of chromosome pairs) is increased in atherogenic plaques. Under these circumstances, increased protein synthesis and cellular hypertrophy appear to be sequelae of the increased number of active genes present.

The Extracellular Matrix

Many mitogens, such as angiotensin II and vasopressin, stimulate VSMC growth and also enhance deposition of extracellular matrix proteins (collagens, elastins, laminins, etc), adding to vascular intimal mass. Degradation of such extracellular matrix proteins via a family of metalloproteinases results in high concentrations of interstitial fluid protein fragments with high affinity for myriad integrin receptors and focal adhesion proteins. Upon binding to such receptors, these peptides regulate ion transport systems, gene expression, cellular pH, and a variety of other physiological variables, which impact VSMC growth. Overexpression of such protein docking sites and enhanced degradation rates of key extracellular matrix proteins have added yet another dimension to the complex interplay of multiple mechanisms that result in the abnormal vascular growth seen in pathological states.

Antihypertensive Therapies and Vascular Growth

Various antihypertensive treatment modalities inhibit VSMC growth. For example, treatment of hypertensive humans and animals with ACE inhibitors and angiotensin receptor blockers leads to diminished VSMC mass, attenuated levels of extracellular matrix proteins, a diminution in vascular media:lumen ratio, normalization of elastin:collagen ratio, enhanced vascular NO synthase expression/activity, and an overall increase in compliance of large and small arteries. In vivo, these effects may come about partially in response to blood pressure attenuation. In vitro, where pressure gradients are absent, VSMC proliferation and extracellular matrix protein deposition are similarly blunted, suggesting involvement of a VSMC autocrine renin–angiotensin II mechanism. Calcium channel blockade (verapamil, isradipine, etc), also causes a pressure-independent reduction of normal cellular growth.

SUGGESTED READING

1. Itoh H, Mukoyama M, Pratt RE, Gibbons GH, Dzau VJ. Multiple autocrine factors modulate vascular smooth muscle cell growth response to angiotensin II. *J Clin Invest.* 1993;91:2268–2274.
2. Osol G. Mechanotransduction by vascular smooth muscle. *J Vasc Res.* 1995; 32:275–292.
3. Owens GK. Role of contractile agonists in growth regulation of vascular smooth muscle cells. *Adv Exp Med Biol.* 1991;308:71–79.
4. Scott-Burden T, Resink TJ, Bühler FR. Growth regulation in smooth muscle cells from normal and hypertensive rats. *J Cardiovasc Pharmacol.* 1988;12(suppl 5):S124-S127.
5. Standley PR, Ram JL, Sowers JR. The vasculature as an insulin-sensitive tissue: implications of insulin and IGF-1 in hypertension, diabetes, atherosclerosis and arterial smooth muscle growth. In: Crass BF, ed. *Calcium Regulating Hormones and Cardiovascular Disease.* Boca Raton, Fla: CRC Press; 1994:273–293.
6. Sumpio BE, Banes AJ. Response of porcine aortic smooth muscle cells to cyclic tensional deformation in culture. *J Surg Res.* 1988;44:696–701.

Chapter 62

Arterial Stiffness and Hypertension

Michael F. O'Rourke, MD, DSc

KEY POINTS

- Arteriosclerosis is diffuse, generalized, and dilatory, whereas atherosclerosis is focal and constrictive.

- Increased large-vessel stiffness in hypertension and arteriosclerosis is caused by reversible and irreversible changes in the architecture of vessel walls.

- Early return of reflected waves in arteriosclerotic arteries exaggerates the ill effects of increased aortic stiffness and augments peak aortic and left ventricular pressure, predisposing to left ventricular hypertrophy.

- In arteriosclerosis, brachial artery pressure underrepresents increases in aortic and ventricular pressures.

See also Chapters 61, 114, 135

The arteries of hypertensive individuals are stiffer (less compliant) than those of normal subjects. Combined with increased peripheral resistance, this causes a disproportionate increase in systolic compared with mean or diastolic pressure, particularly in the ascending aorta and major central arteries. As repeatedly demonstrated in recent years, increased systolic pressure, even with normal or subnormal diastolic pressure, is a major risk factor for cardiac failure and for the arterial rupture or luminal obstruction that occurs in stroke or heart attack. Hence, from both an etiologic and a therapeutic perspective, increased arterial stiffness is an important clinical parameter.

Mechanisms

Arterial stiffness is increased in hypertension by two mechanisms (**Table 62.1**). The first, which is acute, passive, and reversible, relates to the structural fibers in the normal arterial wall. The load-bearing elements in the arterial wall are the elastin lamellae and the collagen fibers located predominantly in the media. The properties of these fibers are modulated by smooth muscle, although to a lesser degree in the aorta and large proximal elastic arteries (eg, brachiocephalic, carotid) than in the more peripheral, predominantly muscular arteries. At low pressure, strains are placed on the elastin fibers, whereas at very high pressure, collagen fibers bear most of the pressure load. At high pressures, a given change in pressure within the artery causes a far smaller increase in diameter than at lower pressures. The elastic behavior of the artery is thus nonlinear, and arteries are more compliant (less stiff) at lower pressures.

The second mechanism is a chronic, largely irreversible consequence that accompanies long-standing hypertension or aging. In this condition, called "diffuse arteriosclerosis" by Osler and by 19th-century pathologists, the aorta and major arteries become diffusely dilated, tortuous, and stiffened (**Table 62.2**). The media of the aorta and elastic arteries loses its orderly lamellar arrangement, with thinning, splitting, and fraying of the elastic fibers. There is subsequent remodeling, with formation of new collagen fibers and deposition of intercellular and interlamellar matrix. In extreme cases, there is complete breakdown of formed elements (sometimes referred to as medionecrosis) within parts of the media.

Arteriosclerosis vs Atherosclerosis

Arteriosclerosis is often associated with atherosclerosis, but it may be seen alone in elderly or hypertensive subjects in the absence of other major risk factors. It is very common without atherosclerosis in countries such as Japan and mainland China.

Diffuse arteriosclerosis is quite different from atherosclerosis. Arteriosclerosis is generalized, diffuse, and dilatory, whereas atherosclerosis is focal and constrictive. Diffuse arteriosclerosis causes problems predominantly upstream as a consequence of arterial stiffening, whereas atherosclerosis causes ischemic problems predominantly downstream as a consequence of arterial obstruction.

Arterial Stiffening and Wave Reflection

Arterial stiffening (decreased compliance) has two adverse effects on the central circulation and on interactions between the left ventricle and the aorta (**Figure 62.1**). First, because of local aortic stiffening, a given ejection of blood from the left ventricle generates a pressure wave of higher amplitude in the aorta than in the ventricle. This is an obvious and direct effect of decreased aortic compliance. But there is an indirect secondary effect of at least equal importance. Increased arterial stiffness causes increased speed of travel of the aortic pulse along the wall of the aorta and major arteries (increased arterial pulse-wave velocity, an index of arterial stiffness). Aging clearly affects pulse-wave velocity, which is ≈5 to 6 m/s in the aorta of a young adult and perhaps 12 to 15 m/s in a hypertensive 60-year-old person. Increased pulse-wave velocity results in early return of reflected pulse waves to the ascending aorta and left ventricle from the periphery. In young and normotensive subjects, wave reflection is apparent in the aortic pressure tracing as a secondary diastolic pressure wave seen immediately after the high-frequency incisura that marks aortic valve closure. When pulse-wave velocity is increased, the reflected wave returns early, in systole rather than diastole, and causes a secondary boost to pressure in the latter part of systole. This

Table 62.1 Hypertension and Arterial Stiffening

Mechanisms
    Acute stretch (passive)
    Chronic and degenerative
Effects on aortic pressure
    Increased characteristic impedance
    Early wave reflection, causing increase in systolic pressure with
    relative decrease in diastolic pressure
Effects on LV
    Increase in LV load
    Increase in LV metabolic demands
    Relative decrease in coronary perfusion pressure
    Predisposition to LV hypertrophy and LV ischemia
Effects on central and peripheral pressure
    Decrease in pressure amplification
    Greater increase in central aortic than in peripheral systolic
    pressure

LV indicates left ventricle.

Table 62.2. Effects of Chronic Hypertension on the Aortic Wall

Mechanism
    Fatiguing effects of cyclic stress
Consequences
    Fracture, breakdown of elastic lamellae
    Stretching of the media
    Remodeling of the media
    Dilation of the artery, increase in stiffness
    Vicious circle:
      ↑ Stresses   →Degeneration   →↑Stresses

increases aortic and left ventricular pressure, increases myocardial oxygen consumption, and promotes ventricular hypertrophy.

The two phenomena, local increase in aortic stiffness (or characteristic impedance) and early return of wave reflection, can be evaluated from change in amplitude and contour of the central arterial pressure waveform or, more precisely, from determinations of ascending aortic impedance.

Effects on Peripheral Pressure

The ill effects of arterial stiffening on central aortic pressure and on ventricular-vascular interaction are often underestimated from conventional recordings of arterial pressure in the brachial (or radial) artery. In a typical healthy, 20-year-old subject, brachial artery systolic pressure is 10 to 15 mm Hg higher than in the ascending aorta and left ventricle (even though mean pressure is ≈2 mm Hg lower than in the aorta). This phenomenon of amplification of the pressure wave is a normal consequence of wave travel and reflection. With stiffening of arteries, amplification is reduced such that the difference between systolic pressure in the brachial artery and central aorta of a 60-year-old hypertensive subject may be <5 mm Hg. New techniques use conventional sphygmomanometry and applanation tonometry for pressure recording, with a generalized transfer function incorporated into a personal computer to synthesize the aortic wave.

Relationship to Left Ventricular Hypertrophy and Coronary Perfusion

The direct (increased proximal aortic stiffness) and indirect (early wave reflection) effects of hypertension lead to an increase in aortic pressure during systole and a relative decrease in aortic pressure during diastole, both of which exert adverse effects on the heart. In hypertension, aortic systolic pressure increases to a greater degree than brachial systolic pressure and to a far greater degree than brachial diastolic pressure. Increased ascending aortic and left ventricular systolic pressures generate increased left ventricular metabolic demands. In the long term, increased left ventricular systolic pressure predisposes to ventricular hypertrophy, impaired diastolic relaxation, and ultimately cardiac failure.

Increased pressure during systole is associated with a relative decrease in pressure maintained during diastole. Because pressure during

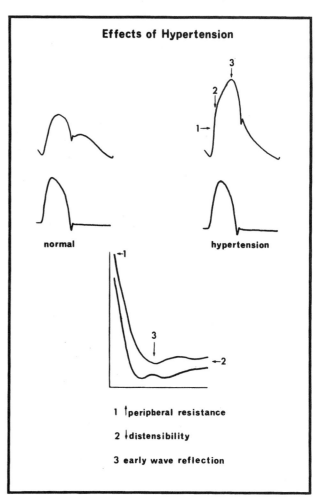

Figure 62.1. Effects of hypertension on aortic pressure-wave contour (top) and on aortic impedance modulus (bottom). Increased peripheral resistance (1) causes increased mean pressure and an increased zero-frequency component of impedance. Decreased arterial distensibility (2) causes increased amplitude of initial pressure peak and increased characteristic impedance. Earlier return of reflected waves from arterial terminations (3) causes late systolic pressure peak and impedance curve to shift to right. Reproduced with permission from O'Rourke MF. Pulsatile arterial hemodynamics in hypertension. *Aust NZ J Med.* 1976;6(suppl 2):40–48.

diastole constitutes the perfusion pressure head for coronary perfusion, increased pulse pressure predisposes to myocardial ischemia. Myocardial ischemia is even more likely to occur in the presence of increased systolic pressure, left ventricular hypertrophy, or impaired ventricular relaxation and may even occur in the subendocardium without significant narrowing of the coronary arteries.

Arterial Degeneration and Cyclic Stress in Hypertension and Aging

The cause of arterial degeneration in hypertension and with aging can be attributed to the fatiguing effects of repetitive cyclic stress on the elastin fibers within the aortic media. These fibers are among the most inert components of the body, with a chemical half-life of several decades. Repeated tensile stresses cause changes in its crystalline structure, such that it becomes more brittle with the passage of time and ultimately fractures at a load it was previously able to withstand. This theory explains why aging (more cycles) and hypertension (higher pressure) have similar effects on the wall of the aorta and elastic arteries. Elastin fiber fracture is thus the basis of arterial dilation and tortuosity, with resulting collagenous remodeling as the basis of increased stiffness.

Implications for Therapy

The importance of arterial stiffness is equal to that of peripheral resistance in raising central aortic systolic pressure and predisposing to cardiac and vascular morbidity and mortality. Stiffness is de-creased passively by any maneuver or drug that reduces mean arterial pressure. The stiffness of major central elastic arteries is not significantly altered directly by most drugs, but some data indicate that ACE inhibition improves abnormal distensibility of the carotid artery. However, early wave reflection can be reduced substantially by nitrates, ACE inhibitors, and calcium antagonists, which can reduce central aortic systolic pressure to a greater degree than brachial artery pressure because of their simultaneous effects of wave transmission.

The beneficial effects of antihypertensive drugs on left ventricular load may be underestimated by reliance on traditional sphygmomanometric measurements of brachial arterial pressure alone. This phenomenon may explain in part the superior effects of drugs such as ACE inhibitors in reduction of left ventricular hypertrophy.

SUGGESTED READING

1. Mahomed FA. On the sphygmographic evidence of arterio-capillary fibrosis. *Trans Pathol Soc.* 1877;28:394–397.
2. Nichols WW, O'Rourke MF. *McDonald's Blood Flow in Arteries.* 4th ed. London, UK: E Arnold; 1998.
3. O'Rourke MF, Safar ME, Dzau VJ, eds. *Arterial Vasodilation: Mechanisms and Therapy.* Philadelphia, Pa: Lea & Febiger; 1992.
4. Sandor B. *Fundamentals of Cyclic Stress and Strain.* Madison, Wis: University of Wisconsin Press; 1972.
5. Virmani R, Avolio AP, Mergner WJ, Robinowitz M, Herderick EE, Cornhill JF, Guo SY, Liu TH, Ou DY, O'Rourke M. Effect of aging on aortic morphology in populations with high and low prevalence of hypertension and atherosclerosis: comparison between occidental and Chinese communities. *Am J Pathol.* 1991;139:1119–1129.

Chapter 63

Oxidative Stress and Hypertension

David G. Harrison, MD; Zorina Galis, PhD; Sampath Parthasarathy, PhD; Kathy K. Griendling, PhD

KEY POINTS

- Reactive oxygen species are produced as a byproduct of numerous cellular metabolic processes.

- Both normal and abnormal cellular processes are influenced by reactive oxygen species, including cellular growth and hypertrophy, inflammation, remodeling, lipid oxidation, and modulation of vascular tone.

- Increased vascular production of superoxide ($O_2{}^{\cdot-}$), which occurs in diseases, modulates the bioactivity of nitric oxide.

- A major source of reactive oxygen species in the vessel wall is a membrane-associated NADH/NADPH-dependent oxidase. The expression and activity of this enzyme system are modulated by angiotensin II. Production of $O_2{}^{\cdot-}$ by this oxidase probably contributes to hypertension caused by chronic elevations of angiotensin II.

See also Chapters 64, 65, 67

Introduction: Redox State, Oxidative Stress, and the Sources of Reactive Oxygen Species

There has been growing interest in the role of "oxidative stress" as a component of many human diseases, particularly vascular diseases, such as hypertension and atherosclerosis. The term "oxidative stress" has been used to imply a state in which cells are exposed to either high concentrations of molecular oxygen or chemical derivatives of oxygen called reactive oxygen species. Cell injury may result from exposure to high levels of molecular oxygen and species called "reactive oxygen species." What are these? In the process of normal cellular metabolism, oxygen undergoes a series of univalent reductions, leading sequentially to the production of the superoxide anion ($O_2{}^{\cdot-}$), hydrogen peroxide (H_2O_2), and H_2O **(Figure 63.1)**. Other important oxidants that have relevance to vascular biology include hypochlorous acid, the hydroxyl radical ($OH^{\cdot}$), reactive aldehydes, lipid peroxides, lipid radicals, and nitrogen oxides. Several of these, including $O_2{}^{\cdot-}$, $OH^{\cdot}$, and the nitric oxide radical ($NO^{\cdot}$), are radicals with an unpaired electron in their outer orbital. Others are oxidants and quite biologically active but are not radicals. Sources of reactive oxygen species include components of mitochondrial electron transport, xanthine oxidase, cyclooxygenase, lipoxygenase, NO synthase, heme oxygenases, peroxidases, hemoproteins such as heme and hematin, and NADH oxidases. One of the best-characterized sources of reactive oxygen species is the phagocytic NADPH oxidase. This enzyme system is capable of producing very large, cytotoxic amounts of radicals. A major source of reactive oxygen species in blood vessels is a membrane-associated NADH/NADPH oxidase expressed by endothelial vascular smooth muscle cells (VSMCs) and fibroblasts, which bears some similarity to the phagocytic oxidase (discussed below).

The terms "oxidative stress" and "redox state" are often used loosely and interchangeably, without attention to their true meaning. The redox state or redox potential of a cell refers to the chemical environment within the cell as it relates to the number of reducing equivalents available. This can be estimated by examining ratios of so-called "redox couples." These include lactate/pyruvate, NADH/NAD$^+$, and the ratio of reduced and oxidized glutathione. Exposure of cells to oxidizing conditions may alter these by consuming reducing equivalents, but redox state may be altered in other ways. For example, exposure of cells to lactate can markedly increase the levels of NADH by conversion of NAD$^+$ to NADH via the action of lactate dehydrogenase. Conversely, exposure to high concentrations of pyruvate can produce the opposite effect. Redox state may also be altered by oxidative stress, but altered redox state may not necessarily change the oxidative environment.

Vascular Processes Affected by Reactive Oxygen Species

Role of Reactive Oxygen Species in Cell Growth

Reactive oxygen species are not simply toxic byproducts of cellular metabolism but also participate in cellular signaling and function in very important ways. Growth of vascular smooth muscle is stimulated by H_2O_2, a process that is dependent on the expression and binding of the transcription factors c-*fos* and c-*jun*. More importantly, hormone- and growth factor–stimulated proliferation and hypertrophy are mediated by and require intracellular H_2O_2. There are probably multiple molecular targets of reactive oxygen species that mediate the growth response, including Ras, p38 mitogen–activated protein kinase, phospholipase D, and protein tyrosine phosphatases. The ways in which these interact and are affected by reactive oxygen species are most likely complex and represent an important area for future investigation.

Regulation of Gene Expression by Oxidative Stress

Oxidative stress is also important as a modulator of gene expression. For example, it seems to play a critical role in initiating expression of proinflammatory molecules such as vascular cell adhesion molecule-1 and monocyte chemotactic protein-1, early events in atherogenesis. An important mediator of transcription of these genes is the transcription factor nuclear factor-κB. This factor exists

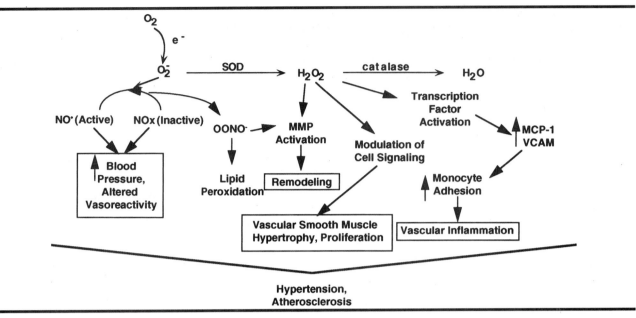

Figure 63.1.   Roles of reactive oxygen species in the vessel wall. Increased production of oxidants may lead to alteration of vasomotor tone, altered gene expression, and inflammatory responses and contribute to remodeling via the mechanisms depicted. Ultimately, these processes, which are activated in hypertension, predispose to formation of atheroma.

in the cytoplasm as a heterotrimer and is stimulated by reactive oxygen species via dissociation of an inhibitory subunit (IκB) from a p50-p65 complex that translocates to the nucleus to mediate gene transcription. Reactive oxygen species also modulate gene expression via transcription factors binding to AP-1, SP-1, antioxidant response elements, and other *cis*-acting elements.

Modulation of Extracellular Matrix

An important component of both vascular growth and remodeling is degradation and resynthesis of extracellular matrix. Specialized enzymes known as matrix metalloproteinases (MMPs) mediate the degradation process. Recent data from our laboratories have shown that two of the MMPs, MMP-2 and MMP-9, involved in degradation of basement membrane and elastin, respectively, are converted from inactive zymogens to their active form by several reactive oxygen species, including H_2O_2 and peroxynitrite. This occurs via a direct effect of the oxidant on the proenzyme, probably via an interaction with a cysteine in the inhibitory domain of the proenzymes. Such an activation process may be quite important in matrix degradation in regions of vessels exposed to high levels of oxidant stress.

Oxidation of Lipoproteins

A particularly important pathophysiological event related to reactive oxygen species is oxidation of lipids, in particular LDL. Under normal circumstances, native LDL cycles in and out of the vessel wall (although its uptake may be enhanced under certain conditions). It is now clear that changes in the oxidative environment in the vessel wall can lead to modification of the LDL particle. These modifications result in formation of a spectrum of oxidized lipoproteins, from minimally modified LDL (mmLDL) to fully oxidized LDL (oxLDL). The LDL receptor is able to differentiate between mmLDL and oxLDL, and each has distinct biological properties. In oxLDL, several

"new" biologically active molecules are formed. oxLDL contains phospholipase A_2–like enzymatic activity, and within the LDL particle, the active conversion of phosphatidylcholine to lysophosphatidylcholine causes numerous untoward biological effects on the endothelium. Linoleic acid and other fatty acids are oxidized to their respective hydroperoxides, which can participate in radical chain reactions, resulting in transfer of electrons to other molecules and the formation of additional radicals.

Modulation of the Biological Activity of NO

Of particular importance to the subject of hypertension and vascular biology is the interaction between $O_2{\cdot}^-$ and NO·. Because $O_2{\cdot}^-$ and NO· are both radicals and contain unpaired electrons in their outer orbitals, they undergo an extremely rapid, diffusion-limited radical/radical reaction, which occurs at a rate of 6.7×10^9 per mol/L per second. This rate is approximately three times faster than the reaction between $O_2{\cdot}^-$ and the superoxide dismutases (SODs) and 10000 times faster than reactions between $O_2{\cdot}^-$ and the common antioxidant enzymes, such as vitamins A, E, and C. The reaction with $O_2{\cdot}^-$ markedly alters the biological activity of NO·.

A major product of this reaction is the peroxynitrite anion ($OONO^-$). Peroxynitrite is a weak vasodilator compared with NO·, and thus, this reaction markedly impairs the vasodilator capacity of NO·. Likewise, many of its other beneficial effects (inhibition of platelet aggregation and smooth muscle cell growth, inhibition of vascular cell adhesion molecule-1 expression, etc) are lost. Peroxynitrite is a strong oxidant and is most likely involved in numerous pathophysiological processes. At physiological pH, peroxynitrite is protonated to form peroxynitrous acid, which can yield nitrogen dioxide and a hydroxyl-like radical, both of which are highly reactive. In the vessel wall, peroxynitrite and peroxynitrous acid may contribute to lipid peroxidation and membrane damage. In the past, it was unclear how scavenging of $O_2^{\cdot-}$ by SOD could be beneficial in biological systems, because the product of this reaction was H_2O_2, a more potent oxidant than $O_2^{\cdot-}$. One currently accepted explanation for this paradox is that SOD prevents the formation of peroxynitrite, which is a much stronger oxidizing agent than H_2O_2.

The rapidity of the reactions between $O_2^{\cdot-}$ and $NO^\cdot$ and $O_2^{\cdot-}$ and SODs would suggest that in compartments in which these three entities coexist, there could be interactions such that alterations in the amounts of either $O_2^{\cdot-}$ or SOD could markedly alter levels of $NO^\cdot$. Indeed, this seems to be the case. In the normal vessel, the balance between $NO^\cdot$ and $O_2^{\cdot-}$ favors the net production of $NO^\cdot$ and permits a state of basal vasodilation and maintenance of normal blood pressure.

The critical balance between $NO^\cdot$ and $O_2^{\cdot-}$ is altered in the setting of numerous common disease states. These include atherosclerosis, hypertension, diabetes, and conditions such as cigarette smoking and aging. In each of these conditions, oxidative stress has been implicated. In hypercholesterolemia, vessels produce excess quantities of $O_2^{\cdot-}$, leading to destruction of $NO^\cdot$ and impaired endothelium-dependent vascular relaxation. Treatment of vessels or animals with membrane-targeted forms of SOD markedly improves endothelium-dependent vascular relaxations. Likewise, infusions of antioxidant vitamins improve endothelium-dependent vasodilation of forearm vessels in human subjects with diabetes and cigarette smokers.

Role of Reactive Oxygen Species in Hypertension

In the past several years, it has become clear that oxidative stress plays an important role in hypertension. One of the first suggestions that $O_2^{\cdot-}$ might contribute to hypertension came from work in spontaneously hypertensive rats (SHRs). Nakazano et al demonstrated that SOD, modified to bind to heparan sulfates in the vessel extracellular matrix, would acutely lower blood pressure in SHRs, while having no effect on blood pressure in normal rats.

Role of Membrane-Bound, NADH/NADPH-Dependent Oxidases as Sources of $O_2^{\cdot-}$ in Vascular Tissues

More recently, studies have focused on the source of $O_2^{\cdot-}$ production in vascular tissues and how they might modulate elevations in blood pressure. Several laboratories have shown that both the endothelium and vascular smooth muscle contain membrane-associated oxidases that utilize NADH and NADPH as substrates for electron transfer to molecular oxygen. The complete molecular structure of the vascular oxidase is unknown. Investigators have focused on potential similarities to the well-characterized neutrophil NADPH oxidase. On a molecular level, the vascular oxidase may share only limited homology to the neutrophil enzyme. Many of the neutrophil components (p67phox, p47phox, and the large subunit of the membrane cytochrome, cytochrome b_{558}) seem to be absent in smooth muscle cells. One component, p22phox, has been cloned in VSMCs and is relatively abundant at the mRNA level. Functionally, it appears that p22phox is critical for function of the oxidase, because antisense inhibition of p22phox expression in VSMCs decreases $O_2^{\cdot-}$ and H_2O_2 production by these cells.

Several functional characteristics of the neutrophil NADPH oxidase are shared by the VSMC enzyme, most notably stimulation by phosphatidic and arachidonic acids, association with the membrane, and sensitivity to the flavin-containing enzyme inhibitor. However, VSMC oxidase differs from neutrophil oxidase in many respects. First and foremost, the time course of stimulation of the oxidase differs dramatically in the two cell types. Superoxide generation by the neutrophil NADPH oxidase is massive and occurs in bursts when the neutrophils are activated, whereas $O_2^{\cdot-}$ production by vascular oxidase is ≈ 0.1 of the amount in phagocytes and is constant in output. The $O_2^{\cdot-}$ generated in VSMCs appears to be mostly intracellular; with only a limited amount of $O_2^{\cdot-}$ being released to the exterior of the cell, as occurs in phagocytes. Finally, the VSMC enzyme appears to utilize NADH to a greater extent than NADPH, which is exactly the opposite of the situation in neutrophils.

Regulation of Oxidase Activity by Angiotensin II: Relevance to Hypertension

A particularly important aspect of the vascular NADH/NADPH oxidase systems is that angiotensin II and certain cytokines regulate their activity. Four-hour treatment of cultured VSMCs with nanomolar levels of angiotensin II markedly increases NADH and NADPH oxidase activity (**Figure 63.2**), resulting in an increased production of both $O_2^{\cdot-}$ and H_2O_2. This increase in production of reactive oxygen species seems essential for the hypertrophy of VSMCs induced by angiotensin II. Cells in which the NADH oxidase expression has been diminished by stable transfection of the full-length antisense against p22phox exhibit a markedly diminished growth in response to angiotensin II.

Recently, these findings were extended to an in vivo model of angiotensin II–induced hypertension. Osmotic minipumps were used to infuse angiotensin II (0.6 mg·kg^{-1}·d^{-1} SC) or norepinephrine in Sprague-Dawley rats. At the end of 5 days, angiotensin II but not norepinephrine infusion increased $O_2^{\cdot-}$ production in the aorta. Even when the endothelium was intentionally removed, there was increased $O_2^{\cdot-}$ production, suggesting that the source of the increase in $O_2^{\cdot-}$ was probably the vascular smooth muscle. Subsequent studies indicated that the membrane-associated NADH oxidase was involved in the increase in $O_2^{\cdot-}$ production.

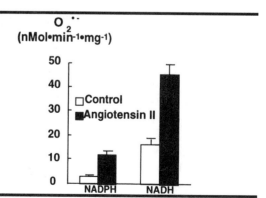

Figure 63.2. Production of $O_2^{\cdot-}$ measured by lucigenin chemiluminescence from homogenates of control and angiotensin II–treated VSMCs upon exposure to NADH or NADPH. Four hours of exposure to angiotensin II markedly increased $O_2^{\cdot-}$ production in response to both NADH and NADPH.

Increased $O_2^{\cdot-}$ Production in Angiotensin II–Induced Hypertension: Changes in Vascular Smooth Muscle

The increase in vascular smooth muscle production of $O_2^{\cdot-}$ caused by angiotensin II treatment was associated with a marked impairment in endothelium-dependent vascular relaxation that was not observed with norepinephrine. In subsequent studies of the resistance circulation, endogenous steady-state levels of vascular $O_2^{\cdot-}$ were lowered by treatment of rats with daily injections of liposome-entrapped SOD. This treatment had no effect on blood pressure in either control or norepinephrine-infused rats, but it lowered blood pressure by 60 mm Hg in rats with angiotensin II–induced hypertension **(Figure 63.3)**. These data suggest that a portion of the hypertension in conditions in which angiotensin II is elevated is associated with an increase in vascular superoxide production.

In these studies, the time course of p22phox expression, oxidase activity, and the onset of hypertension roughly parallel one another during chronic angiotensin II infusion, suggesting that they are closely related. In contrast, the hypertension induced by norepinephrine infusion was not associated with an increase in vascular $O_2^{\cdot-}$ production and did not alter endothelial regulation of vasomotion. Infusion of lower doses of angiotensin II, which had minimal effects on blood pressure, also increased NADH oxidase activity (by $\approx$2-fold). This suggests that hypertension per se is not a stimulus for increased $O_2^{\cdot-}$ production but that conditions in which circulating or local levels of angiotensin II are elevated may have unique effects on the vessel wall independent of elevating blood pressure. Furthermore, these observations are consistent with epidemiological data supporting the supposition that hypertension not associated with increases in angiotensin II may be less likely to produce cardiovascular disease.

It is important to point out that $O_2^{\cdot-}$ and other reactive oxygen species can have effects on vascular reactivity potentially independent of $NO^{\cdot}$. In vascular smooth muscle, intracellular calcium levels may be increased by reactive oxygen species by interference of such species with calcium reuptake by the sarcoplasmic reticulum. It has recently been shown that reactive oxygen species can react with fatty acids in the membrane to produce isoprostanoids, which can be detected in the blood of humans in whom oxidative stress is increased (eg, subjects with hypercholesterolemia, diabetics, and cigarette smokers). These oxidatively modified fatty acids act on prostaglandin H/thromboxane receptors to enhance vasoconstriction.

Another mechanism involved in hypertension caused by angiotensin II relates to endothelin production by the VSMC. It is now clear that angiotensin II can stimulate endothelin-1 (ET-1) gene expression in the vessel wall. ET-1 antagonists can prevent experimental hypertension caused by angiotensin II infusion. The mechanisms whereby increased oxidative stress, loss of $NO^{\cdot}$ bioactivity, and angiotensin II interplay to enhance ET-1 protein production in vivo are unclear but are likely to be quite important in the pathogenesis of hypertension and probably other vascular diseases.

The effect of hypertension on endothelium-dependent vascular relaxation has been somewhat controversial. Furthermore, the cause of altered endothelial regulation of vasomotion in various forms

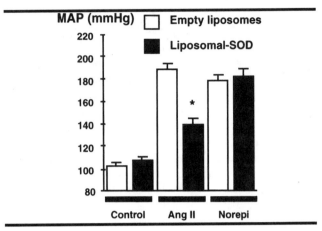

Figure 63.3. Effect of treatment with daily injections of either empty liposomes or liposome-entrapped SOD on mean arterial pressure in conscious rats made hypertensive via either infusion of norepinephrine (Norepi) or angiotensin II. *$P<.05$ vs empty liposome treatment.

of hypertension may vary. On the basis of current findings, it is interesting to speculate that humans with hypertension associated with elevated levels of angiotensin II might exhibit abnormal endothelium-dependent vascular relaxation compared with hypertensives with low-renin/low–angiotensin II states. Beneficial effects on reactive oxygen species may provide insight into why treatment with ACE inhibitors or angiotensin II receptor antagonists may exert favorable effects on target organs that are not matched by other antihypertensive drugs.

SUGGESTED READING

1. Alexander RW. Theodore Cooper Memorial Lecture: Hypertension and the pathogenesis of atherosclerosis: oxidative stress and the mediation of arterial inflammatory response: a new perspective. *Hypertension*. 1995;25:155–161.
2. Griendling K, Masuko U-F. NADH/NADPH oxidase and vascular function. *Trends Cardiovascular Med*. 1997;7:301–307.
3. Harrison DG. Endothelial function and oxidant stress. *Clin Cardiol*. 1997;20(suppl II):II-1-II-17.
4. Diaz MN, Frei B, Vita JA, Keaney JF Jr. Antioxidants and atherosclerotic heart disease. *N Engl J Med*. 1997;337:408–416.
5. Berliner JA, Heinecke JW. The role of oxidized lipoproteins in atherogenesis. *Free Radic Biol Med*. 1996;20:707–727.
6. Parthasarathy S, Santanam N. Mechanisms of oxidation, antioxidants, and atherosclerosis. *Curr Opi Lipidol*. 1994;5:371–375.
7. Freeman, BA, White CR, Guiterrez H, Paler-Martinez A, Tarpey MM, Rubbo H. Oxygen radical-nitric oxide reactions in vascular diseases. *Adv Pharmacol*. 1995;35:45–69.
8. Burdon RH, Superoxide and hydrogen peroxide in relation to mammalian cell proliferation. *Free Radic Biol Med*. 1995;18:775–794.
9. Suzuki YJ, Forman HJ, Sevanian A. Oxidants as simulators of signal transduction. *Free Radic Biol Med*. 1997;22:269–285.
10. Nakazono K, Wantanabe N, Matsuno K, Sasaki J, Sato T, Inoue M. Does superoxide underlie the pathogenesis of hypertension? *Proc Natl Acad Sci USA*. 1991;88:10045-10048.
11. Alderman MH, Madhavan S, Ooi WL, Cohel H, Sealey JE, Laragh JH. Association of the renin-sodium profile with the risk of myocardial infarction in patients with hypertension. *N Engl J Med*. 1991;324:1098–1104.

Chapter 64

Endothelial Dysfunction

James R. Sowers, MD; Joseph L. Izzo, Jr, MD

KEY POINTS

- The endothelium modulates vascular reactivity and also affects growth and remodeling.

- Reductions in endothelial concentrations of nitric oxide (NO) and increased superoxide radical generation promote accelerated atherosclerosis and enhanced expression of vascular growth factors.

- Angiotensin II increases NADH oxidase and vascular $O_2{}^-$ production and impairs NO-mediated vascular relaxation; antioxidants, ACE inhibitors, and estrogen reverse the process.

- Major cardiovascular risk factors such as hypertension, insulin resistance, hypercholesterolemia, tobacco intake, postmenopausal status, and microalbuminuria are associated with systemic endothelial dysfunction.

See also Chapters 63, 65, 67, 75, 118, 145

The endothelium is the largest "organ" in the body, comprising more than 14 000 sq ft of surface area and weighing 2 to 3 kg. Far from being a passive lining, the endothelium is now known to be extremely active functionally and metabolically **(Table 64.1)**.

Vasorelaxant Functions of Normal Endothelium and Nitric Oxide

Furchgott first identified the importance of normal endothelium in maintaining normal vascular function when he realized that removal of aortic endothelial cells caused the usual vasodilatory effect of acetylcholine to be transformed into a paradoxical constrictive effect. Subsequently, others identified a series of vasoactive products of normal endothelium **(Figure 64.1)**. The major endothelial vasodilator substance, initially termed "endothelial-derived relaxing factor" (EDRF), was later identified as nitric oxide (NO). An explosion of recent investigation has revealed that endothelial NO synthesis affects most aspects of vascular function and may modify structural characteristics as well.

Various cellular processes are regulated, in large part, through the release of NO by endothelium, platelets, vascular smooth muscle cells (VSMCs), cardiomyocytes, and other NO-producing cells **(Figure 64.2)**. NO is produced from the endothelium when local physical forces (ie, shear stress) or chemical substances (neurohumoral, paracrine, or pharmacological stimuli) act on endothelial cell receptors to increase intracellular calcium, which then activates endothelial (constitutive) NO synthase. This enzyme catalyzes the oxidation of one of the guanidine nitrogens of arginine to form NO, which is readily permeable across all cell membranes. NO is delivered to target tissues by local production/diffusion or after transport attached to other molecules such as nitrosothiols.

Relationship to Superoxides

Endothelial generation of oxygen-derived free radicals and activation of oxidant-sensitive transcriptional pathways may be an important pathophysiological mechanism mediating abnormal va-

soregulation and cardiovascular damage. It is currently believed that states of increased oxidative stress (hypertension, dyslipidemia, insulin resistance, cigarette smoking, hyperhomocysteinemia) or conditions in which there is activation of the tissue renin-angiotensin system are associated with the induction of redox-responsive genes that encode synthesis of growth factors, cytokines, and adhesion molecules. These substances in turn lead to adverse changes in the structure and function of blood vessels.

Increased production of vascular superoxide ($O_2{}^-$) can result from increased NADH/NADPH oxidase activity. Both endothelial cells and VSMCs manifest extra-mitochondrial or membrane-bound oxidases that use NADH and NADPH as substrates for electron transfer to molecular oxygen. Angiotensin II, in apparent pathophysiological levels, can activate NADH/NADPH oxidase in cultured VSMCs and in vivo. Experimentally, intracellular delivery of superoxide dismutase or the use of angiotensin II receptor antagonists or ACE inhibitors exerts a protective effect on vascular NO action by decreasing oxygen free radical generation. Antioxidants such as ascorbic

---

Table 64.1. Vascular Events Affected by the Endothelium

Thrombosis
   Platelet function
   Clotting factors
Vasoconstriction
   Vascular tone
   Vasoreactivity
Growth
   Vasculogenesis
   Hyperplasia
   Hypertrophy
Vascular injury
   Fibrosis
   Oxidative damage
   Lipid deposition

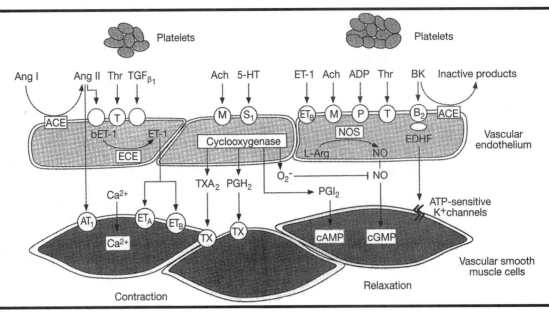

Figure 64.1.   Vasoactive mediators released by the endothelium. The endothelium produces factors that promote both relaxation (right) and contraction (left). Ang indicates angiotensin; ACE, angiotensin-converting enzyme; Ach, acetylcholine; ADP, adenosine diphosphate; ATP, adenosine triphosphate; Bk, bradykinin; cAMP/cGMP, cyclic adenosine/guanosine monophosphate; ECE, endothelin-converting enzyme; EDHF, endothelium-derived hyperpolarizing factor; ET, endothelin-1; 5HT, 5-hydroxytryptamine (serotonin); L-Arg, L-arginine; NO, nitric oxide; NOS, nitric oxide synthase; O_2^-, superoxide; PGH_2, prostaglandin H_2; PGI_2, prostacyclin; $TGF\beta_1$, transforming growth factor β_1; Thr, thrombin; TXA_2, thromboxane A_2. Circles represent receptors (AT indicates angiotensinergic; B, bradykinergic; ET, endothelin receptor; M, muscarinic; P, purinergic; S, serotonergic; T, thrombin receptor; and TX, thromboxane receptor.) From Lüscher TF, Barton M. Biology of the endothelium. *Clin Cardiol.* 1997;20(Suppl II):II-4. Copyrighted and reprinted with the permission of Clinical Cardiology Publishing Company Inc and/or the Foundation for Advances in Medicine and Science Inc, Mahway, NJ 07430-0832, USA.

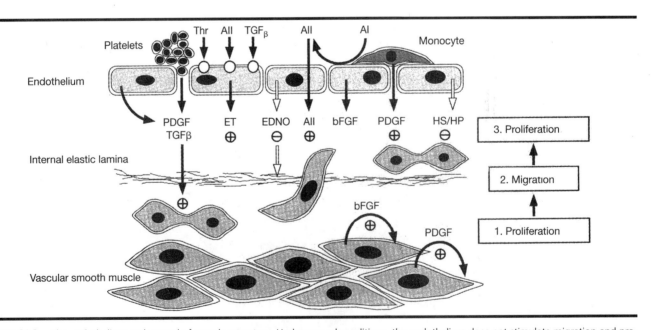

Figure 64.2.   The endothelium and control of vascular structure. Under normal conditions, the endothelium does not stimulate migration and proliferation of vascular smooth muscle cells. With onset of endothelial dysfunction, platelets and monocytes adhere to the vessel wall, and growth factors are released from these cells as well as from the endothelium. AII indicates angiotensin II; bFGF, basic fibroblast growth factor; EDNO, endothelium-derived nitric oxide; HP/HS, heparan sulfates; PDGF, platelet-derived growth factor. Other abbreviations as in Figure 1. From Lüscher TF, Barton M. Biology of the endothelium. *Clin Cardiol.* 1997;20(Suppl II):II-6. Copyrighted and reprinted with the permission of Clinical Cardiology Publishing Company Inc and/or the Foundation for Advances in Medicine and Science Inc, Mahway, NJ 07430-0832, USA.

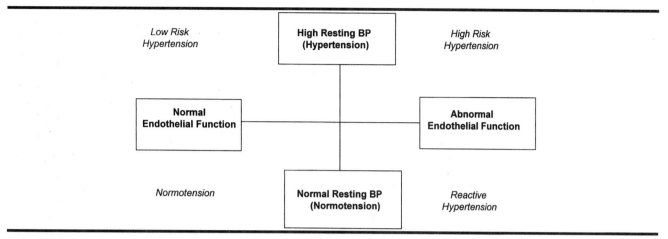

Figure 64.3. Hypothetical model of the interaction of hypertension (defined as increased resting BP) and vasoreactivity (defined as exaggerated stress-induced BP increases). In this model, the two separate axes define two different biological functions (chronic vasoconstriction vs acute vasoreactivity). Factors leading to endothelial dysfunction (smoking, hypercholesterolemia, insulin resistance, male gender, postmenopausal status, etc) cause increased vasoreactivity. The syndrome of high-risk hypertension as identified in the Framingham studies is characterized by both exaggerated BP reactivity and increased baseline vasoconstriction. Reactive BP changes alone (perhaps including the syndrome of white coat hypertension) confer much less overall risk because there is no concomitant endothelial dysfunction.

acid, vitamin E, and probucol may also effectively scavenge superoxide and other reactive oxygen species.

Endothelial Dysfunction and Cardiovascular Risk Factors

Cardiovascular risk factors such as hypertension, tobacco use, hypercholesterolemia, insulin resistance, hyperhomocysteinemia, and postmenopausal status have been found to be associated with endothelial dysfunction, diminished concentrations of vascular NO, and abnormal vasoconstriction. Much current research is centered around the question whether this relative endothelial NO deficiency is caused by decreased production or increased degradation of NO.

When endothelial dysfunction occurs, it appears to be generalized because similar patterns of reduced NO-dependent vasodilation have been demonstrated in multiple vascular beds in the presence of the individual risk factors. Endothelial vasoregulatory function can change acutely as demonstrated by several investigative teams. In a "real-world" experiment, investigators observed that forearm endothelial function was impaired within an hour after ingestion of a high-fat fast-food breakfast (buttered muffin, egg, sausage, fried potatoes).

Fortunately, endothelial dysfunction is reversible with correction of the offending risk factor(s). In hypercholesterolemic individuals, HMG-CoA reductase inhibitors partially normalize abnormal coronary and forearm arterial vasomotion, improve endothelially mediated venorelaxation, and reduce exaggerated blood pressure (BP) responses to mental stress. Use of the insulin sensitizer troglitazone in people with insulin resistance or the use of hormone replacement therapy in postmenopausal women also improves abnormal venous and BP responses. Other data suggest similar beneficial effects of ACE inhibitors and antioxidants.

An Integrated Model: Exaggerated Vasoreactivity and High-Risk Hypertension

A major clinical manifestation of endothelial dysfunction that can be observed clinically seems to be exaggerated vasoreactivity. A model for understanding the implications of exaggerated vasoreactivity is presented in (**Figure 64.3**). In this analysis, persons with endothelial dysfunction are at increased risk for the development of atherosclerotic complications. This model fits the epidemiological data on "standard" risk factors as identified in the Framingham studies (hypertension, cigarette smoking, insulin resistance, hyperhomocysteinemia), which together cause increased cardiovascular risk in those with more than one major risk factor. This idea is also consistent with older insurance industry data that showed that the highest risk group of hypertensives had the largest BP responses to stress (ie, mild exercise, usually the Masters two-step test for 1 minute).

SUGGESTED READING

1. Cooke JP, Dzau VJ. Derangements of the nitric oxide synthase pathway, L-arginine, and cardiovascular diseases. *Circulation.* 1997;96:379–382. Editorial.

2. Griendling KK, Minieri CA, Ollerenshaw JD, Alexander RW. Angiotensin II stimulates NADH and NADPH activity in cultured vascular smooth muscle cells. *Circ Res.* 1994;74:1141–1148.

3. Lüscher TF, Barton M. Biology of the endothelium. *Clin Cardiol.* 1997;20(Suppl II):II-3-II-10.

4. Sowers JR. Impact of lipid and ACE inhibitor therapy on cardiovascular disease and metabolic abnormalities in the diabetic and hypertensive patient. *J Hum Hypertens.* 1997;11:9–16.

5. Sung BH, Izzo JL Jr, Wilson MF. Effects of cholesterol reduction on BP response to mental stress in patients with high cholesterol. *Am J Hypertens.* 1997;10:592–599.

6. Sung BH, Wilson MF, Izzo JL Jr, Ramirez L, Dandona P. Moderately obese, insulin-resistant women exhibit abnormal vascular reactivity to stress. *Hypertension.* 1997;30:848–853.

7. Vogel RA. Coronary risk factors, endothelial function, and atherosclerosis: a review. *Clin Cardiol.* 1997,20:426–432.

Chapter 65

Atherogenesis

John P. Cooke, MD, PhD

KEY POINTS

- Vascular disease begins with endothelial dysfunction caused by hypertension, insulin resistance, tobacco consumption, and other factors.

- Increased intracellular oxidative stress and the activation of oxidant-response genes regulating the expression of adhesion molecules and chemokines causes an abnormal monocyte adhesion and infiltration, platelet adherence, and proliferation of vascular smooth muscle.

- These key processes in atherogenesis are opposed by nitric oxide (NO), which suppresses the expression and signaling of adhesion molecules involved in monocyte adhesion to the vessel wall and inhibits platelet adherence and vascular smooth muscle cell proliferation.

- The NO synthase pathway is perturbed by hypercholesterolemia and other metabolic disorders that predispose to atherosclerosis.

See also Chapters 63, 64, 67, 75, 113, 138, 142

Atherosclerosis is a complex process that is thought to be initiated by a "response to injury" of the endothelium. Risk factors that damage the endothelium include hypercholesterolemia, hypertension, diabetes mellitus, and tobacco use. Another important risk factor, family history of premature atherosclerosis (ie, first-degree relatives who have incurred myocardial infarction or stroke under the age of 60 years), represents predisposing genetic factors that have not yet been elucidated. In addition to these traditional risk factors, evidence is accumulating that elevated plasma levels of lipoprotein(a), homocysteine, and endothelium-derived asymmetric dimethylarginine (ADMA) accelerate the process of atherosclerosis. Finally, obesity, psychosocial factors, and sedentary lifestyle predispose to adverse cardiovascular events.

Pathogenesis of Atherosclerotic Plaques

Elevated LDL cholesterol (particularly oxidized LDL) perturbs the cell membrane, alters permeability and secretion, and is associated with the expression of adhesion molecules, cytokines, and growth factors. Specific glycoprotein adhesion molecules (eg, vascular cell adhesion molecule, or VCAM) and chemokines (eg, monocyte chemotactic protein 1, or MCP-1) elaborated by endothelial cells may participate in monocyte adhesion and infiltration in vessels. Within several days into a high-cholesterol diet, monocytes adhere to the endothelium, particularly at intercellular junctions, then migrate into the subendothelium, where they begin to accumulate lipid and become foam cells. This is the earliest event in the formation of the fatty streak. Activated monocytes (macrophages) then release mitogens and chemoattractants that recruit additional macrophages as well as vascular smooth muscle cells into the lesion. As foam cells accumulate in the subendothelial space, they distort the overlying endothelium and eventually may even rupture through the endothelial surface.

In these areas of endothelial ulceration, platelets adhere to the vessel wall, releasing epidermal growth factor, platelet-derived growth factor, and other mitogens and cytokines that contribute to smooth muscle cell migration and proliferation. These factors induce smooth muscle cells in the vessel wall to proliferate and migrate into the area of the lesion. These activated vascular smooth muscle cells undergo a change in phenotype from "contractile" cells to "secretory" cells, which elaborate extracellular matrix (ie, elastin), which transforms the lesion into a fibrous plaque. Smooth muscle cells may also become engorged with lipid to form foam cells. The lesion grows with the recruitment of more cells, the elaboration of extracellular matrix, and the accumulation of lipid until it is transformed from a fibrous plaque to a complex plaque.

The role of matrix accumulation in the progression of lesions has received little attention. However, recent evidence indicates that the progression of lesions may be affected by the balance between matrix accumulation and degradation. Stromelysin is a member of the matrix metalloproteinase family, which degrades collagen and elastin. In humans with a common genetic variant of the human stromelysin-1 promoter that results in reduced gene expression, serial angiographic studies reveal that progression of old lesions and occurrence of new lesions are more likely to occur, suggesting that reduced matrix degradation may lead to accumulation of extracellular matrix and lesion growth.

The complex plaque typically is characterized by a fibrous cap that overlies a necrotic core composed of cell debris, cholesterol, and a high concentration of thrombogenic tissue factor secreted by macrophages. In later-stage lesions, calcification may occur. Calcifying vascular cells in the vessel wall can transform into osteoblast-like cells and secrete bone proteins such as osteopontin. Microscopic examination of these areas reveals histology very similar to bone tissue. Oxidized lipoprotein stimulates the elaboration of bone protein by these vascular cells.

Pathogenetic Consequences of Plaque Formation

By virtue of its bulk, the complex plaque may limit blood flow. With moderate-sized lesions (ie, occupying ≥50% of the cross-sectional area of the lumen), ischemia occurs only when the tissue supplied by the vessel requires more blood (ie, exercise-induced myocardial ischemia, manifested by exertional angina). As the lesion becomes larger (usually ≥70% of the cross-sectional area), it may limit basal blood flow, causing ischemia at rest (ie, rest angina).

The complicated plaque is the major cause of acute cardiovascular events (eg, unstable angina, myocardial infarction, embolic stroke, and acute arterial occlusion). Hemorrhage into the plaque (secondary to spontaneous rupture of vasa vasorum supplying the lesion) can cause rapid expansion of the plaque and even luminal obstruction. Ulceration or rupture of the fibrous plaque (eg, due to hemodynamic force or balloon angioplasty) exposes the highly thrombogenic necrotic core, leading to local thrombosis and/or distal embolization. Rupture of the complex plaque exposes the flowing blood to the highly thrombogenic constituents of the plaque (the foam cells, which elaborate the highly thrombogenic tissue factor). Microscopic examination of the ruptured plaque generally reveals that the rupture has occurred at the shoulder of the lesion. In this area, the fibrous cap can be seen to be thinned. Immunohistochemical studies reveal an intense concentration of macrophages in the area, which are elaborating copious amounts of metalloproteinases. These macrophages appear to be undermining the fibrous cap, weakening it and predisposing it to rupture under the stress of hemodynamic forces. The fibrous cap, weakened by the degradative action of the macrophages, ruptures under the stress of hemodynamic forces. With rupture of the plaque, thrombus forms in the fissures of the lesion. The thrombus often extends into and may occlude the lumen. Plaque rupture and thrombus formation are the most common causes of heart attack and stroke. Furthermore, as the thrombus organizes, it can contribute to growth of the lesion and increase the patient's symptoms.

New data suggest that plaque formation or disruption may have an infectious etiology. Seroepidemiological links have been made between cytomegalovirus infections and atherosclerosis. There is also histopathological evidence of the presence of cytomegalovirus, herpes simplex virus, and more recently, clamydia trachomatis in atherosclerotic lesions in human vessels. Trials of antibiotics in patients with atherosclerosis are under way in an attempt to test the hypothesis that infection plays a role in the progression of atherogenesis.

Antiatherogenic Effects of Endothelium and Nitric Oxide

The endothelium produces a panoply of paracrine factors that modulate atherogenesis. One of these is endothelium-derived nitric oxide (NO), which not only is a potent vasodilator but also has important effects on circulating blood elements. NO inhibits platelet adherence and aggregation. Together, the endothelial products NO and prostacyclin confer a resistance to platelet–vessel wall interaction. NO exerts its effect on platelet reactivity in part by stimulating intraplatelet production of cGMP, which subsequently phosphorylates proteins that regulate platelet activation and adherence. Platelets themselves contain small amounts of NO synthase (NOS) and are capable of generating NO, which may act as a brake on their activation.

The ability of monocytes to bind to endothelial cells is also inhibited by NO. NO has both acute and chronic effects on monocyte adhesion. Within minutes of exposure to exogenous NO, endothelial cells become more resistant to monocyte adherence. Because of the rapid time course, this effect of NO is most likely due to inhibition of signaling pathways involved in adhesion, perhaps by a cGMP-dependent mechanism. More chronic exposure to NO suppresses gene expression of adhesion molecules (such as VCAM) and chemokines (such as MCP-1) involved in monocyte adhesion and infiltration. NO appears to exert its effects on gene expression by blocking the activation of specific transcriptional proteins (such as nuclear factor-κMB).

NO also regulates the proliferation of vascular smooth muscle cells, an effect that is mimicked by exogenous administration of 8-bromo-cGMP, a stable analogue of the second messenger of NO action. In experimental animal models, chronic inhibition of NO synthesis causes hyperreactivity to vasoconstrictors and medial thickening in the coronary microvasculature. When the release of NO is reduced or abolished, such as in restenosis, hypercholesterolemia, insulin resistance, and hypertension, there is exaggerated vasoreactivity and proliferation of vascular smooth muscle cells within the media and the intima. In experimental angioplasty, restenosis is at least partially inhibited by augmentation of endogenous NO synthesis (either by administration of the NO precursor L-arginine or by gene transfer of a plasmid construct encoding NOS). Parallel data in humans are not yet available.

Proliferation of vascular smooth muscle cells, monocyte adherence and infiltration, platelet adherence and aggregation, all key processes involved in atherogenesis, are inhibited by endothelium-derived NO. Therefore, an endothelial injury or alteration that results in a reduction in NO activity could promote atherogenesis, and accumulating evidence indicates that restoration of NO activity retards progression of the disease. Chronic administration of L-arginine (the NO precursor) to hypercholesterolemic mice or rabbits augments vascular NO synthesis, suppresses superoxide anion generation, inhibits the expression of monocyte chemokine protein, and reduces the accumulation of macrophages in the vessel wall. Enhancement of vascular NO production is associated with reduced progression (and even regression) of intimal lesions, whereas inhibition of NO production accelerates atherogenesis.

The effect of NO on atherogenesis may be mediated in part by apoptosis, or "programmed cell death," of vascular cells, including macrophages, from human atherosclerotic plaques. Factors involved in the initiation and regulation of apoptosis in atherosclerosis have not been fully elucidated, but immunohistochemical studies provide evidence for several proteins known to participate in apoptosis, including p53. Among the myriad pathways that may be involved, there is accumulating evidence to implicate L-arginine/NOS. Cytokine-mediated activation of inducible NOS (iNOS) induces apoptosis of microphages in vitro, which is augmented by additional L-arginine and attenuated by antagonists of NOS. Oral administration of L-arginine to hypercholesterolemic rabbits enhances the production of vascular NO and increases apoptosis of macrophages within intimal lesions of the aorta. When activated cells produce superoxide anion, the product of iNOS is quickly transformed into peroxynitrite anion, a highly reactive free radical that is cytotoxic and induces apoptosis. Peroxynitrite anion can also affect cell function by nitrosylating tyrosine residues that are involved in the signal transduction of transmembrane receptors. Using monoclonal antibodies directed against nitrotyrosine, researchers have detected evidence of peroxynitrite formation in human atherosclerotic plaque.

ADMA: A New Risk Factor for Atherosclerosis?

The mechanism by which hypercholesterolemia impairs the L-arginine/NO pathway is probably multifactorial and dependent on the stage of atherosclerosis. Recently, ADMA, which is present in human endothelium, has been characterized to be an endogenous, competitive inhibitor of NOS. Plasma ADMA is elevated in hypercholesterolemic rabbits as well as in hypercholesterolemic and atherosclerotic humans with impaired endothelial NO elaboration. Incubation of endothelial cells with ADMA (at concentrations that are observed in hypercholesterolemic humans) inhibits NO production and increases endothelial superoxide radical elaboration, MCP-1 expression, and endothelial adhesiveness for monocytes.

Several studies indicate that ADMA is elevated in individuals with atherosclerosis or risk factors for atherosclerosis. Dimethylarginines are the result of degradation of methylated proteins. The specific enzyme S-adenosylmethionine : protein arginine N-methyltransferase (protein methylase I) has been shown to methylate internal arginine residues in a variety of polypeptides, yielding N^G-monomethyl-L-arginine, N^G,N^G-dimethyl-L-arginine, and N^G,N^G-dimethyl-L-arginine upon proteolysis. The metabolism of ADMA occurs via hydrolytic degradation to citrulline by the enzyme dimethylarginine dimethylaminohydrolase (DDAH). Inhibition of DDAH causes a gradual vasoconstriction of vascular segments, which is reversed by L-arginine. This latter finding also suggests that regulation of intracellular ADMA levels affects NOS activity.

SUGGESTED READING

1. Berliner JA, Navab M, Fogelman AM, Frank JS, Demer LL, Edwards PA, Watson AD, Lusis AJ. Atherosclerosis: basic mechanisms: oxidation, inflammation, and genetics. *Circulation.* 1995;91:2488–2496.
2. Cooke JP, Dzau VJ. Nitric oxide synthase: role in the genesis of vascular disease. *Annu Rev Med.* 1997;48:489–509.
3. Cybulsky MI, Gimbrone MA Jr. Endothelial expression of a mononuclear leukocyte adhesion molecule during atherogenesis. *Science.* 1991;251:788–791.
4. Grattan MT, Moreno-Cabral CE, Starnes VA, Oyer PE, Stinson EB, Shumway NE. Cytomegalovirus infection is associated with cardiac allograft rejection and atherosclerosis. *JAMA.* 1989;261:3561–3566
5. Hajjar DP, Pomerantz KB, Falcone DJ, Weksler BB, Grant AJ. Herpes simplex virus infection in human arterial cells: implications in atherosclerosis. *J Clin Invest.* 1987;80:1317–1321.
6. Knox JB, Sukhova GK, Whittemore AD, Libby P. Evidence for altered balance between matrix metalloproteinases and their inhibitors in human aortic disease. *Circulation.* 1997;95:205–212.
7. Moncada S, Higgs EA. Molecular mechanisms and therapeutic strategies related to nitric oxide. *FASEB J.* 1995;9:1319–1330.
8. Parhami F, Morrow AD, Balucan J, Leitinger N, Watson AD, Tintut Y, Berliner JA, Demer LL. Lipid oxidation products have opposite effects on calcifying vascular cell and bone cell differentiation: a possible explanation for the paradox of arterial calcification in osteoporotic patients. *Arterioscler Thromb Vasc Biol.* 1997;17:680–687.
9. Ross R. Cellular and molecular studies of atherogenesis. *Atherosclerosis.* 1997;131(suppl):S3–S4.
10. Ye S, Eriksson P, Hamsten A, Kurkinen M, Humphries SE, Henney AM. Progression of coronary atherosclerosis is associated with a common genetic variant of the human stromelysin-1 promoter which results in reduced gene expression. *J Biol Chem.* 1996;271:13055–13060.

Chapter 66

Microvascular Regulation and Dysregulation

Andrew S. Greene, PhD

KEY POINTS

- Microvascular abnormalities in hypertension include functional (increased vascular sensitivity) and structural (increased vessel wall thickness) changes.

- Microvascular rarefaction, or loss of capillaries in peripheral vascular beds, may cause metabolic abnormalities such as insulin resistance or altered organ function.

- Recent studies suggest that appropriate and aggressive long-term normalization of blood pressure reverses structural changes.

See also Chapters 66, 71, 72, 73

The microcirculation is involved in both the genesis and maintenance of hypertension as well as many of the functional changes that take place in tissues and organs. Because the microcirculation is the site of much of the systemic vascular resistance as well as virtually all of the exchange function, changes in its structure have a significant impact on systemic hemodynamics and organ function (see the **Figure 66.1**). Many of the structural changes that occur in the microcirculation during the development of hypertension may be secondary to the initial elevation in arterial pressure. However, once they occur, they could limit the ultimate effectiveness of current therapeutic strategies that are aimed primarily at vasodilation and reductions in blood volume.

Vascular Structural Changes in Hypertension

Associated with the rise in pressure of hypertension is dramatic remodeling of the microcirculatory architecture, including the vascular connections and the blood vessels themselves. Increased growth of the media of arterioles, due primarily to vascular smooth muscle hyperplasia rather than hypertrophy, results in increased wall-to-lumen ratios. This hypertrophy contributes to increases in peripheral resistance, because these thicker-walled vessels undergo proportionally greater diameter changes than thin-walled vessels for a given level of smooth muscle shortening. Medial hypertrophy also acts to normalize shear stress in arterioles, and it has been hypothesized that shear forces provide a component of the signal for arteriolar remodeling. Increased shear forces in the microcirculation appear to be not only vasodilatory but also angiogenic. In normal situations, neoformation of capillaries promotes a restoration of normal shear forces.

In hypertension, a reverse angiogenesis of small arterioles and capillaries called "rarefaction" may occur. Rarefaction, resulting in a vessel loss of up to 50% of microvessels, may be due either to hemodynamic factors, such as microvascular pressure and flow, or to the action or depletion of locally acting trophic or growth factors, such as angiotensin, insulin, fibroblast growth factor, transforming growth factor-β, platelet-derived growth factor, or others. Ultimately,

this anatomic rarefaction in chronic hypertension is mediated via degenerative changes in microvessels, such as atrophy of vascular smooth muscle cells (VSMCs) through apoptosis and attenuation of the endothelium.

Although hypertension is associated with vascular wall hypertrophy and often with increased vascular tone, alterations in microvessel density alone can cause large increases in tissue vascular resistance, changes in microcirculatory flow distributions, and perhaps most importantly, decreases in tissue oxygen delivery. Substantial decreases in microvessel density greatly diminish the capillary surface area available for transport. The loss of a significant number of parallel branching arterioles and capillaries can increase local vascular resistance to a degree comparable to that of vessel constriction and may be one of the major contributors to elevated systemic vascular resistance in chronic hypertension. The combination of arteriolar remodeling and rarefaction is probably responsible for a structural increase in vascular resistance that is refractory to acute vasodilator therapies. Recent research suggests that with appropriate and aggressive long-term normalization of blood pressure or perhaps with antineurohumoral therapies, these structural changes are fully reversible.

In addition to the postgrowth remodeling of established microvascular networks, morphological abnormalities are also seen. VSMCs may be retracted or atrophic, with extensive rough endoplasmic reticulum and other organelles, suggesting modulation of some VSMCs toward a secretory phenotype. Vessels undergoing hypertrophy have an increased number of polyploid VSMCs. Endothelial cells may be attenuated, separated from VSMCs, or detached from their basement membrane, whereas pericytes are frequently absent from capillaries. These changes in endothelial cell morphology may impact dramatically on the permeability of the microvasculature, resulting in alterations in the transport of metabolites, interstitial matrix injury, and end-organ damage. Thrombi, neutrophils, and prephagocytic cells may also be present in the microcirculatory vessels during the early stages of some experimental forms of hypertension. Interestingly, many degenerative structural changes associated with arteriolar

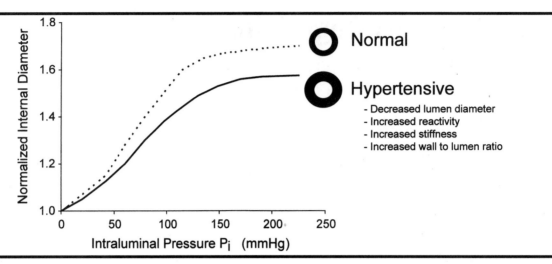

Figure 66.1.   Hypertension results in thickening of vascular wall, which shifts pressure-diameter relationship of arterioles in such a way that internal diameter is reduced. This hypertrophic response to increased pressure results in decreased lumen diameter, increased vascular reactivity, and decreased compliance. Recent studies suggest that only through aggressive long-term normalization of blood pressure can these structural changes be reversed.

rarefaction are similar to those that occur during ischemic injury; however, no inflammatory phagocytic response is observed during the development of hypertension compared with that normally seen in ischemic injury.

Functional Changes in Target Organs

Some vascular alterations found in hypertension are functional in nature. Increased levels of adrenergic stimulation and of circulating pressor hormones contribute to increased peripheral resistance during the development of essential hypertension. Changes in the population of hormone receptors on VSMCs and endothelial cells can augment the constrictor and hypertrophic effects of endocrine, paracrine, and autocrine factors. In addition to the enhanced sensitivity to vasoconstrictor agents, the arterioles of hypertensive individuals appear to be more sensitive to increased levels of oxygen and less responsive to vasodilatory stimuli, including hypoxia, than those of normotensive control subjects. The enhanced constriction of arterioles in response to increased oxygen availability may indicate heightened autoregulatory responsiveness, whereby small increases in total blood volume or decreases in vascular compliance could result in chronic elevation of systemic resistance.

In addition to increased autoregulatory tone, microvascular diameters may also be decreased because of elevated sympathetic nerve activity. Although much of the evidence for participation of a neural component in high systemic resistance has been obtained by indirect approaches, such as neural ablation, experimental evidence suggests that a primary genetic abnormality may exist in control of the peripheral sympathetic outflow, resulting in increased sympathetic drive in many forms of hypertension.

Functional abnormalities of the microcirculatory vessels arise in part from anatomic changes. Microvascular compliance and capacity are reduced because of an increased collagen-to-elastin ratio in microvessels as well as a reduced number of vessels. Increased myo-

genic tone, which contributes to reduced capacity, is due in part to vascular wall hypertrophy. Abnormal responses to constrictor and dilator stimuli are exacerbated by impairment in endothelial function. Permeability of capillaries is increased throughout the body, with a resulting redistribution of protein and water from plasma to the interstitial space. Finally, damage to the blood-brain barrier, which occurs primarily in capillaries and small venules, may be linked to increases in central sympathetic drive.

One of the often-overlooked aspects of hypertension is the impact of microvascular abnormalities on tissue and organ function. For example, a decrease in microvessel density alone causes increased diffusion distances for substances such as oxygen, glucose, and insulin. The functional implications of these increased diffusion distances are many and include reductions in oxygen delivery to skeletal and cardiac muscle, which could contribute to muscle fatigue and the risk of ischemic heart disease in cardiac overload, as well as diminished transport of insulin and glucose to skeletal muscle, which may provide a link between impaired insulin sensitivity and hypertension.

SUGGESTED READING

1. Cannon RO III. The heart in hypertension: thinking small. *Am J Hypertens.* 1996; 9:406–408.
2. Cowley AW Jr. Long-term control of arterial blood pressure. *Physiol Rev.* 1992;72: 231–300.
3. Draaijer P, Le Noble JL, Leunissen KM, Struyker-Boudier HA. The microcirculation and essential hypertension. *Neth J Med.* 1991;39:158–169.
4. Drexler H. Endothelial dysfunction: clinical implications. *Prog Cardiovasc Dis.* 1997;39:287–324.
5. Hutchins PM, Lynch CD, Cooney PT, Curseen KA. The microcirculation in experimental hypertension and aging. *Cardiovasc Res.* 1996;32:772–780.
6. Rieder MJ, Roman RJ, Greene AS. Reversal of microvascular rarefaction and reduced renal mass hypertension. *Hypertension.* 1997;30:120–127.
7. Schiffrin EL. The endothelium of resistance arteries: physiology and role in hypertension. *Prostaglandins Leukot Essent Fatty Acids.* 1996;54:17–25.

Chapter 67

Pathogenesis of Coronary Artery Disease

Charles K. Francis, MD

KEY POINTS

- Ischemic heart disease commonly occurs in association with essential hypertension, but it is useful clinically to separate the pathogenesis of the two conditions.

- The level of systolic and diastolic blood pressure is directly related to coronary artery disease symptoms, morbidity, and mortality.

- Myocardial ischemia (coronary insufficiency) can be caused by blockage of epicardial coronary vessels or by increased metabolic demand in the presence of an inadequate response of coronary blood flow.

- The syndrome of angina-like chest pain in the absence of angiographically demonstrable coronary artery disease (the cardiologist's syndrome X) has been attributed to abnormal constriction of the coronary microcirculation due to endothelial dysfunction.

See also Chapters 63, 64, 65, 138

Hypertension and coronary artery disease (CAD) are intimately interrelated, and the prevalence of essential hypertension is >60% in patients with chronic angina pectoris. Patients with hypertension have an increased incidence of unrecognized myocardial infarction, an increased likelihood of complications, a reduced acute and 5-year survival after myocardial infarction, and a high risk of sudden cardiac death.

Interdependence of Hypertension and CAD

The most direct association of hypertension with acute and chronic coronary syndromes is enhancement or acceleration of the atherosclerotic process in the epicardial coronary vessels. The contribution of elevated blood pressure to the formation, progression, and rupture of atherosclerotic plaque is of major importance. In the hypertensive patient, however, another mechanism is also at work. The increased incidence of myocardial ischemia can result from a supply-demand imbalance in which the metabolic demands of the hypertrophied ventricle exceed coronary blood flow. Myocardial ischemia or coronary insufficiency not directly related to the atherosclerotic process may be the result. Because atherosclerosis is a diffuse process that involves the entire arterial circulation, it is conceivable that atherosclerosis may be a fundamental pathogenetic contributor to the development or maintenance of hypertension or other syndromes of excess vasoreactivity. Conversely, abnormalities of vascular tone and reactivity, which occur in hypertension, may be the result rather than the primary cause of endothelial dysfunction and atherosclerosis.

Clinically, it is useful to consider hypertension and atherosclerosis as distinct conditions that develop in response to shared pathogenetic factors and occur concurrently as well as independently. The clinical manifestations of these separate pathological processes depend on the confluence of multiple genetic and environmental risk factors and the characteristics of each distinctive vascular bed. Com-bined treatment of hypertension and hypercholesterolemia is required for optimal reduction in cardiovascular events, either as primary or secondary (postinfarction) protection.

Risk Factors, Endothelial Dysfunction, and Myocardial Ischemia

Angina pectoris, defined as chest pain precipitated by exercise, environment, or stress (although sometimes occurring at rest), is considered the classic manifestation of myocardial ischemia. Myocardial ischemia is caused by reduced epicardial coronary blood flow or by increased myocardial oxygen demand that outstrips flow reserve. Abnormalities in coronary arterial reactivity may occur before or in the absence of angiographically demonstrable atherosclerotic lesions.

The coronary endothelium, which regulates arterial vasomotion and maintains a nonthrombogenic luminal lining, plays a fundamental role in the pathogenesis of coronary events. Diverse endothelial factors (eg, nitric oxide, prostacyclin, thromboxane A_2) have been shown to be important to the regulation of coronary vasorelaxation and vasoconstriction, the modulation of vasomotor tone, and the balancing of myocardial oxygen supply-and-demand relationships. Defects in endothelial function may also be fundamental to the derangements of peripheral resistance in hypertension, as well as in atherosclerotic and nonatherosclerotic forms of myocardial ischemia.

Abnormalities in coronary vascular reactivity and endothelial dysfunction have been observed in hypertensive patients independent of coronary atherosclerosis or left ventricular hypertrophy. Hypertensive patients also have been shown to have reduced coronary flow reserve in the absence of left ventricular hypertrophy or angiographic CAD. The syndrome of angina-like chest pain in the absence of angiographically demonstrable CAD (the cardiologist's syndrome X) has been attributed to abnormal constriction of the coronary microcirculation due to endothelial dysfunction and with associated defects in platelet aggregation or thrombus formation.

Abnormalities in coronary endothelial function have now been observed in populations at risk for atherosclerotic vascular disease, including smokers, men, and those with obesity, insulin resistance, hypercholesterolemia, and hypertension (the endocrinologist's syndrome X). Atherogenesis begins early in life, progresses slowly over several decades, and ultimately results in the development of mature atherosclerotic plaques at lesion-prone sites, such as bifurcation points and areas of increased wall stress. Hypertension may accelerate the atherosclerotic process through increased transmural pressure, augmentation of mechanical stress, and greater wall tension in the coronary vessel. Enhanced proliferation, hypertrophy, and hyperplasia of smooth muscle cells, fibromuscular thickening, and excess coronary vasoconstriction also contribute.

Coronary Artery Syndromes

Chronic Angina Pectoris

Progression of the atherosclerotic process generally occurs sporadically through plaque extension and growth of the lipid-rich core, as well as thickening of the collagen-rich fibrous cap, gradually eventuating in diffuse involvement of the arterial circulation with confluent plaque. The gradual encroachment of atherosclerotic plaque on the arterial lumen is responsible for the chronic coronary ischemic syndromes, typically angina pectoris.

Stable angina pectoris, ie, the presence of nonprogressive, effort-induced, symptomatic myocardial ischemia, is usually indicative of the presence of a typical cholesterol-laden atherosclerotic plaque in at least one major epicardial coronary artery. Chronic angina is usually quite predictable, occurring with the same level of exertion or degree of emotional stress. This condition can be present for many years and confers only a relatively small increase in mortality rates compared with angina-free individuals.

Acute Coronary Syndromes: Unstable Angina, Myocardial Infarction, and Sudden Death

The acute coronary syndromes (unstable angina pectoris, myocardial infarction, and sudden coronary death) are initiated by fissuring of an atherosclerotic plaque, hemorrhage into the lipid core, platelet aggregation, superimposition of luminal coronary thrombus, and subtotal or total acute occlusion of the coronary artery. Although plaque rupture contributes the thrombogenic substrate, regional flow disturbances are determined by the severity of coronary artery narrowing. Local thrombogenic and vasoconstrictor stimuli, such as increased platelet adherence, decreased fibrinolytic activity, and enhanced smooth muscle reactivity, are also important in the development of acute coronary syndromes.

Clinically, unstable angina represents the last opportunity to restore adequate blood flow to the at-risk region of the myocardium. Often, discrete ECG (ST-segment elevation), echocardiographic (diminished or absent regional wall motion), or nuclear imaging abnormalities offer guides to therapeutic intervention. The presence of ventricular systolic dysfunction (heart failure) in particular is an indication for aggressive management strategies, such as thrombolysis, angioplasty, or coronary artery bypass graft surgery.

In general, two types of acute infarction are recognized: non–Q-wave (nontransmural) and Q-wave (transmural) infarctions. In both syndromes, cell damage results from prolonged ischemia. In both syndromes, there are usually acute ECG changes (ST-segment elevation) and increases in blood levels of cardiac muscle enzymes (creatine kinase MB fraction or troponin). In the "non–Q-wave" infarction, there is loss of subendocardial muscle, with some preservation of the outer layers of myocytes. The presence of a Q wave indicates a wider transmural area of injury, with patchy or incomplete loss of myofibrils. The development of a Q wave generally indicates an irreversible loss of myofibrils as part of a "completed infarction."

SUGGESTED READING

1. Abrams J. Role of endothelial dysfunction in coronary artery disease. *Am J Cardiol.* 1997;79:2–9.
2. Bonow RO, Bohannon N, Hazzard W. Risk stratification in coronary artery disease and special populations [published erratum appears in *Am J Med.* 1997;102:322]. *Am J Med.* 1996;101(suppl 4A):17S–24S.
3. Brush JE Jr, Faxon DP, Salmon S, Jacobs AK, Ryan TJ. Abnormal endothelium-dependent coronary vasomotion in hypertensive patients. *J Am Coll Cardiol.* 1992;19:809–815.
4. Brush JE Jr, Cannon RO III, Shenke WH, Bonow RO, Leon MB, Maron BJ, Epstein SE. Angina due to coronary microvascular disease in hypertensive patients without left ventricular hypertrophy. *N Engl J Med.* 1988;319:1302–1307.
5. Doyle AE. Does hypertension predispose to coronary disease? Conflicting epidemiological and experimental evidence. In: Laragh J II, Brenner BM, eds. *Hypertension: Pathophysiology, Diagnosis and Management.* 2nd ed. New York, NY: Raven Press; 1995:119–125.
6. Fuster V. Lewis A. Conner Memorial Lecture: Mechanisms leading to myocardial infarction: insights from studies of vascular biology [published erratum appears in *Circulation.* 1995;91:256]. *Circulation.* 1994;90:2126–2146.
7. MacMahon S, Peto R, Cutler J, Collins R, Sorlie P, Neaton J, Abbot R, Godwin J, Dyer A, Stamler J. Blood pressure, stroke, and coronary heart disease, I: prolonged differences in blood pressure: prospective observational studies corrected for the regression dilution bias. *Lancet.* 1990;335:765–774.
8. Mark DB, Nelson CL, Califf RM, Harrell FE Jr, Lee KL, Jones RH, Fortin DF, Stack RS, Glower DD, Smith LR, et al. Continuing evolution of therapy for coronary artery disease: initial results from the era of coronary angioplasty. *Circulation.* 1994;89:2015–2025.
9. Solomon AJ, Gersh BJ. Management of chronic stable angina: medical therapy, percutaneous transluminal coronary angioplasty, and coronary artery bypass graft surgery: lessons from the randomized trials. *Ann Intern Med.* 1998;128:216–223.

Chapter 68

Pathogenesis of Left Ventricular Hypertrophy and Diastolic Dysfunction

Joseph L. Izzo, Jr, MD

KEY POINTS

- The concentric increase in left ventricular mass that occurs in hypertension, which is loosely termed left ventricular hypertrophy (LVH), includes an increase in cardiac mass, myocyte size, and extracellular matrix.

- LVH is caused by genetic, mechanical (increased systolic BP and decreased vascular compliance), and hormonal (angiotensin II, etc) mechanisms.

- Diastolic dysfunction can predate the development of systemic hypertension or be the result of hypertension-induced LVH.

See also Chapters 69, 77, 139

Role of Mechanical Forces in Left Ventricular Hypertrophy (LVH)

Mechanical forces are thought to be the principal determinants of cardiac hypertrophy (**Table 68.1**). Increased systolic blood pressure (BP) stretches or "loads" cardiac myofibrils, which respond according to Frank-Starling principles by lengthening and contracting more forcefully against the increased impedance to ventricular outflow. If the systolic BP returns to normal, the myofibrils rapidly reassume their "unloaded" characteristics and return to a normal length and functional range. If the impedance remains elevated, however, cardiac myocytes respond with a more permanent adaptive change in which there is an increase in actinomycin synthesis and cell size.

These hypertrophic cellular changes contribute to an overall concentric increase in myocardial wall thickness. There is a corresponding increase in extracellular protein, principally collagen and osteopontin, that accompanies the increase in myocyte size. The entire process of cellular growth and extracellular matrix increase is loosely termed left ventricular hypertrophy or LVH. In hypertension, hypertrophy is usually concentric with relatively uniform increases in thickness of the septum and free wall. Other forms of LVH such as idiopathic hypertrophic subaortic stenosis (asymmetric cardiac hypertrophy) or exercise-induced hypertrophy are eccentric, with predominant septal hypertrophy. In the case of exercise-induced hypertrophy, there is also relative dilation of the left ventricle, which represents advantageous use of Frank-Starling forces to achieve greater efficiency of energy use (greater stroke volume, lower heart rate). In contrast, concentric hypertrophy causes a relative restriction of diastolic filling, a smaller ventricular chamber size, and a blunting of the heart's ability to efficiently use energy.

Role of Aging and Aortic Stiffness

Early in the process of LVH, increased systemic vascular resistance is the primary mechanical contributor that increases cardiac "afterload" and promotes LVH. With aging, and in particular with the "accelerated vascular aging" found in hypertension, decreased aortic compliance becomes a second major promoter of LVH. As the aorta loses elasticity and compliance, it begins to reflect each systolic pulse wave *backward* toward the left ventricle, substantially augmenting peak systolic BP. Pulse-wave augmentation and hypertension create a vicious cycle requiring increasing force of ventricular emptying and cardiac hypertrophy, which together cause increased transmural stress on the aorta and accelerated aortic sclerosis, which in turn promote further LVH.

Neurohumoral Contributions

It is now known that the mechanical forces favoring hypertrophy work in tandem with a series of potent neurohumoral factors that have independent stimulatory effects on protein synthesis, interstitial matrix formation, and myofibrillar size. At the top of the list of these trophic factors is angiotensin II, but such hormones as norepinephrine and insulin also directly promote myocyte hypertrophy and matrix deposition independent of their effects on systemic BP. These trophins stimulate production of a series of cytokines and growth factors including transforming growth factor-β, fibroblast growth factor, and insulin growth factor that directly stimulate cardiac protein synthesis and hypertrophy.

The clinical importance of these potential "prohypertrophic" actions of angiotensin II is that ACE inhibitors may theoretically allow regression of LVH to a greater degree than agents that do not block the renin-angiotensin system. A meta-analysis (**Figure 68.1**) that suggests superiority of ACE inhibitors over other agents requires clinical trial confirmation. It will also be important for future trials to investigate whether arterial dilators actually increase LV mass in humans as they do in animal models.

Effect on Myocardial Blood Flow

Coronary hemodynamics are also significantly affected in the hypertrophied heart. Pathophysiological changes include increased vascular wall thickness of epicardial coronary arteries, increased coronary vascular resistance, decreased coronary vasodilator capac-

Table 68.1. Factors Promoting Cardiac Hypertrophy

Genetic influences
Mechanical forces
   Impedance-related
     Systemic vasoconstriction
     Arteriosclerosis (pulse-wave augmentation)
   Preload-related
Neurohumoral factors (growth stimulation)
   Renin-angiotensin system
   Sympathetic nervous system
   Insulin and other growth factors

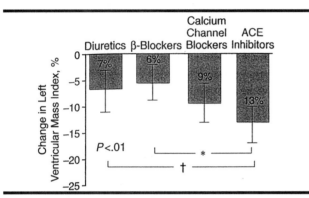

Figure 68.1.   Percentage of change in left ventricular mass index with the 4 antihypertensive drug classes. Mean values and 95% confidence intervals adjusted for duration are given. ACE indicates angiotensin-converting enzyme. *$P<.01$ between drug classes; †$P<.10$ between drug classes (Bonferroni correction) (Used with permission from Schmieder RE, Martus P, Klingbeil A. Reversal of left ventricular hypertrophy in essential hypertension: a meta-analysis of randomized double-blind studies. *JAMA.* 1996;275:1507–1513).

ity, and decreased coronary flow reserve. Small blood vessel flow is affected as well, such that the increased extraluminal pressure caused by LVH can act together with changes in the epicardial circulation to decrease overall blood flow to the myofibrils. These "ischemic" changes probably contribute to the increased incidence of arrhythmias seen in LVH.

Diastolic Dysfunction

Relaxation of the heart is both active and passive. At a cellular level, calcium extrusion is required, and there is evidence that verapamil may have favorable effects on diastolic relaxation by helping to reduce intracellular calcium during diastole. At a systemic level, ventricular filling does not begin until LV pressure is less than atrial pressure. The phase of rapid filling that occurs early in diastole accounts for the majority of diastolic filling and is the phase most affected by LVH. As hypertrophy of the LV wall causes the ventricle to become less compliant, the stiffer ventricle requires increased distending pressure. Compensatory atrial enlargement progresses to atrial hypertrophy as the heart attempts to optimize its overall Frank-Starling relationships in both atria and ventricles. Clinically, inverted P waves in anterior precordial ECG leads, a fourth heart sound, and increased late diastolic mitral flow ("E-A reversal") indicate atrial enlargement and increased LV end-diastolic pressure.

If hypertrophy continues, a series of additional adaptations occurs. The restricted ability of the heart to increase stroke volume in response to stress-induced demands further increases LV end-diastolic pressure over time. At some point, ventricular end-diastolic volume begins to increase, and progression begins toward the syndrome of systolic dysfunction and dilated cardiomyopathy. By restricting cardiac stretch mechanisms, LVH may also blunt the inhibitory influence of cardiopulmonary baroreceptors on sympathetic vasoconstriction, further reducing ventricular performance.

Severe LVH

In patients with severe LVH and diastolic dysfunction, a unique syndrome of "restrictive cardiomyopathy" can occur. The failure of diastolic relaxation can contribute directly to pulmonary vascular congestion, often in the form of "flash pulmonary edema," which can occur despite normal or supranormal ventricular emptying (ie, normal or increased ejection fraction). The pathogenesis of this syndrome is not fully understood, but it is critical for the clinician to recognize that in long-standing hypertension with LVH, any maneuvers that lower cardiac preload precipitously can cause circulatory collapse and death. Volume depletion with diuretics or acute venodilation with nitrates, α-blockers, and sometimes ACE inhibitors are particularly problematic in this group. In general, tachycardia also worsens the hemodynamics of LVH because decreased diastolic filling time further compromises the ability of the stiff heart to increase stroke volume in response to stress.

Therapeutic recommendations in this special case include heart rate control and avoidance of acute reductions in preload and afterload. If accelerated hypertension is present, it seems prudent to lower BP more slowly, stopping at an intermediate value (perhaps 160/100 mm Hg) for a period of time. Specific therapy with β-blockers may be beneficial, especially for heart rate control. Digoxin should generally be avoided. If there is atrial fibrillation, rate control with diltiazem or verapamil can be considered. Although verapamil may facilitate ventricular relaxation in hypertrophic cardiomyopathy, no controlled clinical trials are yet available to identify the clinical impact of the phenomenon.

Sequelae of LVH

The Framingham investigators have clearly established that LVH is an independent risk factor for cardiovascular morbidity and mortality. The increased incidence of ventricular arrhythmias in people with LVH is thought to contribute to overall increases in mortality in this group. LVH also contributes to the development of diastolic and systolic dysfunction and the syndrome of congestive heart failure.

SUGGESTED READING

1. Koren MJ, Devereux RB, Casale PN, Savage DD, Laragh JH. Relation of left ventricular mass and geometry to morbidity and mortality in uncomplicated essential hypertension. *Ann Intern Med.* 1991;114:345–352.
2. Levy D, Garrison RJ, Savage DD, Kannel WB, Castelli WP. Prognostic implications of echocardiographically determined left ventricular mass in the Framingham Heart Study. *N Engl J Med.* 1990;322:1561–1566.
3. Jalil JE, Doering CW, Janicki JS, Pick R, Shroff SG, Weber KT. Fibrillar collagen and myocardial stiffness in the intact hypertrophied rat left ventricle. *Circ Res.* 1989;64:1041–1050.
4. Marcus ML, Harrison DG, Chilian WM, Koyanagi S, Inou T, Tomanek RJ, Martins JB, Eastham CL, Hiratzka LF, et al. Alterations in the coronary circulation in hypertrophied ventricles. *Circulation.* 1987;75(Suppl I):I-19-I-25.

5. Messerli FH, Ventura HO, Elizardi DJ, Dunn FG, Frohlich ED. Hypertension and sudden death: increased ventricular ectopic activity in left ventricular hypertrophy. *Am J Med.* 1984;77:18–22.

6. Ruzicka M, Leenen FH. Renin-angiotensin system and minoxidil-induced cardiac hypertrophy in rats. *Am J Physiol.* 1993;265:H1551–H1556.

7. Schelling P, Fischer H, Ganten D. Angiotensin and cell growth: a link to cardiovascular hypertrophy? *J Hypertens.* 1991;9:3–15. Editorial.

8. Dahlöf B, Pennert K, Hansson L. Reversal of left ventricular hypertrophy in hypertensive patients: a metaanalysis of 109 treatment studies. *Am J Hypertens.* 1992;5:95–110.

9. Devereux RB. Hypertensive cardiac hypertrophy: pathophysiologic and clinical characteristics. In: Laragh JH, Brenner BM, eds. *Hypertension: Pathophysiology, Diagnosis, and Management.* New York, NY: Raven Press Ltd;1990:359–377.

10. Topol EJ, Traill TA, Fortuin NJ. Hypertensive hypertrophic cardiomyopathy of the elderly. *N Engl J Med.* 1985;312:277–283.

Chapter 69

Pathogenesis of Congestive Heart Failure

Edmund H. Sonnenblick, MD; Thierry H. LeJemtel, MD

KEY POINTS

- Two main mechanisms, ventricular hypertrophy and ischemic heart disease, cause accelerated, age-related irreversible loss of myocytes.

- In response to an increase in systolic load, cardiac myocytes hypertrophy; as the myocardial mass increases, characteristic alterations in ventricular performance lead to diastolic dysfunction and eventually cardiac failure.

- As ventricular dysfunction progresses, compensatory vasoconstrictive mechanisms are activated in the general circulation, including the sympathetic nervous system and the renin-angiotensin system; the resulting maladaptive peripheral vasoconstriction is the target of therapy with vasodilator drugs.

- Systemic vascular remodeling is believed to be a major determinant of the functional status (ie, the presence and severity of symptoms) in patients with left ventricular systolic dysfunction.

See also Chapters 68, 77, 140

Left Ventricular Hypertrophy and Diastolic Dysfunction

In response to hypertension, which produces an increase in systolic load, cardiac myocytes hypertrophy, ie, enlarge in their lateral dimension, to normalize the load. Generally, the load is expressed in terms of the fundamental Laplace relation, in that the tension generated within the wall of the heart (T) is directly related to the pressure (P) times the radius of the ventricular cavity (r) and inversely related to two times the wall thickness (h), ie, $T = P \cdot r/2h$. Within broad limits, the tension in the wall is normalized by increasing wall thickness approximately in proportion to the increase in mean systolic stress. The increase in myocyte volume is largely due to an increase in synthesis of contractile mass with an increase in sarcomere mass. As myocardial mass increases, alterations occur in contractile behavior. Characteristically, there is a slowing down and prolongation of contraction and a delay in relaxation. These changes are a result of the load-induced synthesis of "slow" myosin and an altered activation system. Nevertheless, force development of the myocardium is maintained.

When these changes in myocardial performance are translated into ventricular function, one observes preservation of the ventricle's capacity to empty; diastolic volume and ejection fraction are normal, although systolic time is prolonged and diastolic time for a given heart rate is abbreviated. Moreover, because the thickness of the ventricular wall is increased, diastolic pressures tend to rise. With the abbreviation of diastole and elevated filling pressures, pulmonary congestion and even pulmonary edema may occur, although systolic emptying of the heart remains normal. This is worsened by tachycardia, which further reduces the duration of diastole, the loss of the atrial kick with the development of atrial fibrillation, or any degree of salt overload. These alterations in ventricular performance form the basis of what has been called diastolic dysfunction or diastolic failure, as observed in humans during the course of hypertension.

Myocyte Loss and Systolic Dysfunction

Any process that leads to the loss of myocytes places a larger load on the remaining myocytes and may ultimately lead to deterioration of ventricular function. The two principal etiologies for myocyte loss are hypertension and myocardial infarction. The loss of myocytes that occurs as a function of aging per se is $\approx 0.5\%$ of the myocardial cells per year. When individual myocytes are lost, they are replaced by connective tissue, and further hypertrophy occurs in the remaining myocytes. Some further stiffening of the ventricle also occurs in this process ("remodeling"). The other major event that leads to cell loss is ischemic heart disease.

If an excessive systolic overload is maintained for very long periods and if myocyte loss is added to this process, the steady state of compensated function cannot be maintained, and ventricular deterioration begins. This is characterized by an enlargement of diastolic ventricular volume to maintain the stroke volume and a progressive lowering of the ejection fraction. In this sense, systolic dysfunction now becomes added to diastolic dysfunction. As the diastolic size of the heart continues to increase, added stress is placed on the wall as a result of the Laplace phenomenon, and further hypertrophy and remodeling become necessary to sustain normal systolic stress in the ventricular wall. Ultimately, this can progress to gross ventricular dilatation and failure. Dysfunction of the left ventricle also affects the right ventricle by increased pulmonary pressures, hypertrophy of the septum, and transmission of elevated filling pressures to the right side of the circulation.

Systemic Malcompensation: Neurohumoral Activation

As ventricular dysfunction progresses to systolic dysfunction, compensatory mechanisms are activated in the general circulation, including activation of the sympathetic nervous system and the renin-angiotensin system, which can be further activated by the use of diuretics. These neurohumoral systems cause further ventricular deterioration through direct and indirect mechanisms. With progressive cardiac dilatation, in which myocardial cell loss and fibrosis are also observed, decompensated cardiomyopathy ensues. The late stages, when ventricular hypertrophy evolves into ventricular dilatation, can be viewed as progressive ventricular remodeling, in which the diastolic loads adversely affect the shape and function of the heart. Whereas myocyte contractility in terms of force development may be normal in early hypertension and hypertrophy, in the late stages, when cardiomyopathy ensues, myocyte contractility also becomes depressed and adds to the end-stage process. At these late stages, alterations occur in the peripheral circulation that further limit blood flow to peripheral organs and result in not only central congestion but also a lack of peripheral organ perfusion, with decreased exercise performance and fatigue accompanied by edema; namely, congestive heart failure (CHF). All of these changes are shown in the **Figure 69.1**.

Systemic Vascular Adaptations

When the compensatory limit of left ventricular (LV) dilatation is reached, the heart becomes unable to maintain an adequate output and thus to meet the metabolic demands of the body. Compromised regional blood flow promotes vascular endothelial dysfunction by chronically exposing the vasculature to reduced shear stress. It also results in areas of focal ischemia that, in turn, activate the local tissue renin-angiotensin system, growth factors, and cytokines. These local factors are responsible for further alterations in the coronary and peripheral circulation and thus contribute to the vascular re-

modeling that occurs at the late stage of LV systolic dysfunction. Vascular remodeling is believed to be a major determinant of the functional status (ie, the presence and severity of symptoms) in patients with LV systolic dysfunction.

Coronary Circulatory Abnormalities

Most of the alterations documented in the peripheral and coronary circulation of patients with LV systolic dysfunction appear to be functional rather than structural in nature. Coronary blood flow reserve is reduced in patients with dilated cardiomyopathy in the absence of epicardial coronary artery disease. When the metabolic demands are increased by administration of a positive inotropic agent such as dobutamine, the demand in oxygen can outstrip its delivery and myocardial ischemia can occur even in the absence of coronary artery disease. Of interest, coronary blood flow reserve appears to be similarly decreased in patients with dilated LVs independent of coronary artery disease. The mechanisms responsible for lowering coronary blood flow reserve in patients without coronary artery disease are incompletely understood but appear to include a reduction in endothelium-mediated vasodilatation.

Systemic Circulatory Abnormalities

Abnormal behavior of the skeletal muscle vasculature is the major determinant of reduced peak aerobic capacity in patients with severe CHF. Strenuous physical activity is limited in these patients by a blunted or fixed vasodilatory response of the skeletal muscle beds during exercise. A particular problem is lower limb fatigue.

The mechanisms that mediate functional abnormalities of the skeletal muscle vasculature are still poorly understood in patients

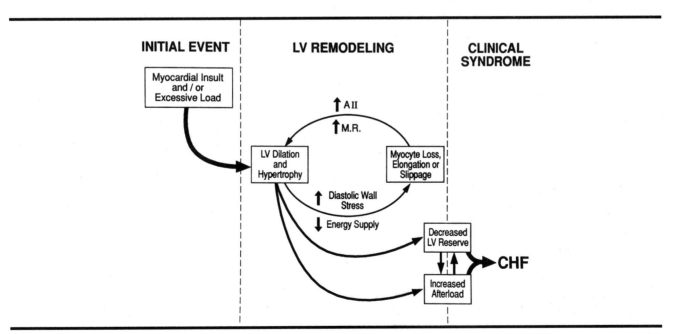

Figure 69.1.   Three stages in the evolution from initial overload to congestive heart failure (CHF). In response to the initial systolic load, LV remodeling occurs, with myocyte hypertrophy. This augments diastolic tensions and, with further myocyte loss and compensatory ventricular dilatation, a vicious circle is created. Secondary activation of the renin-angiotensin system occurs, with increased angiotensin II (A II). Increased ventricular volume produces functional mitral valve regurgitation (M.R.), and further ventricular dilatation occurs. This leads to a decrease in ventricular emptying and an increased afterload for the myocardium, producing end-stage CHF.

with severe CHF. As noted for the coronary circulation, endothelium-mediated dilatation is depressed in the skeletal muscle vasculature of patients with systolic dysfunction. Reduced response of the skeletal muscle vasculature to endothelium-independent dilators indicates that vascular smooth muscle cell relaxation may also be impaired in these patients. Of note, long-term but not acute ACE inhibition improves the vasodilatory response of skeletal muscle beds to exercise. This delayed response to ACE inhibition implies that activation of the renin-angiotensin system may induce favorable alterations in vascular smooth muscle cells and also suggests that the favorable effects are not due to enhancement in endothelium-dependent vasodilatation, which occurs immediately.

SUGGESTED READING

1. Jondeau G, Katz SD, Zohman L, Goldberger M, McCarthy M, Bourdarias JP, LeJemtel TH. Active skeletal muscle mass and cardiopulmonary reserve: failure to attain peak aerobic capacity during maximal bicycle exercise in patients with severe congestive heart failure. *Circulation.* 1992;86:1351–1356.
2. Katz SD. The role of endothelium-derived vasoactive substances in the pathophysiology of exercise intolerance in patients with congestive heart failure. *Prog Cardiovasc Dis.* 1995;38:23–50.
3. LeJemtel TH, Sonnenblick EH, Frishman WHG. Diagnosis and management of heart failure. *Prog Cardiovasc Dis.* 1995;37:745–781.
4. Mancini DM, Davis L, Wexler JP, Chadwick B, LeJemtel TH. Dependence of enhanced maximal exercise performance on increased peak skeletal muscle perfusion during long-term captopril therapy in heart failure. *J Am Coll Cardiol.* 1987;10:845–850.
5. Nakamura M, Funakoshi T, Arakawa N, Yoshida H, Makita S, Hiramori K. Effect of angiotensin-converting enzyme inhibitors on endothelium-dependent peripheral vasodilation in patients with chronic heart failure. *J Am Coll Cardiol.* 1994;24:1321–1327.
6. Olivetti G, Capasso JM, Sonnenblick EH, Ricci R, Puntillo E, Anversa P. Differences in the temporal effects of aging on the structure and function of rat myocardium. *Coron Artery Dis.* 1990;1:240–250.
7. Olivetti G, Melissari M, Capasso JM, Anversa P. Cardiomyopathy of the aging human heart: myocyte loss and reactive cellular hypertrophy. *Circ Res.* 1991;68:1560–1568.
8. Rosendorff C. The renin-angiotensin system and vascular hypertrophy. *J Am Coll Cardiol.* 1996;28:803–812.
9. Schlant RC, Sonnenblick EH, Katz AM. Pathophysiology of heart failure. In: Alexander RW, et al, eds. *Hurst's The Heart.* New York, NY: McGraw Hill; 1997: 687–726.
10. Treasure CB, Vita JA, Cox DA, Fish RD, Gordon JB, Mudge GH, Colucci WS, St John Sutton MG, Selwyn AP, Alexander RW, Ganz P. Endothelium-dependent dilation of the coronary microvasculature is impaired in dilated cardiomyopathy. *Circulation.* 1990;81:772–779.

Chapter 70

Pathogenesis of Stroke

Patrick Pullicino, MD, PhD

KEY POINTS

- Cerebral ischemic injury is caused by cerebral hypoperfusion secondary to arterial embolism, arterial thrombosis, or hemodynamic insufficiency.

- Ceberal ischemic injury is not an "all or none" phenomenon and both the degree and duration of cerebral hypoperfusion are important in determining its severity.

- Clinical features help localize the cerebral ischemic injury but are not a reliable indicator of underlying pathogenesis.

- An understanding of the pathogenesis of cerebral ischemia is important for the appropriate management of a patient with a stroke.

See also Chapters 71, 72, 76, 108, 137

The term "brain attack" has recently been proposed to replace "stroke," to stress the similarity of brain and heart ischemia. Although it is important to underscore the need to treat brain ischemia as urgently as cardiac ischemia, there are three main differences between stroke and heart attack: (1) Embolism from the heart is a major cause of stroke (<20%) but an uncommon cause of heart attack, (2) occlusion of carotid or large intracranial arteries produces focal ischemic necrosis less frequently in the brain than coronary occlusion does in the heart because of brain collateral circulation through the circle of Willis or cortical anastomoses, and (3) hemorrhage secondary to rupture of arteries is a frequent cause of stroke (<10%) but not of heart attack.

Stroke occurs in older patients than does heart attack, because cervical and cerebral atheroscleroses occur more in older patients than does coronary atherosclerosis. Cardiac ischemia can give rise to later cerebral embolism by producing disorders of cardiac function, such as atrial fibrillation and low cardiac output, that predispose to cerebral embolism.

Arterial Occlusion, Cerebral Perfusion, and Clinical Features

It is increasingly realized that ischemic stroke is not an "all-or-none" phenomenon, as was once thought. Reduction of cerebral blood flow due to arterial stenosis or occlusion may produce any degree of tissue injury, varying from isolated neuronal dropout to rarefaction of all tissue elements or to complete cavitary necrosis. The two factors that appear to be most important in determining the severity of injury secondary to arterial occlusion are the efficiency of the collateral circulation and the cardiac output. The clinical manifestations of occlusion of a specific artery vary according to how the interplay of these factors affects local brain perfusion. A minor degree of hypoperfusion is asymptomatic **(Figure 70.1)**, a more severe degree results in a reversible symptomatic loss of function but not tissue injury, and marked hypoperfusion will cause tissue necrosis with persistent clinical sequelae. Because the interplay between site of arterial stenosis or occlusion, cardiac function, and efficiency

of collaterals is different in each patient, clinical deficits produced by cerebral ischemia are not reliable indicators of underlying pathogenesis. Also, the time course of deficits (transient ischemic attack, progressing stroke) is not a good indicator of pathogenesis. Imaging of the brain ischemic lesion (by MRI), of the extent of intracranial and cervical arterial disease (by magnetic resonance angiography [MRA]), and of the state of cerebral perfusion (by single-photon emission computed tomography or transcranial Doppler) may be important in determination of correct therapy.

Watershed, Border-Zone, or Low-Flow Ischemia

When cerebral injury arises secondary to hypoperfusion, it occurs preferentially in border zones or "watershed zones" between arterial territories. Low-flow infarcts are a particular type of border-zone infarcts occurring in the deep white matter adjacent to the lateral ventricle and are frequently associated with an ipsilateral carotid occlusion.

Cerebral Embolism

Emboli arise either from the heart or from proximal arteries. Cardiac emboli arise either from cardiac thrombi arising in the left side of the heart secondary to abnormal intracardiac hemodynamics (eg, dilated left atrium in atrial fibrillation) or from paradoxical embolism due to thrombi arising in the systemic veins and traversing to the left side of the heart through a patent foramen ovale. Arterial emboli are either dislodged fragments of atherosclerotic debris or thrombi arising in an area of stagnant flow distal to a stenosis or secondary to atherosclerosis or dissection. Arteriogenic embolism also frequently arises from the internal carotid artery near the carotid bifurcation and from the vertebral artery near its origin or termination. A hemodynamically tight stenosis can give rise to tiny arteriogenic emboli formed of platelet clumps that may produce recurrent transient focal cerebral or ocular ischemia.

The increased resolution of small cardiac structures by trans-

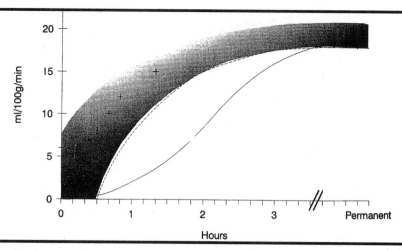

Figure 70.1. Graph showing time-intensity relationship of ischemia and incomplete infarction. Area above curves represents combination of duration and intensity of ischemia that is tolerated without development of infarction, whereas points below curves will result in infarction. Shaded area represents ischemic injury without infarction. Reproduced with permission from Helgason CM, Wolf PA. American Heart Association Prevention Conference IV: prevention and rehabilitation of stroke. *Stroke.* 1997;28:1498–1526.

esophageal echocardiography (TEE) allows the identification of many potential causes of cardiogenic embolism (**Table 70.1**). It also allows the identification of aortic atherosclerosis, which, when >4 mm thick, carries a high relative risk of stroke (due to arteriogenic embolism). TEE may confirm the diagnosis in patients in whom embolism is suspected by clinical features but cannot by itself be used to rule out embolic disease.

Atherosclerosis

Atherosclerosis may become symptomatic by (1) producing arteriogenic embolism, (2) causing hemodynamic obstruction and producing distal cerebral hypoperfusion, or (3) occluding small (penetrating) arteries that arise in the vicinity of the atherosclerotic lesion. Atherosclerosis frequently affects small penetrating arteries <1 mm in diameter (this is called "microatheroma"), may occlude the small artery, and may give rise to a small cavitary ("lacunar") infarct. Critical narrowing of a small penetrating artery may also cause recurrent episodes of transient hypoperfusion distally, presenting clinically as transient ischemic attacks.

Hypertension and Arterial Disease

Hypertension is the most potent risk factor for stroke and contributes to the occurrence of stroke in several ways (**see Table 70.2**).

1. Hypertension accelerates atherosclerosis in large arteries and in this way increases the frequency of stroke related to atherosclerosis.
2. Hypertension causes hypertrophy and thickening of the media of small intracerebral arteries. This may lead to a widespread narrowing of small intracerebral arteries, leading to hypoperfusion and ischemic rarefaction of white matter in the periventricular watershed areas of the brain. This white matter ischemic rarefaction (or subcortical arteriosclerotic encephalopathy) is present in almost all patients with long-standing hypertension and may give rise to a dementia syndrome called Binswanger's disease.

Table 70.1. Trial of Org 10172 in Acute Stroke Treatment (TOAST) Classification of High- and Medium-Risk Sources of Cardioembolism

High-risk sources
  Mechanical prosthetic valve
  Mitral stenosis with atrial fibrillation
  Atrial fibrillation (other than lone atrial fibrillation)
  Left atrial/atrial appendage thrombus
  Sick sinus syndrome
  Recent myocardial infarction (<4 weeks)
  Left ventricular thrombus
  Dilated cardiomyopathy
  Akinetic left ventricular segment
  Atrial myxoma
  Infective endocarditis
Medium-risk sources
  Mitral valve prolapse
  Mitral annulus calcification
  Mitral stenosis without atrial fibrillation
  Left atrial turbulence (smoke)
  Atrial septal aneurysm
  Patent foramen ovale
  Atrial flutter
  Lone atrial fibrillation
  Bioprosthetic cardiac valve
  Nonbacterial thrombotic endocarditis
  Congestive heart failure
  Hypokinetic left ventricular segment
  Myocardial infarction (>4 weeks, <6 months)

Reproduced from Adams HP Jr, Bendixen BH, Kappelle LJ, Biller J, Love BB, Gordon DL, Marsh EE III, and the TOAST Investigators. Classification of subtype of acute ischemic stroke: definitions for use in a multicenter clinical trial. *Stroke.* 1993;24:35–41 with permission.

3. Hypertension may cause focal damage to small intracerebral arteries (known as lipohyalinosis), causing them to occlude. This gives rise to small ischemic cavities in the brain known as lacunar infarcts.

Table 70.2. Arterial Mechanisms of Hypertensive Brain Attacks (Stroke)

Accelerated atheroscleroses (thrombotic or embolic cerebral infarct)
Arteriolar medial hypertrophy with ischemic rarefaction
Lipohyalinosis (lacunar infarcts)
Microaneurysm formation (intracerebral hemorrhage)
Berry aneurysm (subarachnoid hemorrhage)

4. Hypertension is the main cause of intracerebral hemorrhage; this is probably secondary to small aneurysms (microaneurysms) that arise on small intracerebral arteries, and they appear to be part of the pathology of lipohyalinosis.

5. Hypertension is also a risk factor for larger berry aneurysms and subarachnoid hemorrhage.

Clinical Imaging Correlations in Stroke

Clinical history and examination are important to determine the presence of a stroke, to attempt to localize the ischemic lesion, and also to help determine the pathogenesis (subtype of stroke). Different types of strokes have classic presentations. Embolic cerebral infarction is typically very sudden in onset; cerebral hemorrhage is also sudden, but the deficit is progressive, and the patient frequently has headache; and hypoperfusion strokes tend to have a slower, often stuttering, onset. Subarachnoid hemorrhage gives a sudden, very severe headache at onset.

Increasing availability of MRI and MRA has diminished reliance on clinical data to determine pathogenesis and treatment. The importance of accurate localization of a cerebral infarct is to assist determination of the underlying arterial lesion or pathogenesis. MRI, particularly diffusion-weighted imaging, is more accurate than clinical findings and should be used preferentially. If the imaging localization appears to be incompatible with the clinical localization, this may indicate the presence of multiple infarcts or possibly seizures.

Acute Stroke and the Ischemic Penumbra

As pointed out earlier, stroke is not an all-or-none phenomenon, and slight reductions of cerebral blood flow may cause temporary loss of function without injury. It has recently been realized that moderate reduction of blood flow may not produce injury if reversed quickly but will progress to infarction if allowed to persist for 2 to 3 hours (**Figure 70.1**). Many strokes have a central core of severe reduction of blood flow with permanent infarction surrounded by a rim of tissue with moderate reduction of blood flow in which the dysfunction is potentially reversible. This surrounding area is called the "ischemic penumbra." Restoration of normal flow to the penumbra within a few hours can result in restoration of function to the area and clinical improvement. The ability of thrombolytics and brain protective agents to improve outcome after a stroke appears to depend on the presence of an ischemic penumbra.

SUGGESTED READING

1. Adams HP Jr, Bendixen BH, Kappelle LJ, Biller J, Love BB, Gordon DL, Marsh EE III, and the TOAST Investigators. Classification of subtype of acute ischemic stroke: definitions for use in a multicenter clinical trial. *Stroke.* 1993;24:35–41.

2. Bronner LL, Kanter DS, Manson JE. Primary prevention of stroke. *N Engl J Med.* 1995;333:1392–1400.

3. Caplan LR. *Stroke: A Clinical Approach.* Boston, Mass. Butterworth-Heinemann; 1993.

4. Culebras A, Kase CS, Masdeu JC, Fox AJ, Bryan RN, Grossman CB, Lee DH, Adams HP, Thies W. Practice guidelines for the use of imaging in transients ischemic attacks and acute stroke: a report of the Stroke Council, American Heart Association. *Stroke.* 1997;28:1480–1497.

5. Garcia JH, Lassen NA, Weiller C, Sperling B, Nakagawara J. Ischemic stroke and incomplete infarction. *Stroke.* 1996;27:761–765.

6. Helgason CM, Wolf PA. American Heart Association Prevention Conference IV: prevention and rehabilitation of stroke. *Stroke.* 1997;28:1498–1526.

7. Khaw K-T. Epidemiology of stroke. *J Neurol Neurosurg Psychiatry.* 1996;61:333–338.

8. Pullicino PM, Caplan LR, Hommel M. *Cerebral Small Artery Disease.* New York, NY. Raven Press; 1993.

9. Whisnant JP. Effectiveness versus efficacy of treatment of hypertension for stroke prevention. *Neurology.* 1996;46:301–307.

Chapter 71

Pathogenesis of Acute Hypertensive Encephalopathy

Donald D. Heistad, MD; William J. Lawton, MD

KEY POINTS

- Hypertensive encephalopathy, a medical emergency characterized by hypertension, headache, and other neurological symptoms, usually in the setting of severe hypertension, responds clinically to blood pressure reduction.

- Hypertensive encephalopathy apparently is due to marked cerebral vasodilatation and disruption of the blood-brain barrier, particularly in postcapillary venules.

- Sympathetic nerves and local myogenic tone protect the cerebral microvasculature from hypertensive damage.

See also Chapters 38, 66, 70, 72, 151

Hypertensive encephalopathy is a syndrome of severe hypertension, cerebrovascular dysfunction, and neurological impairment. The diagnosis may be in doubt until neurological improvement occurs after reduction of arterial pressure (**Table 71.1**).

Pathophysiology

It was thought in the past that hypertensive encephalopathy is the result of spasm of cerebral blood vessels. This hypothesis was based in part on the finding that, during acute hypertension in experimental animals, cerebral arterioles may resemble a "sausage string," with segments of constricted and dilated blood vessels. A similar sausage-string appearance may be seen in retinal vessels of patients with hypertensive encephalopathy. These observations led to the hypothesis that constricted segments of retinal and cerebral blood vessels were in spasm and that vasospasm produces cerebral ischemia and hypertensive encephalopathy.

There is now considerable evidence that, in arterioles that have a sausage-string appearance, the constricted portions are the normal segments of the vessels. The normal response of cerebral arterioles to acute hypertension is constriction, as the vessels "autoregulate" and prevent increases in blood flow during periods of increased blood pressure. When the autoregulatory capacity of vessels is exceeded during severe hypertension, segments of the vessels dilate, and a sausage-string appearance may occur.

The initial site of disruption of the blood-brain barrier during acute hypertension appears to be cerebral venules, not capillaries or arterioles. When the autoregulatory capacity of cerebral vessels is exceeded, small arteries and arterioles dilate, blood flow increases, and microvascular pressure increases throughout the cerebral microcirculation. Cerebral arterioles are protected by a layer of smooth muscle cells, and wall stress in capillaries may not increase greatly because their diameter is small. In contrast, cerebral venules may be most vulnerable to increases in wall stress during acute hypertension because their diameters are rather large and because venules do not have a layer of smooth muscle cells.

Sympathetic neural discharge, which normally has little effect on cerebral blood vessels, constricts cerebral vessels during acute hypertension. Thus, sympathetic nerves attenuate increases in cerebral blood flow during acute hypertension and protect against disruption of the blood-brain barrier in downstream vessels. During chronic hypertension, hypertrophy of vessels (augmented by a trophic effect of sympathetic nerves) reduces vascular wall stress and protects the vessels.

It now is thought that hypertensive encephalopathy is produced by cerebral vasodilatation, accompanied by disruption of the blood-brain barrier, rather than by cerebral vasospasm. Encephalopathy after disruption of the blood-brain barrier may be related to focal cerebral edema or to local changes in ions and neurotransmitters, with impairment of normal neuronal function.

Clinical Features and Treatment

Hypertensive encephalopathy, which commonly occurs with a background of malignant hypertension, is a triad of severe hypertension, encephalopathy, and rapid resolution during treatment of hypertension.

In most patients with hypertensive encephalopathy, arterial pressure is either extraordinarily high (often >250/150 mm Hg) or of recent onset. In patients with chronic hypertension, there is a shift in the autoregulatory curve, and encephalopathy occurs only at very high levels of pressure. In contrast, in patients with rapid development of hypertension, such as occurs during acute glomerulonephritis or eclampsia, there is not sufficient time for a shift in the autoregulatory curve. In these circumstances, encephalopathy may occur during relatively acute but quantitatively modest elevations of arterial pressure (perhaps 150/100 mm Hg), especially in children.

Encephalopathy may be manifested by a variety of symptoms. Headache, sometimes with restlessness, typically occurs early in the syndrome. Nausea, projectile vomiting, and visual blurring may be followed by drowsiness, confusion, and seizures. Papilledema, usually with retinal hemorrhages and exudates, may be observed, and

Table 71.1. Hypertensive Encephalopathy

Triad
  Severe hypertension
  Encephalopathy
  Rapid resolution with treatment
Usually associated with malignant hypertension
Pathophysiology
  Cerebral vasodilatation
  Disruption of blood-brain barrier
Etiology
  Untreated essential hypertension
  Renal disease
  Renal vascular disease
Pheochromocytoma
Differential diagnosis
  Central nervous system lesion, including tumor and stroke
  Drugs, vasculitis, uremia

retinal arteries may exhibit a sausage-string appearance. Compression of the lateral ventricles on computerized tomographic (CT) scans or magnetic resonance imaging suggests cerebral edema; the presence of cerebellar and brainstem edema may indicate hypertensive encephalopathy. Hypodense areas in white matter, presumably secondary to edema, have been observed during hypertensive encephalopathy and typically clear after treatment. Lumbar puncture probably is not necessary unless other causes of encephalopathy are being considered. Lumbar puncture should be avoided if a mass lesion is suspected.

Patients with hypertensive encephalopathy usually have other findings that are suggestive of malignant hypertension. In addition to papilledema, they may have left ventricular hypertrophy and dysfunction, congestive heart failure, or renal insufficiency. Urinalysis may reveal hematuria, proteinuria (sometimes >3 g protein), and casts. Microangiopathic hemolytic anemia also may be present.

Reduction in blood pressure usually produces rapid clinical improvement. Headache, confusion, and focal neurological deficits may improve within hours, or improvement may take several days. The approaches to antihypertensive therapy include intermediate target values for blood pressure and appropriate pharmacological agents, as discussed elsewhere. Anticonvulsant agents are not necessary for hypertensive encephalopathy.

Differential Diagnosis

Hypertension and generalized or focal cerebral symptoms may be produced by intracerebral hemorrhage, subarachnoid hemorrhage, brain tumor, subdural hematoma, cerebral infarction, or seizures. These disorders often are characterized by localizing or suggestive neurological findings and, with the exception of acute stroke or seizures, generally can be distinguished from hypertensive encephalopathy by CT scan. Antihypertensive therapy should not be delayed for CT scan if the diagnosis of hypertensive encephalopathy is probable. If acute stroke is likely, however, precipitous reduction of blood pressure should be avoided.

The most common underlying cause of hypertensive encephalopathy is untreated essential hypertension. In many patients, however, hypertensive encephalopathy and malignant hypertension are due to underlying treatable diseases such as parenchymal renal disease, renal vascular hypertension, pheochromocytoma, and eclampsia. These possibilities should be evaluated after the clinical condition of the patient becomes stable.

Drugs, especially intravenous amphetamines and cocaine, can produce vasculitis and hypertension with symptoms that are similar to hypertensive encephalopathy. In patients who are taking monoamine oxidase inhibitors, such foods as cheddar cheese that contain tyramine may produce acute hypertension with stroke or signs that resemble hypertensive encephalopathy. Oral contraceptives have been associated with malignant hypertension. Withdrawal from clonidine treatment may produce similar symptoms and signs. Vasculitis from lupus erythematosus or polyarteritis may be associated with moderate or severe hypertension and cerebritis. Uremic encephalopathy may occur when serum creatinine exceeds 10 mg/dL, with clinical presentation similar to hypertensive encephalopathy.

SUGGESTED READING

1. Baumbach GL, Heistad DD. Cerebral circulation in chronic arterial hypertension. *Hypertension.* 1988;12:89–95.
2. Healton EB, Brust JC, Feinfeld DA, Thomson GE. Hypertensive encephalopathy and the neurologic manifestations of malignant hypertension. *Neurology.* 1982;32:127–132.
3. Mayhan WG, Heistad DD. Permeability of blood-brain barrier to various sized molecules. *Am J Physiol.* 1985;248:H712–H718.
4. Strandgaard S, Paulson OB. Hypertensive disease and the cerebral circulation. In: Laragh JH, Brenner BM, eds. *Hypertension: Pathophysiology, Diagnosis, and Management.* New York, NY: Raven Press; 1990;1:399–416.
5. Wright RR, Mathews KD. Hypertensive encephalopathy in childhood. *J Child Neurol.* 1996;11:193–196.

Chapter 72

Pathogenesis of Vascular Disease and Mixed Dementia

Linda A. Hershey, MD, PhD

KEY POINTS

- Vascular dementia is a general term that includes radiographic subtypes, such as multi-infarct dementia and subcortical arteriosclerotic encephalopathy.

- Age, hypertension, hyperlipidemia, and diabetes are risk factors for stroke and vascular dementia.

- Vascular and mixed dementia (a combination of Alzheimer's and vascular changes in the brain) account for 30% to 40% of all patients with dementing illnesses in North America and Europe.

- Aspirin, pentoxifylline, and blood pressure control have been shown to reduce stroke risk and to slow progression of cognitive decline in patients with vascular dementia.

See also Chapters 66, 70, 71, 76, 108, 137

Hypertension and Dementia

Chronic hypertension contributes to the development of both large-vessel disease (atherosclerosis) and small-vessel disease (arteriolosclerosis) in the brain. Multiple atherothrombotic strokes can lead to the condition known as multi-infarct dementia (MID). Arteriolosclerosis and the resultant subcortical hypoperfusion can produce demyelination of white matter and dementia in the condition referred to as subcortical arteriosclerotic encephalopathy (SAE). Because radiographic findings of MID and SAE can coexist in some individuals, we will use the general term "vascular dementia" in this chapter.

Hypertension, aging, hyperlipidemia, and diabetes are major risk factors for stroke and vascular dementia. Hyperlipidemia slows blood flow in the brain by increasing serum viscosity and may also decrease vasoreactivity. Decreased cerebral blood flow may also result from the drugs that are used to treat chronic hypertension. Blood-brain barrier disruption in conjunction with drug-induced vasodilation may contribute to the subcortical white matter changes seen on brain imaging studies of patients with SAE.

Epidemiology

When Rothschild studied the prevalence of the three most common dementing illnesses in 1941, two thirds of his 60 autopsy-proven cases had vascular or mixed dementia (**Table 72.1**) and high systolic blood pressures ($\geq$150 mm Hg) during life. More recent pathological studies have shown that 30% to 35% of demented patients have vascular or mixed dementia. Alzheimer's disease (AD) is now the most prevalent dementing illness in North America and Western Europe, whereas vascular dementia is the most common dementing process in the Orient.

Dementia will be documented within 3 months of stroke onset in ≈25% of all acute ischemic stroke patients, but only 10% to 15% have cognitive impairment that is directly attributable to the most recent stroke. In 120 ischemic stroke patients, we identified 10 with stroke-related dementia, 4 with SAE by computed tomography (CT), 5 with MID, and only 1 with a single large infarct.

Clinical Diagnosis

The memory impairment of vascular dementia usually develops abruptly and tends to progress in a stepwise fashion over time. In contrast, the onset of AD is insidious, and the progression is gradual (**Table 72.2**). Somatic complaints such as syncope, seizures, dizziness, and headaches are more commonly seen in patients with vascular dementia than in those with AD.

Caplan and Schoene found that SAE patients with good blood pressure control fluctuated cognitively over time, whereas those with poor control seemed to deteriorate rapidly. Hershey and others found that a fluctuating course was common to both subtypes (SAE and MID) of vascular dementia. A few of the patients in this series improved cognitively during the first year after their ischemic stroke, just as their motor deficits improved.

Rothschild found that depression was more prevalent among vascular and mixed dementia patients than among those with autopsy-verified AD. This has since been confirmed in a prospective clinical series in which 60% of the vascular dementia patients reported depressive symptoms, compared with only 17% of the AD patients. None of the AD patients in that series had severe depression, whereas 26% of the vascular dementia patients met criteria for major depression.

Emotional lability, or pseudobulbar affect, is a frontal lobe sign that is more prevalent in vascular dementia patients (30% to 40%) than in those with AD (4%). This sign is often associated with other features of pseudobulbar palsy, such as bradykinesia, gait unsteadiness, urinary incontinence, dysarthria, dysphagia, and loss of executive function.

Pathophysiology

Binswanger was the first to link vascular dementia with arteriosclerotic kidney disease and cardiomegaly. Caplan and Schoene subsequently demonstrated that the pathological changes in small vessels

Table 72.1. Autopsy Studies of Dementing Illnesses

AUTHOR (YEAR)	AD	MIX	IVD	OTHER	TOTAL, N
Rothschild (1941)	20	18	22	0	60
Tomlinson et al (1970)	25	9	8	8	50
Wade et al (1987)	39	16	4	6	65

AD indicates Alzheimer's disease; Mix, coexistence of both AD and IVD; and IVD, ischemic vascular dementia.

Table 72.2. Clinical Features of Vascular and Alzheimer's Dementia

FEATURES	VASCULAR OR MIXED DEMENTIA	ALZHEIMER'S DEMENTIA
Onset	Abrupt	Insidious
Course	Fluctuations, stepwise progression, or long plateaus	Gradual progression
Symptoms and signs	Gait disorder	Language disorder
	Urinary incontinence	Motor apraxia
	Depression	Visual agnosia
	Emotional lability	Delusions
	Focal signs	Constructional apraxia
	Syncope	

of SAE patients are the same as those of chronic hypertensive patients with multiple small, deep infarcts. The replacement of smooth muscle cells in small vessels by fibrohyaline material may explain why there is loss of autoregulation in hypertensive patients with SAE.

Yao and others used positron emission tomography to compare chronic hypertensive patients with and without dementia. All of their subjects had severe subcortical white matter changes on brain imaging studies. Their data support the hypothesis that the pathological changes produced by chronic hypertension in small, deep arteries of the brain can result in subcortical white matter hypoperfusion. Dementia develops in the patients who cannot compensate for chronic hypoperfusion by increasing the rate of oxygen extraction from the blood.

Neuroimaging

Vascular dementia patients differ from multi-infarct control subjects in that they have more cerebral infarcts on brain imaging studies, such as CT and magnetic resonance imaging (MRI). Using CT, Gorelick and others also showed that MID patients have larger ventricles and a higher prevalence of periventricular white matter changes than nondemented stroke controls. MRI is more sensitive than CT for detecting cerebral infarction, but some of the white matter changes on MRI are due to enlarged perivascular spaces and periventricular gliosis, not ischemia. The most reliable way to identify patients with vascular dementia is to combine head CT results with clinical diagnostic criteria.

Treatment

Good control of systemic blood pressure in chronic hypertensive patients has been shown to improve cerebral perfusion (subcortical hypoperfusion has been documented in neurologically normal but untreated hypertensive subjects). Excessive reduction of blood pressure is not always advised in patients with vascular dementia, because cognitive decline can occur when systolic pressures are acutely lowered to below the 135 to 150 mm Hg range. β-Blockers and ACE inhibitors are preferred over calcium channel blockers, loop diuretics, or thiazide diuretics for the management of hypertension in those >65 years old.

In addition to appropriate treatment of hypertension, aspirin and pentoxifylline may be useful in patients with vascular dementia. Aspirin (325 mg QD) reduces the risk of stroke and death by ≈25% in patients who have experienced transient ischemic attack or stroke and has been shown to stabilize the course of vascular dementia. Pentoxifylline (400 mg TID) may slow the rate of cognitive decline in vascular dementia patients by its ability to reduce serum viscosity.

SUGGESTED READING

1. Caplan LR, Schoene WC. Clinical features of subcortical arteriosclerotic encephalopathy (Binswanger disease). *Neurology.* 1978;28:1206–1215.
2. Gorelick PB, Chatterjee A, Patel D, Flowerdew G, Dollear W, Taber J, Harris Y. Cranial computed tomographic observations in multi-infarct dementia: a controlled study. *Stroke.* 1992;23:804–811.
3. Heckbert SR, Longstreth WT Jr, Psaty BM, Murros KE, Smith NL, Newman AB, Williamson JD, Bernick C, Furberg CD. The association of antihypertensive agents with MRI white matter findings and with Modified Mini-Mental State Examination in older adults. *J Am Geriatr Soc.* 1997;45:1423–1433.
4. Hershey LA, Modic MT, Jaffe DF, Greenough PG. Natural history of the vascular dementias: a prospective study of seven cases. *Can J Neurol Sci.* 1986;13(suppl): 559–565.
5. Pullicino P, Benedict RHB, Capruso DX, Vella N, Withiam-Leitch S, Kwen PL. Neuroimaging criteria for vascular dementia [published correction appears in *Arch Neurol.* 1996;53:1146]. *Arch Neurol.* 1996;53:723–728.
6. Román GC, Tatemichi TK, Erkinjuntti T, Cummings JL, Masdeu JC, Garcia JH, Amaducci L, Orgogozo JM, Brun A, Hofman A, et al. Vascular dementia: diagnostic criteria for research studies. Report of the NINDS-AIREN International Workshop. *Neurology.* 1993;43:250–260.
7. Rothschild D. The clinical differentiation of senile and arteriosclerotic psychosis. *Am J Psychiatry.* 1941;98:324–333.
8. Tomlinson BE, Blessed G, Roth M. Observations on the brains of demented old people. *J Neurol Sci.* 1970;11:205–242.
9. Wade JPH, Mirsen TR, Hachinski VC, Fisman M, Lau C, Merskey H. The clinical diagnosis of Alzheimer's disease. *Arch Neurol.* 1987;44:24–29.
10. Yao H, Sadoshima S, Ibayashi S, Kuwabara Y, Ichiya Y, Fujishima M. Leukoaraiosis and dementia in hypertensive patients. *Stroke.* 1992;23:1673–1677.

Chapter 73

Pathogenesis of Hypertensive Renal Damage

Sharon Anderson, MD

KEY POINTS

- Hypertension is both a cause and a consequence of glomerulosclerosis, the hallmark lesion of progressive renal disease.

- Hypertensive nephrosclerosis cannot be easily distinguished from other forms of glomerulosclerosis.

- Elevated glomerular capillary pressure and glomerular ischemia lead to glomerulosclerosis.

- Elevated cholesterol, cigarette smoking, and hypertension act synergistically to accelerate renal failure.

See also Chapters 52, 66, 78, 112,141

Progressive sclerosis of glomeruli is the final common pathway of a number of otherwise dissimilar renal diseases. The gross and microscopic appearance of the end-stage kidney with almost every renal disease is that of a shrunken and scarred mass of sclerotic glomeruli with tubulointerstitial fibrosis. At end stage, the initial renal insult often cannot be identified. Hypertension is integrally related to this process, and hypertensive nephrosclerosis often cannot be distinguished from other forms of glomerulosclerosis. It is thus useful to consider these sclerotic disease processes together.

Hypertension and Progressive Renal Disease

Hypertension is both a cause and a consequence of renal disease, and systemic hypertension is one of the most important risk factors for progressive loss of renal function. Moreover, previously normotensive patients usually develop systemic hypertension as renal function fails, leading to the vicious circle of end-stage renal disease (ESRD). Hypertension is associated with faster loss of renal function in patients with intrinsic renal diseases and accelerated age-related loss of renal function in individuals with otherwise normal kidneys. In chronic renal failure and in diabetic nephropathy, patients not only exhibit higher blood pressures but also lose the usual nocturnal decline in blood pressure, so that the hypertensive burden is more continuously present in these patients.

Although hypertension may initiate renal disease, the incidence of hypertensive nephropathy, defined as renal insufficiency in which hypertension is the only known etiologic factor, is difficult to quantify. Often, the coexistence of hypertension and chronic renal disease leads to a *presumptive* diagnosis of hypertensive nephropathy when the underlying problem may be renovascular or parenchymal renal disease.

Most hypertensive patients escape serious renal complications. Nevertheless, the incidence and prevalence of ESRD presumably secondary to essential hypertension are considerable (**Figure 73.1**) and are particularly high in blacks (**Figure 73.2**). The incidence of hypertension as a presumptive cause of ESRD is increasing, with highest rates seen in elderly patients and in blacks. Because ESRD data come from analyses of persons receiving dialysis or kidney transplantation, changes in rates may reflect, in part, changing patterns of

referral to ESRD therapy. Higher ERSD rates may also reflect poor control of hypertension or failure of antihypertensive treatment to limit target-organ damage. Of note, the impressive reductions in morbidity and mortality from stroke and coronary artery disease resulting from modern antihypertensive therapy have not been reflected in commensurate reductions in morbidity and mortality of ESRD.

Benefits of Antihypertensive Therapy

Epidemiological and retrospective studies provide strong evidence that lowering blood pressure slows the age-related loss of renal function. For example, a retrospective study of patients coming to ESRD found that those patients whose diastolic blood pressures were above >90 mm Hg, regardless of presence or absence of antihypertensive therapy, lost renal function at a faster rate than those whose diastolic pressures were <90 mm Hg. Similarly, retrospective analyses of data from both the Hypertension Detection and Follow-up Program Cooperative Group and the Multiple Risk Factor Intervention Trial (MRFIT) studies found accelerated loss of renal function in patients with persistent diastolic hypertension.

Diagnosis of Hypertensive Nephropathy

Although a number of clinical features support a diagnosis of hypertensive nephrosclerosis (**Table 73.1**), this diagnosis can seldom be made with confidence. Prospective clinical follow-up, with observed progression from normal to impaired renal function over many years, improves diagnostic accuracy. Urinalysis is helpful to exclude other conditions. A low degree of proteinuria (usually <1.5 to 2 g/d) may be found, but there should not be evidence of active renal disease (cells or casts). Recently, it has been recognized that a subset of patients (perhaps 15%) with essential hypertension exhibit microalbuminuria (eg, >20 mg/d), which is below that detected by standard dipstick. Microalbuminuria predicts increased cardiovascular risk, but its prognostic value in essential hypertension is not yet known, and its presence does not confirm the diagnosis of hypertensive nephropathy.

Renal imaging studies are also not helpful, other than to exclude alternative causes, such as obstruction, kidney stones, and renal artery stenosis. Even renal biopsy may not confirm the diagnosis be-

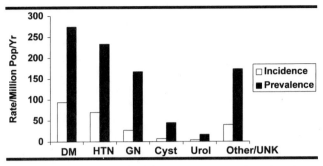

Figure 73.1.   Total treated ESRD incidence and prevalence by primary diagnoses, 1993–1995. DM indicates diabetes; HTN, hypertension; GN, glomerulonephritis; Cyst, cystic diseases; Urol, other urological diseases; and Other/UNK, other or unknown. Adapted from data in The 1997 USRDS Annual Data Report.

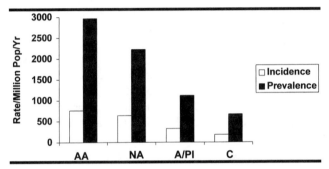

Figure 73.2.   Total treated ESRD incidence and prevalence by race (adjusted for sex and age), 1993–1995. AA indicates African-American; NA, Native American; A/PI, Asians and Pacific Islanders; and C, Caucasian. Adapted from data in The 1997 USRDS Annual Data Report.

Table 73.1. Clinical Features Consistent With Hypertensive Nephrosclerosis

Black race
Positive family history; onset of hypertension between ages 25 and 45 y
Long-standing or very severe hypertension
Evidence of hypertensive retinal damage
Evidence of hypertensive left ventricular hypertrophy
Onset of hypertension before development of proteinuria
Absence of any cause for primary renal disease
Biopsy evidence: degree of glomerular ischemia and fibrosis compatible with degree of arteriolar and small arterial vascular disease

cause the morphological findings are not pathognomonic. Accordingly, the diagnosis of hypertensive nephropathy is usually only presumptive and can be made with reasonable confidence only when other causes of chronic renal failure are excluded.

Morphology of Hypertensive Renal Injury

Classically, the kidney in hypertensive nephrosclerosis is shrunken, scarred, and coarsely granular. Vascular lesions are most notable, including intimal thickening and fibrosis, reduplication of the internal elastic lamina in arcuate and interlobular arteries, and hyalinization of the arterioles (arteriolosclerosis). Glomerular injury is initially

focal in nature and consists of tuft shrinkage with loss of cellularity. Eventually, sclerosis becomes more generalized, and associated tubules are frequently atrophic.

Mechanisms of Hypertensive Renal Injury
Hemodynamic Mechanisms

Hypertension causes renal damage by multiple mechanisms, which may differ in various forms of renal injury. One such mechanism is ischemia, with glomerular hypoperfusion causing glomerulosclerosis. It is likely that this mechanism is operative in patients with renovascular hypertension and may occur in patients with hypertensive renal disease as well. In contrast, in hypertension secondary to intrinsic renal disease, experimental evidence suggests that glomerular capillary hyperperfusion and hypertension, rather than ischemia, are important pathogenetic mechanisms.

Afferent arteriolar resistance determines the degree of transmission of systemic pressure to the glomerular capillary network. The autoregulatory response of the normal kidney to increased perfusion pressure is an increase in afferent arteriolar (preglomerular) resistance, so that the increased systemic pressure is not fully transmitted to the glomerulus **(Figure 73.3)**. However, if reflex afferent arteriolar constriction is impaired by disease or by drugs, the kidney cannot protect itself from increased systemic pressure, which is then freely transmitted into the glomerular capillary network, resulting in glomerular capillary hypertension. Several studies are ongoing to test whether calcium antagonists (afferent arteriolar dilators) protect (of fail to protect) the kidney from focal glomerulosclerosis.

Renal manifestations of essential hypertension may be similar to those in the spontaneously hypertensive rat (SHR). In the SHR, despite very high systemic blood pressure, afferent arteriolar vasoconstriction prevents excessive transmission of flow and pressure into the glomerular capillary network, and glomerular capillary pressure (P_{GC}) remains nearly normal. Despite high pressures, renal injury is modest and late to develop. In humans, a similar physiological situation of high systemic pressures with normal intraglomerular capillary pressures may explain the relatively low incidence of ESRD among the millions of patients with essential hypertension, particularly when hypertension is not severe.

The importance of afferent arteriolar vasoconstriction in conferring protection to the glomerular microvasculature is clearly demonstrated by uninephrectomy in the SHR, which results in lowering of afferent arteriolar resistance in the remaining kidney and elevation of P_{GC}. This latter hemodynamic alteration is associated with a large increase in proteinuria and acceleration of glomerular sclerosis.

Glomerular Capillary Hypertension

In contrast to the protective afferent arteriolar vasoconstriction in the SHR, other forms of renal disease are characterized by primary afferent arteriolar vasodilation and elevation of P_{GC} with coexisting systemic hypertension. This persistent afferent vasodilation can sometimes lead to glomerular hypertension, even when systemic blood pressure is normal, as in the rat with early diabetes.

In animals with chronic renal failure, both afferent and efferent arteriolar resistances are reduced. Because the reduction in afferent resistance exceeds that in efferent resistance, however, there are net increases in P_{GC} and persistent glomerular capillary hypertension.

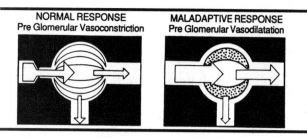

Figure 73.3. Preglomerular adaptations to increased systemic blood pressure. Reproduced with permission from Keane et al. *Ann Intern Med.* 1989;111:503.

Reduction of P_{GC} by dietary protein restriction or pharmacological intervention consistently slows the rate of loss of renal function and limits development of proteinuria and glomerulosclerosis. Indirectly, clinical studies are consistent with the notion that afferent arteriolar vasodilation and consequent glomerular capillary hypertension are present in diabetes and other progressive renal disease. Increased glomerular pressures or renal plasma flow rates affect the growth and activity of glomerular component cells, inducing the elaboration or expression of cytokines and other mediators, which then stimulate mesangial matrix production and promote structural injury.

Other Mechanisms of Injury

Additional mechanisms of injury act synergistically with high systemic and glomerular capillary pressures to accelerate glomerulosclerosis. Although they are well described in experimental models, the role of these factors in clinical hypertensive renal disease is not yet well understood. Their clinical importance is likely to become more clear in the next few years.

Cholesterol

Recent attention has been directed to the potential role of hypercholesterolemia as a risk factor for progression of renal disease. Dietary cholesterol supplementation accelerates glomerular injury in experimental animals, and pharmacological antihyperlipidemic therapy slows disease progression. When systemic hypertension and hyperlipidemia coexist, the combination induces more glomerular injury than either risk factor alone. As with atherosclerosis, oxidation of low-density lipoprotein may be a critical injury-promoting step. It is widely postulated that reactive oxygen species contribute to glomerulosclerosis.

Cigarette Smoking

Epidemiological studies confirm that cigarette smoking is a risk factor for progressive renal disease, particularly in patients with diabetes. Not surprisingly, the mechanisms and risk factors relevant to atherosclerosis appear to be equally relevant to glomerulosclerosis and equally aggravated by cigarette smoking.

Endothelial Cell Dysfunction

Fibrinoid material is found within the glomerulus in many forms of injury, suggesting that glomerular injury is promoted by endothelial cell dysfunction, a process similar to systemic atherogenesis. Abnormal hemodynamic stresses and intracapillary thrombosis also occur and may be triggered by endothelial dysfunction. The vascular endothelial cell is an important source of vasoactive peptides (eg, endothelin) and nitric oxide, which modulate the tone of the subjacent vascular smooth muscle, affect vascular reactivity, and influence cellular injury. Experimental renal disease is slowed by heparin or antiplatelet agents, and a few preliminary clinical studies suggest potential efficacy.

Proteinuria

Elevated P_{GC} leads to enhanced traffic of macromolecules into the mesangial region and the urinary space. Increased macromolecular flux into the mesangium may stimulate the synthesis of matrix components by these cells. It has been suggested that persistent proteinuria may accelerate glomerular and tubular cell injury, consequently accelerating glomerulosclerosis. Indirect evidence in support of this notion derives from intervention trials in which antiproteinuric therapy is associated with slowing of disease progression.

Role of Antihypertensive Therapy

Therapeutic recommendations for patients with hypertensive nephrosclerosis and patients with hypertension secondary to intrinsic renal disease is discussed elsewhere in this book. Given that hypertension hastens loss of kidney function, however, aggressive antihypertensive therapy is clearly mandatory. The older standard World Health Organization definition of hypertension (160/95 mm Hg) has been clearly shown to be too high for the kidney at risk. More current opinion, as outlined in JNC VI, places renal insufficiency in a category requiring more aggressive treatment and lower target blood pressure. That consensus statement recommends that blood pressure should be controlled to ≤130/85 mm Hg, particularly in diabetic patients with proteinuria >1 g/d and suggests that a target of 120/175 mm Hg may be even more appropriate. With regard to safety, a well-designed retrospective study of 150 patients with renal disease found no evidence of a "J" curve; cardiovascular events were decreased when diastolic blood pressures were reduced to <80 mm Hg. The importance of 24-hour blood pressure control has also not been well defined in this population. However, the absence of the usual decline in nocturnal blood pressure in such patients may suggest additional need for round-the-clock antihypertensive therapy.

Different antihypertensive drug classes differ in their ability to lower proteinuria and slow the progression of renal disease in hypertensive patients with renal disease. Of the available agents, ACE inhibitors are the most potent antiproteinuric agents. ACE inhibitors in diabetics with renal disease also prolong the time to death, dialysis, and transplantation. Thus, in hypertensive patients with diabetes and proteinuria or early renal insufficiency, the JNC-VI recommends first-line therapy with ACE inhibitors.

SUGGESTED READING

1. Helmchen U, Wenzel UO. Benign and malignant nephrosclerosis and renovascular hypertension. In: Tisher CC, Brenner BM, eds. *Renal Pathology.* 2nd ed. Philadelphia, Pa: JB Lippincott; 1994:1201–1236.

2. Joint National Committee. The sixth report of the Joint National Committee on Prevention, Detection, Evaluation, and Treatment of High Blood Pressure (JNC VI). *Arch Intern Med.* 1997;157:2413–2446.

3. Luke RG, Curtis JJ. Nephrosclerosis. In: Schrier RW, Gottschalk CW, eds. *Diseases of the Kidney.* 5th ed. Boston, Mass: Little Brown; 1993:1433–1450.

4. Mountokalakis TD. The renal consequences of arterial hypertension. *Kidney Int.* 1997;51:1639–1653.

5. Remuzzi G, Bertani T. Is glomerulosclerosis a consequence of altered glomerular permeability to macromolecules? *Kidney Int.* 1990;38:384–394.

6. Rennke HG, Anderson S, Brenner BM. Structural and functional correlations in the progression of renal disease. In: Tisher CC, Brenner BM, eds. *Renal Pathology.* 2nd ed. Philadelphia, Pa: JB Lippincott; 1994:116–142.

7. Schulman NB, Ford CE, Hall WD, et al. Prognostic value of serum creatinine and effect of treatment of hypertension on renal function: results from the Hypertension Detection and Follow-up Program. *Hypertension.* 1989;13(suppl I):I-80-I-93.

8. Silverman M, Bakris GL. Treatment of renal failure and blood pressure. *Curr Opin Nephrol Hypertens.* 1997;6:237–242.

9. Whelton PK, He J, Perneger TV, Klag MJ. Kidney damage in benign essential hypertension. *Curr Opin Nephrol Hypertens.* 1997;6:177–183.

10. Weisstuch JM, Dworkin LD. Does essential hypertension cause end-stage renal disease? *Kidney Int.* 1992;41(suppl 36):S-33-S-37.

Chapter 74

The Eye in Hypertension

Robert N. Frank, MD

KEY POINTS

- The three circulations of the posterior portion of the eye (retinal, choroidal, and optic nerve) all can be affected by hypertension.

- Diabetes and other disease processes also affect the ocular circulations, often in ways similar to hypertension.

- Clinical descriptions of ophthalmoscopic changes in hypertension are important and should include specific observations about the three ocular circulations rather than a nonspecific grade.

- Although the classic changes of hypertension in the retina, choroid, and optic nerve have become less common, hypertension may accelerate other retinal disease processes, including diabetic retinopathy, retinal vein occlusions, and neovascular age-related macular degeneration.

See also Chapters 66, 78, 146

Figures in this chapter are located on the back cover.

The retina is the only tissue in the body in which the blood vessels can be observed directly. Examination of the ocular fundi therefore provides an opportunity to observe the effects of hypertension in a unique vascular bed. In humans and other species with vascularized retinas, the rates of glucose consumption and oxygen utilization are 3-fold higher in the retina than in any other tissue in the body. The retinal circulation is therefore highly sensitive to local tissue metabolic needs and is susceptible to damage from circulatory dysfunction.

The Ocular Circulations and Hypertensive Changes

The retina and optic nerve in humans are supplied by three circulations, all of which derive from branches of the ophthalmic artery.

Retinal Circulation

The retinal circulation is composed of the central retinal artery, the central retinal vein, and their branches. The central retinal artery supplies the inner retinal layers and usually divides into four principal branches at the anterior surface of the optic nerve. Anterior to the lamina cribrosa of the optic nerve head, the retinal arteries and veins have no autonomic innervations but are controlled by autoregulation in response to local metabolic signals, in particular P_{O_2} P_{CO_2}, and intraocular pressure. Tight junctions between adjoining endothelial cells in the retinal vessels form one part of the blood-retinal barrier, which strictly governs the passage of molecules into the neural tissue of the retina. Breakdown of this barrier is an important pathological change.

Changes in the retinal blood vessels are the commonest vascular lesions of systemic hypertension in the eye. There have been a number of classifications of hypertensive retinopathy, of which the best known are those of Keith, Wagener, and Barker first proposed in 1939 and of Schele in 1953. While these classifications are undoubtedly of historic interest, they are less useful clinically than a careful description of the lesions existent in the eye.

Hypertensive retinopathy is a continuum, and certain types of lesions may be found in various combinations. Some lesions are relatively specific for hypertensive retinopathy (eg, "copper wiring" of arterioles, "arteriovenous [A-V] nicking" and related crossing changes, and arterial macroaneurysms). Other "hypertensive" lesions found in a number of disorders include the "cotton wool spots" of diabetic retinopathy, systemic lupus erythematosus, retinal vein occlusions, and AIDS. Flame-shaped intraretinal hemorrhages occur also in diabetic retinopathy, retinal vein occlusions, profound anemia, the leukemias, and other blood dyscrasias. Arterial "silver wiring" may occur in diabetic retinopathy, colllagen-vascular diseases, and arterial occlusive diseases.

Choroidal Circulation

The choroidal circulation includes the short posterior ciliary arteries and their branches in the choroid. In humans, there are two external layers of arteries and veins and an inner layer, the choriocapillaris, which lies just outside the pigment epithelium of the retina. The portion of the choriocapillary endothelium immediately adjacent to the pigment epithelium is thin and fenestrated, and small molecules and even larger proteins readily pass in and out of these vessels. However, tight junctions connecting the cells of the retinal pigment epithelium form the second part of the blood-retinal barrier, governing the ingress of nutrient molecules and the egress of waste products. The choroidal vessels have an autonomic nerve supply that can regulate choroidal blood flow, which is substantially greater than that of the retina. The choroidal circulation supplies the retinal pigment epithelium and the photoreceptor layers of the retina, which are rich in mitochondria and contain the major portion of the very active metabolism of that tissue.

Hypertensive choroidopathy occurs most frequently in younger individuals with acute, severe hypertensive episodes such as "malignant" hypertension or toxemia of pregnancy. Hypertensive changes in the choroidal vessels are observed much less frequently than hypertensive changes in the vessels of the retina. In theory, hypertensive choroidopathy occurs because the short choroidal arteries, which are most commonly affected by hypertensive changes, feed at right angles into the choroidal capillaries, allowing direct transmission of systemic blood pressure to the capillaries.

Initial changes may include focal regions of choriocapillary nonperfusion due to fibrinoid necrosis of the vessels. Clinically, this may be recognized initially only by special techniques such as intravenous fluorescein angiography. Subsequently, the retinal pigment epithelium over these nonperfused regions may develop a yellowish coloration, the "Elschnig spot," which later becomes a scar with a pigmented center and an atrophic, surrounding halo.

Optic Nerve Circulation

Anteriorly, the optic nerve circulation is composed of branches of the central retinal artery, and posteriorly of branches of the short posterior ciliary vessels and of vessels supplying the pia mater. Blood flow in these vessels is highly influenced anteriorly by the intraocular pressure and posteriorly by intracranial pressure transmitted through the subarachnoid space.

Hypertensive changes in the optic nerve are also relatively uncommon at the present time. The principal optic nerve lesion of hypertension is disc edema **(Figure 74.1)**. The cause of this lesion is unclear because, as noted earlier, the optic nerve in the orbit receives a different blood supply in its anterior and posterior portions. Some investigators believe that a combination of ischemia caused by vascular changes and increased intraocular or intracranial pressure and diminished axoplasmic flow in the optic nerve fibers causes hypertensive optic nerve swelling.

Opthalmoscopy in Hypertension
Arterial Changes

The initial visible change in the retinal vessels in hypertension is arterial and arteriolar narrowing. By convention, the central retinal artery and its four major branches are called "arteries," while smaller branches are termed "arterioles," irrespective of the actual microscopic anatomy of these vessels. However, this terminology is not used by all writers. The normal ratio of retinal artery:vein diameters is 2:3.

Changes in the retinal arterial wall in hypertension represent true arteriosclerosis, with thickening of the wall represented histopathologically by multiple internal elastic laminae and replacement of the muscle layer by collagen. Arteriosclerotic changes produce an increase in the central light reflex and a decrease in the width of the blood column seen on either side of the light reflex. As these changes progress, the normally yellowish-white light reflex becomes reddish-brown, giving rise to the term "copper wire" change. As thickening of the wall progresses, visibility of the blood column diminishes and eventually disappears, leading to the appearance of the artery as a white thread, the "silver wire" change **(Figure 74.2)**. Arterial silver wiring does not always mean that the vessel is no longer perfused, since blood flow can often be demonstrated by fluorescein angiography.

By contrast, atherosclerosis is demonstrated in the retinal vessels only when cholesterol emboli lodge in the central retinal artery or one of its branches, where they may become visible ophthalmoscopically **(Figure 74.3)**.

An additional ophthalmoscopically visible change produced in the retinal vessels by hypertension and arteriosclerosis is "A-V nicking." Ocular vessels are contained in an adventitial sheath. At those points where branch arteries cross over veins, the sheaths are essentially shared. The artery with its thickened wall and increased lumenal pressure, together with proliferation of perivascular glia, externally compresses the low-pressure, thin-walled vein. Sometimes the vein may also change direction where the artery crosses it, producing a right-angled bend. The most serious consequence of A-V nicking is actual occlusion of the vein.

Central Vein Occlusion

Central retinal vein occlusion occurs where the central retinal artery and vein come in continuity with one another within the substance of the optic nerve. It is characterized by sudden, severe loss of vision and a "blood and thunder" fundus appearance, with dilated and tortuous veins and extensive hemorrhages in all four quadrants around the nerve head **(Figure 74.4)**. Branch vein occlusion may cause vision loss if the central portion of the retina (the macula) is affected. A wedge-shaped cluster of hemorrhages, with its apex pointing at the responsible A-V crossing, is always present.

After diabetic retinopathy, retinal vein occlusion is the second most common vascular disorder of the retina. It is an important cause of visual loss. Although several causal factors may be involved, systemic hypertension is one of the most important.

Cotton Wool Spots

Reduced blood flow produced by sclerosis or fibrinoid necrosis of small retinal arterioles may lead to regions of infarction, which eventually become evident as round to oval white patches with soft borders, the so-called 'cotton wool spots,' or cytoid bodies **(Figure 74.5)**. Because these lesions are the result of infarction, not exudation, they should not be termed "soft exudates."

Aneurysms

Lesions induced by excessive transmural pressure in the retinal vascular wall in hypertensive retinopathy include capillary microaneurysms and arterial (or arteriolar) macroaneurysms. Capillary microaneurysms are fusiform or berry-shaped outpouchings of the retinal capillaries. Although they are usually considered classic lesions of diabetic retinopathy, they may also occur in hypertensive retinopathy, in retinal vein occlusions even in the absence of hypertesnion, and in the retinopathy produced by leukemias and other blood dyscrasias. Arteriolar macroaneurysms, however, are characteristic of hypertension alone. They are berry-shaped dilations of a retinal artery or arteriole **(Figure 74.6)**, which may be surrounded by hemorrhage or retinal edema with a circumferential ring of lipid exudate. Although macroaneurysms are dramatic in appearance, they are usually benign in behavior, since they often thrombose spontaneously. Evidence of hemorrhage or substantial retinal edema may be indications for laser photocoagulation.

Flame Hemorrhages

Hypertensive retinopathy may also lead to a breakdown in the blood-retinal barrier, as demonstrated by intraretinal hemorrhages that are often flame shaped. In the retinopathy of malignant hypertension, there is profound leakage of plasma from the capillaries within the macula. This condition may lead to loss of vision from the resultant macular edema and to the precipitation of lipid exudate in the form of radial deposits, the so-called "macular star figure" surrounding the fovea at the center of the macula.

Clinical Significance

The ocular lesions of systemic hypertension convey important information about the duration and severity of the hypertensive state and the efficacy of treatment. Because several of these lesions may have adverse consequences, the clinician should carefully examine the ocular fundi of all hypertensive patients as a regular part of the initial examination and of periodic follow-up visits. Individuals with suspicious regions of the fundus or those with acute, severe hypertensive episodes or with accelerated or malignant disease merit consultation with an ophthalmologist.

Systemic Hypertension and Other Retinal and Choroidal Diseases

Classic hypertensive retinopathy in its malignant stages has become less frequent due to more effective treatment of systemic hypertension. Systemic hypertension, however, is now recognized as contributory to several other vision-threatening ocular disorders. In addition to retinal vein occlusion, diabetic retinopathy progresses more rapidly in individuals whose blood pressures are not controlled. The Macular Photocoagulation Study, a national randomized, controlled clinical trial of laser photocoagulation for the neovascular form of age-related macular degeneration, showed better outcomes in normotensive patients than in hypertensives.

SUGGESTED READING

1. Frank RN. Vascular disease of retina. In: Tso MOM, ed. *Retinal Diseases.* Philadelphia, Pa: JB Lippincott; 1987:138–164.
2. Keith NM, Wagener HP, Barker NW. Some different types of essential hypertension: their course and prognosis. *Am J Med Sci.* 1974;268:336–345.
3. Knowler WC, Bennett PH, Ballintine EJ. Increased incidence of retinopathy in diabetics with elevated blood pressure: a six-year follow-up study in Pima Indians. *N Engl J Med.* 1980;302:645–650.
4. Macular Photocoagulation Study Group. Laser photocoagulation for juxtafoveal choroidal neovascularization: five-year results from randomized clinical trials. *Arch Ophthalmol.* 1994;112:500–509.
5. Rath EZ, Frank RN, Shin DH, Kim C. Risk factors for retinal vein occlusions: a case-control study. *Ophthalmology.* 1992;99:509–514.
6. Scheie HG. Evaluation of ophthalmoscopic changes of hypertension and arteriolar sclerosis. *Arch Ophthalmol.* 1953;49:117–138.
7. The Eye Disease Case-Control Study Group. Risk factors for branch retinal vein occlusion. *Am J Ophthalmol.* 1993;116:286–296.
8. The Eye Disease Case-Control Study Group. Risk factors for central retinal vein occlusion. *Arch Ophthalmol.* 1996;114:545–554.
9. Tso MOM, Jampol LM. Pathophysiology of hypertensive retinopathy. *Ophthalmology.* 1982;89:1132–1145.
10. Wagener HP, Clay GE, Gipner JF. Classification of retinal lesions in presence of vascular hypertension: report submitted by committee. *Trans Am Ophthalmol Soc.* 1947;45:57–75.

Part B

POPULATION SCIENCE

Section Editors: *Jeffrey A. Cutler, MD*
Theodore A. Kotchen, MD

Cardiovascular Risk and Hypertension
Impact of Hypertension: Globally and Special Populations
Lifestyle Factors and Blood Pressure
Prevention and Control

Dr. Cutler's chapters in this section were edited by Dr. Jeffrey A. Cutler in his private capacity. No official support or endorsement by the NIH is intended and none should be inferred.

Chapter 75

Cardiovascular Risk Factors and Hypertension

William B. Kannel, MD; Peter W.F. Wilson, MD

KEY POINTS

- Hypertension generally doubles the risk of cardiovascular diseases.

- Systolic and diastolic pressure levels are associated with atherosclerotic events in a continuous, graded fashion.

- Elevated systolic pressure levels are highly associated with atherosclerotic disease even in the presence of normal diastolic pressure.

- Hypertension is usually accompanied by other risk factors and seldom occurs in isolation.

See also Chapters 76, 77, 82, 83, 97, 98

Hypertension is a well-established risk factor for the development of all of the clinical manifestations of atherosclerosis. Elevated blood pressure is a common and powerful predisposing factor for the development of coronary disease, strokes, peripheral artery disease, and heart failure. The high prevalence of this condition, its powerful impact on the incidence of cardiovascular disease, and its controllability justify giving it a high priority for detection and treatment by physicians and health officials. Hypertension may directly induce encephalopathy and renal insufficiency, whereas the accelerated atherogenesis it induces is a more complex process that is greatly influenced by other coexistent atherogenic traits.

Atherosclerotic Hazards

Atherosclerotic sequelae imposed by hypertension occur at a 2-fold to 3-fold increased rate compared with normotensive persons of the same age. The risk ratio imposed is greatest for heart failure and least for coronary disease, but coronary disease is the most common hazard of hypertension because of its greater incidence in the general population (**Table 75.1**). The lower-than-expected efficacy of antihypertensive therapy for the prevention of coronary disease in trials has led to unjustified doubt about the etiologic role of hypertension in the development of coronary disease. However, the risk of development of all clinical manifestations of coronary disease has been shown to be related to the severity of antecedent hypertension in the Framingham Study and elsewhere. Blood pressure appears to be critical to the atherosclerotic process because atherosclerosis seldom occurs in low-pressure segments of the circulation, such as the pulmonary arteries or veins, unless disease induces a raised blood pressure in these segments of the circulation. Also, animal experiments have shown that lipid-induced atherogenesis can be accelerated or retarded by manipulating the blood pressure. Elevated blood pressure has been found to be related to the development of cardiovascular disease in a continuous, graded fashion, with no indication of a critical value. The risk of cardiovascular sequelae increases with each increment in blood pressure, even within the high-normal range (**Figure 75.1**). Mild hypertension is a significant contributor to atherosclerotic cardiovascular disease, and because it is so much more prevalent than severe grades of hypertension, a large proportion of the cardiovascular disease attributable to hypertension derives from this apparently innocuous mild hypertension.

Blood Pressure Components

Comparison of the impacts of the systolic and diastolic blood pressure components gives no indication of a greater influence of the diastolic pressure for any sequela of hypertension, and isolated systolic hypertension has been shown to be distinctly hazardous at all

Table 75.1. Risk of Cardiovascular Events in Subjects With Hypertension: 36-Year Follow-up in Framingham Heart Study Participants 35 to 64 Years Old

CARDIOVASCULAR EVENTS	AGE-ADJUSTED BIENNIAL RATE PER 1000		AGE-ADJUSTED RISK RATIO		EXCESS RISK PER 1000	
	MEN	WOMEN	MEN	WOMEN	MEN	WOMEN
Coronary heart disease	45	21	2.0*	2.2*	23	12
Stroke	12	6	3.8*	2.6*	9	4
Peripheral arterial disease	10	7	2.0*	3.7*	5	
Cardiac failure	14	6	4.0*	3.0*	10	4
Cardiovascular events	65	35	2.2*	2.5*	36	21

*P<0.001.

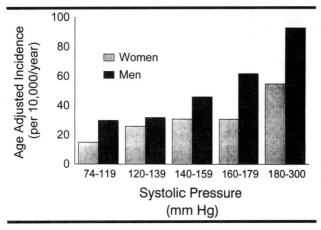

Figure 75.1. Risk of cardiovascular events by level of systolic blood pressure: 38-year follow-up for Framingham subjects 65 to 94 years old.

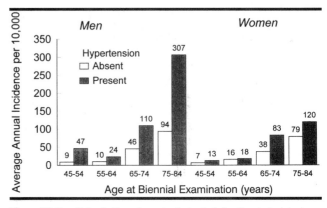

Figure 75.2. Risk of atherothrombotic brain infarction in isolated systolic hypertension: experience of Framingham men and women 45 to 84 years old over 24 years of follow-up. Adapted from Kannel WB. *J Cardiovasc Pharmacol.* 1993;21:527.

ages, including in the elderly **(Figure 75.2)**. Systolic hypertension has been shown to be a persistent risk factor even when arterial compliance has been taken into account, and treatment of this variety of hypertension has been shown to greatly reduce the risk of cardiovascular disease. Overreliance on diastolic pressure to assess hypertensive risk can be misleading, particularly in advanced age, when the predominant type of hypertension is of the isolated systolic variety.

Risk Factor Clustering

Hypertension seldom occurs in isolation from other atherogenic risk factors. It tends to occur in association with other atherogenic risk factors that both promote its occurrence and greatly influence its impact on cardiovascular disease. It appears to be metabolically linked to dyslipidemia, glucose intolerance, abdominal obesity, hyperinsulinemia, and hyperuricemia, among others. Clustering of these risk factors with hypertension was investigated in the Framingham Study, and hypertension was found to occur in isolation only ≈20% of the time. Clusters of two or three of these risk factors with hypertension was found to occur ≈50% of the time, a rate twice that expected by chance **(Table 75.2)**. Approximately 63% of the cases of coronary disease that occurred in hypertensive Framingham Study men had two or more additional risk factors. It is evident from these data that in evaluating a patient with an elevated blood pressure, it is imperative that the presence of the other atherogenic risk factors be anticipated and tested for. This is an important consideration, because the risk of cardiovascular sequelae in general and of coronary disease in particular varies widely, depending on the burden of the associated risk factors **(Figure 75.3)**. The risk of coronary events in the Framingham Study participants increased with the degree of risk factor clustering with hypertension, so that 39% of the coronary events in men with elevated blood pressure were attributable to having two or more additional risk factors. This is particularly important in those with mild hypertension, in whom the average risk is modest, and many would have to be treated to prevent one cardiovascular event.

The same cluster of atherogenic risk factors that often accompanies hypertension also influences the hazard of developing a stroke, peripheral artery disease, or heart failure. For stroke, atrial fibrillation, coronary disease, and left ventricular hypertrophy also play an important role. For heart failure, coronary disease, heart murmurs,

Table 75.2. Number of Other Risk Factors: Framingham Heart Study Offspring With Elevated Blood Pressure 18 to 65 Years Old

NUMBER OF RISK FACTORS	PERCENT WITH SPECIFIED NUMBER OF RISK FACTORS		OBSERVED/EXPECTED RATIO	
	MEN	WOMEN	MEN	WOMEN
0	24.4%	19.5%	0.74	0.59
1	29.1%	28.1%	0.71	0.69
≥2	46.5%	52.4%	1.8	2.01

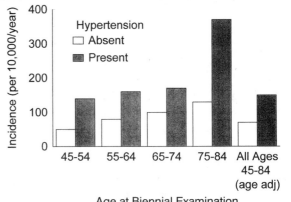

Figure 75.3. Risk of myocardial infarction in isolated systolic hypertension: experience of Framingham men and women 45 to 84 years old over 24 years of follow-up. Adapted from Kannel WB. *J Cardiovasc Pharmacol.* 1993;21:527.

cardiomegaly, a low vital capacity, and a rapid heart rate are the additional features of the risk profile.

A rapid resting heart rate is more common in persons with hypertension and also predisposes to its occurrence. Hypertension associated with a rapid resting heart rate has been found to be associated with a higher mortality rate from cardiovascular disease in general and from coronary disease in particular. A rapid resting heart

Table 75.3. Risk Factor Clustering in the Framingham Study Offspring With Elevated Blood Pressure According to the Body Mass Index: Subjects 18 to 74 Years Old

MEN		WOMEN	
BODY MASS INDEX, KG/M²	**AVERAGE NO. OF RISK FACTORS**	**BODY MASS INDEX, KG/M²**	**AVERAGE NO. OF RISK FACTORS**
<23.7	1.68±0.91	<20.8	1.80±0.87
23.7–25.5	1.85±0.95	20.8–22.3	2.00±1.02
25.6–27.2	2.06±1.05	22.4–23.9	2.22±1.06
27.3–29.5	2.28±1.09	24.0–26.8	2.20±0.99
≥29.5	2.35±1.08	≥26.8	2.66±1.09

Elevated blood pressure was defined as systolic pressure ≥138 mm Hg (men) and ≥130 mm Hg (women). Other risk factors included the top quintiles for the factors total cholesterol, body mass index, triglycerides, and glucose and bottom quintile for HDL cholesterol.

rate, low vital capacity, proteinuria, left ventricular hypertrophy, and silent myocardial infarction often signify organ damage in hypertensive persons and escalate hypertensive risk of overt cardiovascular sequelae 2-fold to 3-fold.

Determinants of Clustering

Postulated determinants of metabolic clustering of hypertension with dyslipidemia (elevated triglyceride and reduced HDL cholesterol), glucose intolerance, obesity, left ventricular hypertrophy, and hyperuricemia include insulin resistance and autonomic imbalance. Some consider that essential hypertension is predominantly an insulin-resistant disorder composed of these atherogenic abnormalities plus hyperinsulinemia. Abdominal obesity appears to be a promoter of this syndrome both in hypertension and in general. The tendency for these atherogenic traits to cluster with elevated blood pressure was found in the Framingham Study to increase stepwise with the degree of obesity at baseline and the amount of weight gained on follow-up (**Table 75.3**). A 5-lb weight increase was associated with a 30% increment in the extent of clustering of atherogenic risk factors in persons with hypertension.

Global Cardiovascular Risk

The impact of hypertension (without regard to hypertensive medication) status on coronary heart disease (CHD), atherothrombotic brain infarction, intermittent claudication, heart failure, and all cardiovascular disease in Framingham participants 35 to 64 and 65 to 94 years old is shown for men (**Figure 75.4**). In all instances, definite hypertension (blood pressure ≥160/95 mm Hg) is associated with greater risk of vascular disease compared with persons with normal blood pressure (blood pressure <140/90 mm Hg).

Blood Pressure, Other Factors, and Coronary Risk

Arterial pressure should not be considered alone, because an individual's age, sex, blood cholesterol, cigarette smoking, and diabetes also contribute to increased CHD risk (**Figure 75.5**). In both men and women, CHD risk rises according to the presence of other risk factors. Figure 5 shows the risks for hypothetical 55-year-old Framingham men and women with various combinations of cardiovascular risk factors. Individuals with multiple risk factors typically experience the highest rates of CHD. As shown in Figure 4, an individual

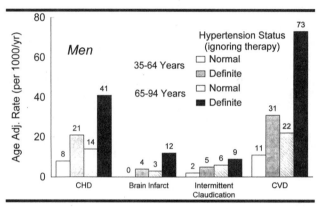

Figure 75.4. Age-adjusted annual rate of coronary heart disease (CHD) according to hypertension status in Framingham cohort men followed up for 30 years, with examinations and reclassification of blood pressure every 2 years. CHD indicates coronary heart disease; CVD, cardiovascular disease.

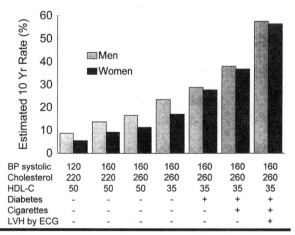

Figure 75.5. Estimated 10-year coronary heart disease risk in hypothetical 55-year-old adult according to levels of various factors. BP indicates blood pressure; HDL-C, HDL cholesterol; and LVH, left ventricular hypertrophy.

with diabetes who smokes cigarettes and has left ventricular hypertrophy in the presence of systolic pressure of 160 mm Hg and low HDL cholesterol has an estimated 10-year risk of CHD that exceeds 55% for both sexes. Predicted CHD rates for men are typically greater than those for women by 1.3 to 1.5 times when only a few risk factors are present. Conversely, the male-to-female difference is small when risk factor levels are high and diabetes, smoking, and left ventricular hypertrophy by ECG are all present in an individual.

Preventive Implications

Optimal cardiovascular protection in hypertension requires more than simply lowering the blood pressure. The potential for development of cardiovascular disease in general and coronary disease in particular and the best choices for therapy are revealed by determining the multivariate risk of the hypertension, taking into account the associated risk factors. This can be conveniently done for estimating the risk of strokes and coronary disease by use of risk factor scoring profiles based on Framingham Study data. Only ordinary office procedures and simple laboratory tests are required for this multivariate assessment.

In this way, hypertensive persons can be more effectively targeted for treatment and more optimal therapeutic choices can be made to maximize the benefit and cost-effectiveness of therapy. The antihypertensive therapy should be tailored to take into account the often associated dyslipidemia, glucose intolerance, and any associated cardiovascular condition as well as the severity and character of the blood pressure elevation.

SUGGESTED READING

1. Anastos K, Charney P, Charon RA, Cohen E, Jones CY, Marte C, Swiderski DM, Wheat ME, Williams S. Hypertension in women: what is really known? *Ann Intern Med.* 1991;115:287–293.
2. Anderson KM, Wilson PWF, Odell PM, Kannel WB. An updated coronary risk profile: a statement for health professionals. *Circulation.* 1991;83:356–362.
3. Dustan HP. Role of nutrition in hypertension and its control: experimental aspects. *Prog Biochem Pharmacol.* 1983;19:177–191.
4. Gillman MW, Kannel WB, Belanger A, D'Agostino RB. Influence of heart rate on mortality among persons with hypertension: the Framingham Study. *Am Heart J.* 1993;125:1148–1154.
5. Gillum RF. Cardiovascular disease in the United States: an epidemiologic overview. In: Saunders E, ed. *Cardiovascular Diseases in Blacks.* Philadelphia, Pa: FA Davis; 1991:1–16.
6. Kannel WB, Gordon T, Schwartz MJ. Systolic versus diastolic blood pressure and risk of coronary heart disease: the Framingham Study. *Am J Cardiol.* 1971;27:335–346.
7. Kannel WB, Wolf PA, McGee DL, Dawber TR, McNamara P, Castelli WP. Systolic blood pressure, arterial rigidity, and risk of stroke: the Framingham study. *JAMA.* 1981;245:1225–1229.
8. Kannel WB. Blood pressure as a cardiovascular risk factor: prevention and treatment. *JAMA.* 1996;275:1571–1576.
9. Reaven GM. Insulin resistance and compensatory hyperinsulinemia: role in hypertension, dyslipidemia, and coronary heart disease. *Am Heart J.* 1991;121:1283–1288.
10. Systolic Hypertension in the Elderly Program Cooperative Research Group. Prevention of stroke by antihypertensive drug treatment in older persons with isolated systolic hypertension: final results of the Systolic Hypertension in the Elderly Program (SHEP). *JAMA.* 1991;265:3255–3264.
11. Wolf PA, D'Agostino RB, Belanger AJ, Kannel WB. Probability of stroke: a risk profile from the Framingham Study. *Stroke.* 1991;22:312–318.

Chapter 76

Cerebrovascular Risk

Philip A. Wolf, MD

KEY POINTS

- Hypertension is the premier risk factor for stroke (both cerebral infarction and hemorrhage).

- The incidence of stroke increases in proportion to increases in blood pressure.

- The incidence of stroke in the elderly is more clearly related to the level of systolic than diastolic blood pressure.

- Treatment of hypertension reduces stroke incidence and may be the basis for the remarkable reduction in US stroke mortality rates.

See also Chapters 70, 72, 75, 77, 108, 137

Death and disability from cardiovascular disease increase steadily with age. Above the age of 65 years, cardiovascular disease accounts for nearly 50% of all deaths. Fully 20% of all cardiovascular disease deaths in the elderly are attributable to stroke. Although cerebrovascular disease is the third-leading cause of death in the United States, stroke is 4 times more likely to produce disability than death and is the leading cause of neurological disability in the elderly. The American Heart Association estimated that in 1995, 500 000 Americans sustained an initial stroke, and 158 061 of them died of it, corresponding to 1 death every 3.4 minutes. However, death statistics fail to communicate the toll in human suffering experienced by stroke survivors and their families, whose lives are irrevocably altered by this neurological catastrophe. There are currently ≈3 890 000 stroke survivors in the United States, many of whom require chronic care.

Stroke is not limited, however, to the elderly; nearly 20% occur in persons <60 years old. Among those <65 years old who are employed at the time of stroke, one third will never work again. To the functionally independent individual, stroke represents a condition that many consider worse than death itself. To them, the attendant loss of function and independence signals the end of worthwhile life.

Etiology of Stroke

Unlike coronary heart disease, in which atherosclerosis of the arteries supplying the myocardium is the underlying disease process, stroke is a heterogeneous condition. Approximately 85% of strokes are due to cerebral infarction, a consequence of interruption of the blood supply to the brain. The remainder are due to hemorrhage, half from intracerebral hemorrhage and half from subarachnoid hemorrhage. Hemorrhage is easy to distinguish from infarction by CT scan of the brain, whereas it is often more difficult to determine the mechanism of infarction. With the exception of embolism from a cardiac source, most brain infarctions result from thrombotic occlusion of large and small arteries in the intracranial and extracranial circulation. Hypertension is the most common and potent risk factor for ischemic stroke, and reduction of elevated blood pressure clearly prevents stroke regardless of infarct subtype.

Incidence of Stroke

In the general population sample at Framingham, Mass, after 40 years of follow-up, stroke occurred in 718 persons, 312 in men and 406 in women. Incidence increased with age, approximately doubling in each successive decade above age 55 years **(Table 76.1)**. Because the most common type, atherothrombotic brain infarction (ABI), may be considered to be analogous to myocardial infarction (MI), it is informative to compare the incidence, by age and sex, of these two manifestations of cardiovascular disease **(Figure 76.1)**. Although both increase with age, approximately doubling in successive decades, there are clear differences. Below the age of 65 years, MI has a striking male predominance; the male-to-female ratio is 4:1. The incidence of MI in women lags 20 years behind that of men; the rate of MI in women 65 to 74 years old approximates that of men 45 to 54 years old. Although ABI incidence is ≈30% higher in men, the ratio is relatively constant across the adult age span, with no striking male predominance at younger ages.

Among stroke subtypes, the most prevalent was ABI resulting from atherosclerosis and thrombosis without a cardiac source for embolism, accounting for 60.9% of cases **(Table 76.2)**. ABI includes infarction

Table 76.1. Annual Incidence of Completed Strokes in Men and Women Ages 35 to 94 years

AGE, Y	MEN		WOMEN	
	NO.	RATE/1000	NO	RATE/1000
35–44	3	0.40	4	0.44
45–54	26	1.79	18	0.99
55–64	64	3.50	62	2.60
65–74	122	8.43	129	6.12
75–84	90	16.17	137	13.46
85–94	7	. . .	56	24.34
Total	312	6.03*	406	4.53*

Data are from the Framingham Study: 40-year follow up.
* Age adjusted, 45–84 years.

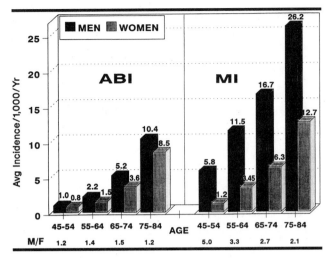

Figure 76.1. Incidence of ABI and MI, 40-year follow-up, the Framingham Study.

Table 76.2. Frequency of Completed Stroke by Type in Men and Women 35–94 Years Old

COMPLETED STROKE	MEN	WOMEN	TOTAL	%
Atherothrombotic brain infarction	194	243	437	60.9
Cerebral embolus	69	101	170	23.7
Intracerebral hemorrhage	25	28	53	6.7
Subarachnoid hemorrhage	20	28	48	7.3
Other	4	6	10	1.4
Total	312	406	718	100.0

Data are from the Framingham Study: 40-year follow up.

resulting from large-vessel atherothrombosis, lacunar infarction, and infarct of undetermined cause. Stroke from cerebral embolus occurred in 23.7%, chiefly from a left atrial clot in the presence of atrial fibrillation and from left ventricular thrombus after acute MI.

Hypertension and the Risk of Stroke

Among stroke risk factors, hypertension is clearly preeminent and is of importance for all stroke types, infarction as well as hemorrhage. The incidence of ABI, the most frequent stroke subtype, was ≈3 times greater in persons with stage 2 or 3 hypertension (≥160 and ≥180 mm Hg systolic, respectively) and 50% higher in stage 1 hypertension (140 to 159 mm Hg systolic) than in persons with high-normal blood pressure and normotensives (<140 mm Hg systolic; **(Figure 76.2)**. This was true in both sexes and in all age categories, including 75 to 84 years of age. There was no evidence that women tolerated hypertension better than men did or that hypertension was unimportant in the elderly. Hypertension made a powerful and significant independent contribution to incidence of ABI even after age and other pertinent risk factors had been taken into account.

Systolic Versus Diastolic Pressure Level

Although hypertension increases the incidence of stroke and ABI, the level of risk is clearly related to the level of blood pressure. Traditionally, greater importance has been ascribed to the diastolic than the systolic pressure level, and although most clinical trials of hyperten-

sion treatment have classified subjects by the diastolic level, evidence for the ascendancy of diastolic blood pressure over systolic is lacking. The opposite is probably true. With advancing age, systolic blood pressure continues to rise into the 70s, whereas diastolic pressures decline after reaching a plateau in the early 50s. Systolic pressure level is clearly directly related to risk of stroke, particularly after age 65 years.

Isolated Systolic Hypertension

In the elderly, stages 2 and 3 isolated systolic hypertension, ≥160/<90 mm Hg, becomes highly prevalent, affecting ≈25% of persons >80 years old. Although common, it is not innocuous. Elderly subjects in Framingham with isolated systolic hypertension, 65 to 84 years of age, have an ≈2-fold increased risk of stroke in men and 1.5-fold increased risk in women. Because isolated systolic hypertension is a consequence of reduced elasticity of the great arteries, it had been suggested that the arterial rigidity per se, rather than the systolic blood pressure, was responsible for the increased stroke rate. However, data from Framingham showed that the risk of stroke was increased in persons with isolated systolic hypertension even after the arterial rigidity was taken into account, and incidence of stroke rose in direct relation to the level of systolic pressure. Furthermore, in two large clinical trials, reduction of increased systolic blood pressure levels was followed by a 40% to 50% reduction in stroke incidence rates.

Treatment Trials in Hypertension

Multiple clinical trials have shown that reduction of elevated blood pressure in hypertensives in middle and advanced age with systolic as well as diastolic hypertension incontrovertibly reduces stroke incidence. Beginning in 1967, stroke and other hypertensive outcomes were clearly reduced by drug treatment of patients with very elevated levels of blood pressure (stages 2 and 3). Since then, a host of clinical trials have consistently demonstrated that stroke can be prevented in those with stage 1 hypertension, regardless of age.

Isolated systolic blood pressure elevations were not as resistant to antihypertensive medications as had been previously thought. Treatment did not precipitate stroke, as had been feared, but rather significantly prevented stroke. Nor did antihypertensive therapy result in

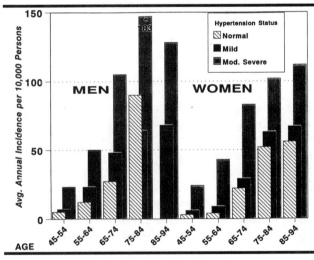

Figure 76.2. Incidence of ABI and hypertensive status, 40-year follow-up, the Framingham Study.

syncope, confusion, falls, or depression. The Systolic Hypertension in the Elderly Program (SHEP) was a randomized trial comparing stroke incidence between elderly persons whose systolic blood pressure levels were treated with a diuretic-based stepped-care regimen and those receiving a placebo. The SHEP trial proved that treatment was safe and feasible and significantly reduced stroke incidence. Of particular interest, subjects in the treatment group of the SHEP trial had lower rates of stroke of all types, of brain infarction, and of both intracerebral and subarachnoid hemorrhage. A second randomized trial, the Systolic Hypertension in Europe Trial (Syst-Eur), in persons ≥60 years old, found a 42% decrease (95% CI, −60 to −17) in stroke incidence after a median of 2 years of follow-up. Nitrendipine, a dihydropyridine calcium channel blocker, was the principal antihypertensive drug used and was quite effective in stroke prevention, with no apparent increase in cardiac end points.

Optimal Blood Pressure

The optimal level to which elevated blood pressure should be reduced for stroke prevention remains undefined, but it is clearly lower than had previously been thought. Fears that overzealous blood pressure reduction would reduce cerebral blood flow in persons with cerebral atherosclerosis and precipitate stroke have not been borne out. Analysis of a large number of clinical trials suggests that systolic pressure should be reduced to <125 mm Hg and diastolic pressure

to <85 mm Hg (**Figure 76.3**). However, this issue of target blood pressure levels has yet to be definitively resolved and is still under study. Because the bulk of the population has blood pressure levels in the high normal and stage 1 ranges, the major effort in stroke prevention must be focused here (**Figure 76.4**).

Secular Trends in Stroke Incidence and Mortality

Since 1972, stroke death rates in the United States have fallen by ≈60% and rates of death from CHD by 46%, whereas noncardiovascular death rates have remained unchanged. Similar improvement in stroke and CHD mortality has occurred in other industrialized nations. The acceleration of a 1% annual decline in stroke death rates from 1915 to 1965, to 5% per year since then, strongly highlights the role of modifiable environmental factors in stroke mortality. Stroke death rates have declined as part of the decrease in total death rates and in deaths from cardiovascular disease.

In some populations, the incidence of stroke has declined, with hemorrhage incidence declining more strikingly than that of cerebral infarctions. In other studies, no decline in incidence has occurred, although most found a decrease in stroke severity. Unfortunately, the age-adjusted death rate for stroke reached a nadir in 1992–1993 and is now rising for the first time since 1915 (**Figure 76.5**). With a growing number of elderly people, it is likely that the

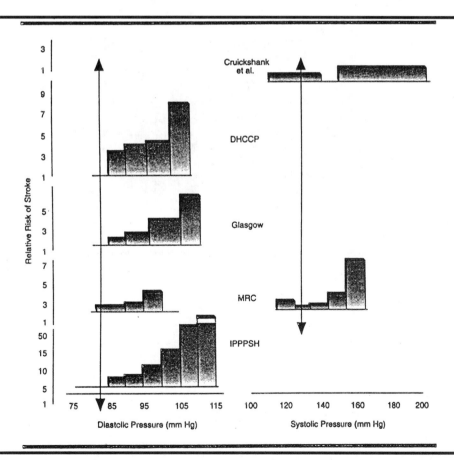

Figure 76.3. Relative risks of stroke according to blood pressure during treatment for hypertension in 8 studies and meta-analyses. Arrows indicate levels of treated systolic and diastolic blood pressure associated with lowest risks of stroke. Reprinted with permission from Fletcher and Bulpitt, copyright 1992 Massachusetts Medical Society. All rights reserved.

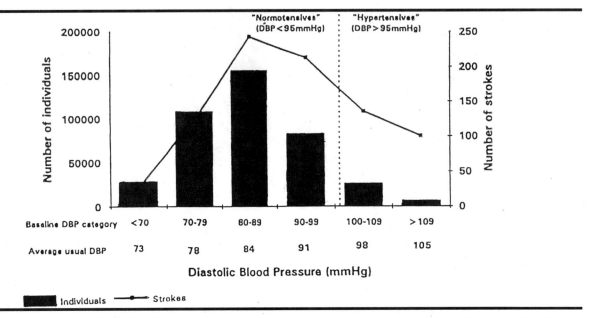

Figure 76.4. Absolute numbers of individuals and numbers of strokes in 7 prospective observational studies, subdivided by baseline diastolic blood pressure category (405 000 individuals and 843 strokes total). Approximately 80% of all strokes occurred among the 95% of individuals classified as "normotensive" (usual DBP <95 mm Hg).

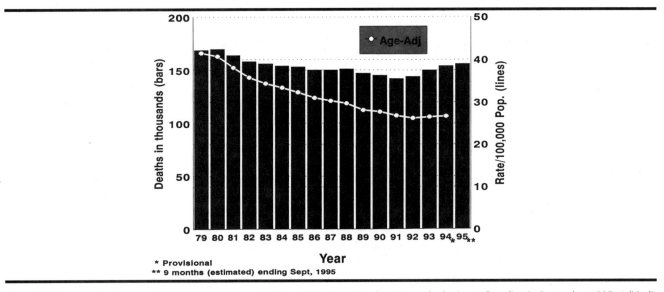

Figure 76.5. Mortality from stroke in the United States, 1979 to 1995. *Provisional; **9 months (estimated) ending in September 1995. Adj indicates adjusted; Pop., population. Data from Vital Statistics of United States, National Center for Health Statistics.

number of persons who will die of or be disabled by stroke will increase during the next century.

Preventive Implications

The demonstration of the benefits of treatment and control of hypertension in stroke prevention in the elderly with diastolic and with isolated systolic hypertension suggests that considerable progress remains to be achieved. It has been estimated that of the 50 million hypertensives in the United States, only 32.5 million were aware of their condition and 24.5 million were being treated. Unfortunately, only

10.5 million of the hypertensives had their blood pressure controlled, leaving nearly 40 million either unaware, untreated, or treated but uncontrolled. Because clinical trial data suggest an ≈40% reduction in stroke incidence even with trials lasting <5 years, a great deal of stroke prevention could be achieved by better control of hypertension. It has been estimated that nearly 250 000 new strokes could be prevented each year by such efforts. In light of the end of the decline in stroke mortality, it is imperative that such preventive efforts be redoubled. Effective programs to detect, treat, and control hypertension, particularly in those at greatest risk of stroke, those >65 years old, hold promise that stroke incidence and mortality may be reduced still further. When these measures are combined with a long-term sustained program of risk factor modification, the tools for achieving further substantial reduction in death and disability from stroke are already available.

SUGGESTED READING

1. Amery A, Birkenhäger W, Brixko P, Bulpitt C, Clement D, Deruyttere M, De Schaepdryver A, Dollery C, Fagard R, Forette F, et al. Mortality and morbidity results from the European Working Party on High Blood Pressure in the Elderly trial. *Lancet.* 1985;1:1349–1354.
2. Dahlof B, Lindholm LH, Hansson L, Schersten B, Ekbom T, Wester P-O. Morbidity and mortality in the Swedish Trial in Old Patients with Hypertension (STOP-Hypertension). *Lancet.* 1991;338:1281–1285.
3. Fletcher AE, Bulpitt CJ. How far should blood pressure be lowered? *N Engl J Med.* 1992;326:251–254.
4. Garraway WM, Whisnant JP. The changing pattern of hypertension and the declining incidence of stroke. *JAMA.* 1987;258:214–217.
5. Howard G, Toole JF, Becker C, Lefkowitz DS, Truscott BL, Rose L, Evans GW. Changes in survival following stroke in five North Carolina counties observed during two different periods. *Stroke.* 1989;20:345–350.
6. MacMahon S, Rodgers A. The epidemiological association between blood pressure and stroke: implications for primary and secondary prevention. *Hypertens Res.* 1994;17(suppl I):S23–S32.
7. SHEP Cooperative Research Group. Prevention of stroke by antihypertensive drug treatment in older persons with isolated systolic hypertension: final results of the Systolic Hypertension in the Elderly Program (SHEP). *JAMA.* 1991;265:3255–3264.
8. Staessen JA, Fagard R, Thijs L, Celis H, Araabidze GG, Birkenhager WH, Bulpitt CJ, de Leeuw PW, Dollery CT, Fletcher AE, Forette F, Leonetti G, Nachev C, O'Brien ET, Rosenfeld J, Rodicio JL, Tuomilehto J, Zanchetti A, for the Systolic Hypertension in Europe (Syst-Eur) Trial Investigators. Randomised double-blind comparison of placebo and active treatment for older patients with isolated systolic hypertension. *Lancet.* 1997;350:757–764.
9. Wolf PA, D'Agostino RB, O'Neal MA, Sytkowski P, Kase CS, Belanger AJ, Kannel WB. Secular trends in stroke incidence and mortality: the Framingham study. *Stroke.* 1992;23:1551–1555.

Chapter 77

Left Ventricular Hypertrophy Prognosis

Daniel Levy, MD

KEY POINTS

- Left ventricular hypertrophy on the electrocardiogram or the echocardiogram is associated with increased risk for cardiovascular disease events.

- Aggressive hypertension treatment can promote reversal of left ventricular hypertrophy.

- Observational studies have suggested that reversal of left ventricular hypertrophy confers a reduction in risk for cardiovascular disease events.

- Clinical trials are needed to determine whether some drugs are better than others in reversing left ventricular hypertrophy and whether reversal leads to a reduction in cardiovascular disease risk.

See also Chapters 68, 139, 140

Left Ventricular Hypertrophy on the Electrocardiogram

The first studies to document the cardiovascular disease (CVD) hazards associated with left ventricular hypertrophy (LVH) were based on its electrocardiographic (ECG) detection. The ECG hallmarks of LVH are increased R-wave and S-wave voltage, reflecting left ventricular forces; a widened QRS complex; a leftward frontal plane axis shift; ST- and T-wave repolarization abnormalities; and P-wave abnormalities reflecting left atrial enlargement. Several reports from the Framingham Heart Study and elsewhere found that individuals with ECG LVH were at increased risk for coronary heart disease, stroke, congestive heart failure, and sudden death. The CVD risks associated with LVH are greatest when increased QRS voltage is accompanied by repolarization abnormalities.

Nearly 30 years ago, investigators reported that among more than 5000 original participants in the Framingham Heart Study, the development of LVH on the ECG (increased voltage with accompanying major repolarization abnormalities) carried a relative risk for developing coronary heart disease (CHD) of 2.2 to 5.1 in men and 1.4 to 2.5 in women. A more recent investigation from Framingham examined the separate contributions of increased voltage and repolarization abnormalities to CVD risk in those with ECG LVH. That study was based on follow-up of 524 subjects who exhibited ECG LVH during nearly 40 years of observation. Among persons free of CVD at baseline, the relative risk for developing CVD, comparing subjects in the top quartile of ECG voltage (sum of R wave in aVL plus S wave in V_3) with those in the bottom quartile, was 3.08 (95% confidence interval [CI], 1.87 to 5.07) in men and 3.29 (95% CI, 1.78 to 6.09) in women. The presence of major repolarization abnormalities also identified individuals with LVH who were at increased risk for CVD. The **Table 77.1** summarizes the incidence rates for a variety of CVD outcomes as a function of ECG LVH status for men and women in two age groups. For all end points, the risks were substantially higher in those with ECG LVH than in those without it.

LVH on the Echocardiogram
Risks of LVH in the General Population

The advent of echocardiography has provided a new and more sensitive tool for the detection of LVH. Whereas ECG LVH was present in only about 2% of subjects from the Framingham Heart Study, echocardiographic LVH was detected in approximately 15%. The echocardiographic diagnosis of LVH is based on the presence of increased left ventricular mass (LVM). LVH considered as a dichotomous variable (ie, LVH versus no LVH) and LVM examined as a continuous variable are both associated with increased risk for CHD, CVD, stroke, and sudden death.

In a large sample of 3220 subjects $\geq$40 years old from the Framingham Heart Study, 208 subjects developed new CVD events, and 124 died during 4 years of follow-up. As shown in **Figure 77.1**, LVM predicted the incidence of CVD, and the association was continuous and graded. In multivariable models adjusting for age and traditional CVD risk factors (blood pressure, antihypertensive treatment, lipids, diabetes, cigarette smoking, body mass index, and ECG LVH), in men a 50-g/m increment in LVM was associated with a relative risk of 1.49 (95% CI, 1.20 to 1.85) for CVD events. The corresponding relative risk in women was 1.57 (95% CI, 1.20 to 2.04). Increased levels of LVM were also associated with increased risk for CVD death and death from all causes. In a subsequent report from Framingham, an association of LVM with risk for stroke or transient ischemic attack was observed. This finding suggests that the target organ damage identified by echocardiography may be reflective of parallel damage throughout the cardiovascular system.

Risks of LVH in Hypertension

The association of echocardiographic LVH with increased risk for CVD has also been observed in studies of hypertensive patients. Researchers at Cornell Medical Center reported an association of echocardiographic LVH with CVD risk in 140 men with uncompli-

Table 77.1. Two-Year Rates of CVD Events per 1000 Subjects Free of Designated Event at Baseline

| | AGE-ADJUSTED BIENNIAL RATE/1000, MEN | | | | AGE-ADJUSTED BIENNIAL RATE/1000, WOMEN | | | |
| | AGE 35–64 | | AGE 65–94 | | AGE 35–64 | | AGE 65–94 | |
OUTCOME	NO LVH	WITH LVH	NO LVH	WITH LVH	NO LVH	WITH LVH	NO LVH	WITH LVH
CVD	35	164*	83	234*	18	135*	57	235*
CHD	27	79*	52	138*	12	55*	31	94*
CHF	5	71*	20	99*	3	36*	15	84*
Stroke	5	29*	23	71*	3	20*	20	90*

Based on 36-year follow-up of Framingham Heart Study subjects. CHD indicates coronary heart disease; CHF, congestive heart failure; and CVD, cardiovascular disease. *$P<0.0001$.

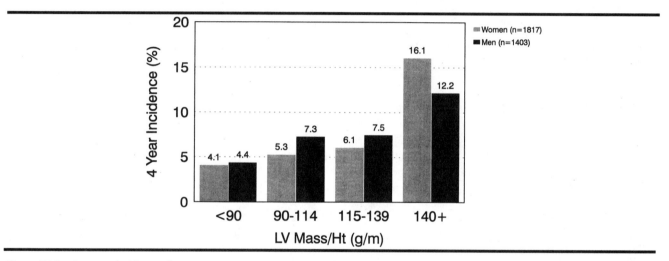

Figure 77.1. Four-year incidence of CVD events in Framingham Heart Study men and women who were free of CVD at baseline as a function of echocardiographic left ventricular (LV) mass (adjusted for height). Used with permission; from Levy D. *N Engl J Med.* 1990;322:1561.

cated hypertension who were followed up for a mean of 4.8 years, during which time there were 14 "hard" CVD events. The definition of LVH was an LVM index >125 g/m². The event rate was 4.6/100 patient-years among men with LVH versus 1.4/100 patient-years in those without LVH (P<.01). In a multivariable analysis adjusting for age, systolic blood pressure, diastolic blood pressure, and left ventricular fractional shortening, LVM index remained predictive of a CVD risk (P=.026) and was the most powerful predictor of events of all the variables examined.

In another study from the Cornell group, 280 patients with uncomplicated hypertension were followed up for an average of 10.2 years, during which time there were 40 incident CVD events. The authors looked at CVD outcome in relation to left ventricular geometry by separating subjects into four mutually exclusive groups on the basis of LVM and relative wall thickness (the ratio of 2 times posterior wall thickness to left ventricular end-diastolic dimension): normal geometry (LVM <125 g/m² and relative wall thickness <0.45), concentric remodeling (LVM <125 g/m² and relative wall thickness >0.45), eccentric LVH (LVM >125 g/m² and relative wall thickness <0.45), and concentric LVH (LVM >125 g/m² and relative wall thickness >0.45). Of the four geometric patterns, concentric LVH

carried the greatest risk for the development of CVD (**Figure 77.2**). It remains to be determined whether concentric LVH contributes causally to the increased risk for CVD events or, as some have suggested, whether the increased risk is a result of the increase in LVM that is also present in patients with this geometric pattern of hypertrophy.

LVH and Coronary Artery Disease

A key question is whether or not the association of LVH with risk for CHD is attributable to the coexistence of subclinical coronary artery disease. Researchers from Cook County Medical Center studied 785 patients who underwent coronary angiography and echocardiography. In this largely black study sample, there were 80 deaths during 4 years of follow-up. Echocardiographic LVH appeared to confer increased risk whether or not coronary artery disease was present. Among patients with documented coronary artery disease, the relative risk for death from any cause among subjects with echocardiographic LVH was 2.14 (95% CI, 1.24 to 3.68) after adjustment for age, sex, and baseline hypertension. Similarly, among subjects without significant coronary artery disease, the adjusted relative risk for death was 4.14 (95% CI, 1.77 to 9.71) among subjects

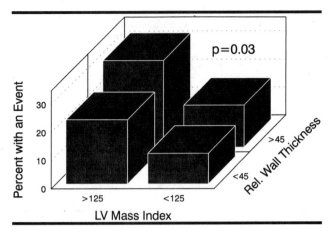

Figure 77.2. Incidence of CVD events in hypertensive subjects according to baseline left ventricular (LV) geometry. Four mutually exclusive groups are defined on the basis of LV mass and relative wall thickness. Used with permission; from Koren et al. *Ann Intern Med.* 1991;114:345.

with echocardiographic LVH. In a subsequent study from the same investigative team, echocardiographic LVH carried the greatest attributable risk for mortality of all risk factors they studied; 37% of deaths were attributed to LVH. Possible explanations for the risk conferred by LVH in patients without epicardial (large-vessel) coronary disease is that it may be associated with malignant ventricular arrhythmias, microvascular coronary disease, and impaired coronary reserve.

Regression of LVH

In hypertensive patients, aggressive blood pressure control can both prevent the development of LVH and reverse or regress it. Numerous clinical trials of antihypertensive drug therapy have documented the occurrence of regression of LVH in response to blood pressure lowering. It remains unresolved whether and to what extent there are differential drug effects on reversing LVH. Two of the largest randomized clinical trials to date, the Treatment of Mild Hypertension Study and the Department of Veterans Affairs Cooperative Study Group on Antihypertensive Agents, have suggested that blood pressure lowering is the key determinant of LVH regression and that differences among drug classes in their ability to reverse LVH are unclear.

In light of the association of LVH with risk for CVD, there has been great interest in studying the impact of LVH regression on CVD

risk. A report from Framingham used serial ECGs to examine the implications of reversal of ECG LVH. In that study, subjects with a serial decline in ECG LVH voltage were at lower risk for CVD than were those with no serial change (men: odds ratio after adjustment for age and baseline voltage, 0.46; 95% CI, 0.26 to 0.84; women: odds ratio, 0.56; 95% CI, 0.30 to 1.04). The results of this investigation suggest that regression of LVH confers an improvement in risk for CVD. The benefits of LVH regression are also supported by studies of hypertensive patients undergoing repeat echocardiographic assessment of LVM; these reports similarly have suggested that regression of LVH is associated with a reduction in CVD risk. The benefits to be derived from regression of LVH must be confirmed in other clinical settings and in larger clinical trials of antihypertensive treatment.

SELECTED READING

1. Bikkina M, Levy D, Evans JC, Larson MG, Benjamin EJ, Wolf PA, Castelli WP. Left ventricular mass and risk of stroke in an elderly cohort: the Framingham Heart Study. *JAMA.* 1994;272:33–36.

2. Casale PN, Devereux RB, Milner M, Zullo G, Harshfield GA, Pickering TG, Laragh JH. Value of echocardiographic measurement of left ventricular mass in predicting cardiovascular morbid events in hypertensive men. *Ann Intern Med.* 1986;105:173–178.

3. Gottdiener JS, Reda DJ, Massie BM, Materson BJ, Williams DW, Andeerson RJ, the Department of Veterans Affairs Cooperative Study Group on Antihypertensive Agents. Effect of single-drug therapy on reduction of left ventricular mass in mild to moderate hypertension: comparison of six antihypertensive agents. *Circulation.* 1997;95:2007–2014.

4. Kannel WB, Gordon T, Castelli WP, Margolis JR. Electrocardiographic left ventricular hypertrophy and risk of coronary heart disease: the Framingham Study. *Ann Intern Med.* 1970;72:813–822.

5. Koren MJ, Devereux RB, Casale PN, Savage DD, Laragh JH. Relation of left ventricular mass and geometry to morbidity and mortality in uncomplicated essential hypertension. *Ann Intern Med.* 1991;114:345–352.

6. Levy D, Salomon MS, D'Agostino RB, Belanger AJ, Kannel WB. Prognostic implications of baseline electrocardiographic features and their serial changes in subjects with left ventricular hypertrophy. *Circulation.* 1994;90:1786–1793.

7. Levy D, Garrison RJ, Savage DD, Kannel WB, Castelli WP. Prognostic implications of echocardiographically determined left ventricular mass in the Framingham Heart Study. *N Engl J Med.* 1990;322:1561–1566.

8. Liao Y, Cooper RS, McGee DL, Mensah GA, Ghali JK. The relative effects of left ventricular hypertrophy, coronary artery disease, and ventricular dysfunction on survival among black adults. *JAMA.* 1995;273:1592–1597.

9. Liebson PR, Grandits GA, Dianzumba S, Prineas RJ, Grimm RH Jr, Neaton JD, Stamler J. Comparison of five antihypertensive monotherapies and placebo for change in left ventricular mass in patients receiving nutritional-hygienic therapy in the Treatment of Mild Hypertension Study (TOMHS). *Circulation.* 1995;91:698–706.

10. Verdecchia P, Schillaci G, Borgioni C, Ciucci A, Gattobigio R, Zampi I, Reboldi G, Porcellati C. Prognostic significance of serial changes in left ventricular mass in essential hypertension. *Circulation.* 1998;97:48–54.

Chapter 78

Renal Risk

Michael J. Klag, MD, MPH

KEY POINTS

- Approximately 90% of persons with end-stage renal disease (ESRD) have a history of hypertension.

- The link between blood pressure (BP) and ESRD has been demonstrated in ecological, case-control, and prospective cohort studies.

- Black men have a greater risk of developing ESRD at every level of BP than do white men.

- Angiotensin-converting enzyme inhibitors appear to offer special renal protection.

See also Chapters 74, 112, 141, 146

In 1836, Bright first described the association of kidney disease, as evidenced by the presence of small kidneys and proteinuria, with hypertension, manifested by left ventricular enlargement and stroke. Bright postulated that kidney disease was the causal factor. In contrast, physicians later in the century argued that high blood pressure (BP) led to the development of kidney disease. This controversy persists to the present day. Renal disease elevates BP; approximately 90% of persons with end-stage renal disease (ESRD) have a history of hypertension. Elevated BP, however, also increases the rate of progression of renal insufficiency and may initiate renal damage. Thus, it is often difficult, both in clinical practice and research, to determine which comes first. Causal inferences are best made from clinical trials of BP lowering where change in renal function is the outcome. This discussion, however, will focus on observational studies of the risk of renal disease associated with BP.

During the last 10 years, the substantial public health impact of renal disease has been recognized. The incidence of ESRD has increased every year since 1973, the first year from which such data are available. In 1994, more than 67 000 persons entered ESRD treatment programs in the United States. In 30% of these cases, the underlying cause of the ESRD was ascribed by the treating nephrologist to hypertension. This number underestimates the importance of the contribution of BP to the burden of ESRD, however, because the etiology of renal disease is multifactorial and higher BP contributes to the incidence of all forms of ESRD. The increasing incidence of ESRD coupled with improvements in patient survival have led to a large number of persons with prevalent ESRD each year. In 1996, for example, almost 290 000 persons received treatment for ESRD in the United States. The economic impact of ESRD is also profound. The cost to Medicare for direct care of patients with ESRD in 1996 was $9.6 billion; for all payers in the United Sates, the cost was $14.5 billion.

Although patient survival after initiation of renal replacement therapy is improving, it is still poor. The most recent survival data indicate that only 37% of persons with ESRD are alive 5 years after beginning treatment, with the most common cause of death being cardiovascular disease. An increased risk of death from cardiovascular disease is also present in persons with milder forms or renal disease without ESRD.

BP and ESRD

The strong association between malignant hypertension and the development of renal failure was first recognized at the beginning of this century. Only within the last 10 years, however, has the risk of developing renal disease associated with less severe hypertension been determined. A link between BP and ESRD has been demonstrated in ecological, case-control, and prospective cohort studies. In an analysis of 26 geographic areas in Maryland, the incidence of hypertensive ESRD correlated closely with prevalence of hypertension, especially severe hypertension. During a 15-year follow-up of 11 912 male hypertensive veterans, pretreatment systolic BP associated with development of ESRD and was more predictive of developing ESRD than was diastolic pressure. Greater decrease in BP with treatment, in an observational analysis, was associated with lower risk of incident ESRD.

ESRD Incidence in MRFIT Men

The risk of ESRD across a wide range of BP was determined in a prospective study of 332 544 men screened for the Multiple Risk Factor Intervention Trial (MRFIT). Between 1973 and 1975, 361 662 men aged 35 to 57 years in 18 US cities were screened for entry into the trial, and 12 866 men entered the trial. Men with evidence of end-organ damage based on medical history or physical examination and a serum creatinine level ≥2.0 mg/dL (176 μmol/L) were excluded from the trial. Excluded from the analysis were 3 men already being treated for ESRD at time of screening and 29 115 men for whom information about systolic BP or income was not available, leaving 332 544 men for analysis.

This large cohort was followed for 16 years; 814 cases of all-cause ESRD, defined as treatment for ESRD or death from renal failure, were identified. Use of all-cause ESRD as the primary outcome precludes misclassification of causes of ESRD. **Figure 78.1** shows cumulative incidence of all-cause ESRD during follow-up by BP assessed at baseline, grouped according to the seven JNC V categories. The incidence of ESRD rose progressively with successively higher BP compared with men with optimal BP. In men with stage 4 hypertension, the highest BP group, the excess incidence was evident within the first 2 years of follow-up. Incidence curves for the other groups did not separate until later in follow-up. The early increase in ESRD incidence in men with the highest BP may reflect pre-existing renal disease in this group.

Table 78.1 gives the number of men in each stratum of BP, number who developed ESRD, age-adjusted incidence rates of ESRD, and multivariate-adjusted relative risk. Of the ESRD cases, 49% occurred at hypertension of stage 1 or higher. The consistency and strength of the association of BP categories with ESRD incidence were impressive. Men with high normal BP have a 2-fold-increased risk of development ESRD compared with men with optimal BP. Stage 4 hypertension imparted a 22-times-greater risk than optimal BP. In men who survived the first 10 years without ESRD, the relative risks of ESRD among those

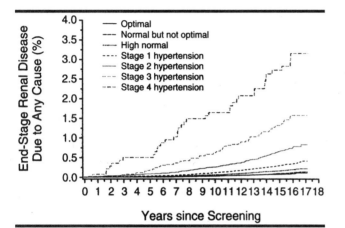

Figure 78.1. Cumulative incidence (%) of all-cause ESRD by JNC V categories of systolic and diastolic BP in 332 544 men screened for the MRFIT Trial. Used with permission from Klag MJ, Whelton PK, Randall BL, Neaton JD, Brancati FL, Ford CE, Shulman NB, Stamler J. Blood pressure and end-stage renal disease in men. *N Engl J Med.* 1996;334:13–18.

with stages 1, 2, 3, and 4 hypertension were 2.8, 5.0, 8.4, and 12.4, respectively, compared with men with optimal BP.

The risk of ESRD associated with BP was strong, positive, and statistically significant both overall in subgroups defined by age and other baseline covariates. However, positive associations were weaker among old men, men with diabetes, and black men.

Black men had a greater risk of developing ESRD at every level of BP than did white men **(Figure 78.2)**. The risk of ESRD associated with BP, however, was similar in the two groups. For every 16 mm Hg higher systolic BP at baseline, the multivariate-adjusted relative risk of ESRD was 1.54 in black men compared to 1.77 in white men. These relative risk estimates were statistically significantly different due to the large numbers of men in the cohort, but the differences were not of clinical importance. Thus, the higher incidence of ESRD in black men compared with white men was not due to a greater sensitivity to the effects of BP in black men. Higher BP in the black men did explain a substantial portion of the excess ESRD risk seen in this group. Adjustment for systolic BP reduced the relative risk of all-cause ESRD in black men compared with white men from 3.20 to 2.56 **(Table 78.2)**.

Systolic and diastolic BP imparted a similar magnitude of ESRD risk. With multivariate adjustment for the covariates listed in the footnotes to Table 78.1, for example, the relative risk of developing ESRD associated with one standard deviation higher BP at baseline was 1.7 (95% confidence interval (CI), 1.7 to 1.8) for systolic BP and 1.7 (95% CI, 1.6 to 1.8) for diastolic BP. However, when systolic and diastolic pressure were considered together in the same proportional hazards model with adjustment for all other variables, systolic BP (relative risk 1.6; 95% CI, 1.5 to 1.7) had more predictive power than diastolic pressure (relative risk 1.2; 95% CI, 1.1 to 1.2). Stratified analyses without use of statistical models also showed that the risk relationships were stronger and more consistent for systolic pressure than diastolic pressure when both were considered together.

Table 78.1. Baseline Blood Pressure and All-Cause End-Stage Renal

BP CATEGORY*	MEN, N	ALL-CAUSE ESRD, N	AGE-ADJUSTED RATE/100 000 PERSON-YEARS†	ADJUSTED RELATIVE RISK‡ (95% CI)
Optimal	61 089	51	5.3	1.0
Normal, but not optimal	81 621	86	6.6	1.2 (0.8 to 1.7)
High normal	73 798	134	11.1	1.9§ (1.4 to 2.7)
Hypertension				
Stage 1	85 684	275	21.0	3.1§ (2.3 to 4.3)
Stage 2	23 459	158	43.6	6.0§ (4.3 to 8.4)
Stage 3	5464	73	96.1	11.2§ (7.7 to 16.2)
Stage 4	1429	37	187.1	22.1§ (14.2 to 34.3)
Overall	332 544	814	15.6	

*Classification of BP is based on the higher of systolic or diastolic pressure according to JNC V: optimal: systolic <120 and diastolic <80 mm Hg; normal, not optimal: systolic 120 to 129 and diastolic <84 mm Hg or diastolic 80 to 84 and systolic <130 mm Hg; high normal: systolic 130 to 139 and diastolic <90 mm Hg or diastolic 85 to 89 and systolic <140 mm Hg; stage 1: systolic 140 to 159 and diastolic <100 mm Hg or diastolic 90 to 99 and systolic <160 mm Hg; stage 2: systolic 160 to 179 and diastolic <110 mm Hg or diastolic 100 to 109 and systolic <180 mm Hg; stage 3: systolic 180 to 209 and diastolic <120 mm Hg or diastolic 110 to 119 and systolic <210 mm Hg; stage 4, systolic ≥210 mm Hg or diastolic <me>≥120 mm Hg.
†Adjusted using the direct method for the age distribution of all men screened.
‡Estimated using proportional hazards regression model stratified by clinic and adjusted for age, ethnicity, income, serum cholesterol, reported cigarettes per day, use of medication for diabetes, and previous myocardial infarction.
§P<.001.
Used with permission from Klag MJ, Whelton PK, Randall BL, Neaton JD, Brancati FL, Ford CE, Shulman NB, Stamler J. Blood pressure and end-stage renal disease in men. *N Engl J Med.* 1996;334:13–18.

Risk associated with BP was similar for ESRD ascribed to hypertension compared with all-cause ESRD; 193 men developed hypertensive ESRD. After adjustment for the covariates listed in Table 78.1, the relative risk of this outcome associated with a one standard deviation higher blood pressure was 2.0 (95% CI, 1.8 to 2.1) for systolic and 1.94 for diastolic (95% CI, 1.8 to 2.2).

Higher BP in men with diabetes is also an important contributor to the risk of ESRD associated with diabetes mellitus. Adjustment for systolic BP reduced the relative risk of all-cause ESRD associated with diabetes by 18%, from 11.4 to 9.3, and the relative risk of diabetic ESRD by 15%, from 11.4 to 9.3.

Results in Men Who Entered the Trial

The relationship between BP and all-cause ESRD was also investigated in the 12 866 men who were screened and who entered the trial.

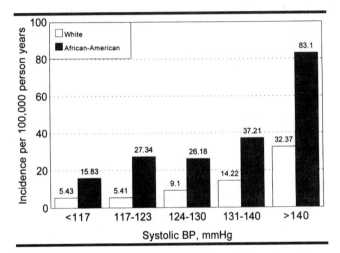

Figure 78.2. Age-adjusted 16-year incidence of all-cause end-stage renal disease by level of systolic blood pressure in 300 645 white men and 20 222 black men screened for the Multiple Risk Factor Intervention Trial. Used with permission from Klag MJ, Whelton PK, Randall BL, Neaton JD, Brancati FL, Stamler J. End-stage renal disease in African-American and white men: 16-year MRFIT findings. *JAMA.* 1997;277: 1293–1298.

In this group, BP was unlikely to be elevated as a consequence of pre-existing renal disease. The availability of serum creatinine measurements and dipstick assessment of urinary protein in these men at entry into the trial also permitted analysis of the relation of BP to incidence of ESRD, taking into account renal function at baseline. Among the men in the trial, an increase in systolic BP of one standard deviation (15.8 mm Hg) was associated with a 2-fold-increased risk of ESRD, similar to the 1.8-fold-increased risk seen in those not in the trial. Risk estimates associated with diastolic BP were also similar in men who entered the trial compared with those who did not. When serum creatinine and urinary protein excretion at time of entry into the trial were included as covariates in multivariate models, the relative risk of ESRD associated with BP was unchanged (2.0; 95% CI, 1.5 to 2.7 for systolic BP; and 2.5; 95% CI, 1.4 to 4.3 for diastolic BP). Moreover, when analysis was confined to the 7817 men with a serum creatinine <1.2 mg/dL (106 µmol/L) and <1+ urinary protein excretion at entry, among whom 19 men developed ESRD, the relative risk estimates were not significantly different from analyses including all 12 866 men (1.8; 95% CI, 1.2 to 2.7 for systolic BP; 1.7; 95% CI, 0.8 to 3.4 for diastolic BP). The similar relationships between BP and all-cause ESRD in the men who were included in the trial and those who were not, the independence of the association of baseline serum creatinine and urinary protein excretion in the men entering the trial, and the persistence of the association after 10 years of follow-up in the screened men argue against prevalent renal disease as an important contributor to the observed associations. The lack of information on renal function at baseline and during follow-up does mean, however, that we cannot say whether the strong association between BP and incidence of ESRD was due to initiation of renal disease or accelerated progression of pre-existing renal disease.

BP and Hypercreatinemia

Several studies have examined hypercreatinemia, an intermediate stage between normal renal function and ESRD, as an outcome. In an analysis of the 10 940 participants with hypertension in the Hypertension Detection and Follow-up Program, the incidence of clinically significant hypercreatinemia (defined as a creatinine ≥2.0 mg/dL and at least 1.25 times the level at entry into the trial) during

Table 78.2. Adjusted Relative Risk (95% Confidence Intervals) of Developing End-Stage Renal Disease for 20 222 Black Men Compared With 300 645 White Men Screened for MRFIT: Cox Proportional Hazards Analysis

	RELATIVE RISK, BLACK COMPARED TO WHITE (95% CI)		
ADJUSTED FOR:	ALL-CAUSE ESRD*	HYPERTENSIVE ESRD†	NONHYPERTENSIVE ESRD‡
Age	3.20 (2.62, 3.91)	5.16 (3.64, 7.31)	2.61 (2.04, 3.35)
Age, systolic BP§	2.56 (2.09, 3.13)	3.84 (2.68, 5.48)	2.14 (1.66, 2.75)
Age, serum cholesterol	3.25 (2.66, 3.98)	5.21 (3.68, 7.40)	2.65 (2.07, 3.40)
Age, cigarettes/d	3.26 (2.67, 3.98)	5.35 (3.77, 7.59)	2.64 (2.06, 3.39)
Age, median income	2.32 (1.82, 2.95)	2.83 (1.80, 4.45)	2.05 (1.53, 2.74)
Age, diabetes	2.73 (2.23, 3.34)	4.83 (3.40, 6.86)	2.16 (1.68, 2.78)
Age, previous MI	3.20 (2.62, 3.91)	5.19 (3.66, 7.35)	2.61 (2.04, 3.35)
All of the above	1.87 (1.47, 2.39)	2.42 (1.52, 3.84)	1.63 (1.22, 2.18)

*All-cause ESRD: Entry into ESRD registry or death from renal disease.
†Hypertensive ESRD: Entry into ESRD registry with renal disease attributed to hypertension or death from hypertensive renal disease.
‡Nonhypertensive ESRD: Entry into ESRD registry with other than hypertensive renal disease or death from renal disease other than hypertensive.
§Systolic BP modeled as a continuous variable.

5 years of follow-up was strongly related to diastolic BP at baseline. Incidence of renal insufficiency in the Stepped-Care group rose from 13.2 per 1000/5 years in the 90 to 104 mm Hg BP stratum, to 34.4 in those with a BP of 105 to 114 mm Hg, and 63.7 per 1000/5 years in the ≥115-mm Hg BP category. The relation of systolic BP to change in renal function was not studied. Smaller clinical observational studies of persons with hypertension have also demonstrated that higher BP is associated with decline in renal function. Such studies also suggest that control of high BP slows loss of renal function, consistent with results of clinical trials.

Summary

Blood pressure measured carefully on a single occasion is a strong independent risk factor for development of renal disease, both hypercreatinemia and ESRD. The increased risk associated with high BP is graded, continuous, and present throughout the entire distribution of BP above optimal. risk estimates are graded for both systolic and diastolic BP, but systolic BP is the stronger measure for prediction of subsequent ESRD. These relations are very similar to the risk of coronary heart disease and stroke associated with BP. Most of the risk estimates are based on BP measured on a single occasion, resulting in an underestimation of the strength of the real association of ESRD with BP due to regression-dilution. Most of the data were generated before the widespread use of ACE inhibitors, a class of antihypertensive drugs that appears to offer special renal protection. Widespread use of these drugs in the population may alter the relation between BP and ESRD observed in studies to date. The results of these studies also suggest that risk of renal disease associated with BP is present in persons without clinical evidence of renal disease. Lastly, the presence of renal disease increases the risk of cardiovascular disease.

Interventions to prevent renal disease need to emphasize prevention and control of high BP. Primary prevention of hypertension by slowing or stopping the rise in BP, from youth to middle age, has the potential to prevent many ESRD cases. In addition, the need to prevent ESRD dictates continued efforts to achieve early detection of hypertension and to ensure effective antihypertensive therapy.

SUGGESTED READING

1. Brancati FL, Whelton PK, Randall BL, Neaton JD, Stamler J, Klag MJ. Risk of end-stage renal disease in diabetes mellitus: a prospective cohort study of men screened for MRFIT. *JAMA.* 1997;278:2069–2074.
2. Klag MJ, Whelton PK, Randall BL, Neaton JD, Brancati FL, Ford CE, Shulman NB, Stamler J. Blood pressure and end-stage renal disease in men. *N Engl J Med.* 1996;334:13–18.
3. Klag MJ, Whelton PK, Randall BL, Neaton JD, Brancati FL, Stamler J. End-stage renal disease in African-American and white men: 16-year MRFIT findings. *JAMA.* 1997;277:1293–1298.
4. Perneger TV, Nieto FJ, Whelton PK, Klag MJ, Comstock GW, Szklo M. A prospective study of blood pressure and serum creatinine: results from the "Clue" Study and the ARIC Study. *JAMA.* 1993;269:488–493.
5. Perry HM Jr, Miller JP, Fornoff JR, Baty JD, Sambhi MP, Rutan G, Moskowitz DW, Carmody SE. Early predictors of 15-year end-stage renal disease in hypertensive patients. *Hypertension.* 1995;25:587–594.
6. Shulman NB, Ford CE, Hall WD, Blaufox, MD, Simon D, Langford HG, Schneider KA. Prognostic value of serum creatinine and effect of treatment of hypertension on renal function: results from the Hypertension Detection and Follow-up Program. *Hypertension.* 1989;13(suppl):I-80-I-93.
7. U.S. Renal Data System. *USRDS 1998 Annual Data Report.* Bethesda, Md: The National Institutes of Health, National Institute of diabetes and Digestive and Kidney Diseases; 1998.
8. Whittle JC, Whelton PK, Seidler AJ, Klag MJ. Does racial variation in risk factors explain black-white differences in the incidence of hypertensive end-stage renal disease? *Arch Intern Med.* 1991;151:1359–1364.

Chapter 79

Peripheral Arterial Disease and Hypertension

Michael H. Criqui, MD, MPH; Julie O. Denenberg, MA; Robert D. Langer, MD, MPH; Arnost Fronek, MD, PhD; Gloria Bensussen, MD, MPH

KEY POINTS

- Cigarette smoking and diabetes appear to be the most important risk factors for peripheral arterial disease (PAD).

- The association of PAD with systolic blood pressure appears to be stronger than the association with diastolic blood pressure.

- People with moderate PAD have a ≥50% increase in hypertension, and persons with severe PAD have nearly twice as much hypertension as normotensives.

- Hypertension is likely to be an important causal factor in the pathogenesis of PAD.

See also Chapters 65, 113, 142

It is generally accepted that the "big three" modifiable risk factors for coronary heart disease (CHD) are cigarette smoking, dyslipidemia, and elevated blood pressure (hypertension). Age and male sex are also major risk factors for CHD, but they are not modifiable. The prevalence of peripheral arterial disease (PAD) increases with age, and the rates are higher among men than women. Similarly, rates of systolic blood pressure (SBP) are higher in the aged and in men. Other important risk factors include diabetes, obesity, and physical inactivity. Because each of the above risk factors is thought to influence atherosclerosis, they should be related to PAD as well as CHD. However, cigarette smoking and diabetes appear to be the most important risk factors for PAD.

The association of hypertension with PAD is examined below. The evidence is stratified by different definitions of PAD.

Intermittent Claudication Prevalence

Intermittent claudication (IC) is the classic symptom of PAD, consisting of ambulatory leg pain not present at rest and relieved by rest. By definition, this criterion excludes asymptomatic and presumably less extensive PAD. However, studies using IC as their definition of PAD have produced somewhat conflicting results. Some studies showed no association, and in some studies showing a positive association, the relationship was stronger for SBP than for diastolic blood pressure (DBP).

Cross-sectional studies such as these could be biased by a number of factors. First, IC is an imprecise end point for PAD. Although IC reflects symptomatic and thus usually significant obstruction, surprisingly, nearly half of the patients reporting IC in a population study had no demonstrable reduction in arterial flow on extensive noninvasive testing. Such misclassification would result in a conservative bias. Second, a conservative bias could also be introduced by diet, lifestyle, or pharmaceutical interventions after the diagnosis of IC. Conversely, it seems possible that cross-sectional studies could be liberally biased by an increase in peripheral resistance secondary to PAD. In this instance, PAD might cause hypertension rather than vice versa.

Ankle-Brachial Index Prevalence

In general, an ankle pressure that is <90% of the brachial pressure is considered indicative of PAD. Studies using this criterion or a more conservative criterion, such as an ankle-brachial index (ABI) of <0.80 or even <0.75, have generally found an association with elevated blood pressure. In several studies, the association with SBP appeared to be stronger than the association with DBP. In the CHS study, there was a gradation of effect, with an inverse relationship of ABI measurement in relation to both percent reported hypertension (SBP >160 mm Hg, DBP >95 mm Hg, or self report of hypertension along with use of antihypertension medications) and SBP. That is, after adjustment for age and sex, as the ABI decreased, the number of persons reporting hypertension and the relative risk of hypertension increased, as did the mean SBP. The trend was highly significant. DBP did not differ significantly with varying levels of ABI. Other studies have shown a similar association between ABI and hypertension. However, these studies may have the limitations of cross-sectional studies, and the use of the ABI as the only criterion for PAD also results in false-positives and false-negatives.

PAD Prevalence by Multiple Noninvasive Tests

A study in an older free-living population in the United States used ratios of SBPs at several levels of the lower extremity to the systolic brachial pressure, as well as flow velocity determination in the femoral and posterior tibial arteries, to define PAD. In addition, a small number of patients who had had PAD surgery were included. Of the nonsurgical patients, only 20% had ambulatory leg pain, and overall, ≈33% of the patients were asymptomatic. This resulted in a broader spectrum of disease, with many more mild cases of PAD than usually found in epidemiological studies. In this study, the extensive use of noninvasive testing minimized the number of false-positive and false-negative cases. In our previously published analyses, we used random-zero arm blood pressures. However, because the random-zero technique has been questioned, we subsequently reanalyzed our data using blood pressures measured with a standard technique. Patients with moderate PAD showed a small increase in SBP, but the difference was not statistically significant. Patients with severe PAD showed a significant increase in SBP (11.7 mm Hg), but the increase in DBP (1.8 mm Hg) was not statistically significant (**Table 79.1**). We also evaluated this association in this population including information on any use of antihypertensive medication. **Table 79.2** shows the results of this analysis. Hypertension was defined either liberally as an SBP >140 mm Hg or a DBP >90 mm Hg or use of hypertensive medications (HTN1), or more conservatively by changing the blood pressure criteria to an SBP >160 mm Hg or a DBP >95 mm Hg or use of medication (HTN2). By either definition, in both sexes there was a stepwise increase in the proportion of hypertensives from normotensives to people with moderate PAD to people with severe PAD. For men and women combined, people with moderate PAD had a ≥50% increase in hypertension, and persons with severe PAD had nearly twice as much hypertension as normotensives. These findings were highly statistically significant and suggest a stronger relationship between hypertension and PAD when antihypertensive medication use is included in the definition of hypertension.

Table 79.1. Age-Adjusted Mean Levels of Blood Pressure (mm Hg) by PAD Status

PAD STATUS	MEN	WOMEN	MEN AND WOMEN (ADJUSTED FOR SEX)
Normal, n	183	225	408
SBP	131.2	128.2	129.2
DBP	77.2	73.9	75.4
Moderate PAD, n	22	27	49
SBP	138.9*	125.4	131.4
DBP	80.0	71.6	75.2
Severe PAD, n	12	6	18
SBP	140.4*	141.9*	140.9†
DBP	78.2	74.8	77.2

*$P \leq 0.05$, †$P \leq 0.01$ vs normal group.

Table 79.2. Age- and Sex-Adjusted Percentages of Hypertensives by PAD Status Using Two Different Definitions of HTN

PAD STATUS		MEN	WOMEN	MEN AND WOMEN (ADJUSTED FOR SEX)
Normal, n		183	225	408
	% HTN1	39.5	46.6	41.6
	% HTN2	24.3	32.8	26.9
Moderate PAD, n		22	27	49
	% HTN1	65.4*	58.5	60.3†
	% HTN2	54.2†	43.8	46.5†
Severe PAD, n		12	6	18
	% HTN1	74.5*	90.0*	81.2‡
	% HTN2	53.8*	61.8	55.7*

HTN1 indicates HTN drugs or SBP ≥140 or DBP ≥90; HTN2, HTN drugs or SBP ≥160 or DBP ≥95.
*$P \leq 0.05$; †$P \leq 0.01$; ‡ $P \leq 0.001$ vs normal group.

In a study of subjects from a vascular laboratory, which used segmental pressures to assess PAD, an SBP >140 mm Hg was highly associated with PAD at all levels in the lower extremity in women and in the two proximal levels in the men (**Table 79.3**).

PAD Prevalence by Angiography

In these studies, PAD was confirmed by angiography or by angiography in combination with other tests or symptoms. Thus, the diagnosis of PAD in these studies is highly reliable, and most patients have disease severe enough to be symptomatic. Nonetheless, as in studies in which prevalent PAD is defined as IC, the results are mixed, ranging from no association to strong associations. An Italian study found a statistically significant, >5-fold increase in the prevalence of hypertension (SBP >160 and/or DBP >95 mm Hg) among patients with PAD compared with age- and sex-matched control subjects. When matching PAD patients and control subjects for mean arterial pressure, Safar found that PAD patients had increased SBP and decreased DBP and thus increased pulse pressure. Pulse pressure was inversely correlated with arterial compliance, presumably because of changes in viscoelastic properties of the arterial wall. Again, data in these studies are subject to the usual cross-sectional study limitations. In addition, unlike population-based epidemiological studies, angiographic studies use clinical samples, which may not be representative of the general population.

Incidence Studies

These studies have the distinct advantage of having blood pressure measurements made before the development of the PAD end point of interest. Each of the studies discussed below had a different design.

IC Incidence

Carefully collected data in the Framingham study showed a steep, more or less linear gradient between the baseline level of SBP and the 26-year incidence of IC. For baseline DBP, the data suggest a threshold effect beginning at the fourth quintile (87 to 94 mm Hg) in women and the fifth quintile (>95 mm Hg) in men. For the fifth quintile of SBP (>180 mm Hg) compared with the first quintile of SBP (<119 mm Hg), the relative risk in men was 2.7 and in women was 5.2. Interestingly, the attributable (or excess) risk in both men and women for the fifth versus the first quintile was the same in both men and women (8/1000 biennial rate). The misclassification inherent in defining PAD by IC would suggest that these strong associations might be conservative.

Table 79.3. Adjusted Odds Ratios* for SBP >140 mm Hg With Presence of Isolated Arterial Lesions

	OR (95% CI)	
	MEN	WOMEN
Aortoiliac	3.0 (1.6–5.4)	5.1 (1.6–16.0)
Femoropopliteal	2.3 (1.3–4.3)	2.4 (1.2–4.9)
Tibioperoneal	0.9 (0.5–1.9)	5.0 (1.7–14.4)

*OR; adjusted for age, current smoker, former smoker, diabetes, history of angina, ischemic heart disease, stroke, and congestive heart failure.

PAD Progression

Palumbo et al reported on the prospective progression of PAD as defined by the rate of change in the postexercise ABI over 4 years, as well as the occurrence of clinical events, such as PAD surgery, including amputation. In multivariate analyses, SBP was independently and significantly predictive of PAD progression. Similar data exist in other studies.

Randomized Controlled Trials

The only way to definitively test whether hypertension is a causal factor in the pathogenesis of PAD would be a randomized clinical trial. Only limited data are available. In the Prevention of Atherosclerosis Complications with Ketanserin (PACK) study, nearly 4000 patients with IC and an ABI <0.85 were randomized, and 46% had hypertension (SBP >160 and/or DBP >95 mm Hg). Above-ankle amputations were reduced 47% (17 versus 32) in the ketanserin group. However, although this finding is consistent with a causal association between hypertension and PAD, it does not represent definitive proof, because ketanserin, in addition to being an antihypertensive agent, also inhibits platelet aggregation and has hemorheological effects.

Conclusions

The majority of studies addressing the association of hypertension and PAD find a positive association, typically stronger for SBP than DBP. Some studies are flawed by inexact definitions of PAD, and cross-sectional studies have the inherent limitation of being unable to determine whether any observed blood pressure differences preceded or followed the development of PAD.

In general, cross-sectional studies with better methodology tend to show more consistent relationships between hypertension and PAD. The limited number of prospective (incidence) studies available all suggest a rather strong relationship between hypertension and PAD. Although the currently available data are not definitive, we conclude that hypertension is likely to be an important causal factor in the pathogenesis of PAD.

SUGGESTED READING

1. Criqui MH, Fronek A, Klauber MR, Barrett-Connor E, Gabriel S. The sensitivity, specificity, and predictive value of traditional clinical evaluation of peripheral arterial disease: results from noninvasive testing in a defined population. *Circulation.* 1985;71:516–522.

2. Criqui MH, Langer RD, Fronek A, et al. The epidemiology of large vessel and isolated small vessel peripheral arterial disease. In: Fowkes FGR, ed. *Epidemiology of Peripheral Vascular Disease.* London, UK: Springer-Verlag; 1991.

3. Fowkes FGR, Housley E, Riemersma RA, Macintyre CC, Cawood EH, Prescott RJ, Ruckley CV. Smoking, lipids, glucose intolerance, and blood pressure as risk factors for peripheral atherosclerosis compared with ischemic heart disease in the Edinburgh Artery Study. *Am J Epidemiol.* 1992;135:331–340.

4. Kannel WB, McGee DC. Update on some epidemiologic features of intermittent claudication: the Framingham Study. *J Am Geriatr Soc.* 1985;33:13–18.

5. Newman AB, Siscovick DS, Manolio TA, Polak J, Fried LP, Borhani NO, Wolfson SK, for the CHS Collaborative Research Group. Ankle-arm index as a marker of atherosclerosis in the Cardiovascular Health Study. *Circulation.* 1993;88:837–845.

6. Palumbo PJ, O'Fallon WM, Osmundson PJ, Zimmerman BR, Langworthy AL, Kazmier FJ. Progression of peripheral occlusive arterial disease in diabetes mellitus: what factors are predictive? *Arch Intern Med.* 1991;151:717–721.

7. Prevention of Atherosclerotic Complications with Ketanserin Trial Group. Prevention of atherosclerotic complications: controlled trial of ketanserin [published correction appears in *BMJ.* 1989;298:644]. *BMJ.* 1989;298:424–430.

8. Safar ME, Laurent S, Asmar RE, Safavian A, London GM. Systolic hypertension in patients with arteriosclerosis obliterans of the lower limbs. *Angiology.* 1987;38:287–295.

9. Strano A, Novo S, Avellone G, Di Garbo V, Abrignani MG, Liquori M, Panno V. Hypertension and other risk factors in peripheral arterial disease. *Clin Exp Hypertens.* 1993;15(suppl 1):71–89.

10. Vogt MT, Wolfson SK, Kuller LH. Segmental arterial disease in the lower extremities: correlates of disease and relationship to mortality. *J Clin Epidemiol.* 1993;46:1267–1276.

Chapter 80

Genetics and Family History of Hypertension

Steven C. Hunt, PhD, Roger R. Williams, MD

KEY POINTS

- Blood pressure levels and hypertension have a strong genetic component, and family history is a useful predictor of hypertension risk.

- The aggregation of hypertension and familial lipid abnormalities was estimated to occur in 12% to 16% of all hypertensive patients and in 1% to 2% of the general population.

- Intermediate phenotypes associated with hypertension include angiotensinogen, glucocorticoid-remediable aldosteronism, Liddle's syndrome, nonmodulation of the renin-angiotensin system, urinary kallikrein, adducin. and sodium-lithium countertransport.

- Genes that significantly increase a person's body weight would tend to increase that person's blood pressure and increase the clustering of hypertension in that family.

See also Chapters 39, 40, 41, 81, 107

There is considerable evidence for genetic determination and control of blood pressure in humans. Mounting data suggest that there are several "intermediate phenotypes" characterized by variables that may control blood pressure and are more directly related to specific genes than are blood pressure levels. These intermediate phenotypes in appropriate combinations should aid in explaining why certain persons develop hypertension.

Family History of Hypertension

A good family history will enumerate all first-degree relatives and their age, sex, and current blood pressure status. A positive family history of hypertension is a commonly used measure of the familial aggregation of hypertension. Family history in close relatives has been used as a surrogate measure for undefined risk factors that may be shared by the family. Family history of hypertension significantly predicts the future onset of hypertension in family members. The strength of the prediction depends on the definition of a positive family history and on the age of the person at risk **(Table 80.1)**, but the finding of a single first-degree relative with hypertension is only a weak predictor of future hypertension. A finding of ≥2 relatives with hypertension at an early age (<55 years) identifies a smaller subset of families who are at much higher risk. Older persons in families with a strong family history of hypertension have risks of developing hypertension similar to those of the general population. This is probably because they do not share the genetic or environmental factors leading to early onset in their family. The presence of stroke or coronary artery disease in family members should also be a modifying factor when the significance of a positive family history of hypertension is evaluated and when the level of aggression in treatment of a patient's blood pressure is determined.

Although these definitions work well for adults, youths generally have first-degree relatives too young to have hypertension. In this setting, children have usually been categorized into family history groups on the basis of number of parents (0, 1, or 2) with hyperten-

sion. In longitudinal studies of children, those with a positive family history of hypertension have higher blood pressures than those without a positive family history. Young adults with a systolic blood pressure reading higher than the age- and sex-specific 90th percentile had a greater prevalence of a positive family history of hypertension, and more relatives had ischemic heart disease and stroke.

Family Aggregation of Blood Pressure

Correlation coefficients of blood pressure are in the 0.1 to 0.3 range in family studies. The correlations between brother pairs are generally similar to those of sister pairs and brother-sister pairs. Parent-offspring correlations tend to be slightly smaller than sib-sib correlations. Heritability estimates cluster at ≈20% for family studies but are much higher (≈60%) when twins are used.

Adoption studies have also provided evidence for the genetic control of blood pressure. In families with natural children, adoptive children, or both natural and adoptive children, the intraclass correlation for systolic blood pressure between adopted siblings was 0.16 compared with 0.38 between natural siblings. For diastolic blood pressure, the adoptee and natural sibling correlations were 0.29 and 0.53, respectively. The parent-adoptee correlations were also much smaller than the parent–natural child correlations.

In isolated populations in which salt intake is low, blood pressure does not seem to increase with age. In most industrialized countries, however, blood pressure does increase with age. It has been suggested that there is an underlying major gene affecting blood pressure and that the increase of systolic blood pressure with age depends on the blood pressure genotype and the sex of the person. In this study, the high blood pressure genotype in women had a larger increase in systolic blood pressure with age than the other two genotypes. This was true in men also, although the increased slope was not as pronounced as it was for women. Studies like this one show the importance of simultaneously investigating environmental and genetic risk factors, because a person's genotype may deter-

Table 80.1. Relative Risks of Hypertension for Different Definitions of a Positive Family History of Hypertension for Men and Women

DEFINITIONS OF +FHX	% WITH +FHX	AGE GROUP				
		20–39	40–49	50–59	60–69	≥70
Men						
≥1 Affected	53	2.5	1.8	1.7	1.2	0.9
≥1 Before age 55 y	32	2.8	2.1	1.8	1.1	0.8
≥2 Affected	24	3.8	2.4	2.3	1.2	0.6
≥2 Before age 55 y	11	4.1	2.5	2.4	1.0	0.8
Women						
≥1 Affected	. . .	2.8	2.0	1.5	1.0	0.8
≥1 Before age 55 y	. . .	3.2	2.3	1.5	1.0	0.8
≥2 Affected	. . .	3.8	2.4	2.3	1.2	0.6
≥2 Before age 55 y	. . .	5.0	3.5	1.5	0.7	0.8

FHx indicates family history of hypertension. Relative risks are based on 13 years of follow-up in a retrospective cohort study of 94 292 persons in 15 200 families and are relative to persons without any first-degree relative with hypertension.

mine different environmental responses that would be missed if genotype were not taken into account.

Several prospective studies have shown that measures of central obesity, particularly subscapular skinfold thickness, are strong predictors of the development of hypertension. Body mass index has also been shown in large population studies to be partially determined by a major gene with large effects. Weight and obesity are responsible for part of the familial aggregation of blood pressure found between siblings and between spouses. Therefore, a gene that significantly increases a person's body weight would tend to increase that person's blood pressure and increase the clustering of high blood pressure in that family.

The clustering of abnormal lipid and insulin levels with elevated blood pressure has been well described in nonobese individuals, and these abnormalities appear to precede the development of increased blood pressure. This metabolic syndrome has also been shown to be familial and to exist in obese individuals. In a population-based sample of hypertensive siblings, the most striking sibling aggregation of risk factors occurred for reduced HDL cholesterol and elevated triglyceride levels. Decreased HDL cholesterol below the appropriate age- and sex-specific 10th percentile of the Lipid Research Clinic tables was found 3.9 times more often than expected. Triglycerides were elevated above the 90th percentile 3.0 times more often than expected. The sibship aggregation of these abnormalities was much higher than expected ($P<0.0001$), with 40% of the 58 sibships showing concordance for ≥1 lipid abnormalities. These hypertensive siblings were also significantly more obese than the general population and had elevated fasting insulin levels, smaller LDL particle size, and increased apolipoprotein B levels. The aggregation of hypertension and familial lipid abnormalities was estimated to occur in 12% to 16% of all hypertensive patients and 1% to 2% of the general population.

The familial aggregation of this syndrome was verified in a large twin study. Very similar estimates of the increased prevalence of lipid abnormalities in hypertensive twins were found. Dyslipidemic hypertension was concordant three times more often among identical twins than among nonidentical twins ($P=0.06$). In identical twin pairs who were discordant for this syndrome, the affected twin was often obese, while the unaffected twin had more normal weight. Thus, a nongenetic (environmental) factor influencing obesity may affect the expression of familial dyslipidemic hypertension. In addition, persons with both hypertension and lipid abnormalities had much greater than expected incidence of future coronary heart death compared with twins with only hypertension or lipid abnormalities. In another study, at least 21% of all sibling pairs with coronary heart disease had this syndrome of hypertension and lipid abnormalities.

Intermediate Phenotypes

If an intermediate phenotype is responsible for the familial aggregation of hypertension, then it must both predict hypertension in independent samples of persons and aggregate within families. Although renin plays an important role in the control of blood pressure, no genetic polymorphisms have yet been found linking any defect in the renin molecule on chromosome 1 to human hypertension. Likewise, genetic linkage of hypertension to the ACE locus on chromosome 17 has not been found in most hypertensive sib-pair analyses.

Angiotensinogen

One of the most consistent genetic findings has been the linkage and association of polymorphisms (different forms of the gene at a single chromosomal location) at the angiotensinogen locus on chromosome 1 to angiotensinogen levels and to hypertension. Genetic linkage implies that the genetic marker is nearly always transmitted from parent to offspring along with the DNA sequence actually responsible for the trait or disease. The angiotensinogen gene seems to predispose individuals to more severe hypertension, because linkage is strongest in the subset of individuals who require two or more antihypertensive drugs to control their blood pressures ($P<0.001$). There appears to be a functional mutation (G to A substitution) in the promoter region of the gene 6 bp before the transcription start site that increases angiotensinogen levels. The frequency of the AA genotype at the −6 locus (associated with hypertension and high angiotensinogen levels) ranges from 12% to 18% in white populations. Frequencies are ≈25% in severely hypertensive patients.

The angiotensinogen gene is also related to increased blood pressure sensitivity to salt. After 3 years of follow-up in a randomized clinical intervention trial, borderline hypertensive patients in the usual care group who had the AA genotype at the −6 locus had a somewhat higher incidence of hypertension than patients with the GG genotype. After sodium reduction, however, the patients with the AA genotype had a lower 3-year incidence of hypertension than patients with the GG genotype. Thus, there was a gene-environment interaction between angiotensinogen genotype, dietary sodium, and blood pressure levels, suggesting that the AA genotype is associated with salt sensitivity.

Adducin

α-Adducin is a cytoskeletal protein that is involved with membrane transport. Markers at this locus have been genetically linked to hypertension, and association studies have found a variant within the gene that is associated with higher blood pressures. Persons with this variant have increased maximal Na,K-ATPase pump velocity, resulting in increased renal tubular sodium reabsorption. Patients with the variant have a greater blood pressure response to diuretic treatment and also have a greater blood pressure decrease after acute sodium depletion by diet and furosemide.

Nonmodulation of the Renin-Angiotensin-Aldosterone System

Nonmodulation of the renin-angiotensin-aldosterone system has been suggested to be an important intermediate phenotype that is found in ≈50% of hypertensive individuals with normal or high renin levels. This phenotype is identified either by the magnitude of the renal blood flow response to an infusion of angiotensin II in subjects on a high-salt diet or by the response of aldosterone to angiotensin II infusion in those on a low-salt diet. Nonmodulators are defined as persons who do not have normal changes in renal blood flow or aldosterone during these maneuvers. Change in renal blood flow in response to either angiotensin II infusion or change in sodium intake (10 to 200 mEq/d) is significantly less in subjects with a positive family history of hypertension. Concordance of the nonmodulation trait in hypertensive sib pairs is 3.5 times higher than expected, whereas concordance for modulating status in these hypertensive sib pairs is one-seventh of the expected value.

Kallikrein

Kallikrein is an enzyme that converts inactive kininogens to kinins, which are potent vasodilators. A major gene has been statistically identified for low urinary kallikrein levels that explains 39% of the variance of urinary kallikrein. A significant gene-environment interaction occurs for the underlying variables represented by urinary kallikrein and potassium levels. This interaction suggests that persons homozygous for the low-kallikrein gene have low levels of renal kallikrein that are not modified by changes in dietary potassium intake. If the kallikrein gene can be shown to be related to hypertension, persons homozygous for high kallikrein levels may be protected from the development of hypertension by their ability to maintain high kallikrein levels regardless of potassium intake. However, the heterozygotes, who constitute 50% of the population from which these pedigrees were selected, showed a very significant positive relation between urinary kallikrein and potassium. In other words, a decrease in dietary potassium in the heterozygotes would result in kallikrein levels similar to those of the low-kallikrein homozygotes, increasing the risk of hypertension. An increase in dietary potassium would be expected to raise kallikrein levels up to the high-kallikrein homozygote mean, reducing the risk of hypertension.

Sodium-Lithium Countertransport

Na-Li countertransport, probably representing in vivo Na^+-H^+ exchange, is significantly different between hypertensive and normotensive patients. Subsequent familial aggregation, twin, and pedigree studies have shown significant genetic control of this cation exchanger. Major gene segregation for Na^+-Li^+ countertransport has been shown in three different populations. A study in Italy suggested possible major gene inheritance of Na^+-K^+ cotransport, especially in hypertensive families.

Polygenic Determinants

Biochemical variables with the strongest polygenic effects (many genes with additive, small effects) include intraerythrocytic sodium, Na^+-Li^+ countertransport, the number of erythrocyte ouabain-binding sites, plasma Mg^{2+} concentration, bilirubin, and platelet aggregation. Some of these phenotypes also show evidence of major gene control. Segregation analysis suggests that intraerythrocytic sodium levels are partially determined by a major gene with four alleles. The major gene explained 29% of the variance, whereas polygenes explained another 55%. Recessive inheritance of a major gene for a higher number of ouabain-binding sites explains 14% of the variance in the number of binding sites, and polygenic inheritance explains another 63%. The major gene was not frequent, with a 1.7% genotype frequency for the high homozygotes, but it was associated with an increased number of sites, 80% above the other two genotypes. Individuals with the major gene had lower intraerythrocytic Na^+ levels in accordance with observations that higher Na^+,K^+-ATPase activity decreases intracellular Na^+ levels. Uric acid has been shown in multivariate analyses to predict the future onset of hypertension, with relative risks in the range of 1.8 to 2.2, and has been strongly related to hypertension and blood pressure in cross-sectional studies. Uric acid correlates significantly within families. Segregation analyses of uric acid suggest that there may be two distributions but that these were not likely to be caused by the segregation of a major gene, because of non-Mendelian estimates of transmission and inability to reject an environmental cause of the two distributions.

Rare Mendelian Forms of Hypertension

Single-gene causes of hypertension also exist, as opposed to the susceptibility genes discussed above. Glucocorticoid-remediable aldosteronism is an autosomal dominant disorder that causes high levels of aldosterone, 18-oxocortisol, and 18-hydroxycortisol and causes early hypertension and strokes. Others, including Liddle's syndrome, are discussed elsewhere. Genes have also been identified that cause low blood pressure (Gitelman's and Bartter's syndromes).

SUGGESTED READING

1. Hunt SC, Williams RR, Barlow GK. A comparison of positive family history definitions for defining risk of future disease. *J Chron Dis.* 1986;39:809–821.

2. Ward R. Familial aggregation and genetic epidemiology of blood pressure. In: Laragh JH, Brenner BM, eds. *Hypertension: Pathophysiology, Diagnosis, and Management.* New York, NY: Raven Press Ltd; 1990:81–100.

3. Annest JL, Sing CF, Biron P, Mongeau J-G. Familial aggregation of blood pressure and weight in adoptive families, II: estimation of the relative contributions of genetic and common environmental factors to blood pressure correlations between family members. *Am J Epidemiol.* 1979;110:492–503.

4. Pérusse L, Moll PP, Sing CF. Evidence that a single gene with gender- and age-dependent effects influences systolic blood pressure determination in a population-based sample. *Am J Hum Genet.* 1991;49:94–105.

5. Williams RR, Hunt SC, Hopkins PN, Stults BM, Wu LL, Hasstedt SJ, Barlow GK, Stephenson SH, Lalouel J-M, Kuida H. Familial dyslipidemic hypertension: evidence from 58 Utah families for a syndrome present in approximately 12% of patients with essential hypertension. *JAMA.* 1988;259:3579–3586.

6. Selby JV, Newman B, Quiroga J, Christian JC, Austin MA, Fabsitz RR. Concordance for dyslipidemic hypertension in male twins. *JAMA.* 1991;265:2079–2084.

7. Jeunemaitre X, Soubrier F, Kotelevtsev Y, Lifton RP, Williams CS, Charru A, Hunt SC, Hopkins PN, Williams RR, Lalouel JM, Corvol P. Molecular basis of human hypertension: role of angiotensinogen. *J Nephrol.* 1997;10:172–178.

8. Manunta P, Cerutti R, Bernardi L, Stella P, Bianchi G. Renal genetic mechanisms of essential hypertension. *J Nephrol.* 1997;10:172–178.

9. Williams GH, Dluhy RG, Lifton RP, Moore TJ, Gleason R, Williams R, Hunt SC, Hopkins PN, Hollenberg NK. Non-modulation as an intermediate phenotype in essential hypertension. *Hypertension.* 1992;20:788–796.

10. Hunt SC, Hasstedt SJ, Wu LL, Williams RR. A gene-environment interaction between inferred kallikrein genotype and potassium. *Hypertension.* 1993;22:161–168.

Chapter 81

Gene-Environment Interactions

Anne E. Kwitek-Black, PhD; Howard J. Jacob, PhD

KEY POINTS

- Primary hypertension is a multifactorial trait, with interactions between environment and genetic susceptibility.

- Two people with the same genetic disposition may or may not get primary hypertension, depending on environmental stimuli.

- Gene-environment interactions have been described for blood pressure responses to sodium/potassium intake, obesity and/or fat intake, and stress.

- Identifying the genes, environmental stimuli, and their interactions may lead to a more targeted approach to the prevention and treatment of hypertension.

See also Chapters 39, 40, 41, 80, 107

Blood Pressure Is Multifactorial

Blood pressure is a quantitative trait with a normal, continuous distribution in the general population. Hypertension is a clinical definition of the upper end of the blood pressure distribution. Blood pressure has both genetic and environmental components, which defines it as a multifactorial trait (**Figure 81.1**). Furthermore, the genetic involvement is polygenic in nature, meaning that several genes affect blood pressure in an additive and/or interactive manner. These interactions affect a complicated set of pathways in the renal, neuroendocrine, and cardiovascular systems. A deviation from homeostasis in these systems can result in increased cardiac output and/or increased total peripheral resistance, leading to high blood pressure (**Figure 81.2**).

The complexity of hypertension makes identifying the mechanistic pathways a challenge. Studies indicate not only that environmental and genetic factors independently affect blood pressure regulation but also that gene-environment interactions are apparent. Individuals who have the same genetic predisposition to hypertension may or may not be hypertensive, depending on their environment; conversely, individuals in the same environment may or may not develop hypertension, depending on their genetic makeup. For instance, in monozygotic twins, in whom genetic makeup is identical, if one twin develops primary hypertension, the other has a 41.6% chance of developing hypertension. Knowledge of gene-environment interactions would further our understanding of the disease pathways and could determine the correct treatment (ie, targeted drug therapy) or help prevent hypertension by reducing or eliminating environmental risk factors.

Determining Genetic and Environmental Contributions

Determining the genetic and environmental components of hypertension promotes understanding of the complex pathways involved in blood pressure regulation. A combination of twin, family, and adoption studies estimates that genetic factors account for 20% to 50% of blood pressure variability; the environmental contribution has been estimated to contribute to ≈20%. Given these values, the

interaction between the two may account for a large portion of blood pressure variability (30% to 60%). If the genetic factors involved in blood pressure can be dissected, understanding of the gene-environment interactions can more easily be realized.

Using molecular genetic technologies, many studies have been performed to identify the genes that play a role in blood pressure regulation. Several genes, including those for angiotensinogen, renin, α_2- and β_2-adrenergic receptors, and adducin, have been reported to be involved in human primary hypertension. It must be noted, however, that studies of these genes have differing results in diverse populations and/or ethnic groups, partly because of etiologic heterogeneity. This means that although two individuals may both have hypertension, the gene combinations leading to it may differ. Conversely, individuals with mutations in the same gene may or may not develop the disease, according to their genetic backgrounds. These discrepant results reflect the multifactorial nature of the disease and explain the incongruity among studies using different populations under different environmental conditions.

Environmental risk factors, such as dietary sodium, potassium, and calcium intake, as well as exercise and stress, are also involved in the development of hypertension. Although the known risk factors are difficult to quantify, it is estimated that 20% of blood pressure variability may be determined by environmental factors. The most studied environmental risk factor for hypertension is dietary sodium. It is clear that excess sodium intake is intimately associated with an increase in blood pressure within the general population; most large population studies identify a significant correlation between excess sodium intake and hypertension. The Intersalt study estimates a 3 mm Hg decrease in systolic blood pressure with a 100-mmol/d decrease in dietary sodium intake.

Although dietary restriction of sodium may be an important, nonpharmacological form of therapy for hypertension, it is clear that individuals differ in how much their blood pressure varies with changes in dietary sodium. A genetic predisposition to sodium sensitivity of blood pressure probably accounts for this variability

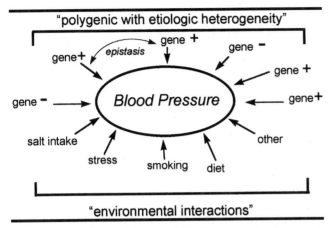

Figure 81.1. Multifactorial nature of blood pressure. Blood pressure is controlled by both genes and environment with both epistatic and gene-environment interactions. Modified with permission from a slide by Dr Allen W. Cowley.

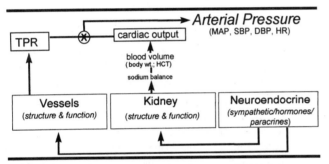

Figure 81.2. Organ systems and pathways involved in blood pressure regulation. Blood pressure is determined by total peripheral resistance (TPR) × cardiac output. Affecting TPR are the neuroendocrine and cardiovascular systems; affecting cardiac output are the kidney and the neuroendocrine systems. Measures of arterial pressure include mean arterial pressure (MAP), systolic blood pressure (SBP), diastolic blood pressure (DBP), and heart rate (HR). Modified with permission from a slide by Dr Allen W. Cowley.

among individuals. It is likely that there is also a genetic susceptibility to the impact of other environmental factors on blood pressure, eg, dietary potassium and calcium, alcohol and fat intake, physical exercise, and psychological stress. Several of these factors have been and will be further studied to evaluate their interactive effects with genes thought to be involved in the regulation of blood pressure.

Gene-Environment Interactions

Studies have clearly shown that the contributing factors leading to hypertension are both environmental and genetic. In general, a single gene or environmental stimulus does not cause primary hypertension. It is more likely that hypertension can be divided into several categories, each of which has a combination of gene variants interacting with environmental stimuli. If the particular combinations were identified, one could feasibly target treatments to patients on the basis of their subtype of hypertension. For instance, if a person were found to have the combination of genes that leads to sodium-sensitive hypertension, a sodium-restricted diet would be an effective treatment, whereas a person with hypertension not due to sodium sensitivity would not be placed on a low-sodium diet. Furthermore, drug therapy could be targeted to a specific mechanistic pathway leading to hypertension. Although pharmacogenetics will not be applicable in hypertension until the various mechanistic pathways are defined, it offers an important goal for the future of hypertension prevention and treatment.

SUGGESTED READING

1. Burke W, Motulsky AG. Hypertension. In: King RA, Rotter JI, Motulsky AG, eds. *The Genetic Basis of Human Diseases.* New York, NY: Oxford University Press; 1992:170–191.
2. Kaplan N.M. *Clinical Hypertension.* 7th ed. Baltimore, MD: Williams & Wilkins; 1998.
3. Williams RR, Hunt SC, Hopkins PN, Wu LL, Hasstedt SJ, Stults BM, Kuida H. Genes, hypertension and early familial coronary heart disease. In: Laragh JH, Brenner BM, eds. *Hypertension: Pathophysiology, Diagnosis, and Management.* Vol 1. New York, NY: Raven Press; 1990:127–136.
4. Williams RR, Hunt SC, Hasstedt SJ, Hopkins PN, Wu LL, Berry TD, Stults BM, Barlow GK, Schumacher MC, Lifton RP, Lalouel JM. Are there interactions and relations between genetic and environmental factors predisposing to high blood pressure? *Hypertension.* 1991;18(suppl I):I-29-I-37.

Chapter 82

Geographic Patterns of Hypertension

A Global Perspective

Richard S. Cooper, MD

KEY POINTS

- Geographic patterns of hypertension primarily reflect the level of economic and social development, as mediated by local cultural practice, rather than climate or natural phenomena.

- Interpreting cross-cultural variation in blood pressure is inherently difficult, given the problems of standardizing survey methods and the overlay of ethnicity and social factors.

- The determinants of geographic variation in hypertension that have been quantified are obesity, sodium and fat intake, and black ancestry.

See also Chapters 75, 83

Abundant Data, Yet Few Explanations

Hypertension is common to all human populations, with the exception of a few thousand individuals surviving in cultural isolation, and accounts for 6% of deaths in adults worldwide. Unlike coronary heart disease, for which studies of "geographic pathology" were so instructive about the underlying cause, regional variation in hypertension remains poorly understood. Although pronouncements regarding global influences, such as a temperature gradient leading away from the equator, have been made, the patterns are determined primarily by social and cultural factors at the local level.

Substantial problems confront the attempt to sort out the causal processes that determine consistent variation among population groups. These include lack of standardization of blood pressure measurements, potential bias introduced by variable treatment rates, and potential confounding effects of age differences. Despite these obvious problems, it is nonetheless surprising that no databases exist that summarize in a standardized manner the prevalence of hypertension in the international context.

The overlay of race and ethnicity with variation in environmental factors has further limited our ability to extract meaningful etiological insights. At the very least, mass migrations over the past century have demonstrated that the role of intrinsic susceptibility is clearly secondary to social conditions. Several of the putative factors that lead to hypertension are also extremely difficult to measure, particularly physical activity and psychosocial stress.

Patterns of Variation

For summary purposes, populations can be separated into groups at 4 levels of risk (**Table 82.1**). Only a handful of "no hypertension" societies still exist, primarily confined to the Amazon basin. In these groups, blood pressure does not rise, and perhaps declines, from age 18 years onward, following the pattern assumed to be "normal" for our species. In other regions of the tropics, where subsis-

tence agriculture remains the way of life, mean systolic pressure rises ≈10 mm Hg over the life course, and hypertension is not uncommon. These moderate rates also characterize most parts of Asia and the Indian subcontinent, with the notable exception of Japan.

Most industrialized countries of Europe, North America, and the Pacific would appear to have rates that are sufficiently similar as to be indistinguishable. Subpopulations within these regions have emerged that experience much greater risk, however. The extraordinary health burden imposed by hypertension on blacks is well recognized. Surprisingly little attention has been given to similar observations in Slavic countries and Finland, however. Local surveys, as well as a major US-USSR cooperative study that used a standardized methodology, demonstrate virtually identical levels of blood pressure and hypertension prevalence among Finns, Russians, Poles, and US blacks. Hypertension at these levels has also been reported from northern rural areas in Japan, variously attributed to high intake of sodium or of alcohol. Cardiovascular sequelae likewise occur at similarly high rates among all these groups.

At the global level, a north-south hypertension gradient is apparent, although this most likely reflects parallel economic and industrial development. Increasing hypertension with distance from the

Table 82.1. Categories of Hypertension Prevalence in Populations

CATEGORY	EXEMPLARY GROUPS	PREVALENCE,* %
Absent	Yanomami, Xingu	0
Low	Rural Africa and South China	7–15
Usual	Europe, US Whites, Japan	15–30
High	US Blacks, Russia, Finland	30–40

*Assumes a population structure with even distribution among 10-year age groups from 25 to 74 years.

equator has also been documented in China. The cause is unlikely to be climate or temperature, given the reverse pattern in the US.

Geographic variation within the US is limited. The exception has always been the rural South, particularly the Southeast, where during the 1950s and 1960s, blacks were found to have among the highest blood pressures in the world. The regional variation in blood pressure has left an indelible imprint on rates of cardiovascular disease, and migrants from the South carry with them a substantial excess risk. Although the survey data lack direct comparability, it appears that blood pressures have declined in the US over the past 3 decades, and this secular trend may have been most prominent in the rural South. No obvious amelioration of risk factors can explain this phenomenon, and for obesity, the trends are in the opposite direction.

Role of Covariation in Risk Factors

Geographic patterns in hypertension are influenced by both the overall variation in risk factors across the spectrum of economic development and specific local conditions. The high-fat diet of Finland and Russia, for example, has been suggested to be the cause of the exceptionally high prevalence of hypertension in that region. Blacks share the excess risk associated with lower socioeconomic status in industrialized societies and are exposed to additional psychosocial stressors. Given these complex patterns, it is virtually impossible to isolate variation in genetic predisposition across groups.

Intrinsic factors have often been postulated as the cause of higher blood pressures among blacks. From the global perspective, however, populations of African origin are predominantly at low risk, given the level of economic development in most of Africa and the Caribbean. The recent International Collaborative Study on Hypertension in Blacks (ICSHIB) documents the wide variation in hypertension prevalence across the course of the African diaspora. Body mass index, as a measure of obesity and a proxy for the industrialized lifestyle, is virtually collinear with hypertension prevalence in community samples from rural West Africa, the Caribbean, and the United States **(Figure 82.1)**. A similar gradient in sodium and potassium intake exists across these populations, and as shown by INTERSALT, also explains some of the population variance. Factors that remain unaccounted for are psychosocial stressors and the direct effect of physical activity. Local variation, for example, among

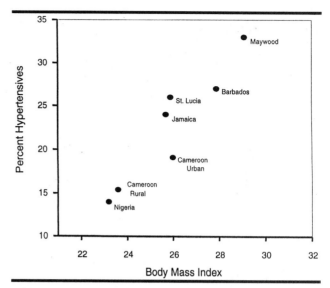

Figure 82.1.   Prevalence of hypertension by body mass index in among seven populations of the African diaspora.

ethnic groups within a society, may reflect various combinations of these risk factors.

SUGGESTED READING

1. Cooper R, Rotimi C, Ataman S, McGee D, Osotimehin B, Kadiri S, Muna W, Kingue S, Fraser H, Forrester T, Bennett F, Wilks R. The prevalence of hypertension in seven populations of West African origin. *Am J Public Health.* 1997;87:160–168.
2. Kaufman JS, Owaje EE, James SA, Rotimi C, Cooper RS. The determinants of hypertension in West Africa: contribution of anthropometric and dietary factors to urban-rural and socio-economic gradients. *Am J Epidemiol.* 1996;143:1203–1218.
3. McDonough R, Garrison GE, Hames CG. Blood pressure and hypertensive disease among Negroes and Whites in Evans County, Georgia. In: Stamler J, Stamler R, Pullman TN, eds. *The Epidemiology of Hypertension.* New York, NY: Grune & Stratton; 1967:167–187.
4. People's Republic of China–United States Cardiovascular and Cardiopulmonary Epidemiology Research Group. An epidemiological study of cardiovascular and cardiopulmonary disease risk factors in four populations in the People's Republic of China. *Circulation.* 1992;85:1083–1096.
5. Tyroler HA, Gasunov IS, Deev AD. A comparison of high blood pressure prevalence and treatment status in selected US and USSR populations. First Joint US-USSR Symposium on Hypertension. Bethesda, Md: NIH DHEW publication 79–1272.

Chapter 83

Geographic Patterns of Hypertension in the United States

W. Dallas Hall, MD

KEY POINTS

- The "stroke belt" is defined as those states with a stroke mortality greater than 10% above the national mean.

- Ten of the 11 states in the stroke belt are in the southeastern United States.

- The prevalence of hypertension is higher in the southeastern United States.

- In the stroke belt, the excess risk of stroke mortality occurs in whites as well as blacks and in women as well as men.

See also Chapters 75, 82

Hypertension in the Southeastern United States

The prevalence of hypertension is relatively high in the southeastern United States. **Table 83.1** compares the rates in the South with those in the rest of the nation, categorized by gender and race. The rates are higher for black men and women, but are also higher for white men and, to a lesser degree, white women residing in the southern region. Among hypertensives, the level of blood pressure is higher in the Southeast.

It is not known whether blood pressure changes after a person moves into or out of the southeastern region. Blacks born in the Southeast have a higher age-adjusted stroke mortality than blacks living in but born outside the Southeast, suggesting that indigenous rather than acquired factors are involved. Southern-born blacks residing in New York City have substantially higher cardiovascular disease mortality than do northeast-born blacks residing in New York City.

Table 83.2 compares the hypertension awareness, treatment, and control rates in the South with those in the nation as a whole, by gender and ethnicity. Hypertension awareness rates are good in the South. Hypertension treatment rates are similar in women, but lower in men residing in the South. Overall hypertension control rates are poor in the South, especially in men.

Consequences of Hypertension in the Southeastern United States

Stroke

Stroke mortality is also relatively high in the southeastern United States. This factor has led to the designation of a stroke belt (**Figure 83.1**), defined as those states with a stroke mortality more than 10% above the national mean. Ten of the 11 states in the stroke belt are in the Southeast. **Table 83.3** provides a summary of the national rank and the absolute stroke mortality rate for these states.

End-Stage Renal Disease

The southeastern area has one of the highest rates of end-stage renal disease (ESRD) in the nation, with 10 of the top 15 states in this area. Hypertension and diabetes are the two leading causes of ESRD. The 1995 sex- and age-adjusted incidence of hypertension-related ESRD is sixfold higher in blacks (237 per million) than in whites (39 per million). Fifty-four percent of US blacks reside in the Southeast, a fact that undoubtedly influences the high prevalence of ESRD in the region.

Racial differences in the incidence of ESRD are confounded by socioeconomic status. For example, in Alabama, a clear relation has been reported between the number of patients with treated ESRD and the number of households with per capita incomes below $7500 within individual zip codes. Others have reported an independent inverse association between socioeconomic status and the incidence of treated ESRD. The high incidence in blacks is only partially explained by lower socioeconomic status.

Congestive Heart Failure

Hypertension is the most important risk factor for heart failure. The prevalence and hospitalization rates for heart failure are increasing annually, and heart failure is now the most common hospital discharge diagnosis among individuals 65 years or older. The five states with the highest age-adjusted 1990 death rates for congestive heart failure are all in the southern region.

All-Cause Mortality

In a 15-year follow-up study of 11,936 hypertensive male veterans, all-cause mortality was 23% higher in the southeastern stroke belt than other regions of the country. Access to medical care was equal for black and white veterans, and no racial difference in mortality was observed.

Possible Causes for the High Prevalence and Poor Control of Hypertension in the Southeastern United States

Obesity

Obesity is a strong and independent risk factor for hypertension in all racial and socioeconomic groups. Weight gain also contributes

Table 83.1. Age-Adjusted Prevalence of Hypertension in the South

	SOUTH	OTHER REGIONS*
Black men	35.0%	33.0%
Black women	34.7%	27.8%
White men	26.5%	24.3%
White women	21.5%	21.0%

*Northeast, Central, and West.

Table 83.2. Awareness, Treatment, and Control Rates (% of Total) for Hypertension in the South

	SOUTH	OTHER REGIONS*
Aware		
White men	61.8	62.9
Black men	68.6	68.8
White women	76.4	74.5
Black women	81.2	74.7
Treated		
White men	43.8	45.0
Black men	44.3	49.5
White women	60.1	59.8
Black women	65.3	65.0
Controlled†		
White men	18.5	19.3
Black men	19.3	22.3
White women	30.1	26.7
Black women	32.3	24.1

*Northeast, Central, and West.
†Blood pressure <140/90.

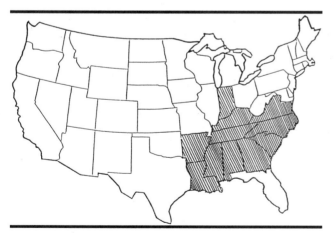

Figure 83.1.

to much of the rise in blood pressure with aging, and obesity may be one of the best predictors for the risk of developing hypertension later in life.

Weight loss reduces blood pressure in normotensive and hypertensive subjects. Even modest weight loss can lower blood pressure or decrease the number of antihypertensive medications necessary for treating hypertensive individuals.

Table 83.3. Age-Adjusted Stroke Mortality in the Southeast, by State, 1986

MORTALITY/100 000	RANK (OF 53)	
South Carolina	1	88.9
Georgia	2	83.7
North Carolina	3	77.9
Alabama	4	75.2
Tennessee	5	75.0
Mississippi	6	74.3
Virginia	7	72.6
Arkansas	8	71.6
Kentucky	11	70.3
Louisiana	12	70.3
District of Columbia	19	62.7
Maryland	25	60.5
Florida	41	51.7
National median	. . .	51.8

National trends in obesity indicate that even after adjustment for age, the prevalence of obesity in US adults has increased from 25% to 33% during the past decade. Obesity is very prevalent in the southeastern region, affecting 24% to 28% of all adults. Regarding the prevalence of obesity, 6 of the top 15 states are in the southeastern region. The highest national prevalence of obesity (44%) occurs in black women, and in the Southeast, 71% of black women are obese.

Physical Inactivity

The prevalence of hypertension is increased in individuals with a low level of physical fitness. Physical inactivity is directly associated with an increase in mortality from cardiovascular disease. Approximately one in four US adults (more so in women) report a sedentary lifestyle with no leisure-time physical activity. Physical inactivity is highly prevalent in the Southeast, affecting 25% to 43% of adults. Seven of the 10 states with the highest reported rates of no leisure-time physical activity are in the southeastern region.

Dietary Factors

Salt. Excessive dietary salt intake has been suspected as a cause of the high prevalence of hypertension in the Southeast, especially in blacks. In the Southeast, the estimated average sodium intake ranges from about 140 to 180 mEq/d (ie, 3200 to 4000 mg/d sodium, or 8 to 10 g/d salt). A high dietary salt intake clearly contributes to the risk of hypertension. High salt intake also antagonizes the blood pressure–lowering effect of most antihypertensive drugs. In the Southeast, where obesity and salt sensitivity are very prevalent, high salt intake might have even greater therapeutic and public health implications than elsewhere in the United States. The INTERSALT study noted an association between high dietary salt intake and stroke mortality that was even stronger than the association between salt intake and the level of blood pressure. These data suggest a direct effect of salt on the vascular wall.

Potassium. In the Southeast, there is a relatively low dietary intake of potassium, ranging from about 34 to 55 mEq/d (ie, 1300 to 2000 mg/d). A low dietary potassium intake might contribute to the risk of hypertension and stroke.

Low Birth Weight

Low birth weights, in particular those less than 2500 to 3000 g, have been associated with a number of cardiovascular risk factors, including hypertension. In the Southeast, about 14% of black babies and 6% of white babies weigh less than 2500 g. These rates of low–birth weight infants are higher than race-matched rates of low–birth weight infants in the United States as a whole.

SUGGESTED READING

1. Burt VL, Whelton P, Roccella EJ, Brown C, Cutler JA, Higgins M, Horan MJ, Labarthe D. Prevalence of hypertension in the US adult population: results from the Third National Health and Nutrition Examination Survey, 1988–1991. *Hypertension.* 1995;25:305–313.

2. Fang J, Madhavan S, Alderman MH. The association between birthplace and mortality from cardiovascular causes among black and white residents of New York City. *N Engl J Med.* 1996;335:1545–1551.

3. Gaines K. Regional and ethnic differences in stroke in the southeastern United States population. *Ethn Dis.* 1997;7:150–164.

4. Hall WD, Ferrario CM, Moore MA, Hall JE, Flack JM, Cooper W, Simmons JD, Egan BM, Lackland DT, Perry M Jr, Roccella EJ. Hypertension-related morbidity and mortality in the southeastern United States. *Am J Med Sci.* 1997;313:195–209.

5. Howard G, Evans GW, Pearce K, Howard VJ, Bell RA, Mayer EJ, Burke GL. Is the stroke belt disappearing? An analysis of racial, temporal and age effects. *Stroke.* 1995;26:1153–1158.

6. Lopes AAS, Port FK. The low birth weight hypothesis as a plausible explanation for the black/white differences in hypertension, non–insulin-dependent diabetes, and end-stage renal disease. *Am J Kidney Dis.* 1995;25:350–356.

7. Moore MA. End-stage renal disease: a southern epidemic. *South Med J.* 1994;87:1013–1017.

8. *NHLBI Data Fact Sheet. The Stroke Belt: Stroke Mortality by Race and Sex.* Washington, DC: US Dept of Health and Human Services, Public Health Service; October 1989. Publication NIH.

9. Perry HM Jr, Gillespie KN, Romeis JC, Smith MM, Virgo KS, Carmody E, Sambhi MP. Effects of "stroke-belt" residence, screening blood pressure and personal history risk factors on all-cause mortality among hypertensive veterans. *J Hypertens.* 1994;12:315–321.

10. Siegel PZ, Frazier EL, Mariolis P, Brackbill RM, Smith C. Behavioral Risk Factor Surveillance, 1991: monitoring progress toward the nation's year 2000 health objectives. *MMWR.* 1993;42:1–21.

Chapter 84

Gender and Blood Pressure

David A. Calhoun, MD; Suzanne Oparil, MD

KEY POINTS

- There is a sexual dimorphism in blood pressure: men tend to have higher blood pressures than women with functional ovaries, while ovariectomy or menopause tends to abolish the sexual dimorphism and cause women to develop a "male" pattern of blood pressure.

- Synthetic estrogens and progestins, found in oral contraceptives, tend to elevate blood pressure, while naturally occurring estrogens lower it or have no effect.

- Women are more likely than men to be aware of their hypertension, to be treated with antihypertensive drugs, and to have their blood pressure controlled.

- Antihypertensive therapy induces similar blood pressure reductions in men and women. However, men experience larger reductions in total cardiovascular risk with successful treatment of high blood pressure, since their absolute risk of coronary events at baseline is so much higher.

See also Chapters 59, 148

Sexual Dimorphism of Blood Pressure

A sexually dimorphic pattern of blood pressure (BP) development is evident in human populations. The Third National Health and Nutrition Examination Survey (NHANES III) found that overall mean arterial pressure is higher in both normotensive and hypertensive men than in women. Gender differences in BP emerge during adolescence and persist through adulthood. In all ethnic groups, men tend to have higher mean systolic BP (SBP) and diastolic BP (DBP) than women (by 6 to 7 mm Hg and 3 to 5 mm Hg, respectively), and through middle age, hypertension is more prevalent among men than among women (**Figure 84.1**). However, NHANES III found that hypertension is more prevalent among women than among men after age 59. Further, the Community Hypertension Evaluation Clinic (CHEC) program, which screened 1 million Americans between 1973 and 1975, found that mean DBP was higher in men than in women at all ages. However, mean SBP was higher in men until age 50 for blacks and age 65 for whites and was higher in women thereafter. The Hypertension Detection and Follow-up Program (HDFP) Cooperative Group screened 158,906 persons aged 30 to 69 in 14 communities between 1973 and 1974 and found that hypertension (DBP≥95 mm Hg) was more prevalent in men than in women of both black and white races.

Whether there is a "crossover" in the relative prevalence of hypertension in men versus women, with younger men and older women having more hypertension, is a point of controversy. A crossover has been reported in a number of cross-sectional studies but was not apparent in the 30-year longitudinal data from Framingham. Mean SBP in older women in Framingham approached but did not exceed that of older men; mean DBP was lower in women at all ages and declined in both sexes after age 65.

The influence of menopause on BP in women is another matter of controversy. Longitudinal studies from Framingham, Allegheny County, and the Netherlands did not document a rise in BP with menopause. In contrast, cross-sectional studies from Belgium and the United States found significantly higher SBP and DBP in postmenopausal than in premenopausal women. Staessen et al reported a fourfold-higher prevalence of hypertension in postmenopausal women than in premenopausal women (40% versus 10%, $P<.001$). After adjustment for age and body mass index, postmenopausal women were still more than twice as likely to have hypertension as premenopausal women. Further, enhanced stress-induced cardiovascular responses and higher ambulatory BPs have been documented in normotensive postmenopausal compared with premenopausal women. A menopause-related increase in BP has been attributed to a variety of factors, including estrogen withdrawal, overproduction of pituitary hormones, weight gain, or a combination of these and other yet undefined neurohumoral influences. Further research is needed to elucidate the effects of the sex hormones and their withdrawal on BP.

There also appears to be a sexual dimorphism in the sensitivity of BP to dietary NaCl in human populations, and this dimorphism appears to be age and/or sex hormone dependent. Studies carried out in different ethnic groups suggest that elderly (postmenopausal) women are more NaCl sensitive than men. Further, a study carried out in postmenopausal Japanese women showed that NaCl sensitivity correlated inversely with levels of circulating ovarian hormones. BP responses to high- and low-NaCl diets were compared in 12 hypertensive postmenopausal women and 7 age-matched normotensive postmenopausal women. Eight of the 12 hypertensive women were NaCl sensitive, but only 1 of the 7 normotensive subjects was NaCl sensitive. Circulating levels of prolactin, estrogen, and progesterone were significantly lower in the hypertensives than in the normotensives. These results were interpreted as suggesting that decreases in sex hormones and increased sensitivity to dietary NaCl are important factors in the genesis of postmenopausal hypertension.

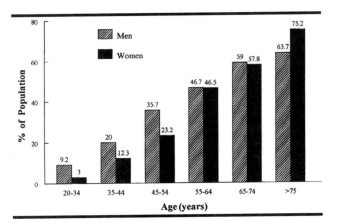

Figure 84.1.   Prevalence of hypertension in the US adult population by gender and age (NHANES III, phase 1, 1988–1991).

Postmenopausal Hormone Replacement Therapy and BP

The conjugated and natural estrogen preparations used for postmenopausal replacement therapy are administered at doses that result in "physiological" levels of circulating estrogen and do not appear to cause hypertension or even a tendency for BP elevation. Prospective studies have shown that administration of conjugated and natural estrogens, alone or in combination with a progestin, to normotensive postmenopausal women generally has no effect on BP or tends to reduce it **(Figure 84.2)**. The finding of significant increases in BP in a small proportion (<2%) of postmenopausal women when starting treatment with natural oral estrogens does not alter this conclusion, since the pressor response occurred so infrequently that it might have been due to chance. Further, the presence of hypertension is not a contraindication to postmenopausal estrogen replacement therapy, because postmenopausal estrogens appear from observational studies to have a beneficial or neutral effect on BP, as well as a beneficial effect on overall cardiovascular risk. However, since interventional studies of hormonal replacement therapy in hypertensive menopausal women have been either retrospective, short-term, small in number of participants, or open in design, some caution should be exercised when treating these patients with hormones. It is recommended that all hypertensive women treated with postmenopausal hormone replacement have their BP monitored at 3- to 6-month intervals.

Oral Contraceptives and BP

Many women taking oral contraceptives experience a small but detectable increase in BP; a small percentage experiences the onset of frank hypertension, which resolves with withdrawal of oral contraceptive therapy. This is true even with modern preparations that contain only 30 μg estrogen. The Nurses' Health Study found that current users of oral contraceptives had a significantly increased (relative risk [RR] = 1.8; 95% confidence interval [CI] = 1.5–2.3) risk of hypertension compared with never users. Of note, absolute risk was small: only 41.5 cases of hypertension per 10,000 person-years could be attributed to oral contraceptive use. Risk decreased quickly with cessation of contraceptive use: past users had only a slightly increased risk (RR = 1.2; 95% CI = 1.0–1.4) compared with never

users. Controlled prospective studies have demonstrated a return of BP to pretreatment levels within 3 months of discontinuing oral contraceptives, indicating that their BP effect is relatively acute and readily reversible. Nevertheless, oral contraceptives occasionally appear to precipitate accelerated, or malignant, hypertension. Genetic characteristics, such as family history of hypertension, as well as environmental characteristics, including preexisting pregnancy-induced hypertension, occult renal disease, obesity, middle age (>35 years), and duration of oral contraceptive use, increase susceptibility to oral contraceptive–induced hypertension.

A family history of hypertension and a personal history of renal disease or pregnancy-induced hypertension are relative contraindications to oral contraceptive use. Women over 35 years of age, particularly if obese, should be cautioned about the risk of developing hypertension while taking oral contraceptives and should be observed closely and their BPs measured on several occasions during the first year of treatment and annually thereafter. Contraceptive-induced hypertension can be diagnosed by documenting the onset of hypertension de novo during contraceptive therapy, along with resolution of the hypertension on drug withdrawal. The mechanism of contraceptive-induced hypertension is unclear but appears to be related to the progestogenic, not the estrogenic, potency of the preparation. The risk of hypertension is greater among users of monophasic combination oral contraceptives than among users of biphasic or

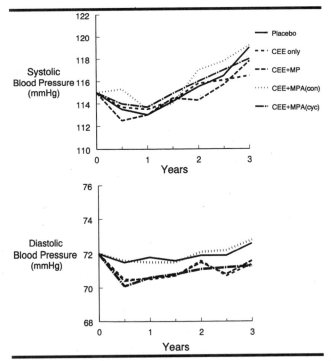

Figure 84.2.   Effect of hormone replacement therapy on systolic and diastolic blood pressure in normotensive postmenopausal women. CEE indicates conjugated equine estrogens; MP, micronized progesterone; MPA, medroxyprogesterone acetate; CEE only, CEE 0.625 mg daily; CEE+MP, CEE 0.625 mg daily plus MP 200 mg, days 1 through 12; CEE+MPA (con), CEE 0.625 mg daily plus MPA 2.5 mg daily; CEE+MPA (cyc), CEE 0.625 mg daily plus MPA 10 mg, days 1 through 12. From the PEPI Writing Group. Effects of estrogen or estrogen/progestin regimens on heart disease risk factors in postmenopausal women: the Postmenopausal Estrogen/Progestin Intervention (PEPI) trial. *JAMA.* 1995; 273:199–208.

triphasic combinations, perhaps because the total dose of progestin delivered is greater with the monophasic preparation.

Gender and Awareness, Treatment, and Control of High BP

Women are more likely than men to be aware that they are hypertensive, to be receiving antihypertensive treatment, and to have their BP controlled **(Figure 84.3)**. In NHANES III, approximately 75% of non-Hispanic black and white women were aware of their high BP, while only 65% of men in these ethnic groups were so informed. Interestingly, awareness rates were 64% for Mexican American women and only 44% for Mexican American men. Similarly, 61% of hypertensive women, but only 44% of men, were being treated with medication. This gender difference held across the three major ethnic groups. Finally, 28% of women and 19% of men overall had their BP controlled (<140/90 mm Hg). A recent survey of the literature revealed that, in developed countries worldwide, hypertensive women were 1.33-fold (95% CI=1.32–1.34) more likely to be treated with antihypertensive drugs than were hypertensive men. On average, 66% of hypertensive women but only 48% of hypertensive men were receiving antihypertensive drugs. The gender difference was greatest in the former USSR, where twice as many women as men were treated for hypertension. The higher antihypertensive treatment rates in women have been attributed to increased numbers of physician contacts because of visits for reproductive health and child care, as well as a lower probability of employment outside the home. Although there is clearly room for improvement, it is encouraging that women are attentive to their own health needs in the area of hypertension and BP control. This finding bodes well for the future cardiovascular health of women in the aging population.

Clinical Trials of Antihypertensive Treatment by Gender

Women, like men, suffer from cardiovascular complications of hypertension, and their lives are shortened if BP is not adequately

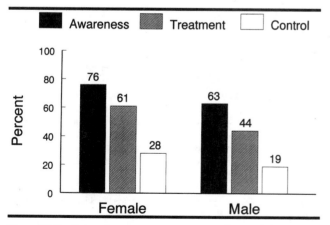

Figure 84.3. Rates of awareness, treatment, and control of hypertension by race and gender (age 18 years and older, NHANES III, phase 1, 1988–1991). The control rate represents the proportion of persons with hypertension who are controlled to < 140/90 mm Hg. From Burt et al. Prevalence of hypertension in the US adult population: results of the Third National Health and Nutrition Examination Survey, 1988–1991. *Hypertension.* 1995;25:305–313. Reproduced by permission.

controlled. Accordingly, the ultimate goal of antihypertensive treatment in women is the prevention of cardiovascular morbidity and mortality. Most of the large multicenter trials of antihypertensive therapy with "hard" end points have included slightly larger numbers of women than men. However, none of these trials included enough women to analyze data from gender subgroups convincingly. Subgroup analyses from individual trials have yielded variable results regarding the risk/benefit ratio of pharmacological treatment of hypertension in women, leading some to conclude that women derive less benefit than men from antihypertensive treatment.

A subgroup meta-analysis of individual patient data according to gender based on seven trials from the INDANA (Individual Data Analysis of Antihypertensive intervention trials) database was recently carried out to quantify treatment effect by sex and determine whether there are gender differences in treatment effect. These trials included 20 802 women and 19 975 men recruited between 1972 and 1990 and treated with thiazide diuretics and/or β-blockers. In women, significant treatment benefits included reductions in strokes (total and fatal) and major cardiovascular events **(Figure 84.4)**. In men, treatment benefits were significant for all seven outcomes considered (Figure 84.4). In terms of relative risk, treatment benefits did not differ between the sexes. Absolute risk reduction, in contrast, is dependent on untreated risk, and untreated risk for stroke was similar in the two sexes; for coronary events, it was greater in men. Accordingly, absolute risk reduction for stroke attributed to treatment was similar in men and women; for coronary events, it was greater in men.

As acknowledged by the authors, these results cannot be extrapolated to the newer classes of antihypertensive drugs without further research. Such a review is planned by the INDANA group for ongoing prospective clinical trials. Nevertheless, since a major benefit of antihypertensive treatment is prevention of stroke and the risk of stroke is similar in both sexes, these data suggest that, in general, the sex of the patient should not play a role in decisions about whether or not to treat high BP. Whether the threshold for pharmacological treatment of hypertension should be higher for young women (minor contributors to the INDANA study population) than for older women and men because of their very low cardiovascular risk is currently being debated.

Gender Considerations in Choice of Antihypertensive Drugs

Women generally respond to antihypertensive drugs similarly to men, but some special considerations may dictate treatment choices for women. β-Adrenergic blockers tend to be less effective than in men. Diuretics are particularly useful in women, particularly elderly women, because their use is associated with decreased risk of hip fracture. Diuretics are the favorite antihypertensive drug class for the treatment of women throughout the world, while β-blockers, angiotensin-converting enzyme inhibitors, and calcium channel blockers are more often prescribed for men. Women are more vulnerable to the adverse effects of some antihypertensive drugs; for example, angiotensin-converting enzyme inhibitor–induced cough, calcium channel blocker–induced edema, and minoxidil-induced hirsutism. Further, angiotensin-converting

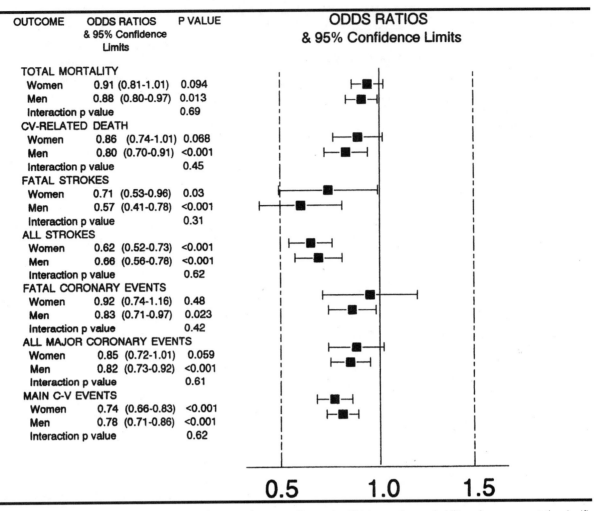

Figure 84.4. Effects of antihypertensive treatment by gender. CV indicates cardiovascular. The interaction probability values represent the significance of difference in odds ratios between men and women.

enzyme inhibitors and AT_1 receptor blockers are contraindicated for women who are or intend to become pregnant because of the risk of fetal developmental abnormalities.

SUGGESTED READING

1. Burt VL, Whelton P, Roccella EJ, Brown C, Cutler JA, Higgins M, Horan MJ, Labarthe D. Prevalence of hypertension in the US adult population: results of the Third National Health and Nutrition Examination Survey, 1988–1991. *Hypertension.* 1995; 25:305–313.

2. Calhoun DA, Oparil S. High blood pressure in women. *Int J Fertil Womens Med.* 1997;42:198–205.

3. Chasan-Taber L, Willett WC, Manson JE, Spiegelman D, Hunter DJ, Curhan G, Colditz GA, Stampfer MJ. Prospective study of oral contraceptives and hypertension among women in the United States. *Circulation.* 1996;94:483–489.

4. Gueyffier F, Boutitie F, Boissel J-P, Pocock S, Coope J, Cutler J, Ekbom T, Fagard R, Friedman L, Perry M, Prineas R, Schron E, for the INDANA Investigators. Effect of antihypertensive drug treatment on cardiovascular outcomes in women and men: a meta-analysis of individual patient data from randomized, controlled trials. *Ann Intern Med.* 1997;126:761–767.

5. Jackson R, Barham P, Bills J, Birch T, McLennan L, MacMahon S, Maling T. Management of raised blood pressure in New Zealand: a discussion document. *BMJ.* 1993;307:107–110.

6. Klungel OH, de Boer A, Paes AH, Seidell JC, Bakker A. Sex differences in the pharmacological treatment of hypertension: a review of population-based studies. *J Hypertens.* 1997;15:591–600.

7. Kotchen JM, McKean HE, Kotchen TA: Blood pressure trends with aging. *Hypertension.* 1982;4(suppl III):III-128-III-134.

8. Lewis CE. Characteristics and treatment of hypertension in women: a review of the literature. *Am J Med Sci.* 1996;311:193–199.

9. PEPI Trial Writing Group. Effects of estrogen or estrogen/progestin regimens on heart disease risk factors in postmenopausal women: the Postmenopausal Estrogen/Progestin Intervention (PEPI) trial [published correction appears in *JAMA.* 1995;274:1676]. *JAMA.* 1995;273:199–208.

10. Royal College of General Practitioners' Oral Contraception Study Group. *Oral Contraceptives and Health.* New York, NY: Pitman.

Chapter 85

Blood Pressure in Children

Alan R. Sinaiko, MD

KEY POINTS

- Blood pressure is considerably lower in children than in adults and increases steadily throughout the first two decades of life.

- Hypertension is defined as an average systolic or diastolic blood pressure (or both), according to the fifth Korotkoff sound, in the 95th percentile or higher for sex, age, and height, with measurements obtained on at least three occasions.

- Certain factors, including weight, height, and family history, are known to be associated with higher levels of blood pressure in children and adolescents.

- No significant differences have been found between ethnic groups until late adolescence.

- Measurement of blood pressure is recommended yearly after the age of 3 years.

See also Chapter 147

Arterial hypertension has a relatively low prevalence in children compared with adults. Nonetheless, in a small number of children, the problem is clinically significant, and guidelines on detection, evaluation, and treatment are of considerable importance in their care. Moreover, because the essential hypertensive adults of tomorrow will emerge in large part from the normotensive, seemingly healthy children of today, it is important from a preventive standpoint to begin thinking of hypertension as a risk factor in the pediatric age group, even before clinical manifestations of the disease become apparent.

The relevance of childhood blood pressure (BP) to pediatric healthcare delivery and the development of adult essential hypertension has undergone substantial conceptual change during the past two decades. From a historical standpoint, the primary orientation of healthcare providers in regard to BP in children and adolescents was toward identification and treatment of secondary forms of hypertension, such as renal parenchymal disease and renal artery stenosis. The incorporation of BP measurement into routine pediatric examination and the publication of the National Health Survey data on BP in children confirmed that mild elevations in BP during childhood were more common than previously recognized, particularly in adolescents (ie, beginning with the second decade of life). As a consequence, important questions were raised by pediatricians, school health personnel, and others active in the care of children about BP patterns in the pediatric age group, the definition of childhood hypertension, and the most appropriate intervention approach by the healthcare professional to the child with early signs of essential hypertension. The First Task Force on Blood Pressure Control in Children was convened in 1977 by the National Heart, Lung, and Blood Institute (NHLBI) in response to these questions, with the primary goal of developing recommendations for the treatment of childhood hypertension. The report was updated in 1987 and 1996.

There continue to be compelling reasons for developing the broadest base of information about BP in children and adolescents.

The prevalence of essential hypertension in the US adult population, defined as BP >140/90 mm Hg or the taking of antihypertensive medication, has been estimated to be 25%, or ≈50 million Americans. Although the prevalence of clinical hypertension is of far lesser magnitude in children than in adults, ample evidence supports the concept that the roots of essential hypertension extend back into childhood. Familial patterns for BP have been established from early infancy, and children with BP in the higher distributional percentiles are more likely to come from families with histories of hypertension. Although it is generally agreed that early essential hypertension poses little immediate risk to most children, evidence from preliminary studies in children and adolescents has shown cardiac ventricular and hemodynamic changes consistent with an adverse effect of mild hypertension before the third decade of life.

Prospective cohort data that could yield precise information about the relationship between childhood BP and cardiovascular risk are only now becoming available. BP is considerably lower in children than adults and increases steadily throughout the first two decades of life. The average systolic BP (SBP) at birth is 70 mm Hg in full-term infants, and it increases to 85 mm Hg by 1 month of age. BP increases at a greater rate in premature infants than full-term infants during the first year of life, and there is a significant inverse relation between birth weight and the risk of hypertension in adulthood.

During the preschool years, BP begins to follow a tracking pattern in which children tend to maintain specific levels of BP distribution relative to their peer group as they age. Tracking has been demonstrated by a number of statistical methods, including both percentile and raw BP data, and may increase in significance in evaluation of groups of subjects selected from the extremes of the BP distribution. Of particular importance is the documentation that BP tracking bridges the gap between childhood and early adulthood.

A number of factors known to be associated with hypertension in adults also have been associated with higher levels of BP in children and adolescents. A direct relation between weight and BP has been documented as early as 5 years of age and is more prominent in the second decade. Height is independently related to BP at all ages. Sex and race do not have the same impact on BP in children as in adults. No significant differences have been found in comparisons of whites, blacks, Hispanics, and Southeast Asians until later childhood or adolescence. Even then, the differences are small and have varied among epidemiological studies. Reference standards for BP in children do not distinguish between ethnic groups, because the differences are not clinically relevant. BP in boys is slightly higher than in girls during the first decade of life. The difference between boys and girls begins to widen around the onset of puberty, and BP is significantly higher in boys by the end of the teenage years.

Children from hypertensive families tend to have BPs that are higher than those of children from normotensive families, and the significant correlation of BP and cardiovascular risk factors between parents and their children is widely recognized. Siblings of children with high BP have significantly higher BP than siblings of children with low BP. The BP correlation is higher between mothers and their children than between fathers and their children, suggesting a direct prenatal influence.

BP Measurement

There are some special features to the measurement and evaluation of BP in children that are not considered when measuring BP in adults. Measurement by usual auscultation methods is not feasible in infants and very young children because of practical problems with anxiety and cooperation. Therefore, automated devices are widely used in this age group, and they are reliable.

Measurement of BP is recommended yearly after the age of 3 years. Use of a BP cuff of appropriate size is necessary to ensure accurate measurement, and the current commercially marketed series of pediatric cuffs along with the regular and oversized adult arm and thigh cuffs provides a sufficiently broad range of sizes. In a busy clinical setting, correctness of cuff size can be determined by use of the manufacturer's suggested markings on the cuff or selection of a cuff size with a width approximately two thirds of the distance between the shoulder and elbow. Choosing an inappropriate cuff size may either falsely elevate the BP, in the case of a small cuff, or falsely reduce the BP, in the case of a large cuff. However, if one must choose between two cuffs, both of which are close in size to the measured width of the arm, the larger cuff should be selected. It is uncommon for a slightly larger cuff to mask true hypertension, whereas it is more likely that use of a small cuff will lead to an elevated reading.

Until recently, the fourth-phase Korotkoff sound (K4) was used to designate diastolic BP (DBP) in children <13 years, and the fifth-phase Korotkoff sound (K5) was used for DBP in children ≥13 years old. With the addition of more childhood epidemiological BP data and reanalysis of the database used to establish previous standards, the 1996 Task Force Report determined that K5 is a reliable measure of DBP for children of all ages.

Definitions and Classification of High BP

As with adults, there are no data to support the rigorous classification of BP as normotensive or hypertensive or to further delineate hypertensive categories. Nonetheless, it becomes a matter of practical necessity to have definitions and classifications of hypertension to determine when and how vigorously hypertension should be treated. Definitions of hypertension are, of necessity, based on clinical experience and consensus rather than on risk data and are determined on the basis of percentile BP distribution within the pediatric population as follows: (1) normal BP: SBP and DBP <90th percentile for age and sex; (2) high-normal BP: average SBP or DBP (or both) between the 90th and 95th percentiles for age and sex; and (3) high BP (hypertension): average SBP or DBP (or both) ≥95th percentile for age and sex, with measurements obtained on at least three occasions.

Table 85.1. SBP and DBP Levels for the 95th Percentile of BP for Boys and Girls 3 to 6 Years old According to Height*

	SBP							
	HEIGHT PERCENTILES							
	BOYS				**GIRLS**			
AGE, Y	**5TH**	**25TH**	**75TH**	**95TH**	**5TH**	**25TH**	**75TH**	**95TH**
3	104	107	111	113	104	105	108	110
6	109	112	115	117	108	110	112	114
10	114	117	121	123	116	117	120	122
13	121	124	128	130	121	123	126	128
16	129	132	136	138	125	127	130	132
	DBP							
3	63	64	66	67	65	65	67	68
6	72	73	75	76	71	72	73	75
10	77	79	80	82	77	77	79	80
13	79	81	83	84	80	81	82	84
16	83	84	86	87	83	83	85	86

*Height percentile is determined from standard growth curves
Reprinted with permission from the *New England Journal of Medicine* as adapted from the Update on the 1996 Task Force Report on High Blood Pressure in Children and Adolescents.

Tables used to classify hypertension in children now take into account the documented effect of body size and differential rates of growth in children by relating BP to both age and height. The average 95th percentile SBP and DBP for boys and girls by height at selected ages are provided **(Table 85.1)**. BP norms for any given age decrease with decreasing height and increase with increasing height. Referring to these published norms should prevent mislabeling of tall, nonoverweight children as hypertensive or missing a diagnosis of high-normal BP or hypertension in shorter, heavier children. Obese children are unlikely to have a cause for their high BP other than their excessive weight. However, obesity is of medical importance because of its known relationship to high BP in children and adults. If a child or adolescent has an average BP greater than the 95th percentile for age but is not tall or heavy, there is greater probability that the elevation is the result of some secondary cause and that the child needs specific evaluation.

Except in cases of severe hypertension with manifest target organ damage, identifying children with high BP requires multiple BP measurements on several visits. On the first visit and during all subsequent visits, elevated BP readings should indicate the need for repeated measurements. Specifically, if the BP is above the 90th percentile, the child is scheduled for repeat BP measurements, usually over several visits. If the average BP is below the 90th percentile, the child returns to continuing health care. If the average BP is between the 90th and 95th percentiles, the child has high-normal BP and should remain under surveillance, with BP measurements at least every 6 months.

Under optimal circumstances, children will be receiving their care from a continuing source, and good records will be kept of their clinical progress, whether in the office of a private practitioner or in a clinic. A record of the patient's BP should be maintained throughout the years and plotted against the BP/age percentile charts. In this way, the healthcare provider will be able to determine at a glance whether the child is trending in a favorable or an unfavorable direction, which will provide guidance for determining how closely the child should be monitored.

SUGGESTED READING

1. Lauer RM, Clarke WR. Childhood risk factors for high adult blood pressure: the Muscatine Study. *Pediatrics.* 1989;84:633–641.
2. *National Health Survey: Blood Pressure Levels of Persons 6–74 years, US, 1971–74.* Hyattsville, Md: National Center of Health Statistics; 1977: US Department of Health, Education, and Welfare publication (HRA) 78–1648 (Vital and Health Statistics; Series 11, No. 203); 1977:37–44.
3. Shear CL, Burke GL, Freedman DS, Berenson GS. Value of childhood blood pressure measurements and family history in predicting future blood pressure status: results from 8 years of follow-up in the Bogalusa Heart Study. *Pediatrics.* 1986;77:862–869.
4. Sinaiko AR, Gomez-Marin O, Prineas RJ. Prevalence of "significant" hypertension in junior high school-aged children. *J Pediatr.* 1989;114:664–669.
5. Sinaiko AR. Hypertension in children. *N Engl J Med.* 1996;335:1968–1973.
6. Task Force on Blood Pressure Control in Children. Report of the Second Task Force on Blood Pressure Control in Children, 1987. *Pediatrics.* 1987;79:1–25.
7. Update on the Task Force (1987) on High Blood Pressure in Children and Adolescents: A working group from the National High Blood Pressure Education Program. *Pediatrics.* 1996;98:649–658.

Chapter 86

The Elderly Patient With Hypertension

William B. Applegate, MD, MPH

KEY POINTS

- From middle age on, elevation of systolic blood pressure is more predictive of subsequent cardiovascular disease (CVD) events than elevation of diastolic blood pressure, and diastolic blood pressure becomes increasingly less important in old age.

- Recent analyses indicate that increased pulse pressure is at least as predictive of future CVD events as is elevation of systolic blood pressure.

- Both a chlorthalidone-based regimen and a nitrendipine-based regimen have been shown to reduce CVD events in older persons with isolated systolic hypertension.

See also Chapter 149

Epidemiology

Elevation of either systolic blood pressure (SBP) or diastolic blood pressure (DBP) is a prevalent problem with major health implications in older patients. In all industrialized countries, average SBP rises throughout the life span, whereas DBP rises until age 55 to 60 years and then levels off or even declines. Therefore, most of the increase in prevalence of high blood pressure in older persons is due to an increase in isolated systolic hypertension (ISH; SBP >140 mm Hg, DBP <90 mm Hg).

Although the treatment of hypertension has classically focused more on DBP levels, epidemiological data indicate that for middle-aged and elderly adults, SBP is more predictive of future cardiovascular disease than DBP. For instance, data from the Multiple Risk Factor Intervention Trial screenees indicate that for middle-aged men, an SBP of 140 mm Hg confers slightly more risk for an individual than does a DBP of 90 mm Hg, and an SBP of 160 mm Hg confers more risk than a DBP of 100 mm Hg. Recent population-based studies from East Boston indicate that as persons approach advanced old age (≥80 years), elevations of SBP continue to be the single strongest cardiovascular risk factor, but elevations of DBP are diminished substantially in terms of associated risk. Recent analyses from the Systolic Hypertension in the Elderly Program (SHEP) show that a pulse pressure >100 mm Hg confers as much risk of future CVD events as an SBP >160 mm Hg.

Estimates of the prevalence of hypertension (both systolic/diastolic hypertension [SDH] and ISH) in people >65 years old vary greatly, depending on the age and race of the group studied, the blood pressure cutoff point used for the definition of hypertension, and the number of measurements made. On the basis of estimates from the Hypertension Detection and Follow-up Program (HDFP), the prevalence of SDH in people >65 years old is ≈15% in whites and 25% in blacks. In screening for the pilot study for SHEP, ISH was found in ≈10% of people ≥70 years old and 20% of people >80 years old in both blacks and whites.

Recent Clinical Trials

Since the results of SHEP were published in 1991, we have known that treating ISH with a stepped-care approach using a low to moderate dose of diuretic, with the next step usually consisting of a β-blocker, lowers the subsequent risk of stroke and coronary artery disease. Shortly after the publication of SHEP, the publication of the Medical Research Council—Elderly (MRC-E) trial found that a diuretic-based regimen in older persons with predominant systolic hypertension decreased the risk of both stroke and coronary artery disease. Also, the first Swedish Trial to Stop Hypertension (STOP-1) showed that lowering very high SDH in the elderly improved total mortality **(Table 86.1)**. The SHEP group recently published two very important papers. In one, these investigators show that the diuretic-based regimen in SHEP was remarkably effective in preventing future episodes of heart failure. In addition, the SHEP investigators have shown that the subgroup of older persons with type II diabetes (those on insulin at the start were excluded) experienced at least as great a reduction in stroke and coronary disease as was seen in the nondiabetics.

The data from the European Trial of Systolic Hypertension in the Elderly (Syst-Eur) replicated and extended the findings of SHEP. A nitrendipine-based regimen resulted in a substantial reduction in rates of fatal and nonfatal stroke. In the Shanghai Trial of Nifedipine in the Elderly (STONE), patients with ISH treated with long-acting nifedipine had lower rates of stroke than those who were given placebo. The levels of prerandomization blood pressure, age, and other demographic and risk factor characteristics were similar between Syst-Eur and SHEP, and the amount of blood pressure lowering was nearly equivalent between the two studies. In Syst-Eur, the reduction of stroke (44%) was slightly greater than in SHEP (37%), but this level of difference is unlikely to be meaningful. SHEP showed a reduction in total coronary heart disease of 25% and in total cardiovascular disease of 32%, and the corresponding numbers for Syst-Eur were reductions of 26% and 31%, respectively. In the Syst-Eur trial, the nitrendipine-based regimen did not have nearly the impact on heart failure (relative risk [RR], 71; 95% CI, 0.47 to 1.10; $P=0.12$) as shown in SHEP (RR, 0.51; 95% CI, 0.37 to 0.71; $P<0.001$). However, some of this difference could be explained by the fact that the

Table 86.1. Effects of Therapy in Older Person With Hypertension

	CLINICAL TRIAL NAME					
	EWPHE	**SHEP**	**SYST-EUR**	**STOP-HYPERTENSION**	**MRC**	**STONE**
No. of patients	840	4736	4695	1627	4396	1632
Age range, y	≥60	≥60	≥60	70–84	65–74	60–79
Mean BP at entry, mm/Hg	182/101	170/77	174/86	195/102	185/91	188/98
Relative risk of event (treated vs control)						
Stroke	0.64	0.67[†]	0.58[†]	0.53[†]	0.75[†]	0.43[†]
CAD	0.80	0.73[†]	0.74[*]	0.87[‡]	0.81	. . .
CHF	0.78	0.45[†]	0.71	0.49[†]	. . .	0.32
All CVD	0.71[†]	0.68[†]	0.69[†]	0.60[†]	0.83[†]	0.40[†]

EWPHE indicated the European Working Party on High Blood Pressure in the Elderly; SHEP, the Systolic Hypertension in the Elderly Program; Syst-Eur, Systolic Hypertension in Europe; STOP-Hypertension, the Swedish Trail in Old Patients with Hypertension; MRC, the Medical Research Council; STONE, Shanghai Trial of Nifedipine in the Elderly (nonrandomized, single-blind); BP, blood pressure; CAD, coronary artery disease; CHF, congestive heart failure; and CVD, cardiovascular disease.
[*]Indicates CHF also.
[†]Statistically significant.
[‡]Myocardial infarction only; sudden deaths decreased from 13 to 4.
Reprinted with modification and permission from National High Blood Pressure Education Program Working Group Report on Hypertension in the Elderly. *Hypertension.* 1994; 23:278.

duration of follow-up in Syst-Eur was substantially shorter than that in the SHEP Trial **(Table 86.1).**

Pathophysiology

The exact causal mechanisms for development of hypertension in the elderly compared with younger persons remain to be fully determined. Because most cases of SDH occur by age 55 years, it is unlikely that the pathophysiology of SDH is much different in the elderly than in the middle-aged. Older persons with hypertension generally have lower renin levels and are more sensitive to sodium repletion or depletion than younger hypertensive persons. Structural changes in the large vessels may play a predominant role in the rise of SBP levels with age. Both a decrease in connective tissue elasticity and an increase in the prevalence of atherosclerosis may result in an increase in peripheral vascular resistance and aortic impedance with age. There is a strong negative correlation between large-vessel compliance and systolic pressure in older patients.

Clinical Evaluation

High blood pressure is usually detected in an asymptomatic older person at a routine office visit or through various programs that offer blood pressure screening examinations to older individuals. However, in ≈10% of older persons, high blood pressure is first diagnosed when an older person presents with a clinical event that was probably triggered by long-standing high blood pressure, such as a stroke, heart failure, or myocardial infarction. At times, older patients will complain of dizziness or headaches that they believe may be associated with elevations of blood pressure, but studies have consistently shown that, unless the blood pressure is either extremely high or extremely low, symptoms are usually absent unless the patient presents with a cardiovascular clinical event. However, as blood pressure increases with age, the baroreceptor reflex is diminished, and patients may also present with either postural hypotension or postprandial hypotension.

Although most older persons who present with high blood pres-

Table 86.2. Indications for Further Evaluation for Secondary Hypertension

New onset of stage 3 hypertension in person >60 years old
Hypertension refractory to three-drug regimen
Clinical or laboratory findings suggest identifiable causes of hypertension
Spontaneous and refractory hypokalemia while on thiazides
Symptoms suggestive of pheochromocytoma
Continued creatinine rise while on appropriate antihypertensive therapy

Adopted with permission from the Sixth Report of the Joint National Committee on Detection, Evaluation, and Treatment of High Blood Pressure.

sure are asymptomatic, it is nonetheless important to question the patient about potential symptoms related to acute rises in blood pressure as well as symptoms related to the vascular complications of high blood pressure. Of course, it is important to question the patient about previous occasions when blood pressure may have been measured and, if possible, to document how long the blood pressure has been elevated and types of medications used. Finally, older patients frequently take multiple prescription or over-the-counter medications, some of which can cause an elevation of blood pressure.

The physical examination should focus on examining the patient for potential signs of organ damage from high blood pressure and an examination for any potential underlying physical abnormalities that might contribute to the rise in blood pressure. Meticulous and accurate measurement of the blood pressure itself is the most critical component of the physical examination in an elderly person with high blood pressure. The diagnosis of high blood pressure should be based on the average of three measurements over two or three visits. In the majority of cases, an older person's blood pressure should be based on office assessment with use of a mercury sphygmomanometer. There is more measurement error in ambulatory blood pressure monitor (ABPM) measurement in older persons than in younger persons. Because the prevalence of postural hypotension increases as the blood pressure increases, older persons with elevations of blood pressure should also regularly have their blood pressure measured in both the supine and standing positions. As many as 10% to 15% of untreated elderly persons with high blood pressure will have a decrease in standing SBP of ≥20 mm Hg. This is rarely associated with symptoms of postural hypotension.

Recommendations for laboratory testing, in general, do not differ in elderly versus middle-aged patients with hypertension. Because risk stratification may be important in deciding how aggressive to be in lowering blood pressure in some older persons, recent reports indicate that assessment of the ankle-arm blood pressure index (AAI) is a good measure of underlying atherosclerosis. Recent population-based studies have shown that an AAI for SBP measured with a hand-held Doppler probe of <0.9 is a very good marker of risk of future atherosclerotic events. In fact, an AAI of <0.9 is a greater predictor of subsequent risk than is an elevation of serum cholesterol or LDL cholesterol.

There is one major type of misclassification, pseudohypertension, that can occur in older persons. Pseudohypertension is thought to occur in elderly persons who have rigid arteries. Rigidity of arteries, on average, increases with age. The indirect sphygmomanometer can overestimate the true intra-arterial pressure, because increased pressure is required for the blood pressure cuff to compress a stiff artery. Unfortunately, the studies of this phenomenon do not contain representative samples of older persons, so it is difficult to assess the potential prevalence of this condition in the general population. Although there may be some increased estimate of blood pressure by indirect sphygmomanometry in older persons, the actual magnitude of measurement error in most patients is not large and often does not alter whether an older person would be classified as having hypertension. Nevertheless, a diagnosis of pseudohypertension should be suspected in older persons who have relatively high blood pressures but have no evidence of target-organ damage or in older persons who have symptoms of excessive low blood pressure on antihypertensive therapy even though their blood pressures appear to be in the normal range. Checking the patient for Osler's sign (a palpable radial or brachial artery after the blood pressure cuff has been inflated above peak SBP) is not advised, because it has low sensitivity and specificity for pseudohypertension.

Probably <1% of older persons have a secondary cause of hypertension amenable to targeted therapy. The most common cause of secondary hypertension in older persons is renovascular hypertension, but this diagnosis is difficult to make, and surgical treatment is often not curative, although the blood pressure may become easier to control. Criteria for considering an evaluation for an underlying secondary cause of hypertension are listed in **Table 86.2.**

Strategies for Optimal Care

Once the diagnosis of high blood pressure is firmly established in an older person, the first step in managing the patient is to assess his or her nutrition and lifestyle. Excessive ethanol use, high sodium in-

take, increased body weight, inactivity, and use of certain drugs, such as oral sympathomimetics or nonsteroidal anti-inflammatory drugs (alone or in combination), may actually be the culprit in raising the blood pressure. At present, it would be prudent to advise weight loss, decreased sodium intake, increased physical activity, and a review of over-the-counter and prescription medications for all older persons before drug treatment for high blood pressure.

The majority of older persons diagnosed with high blood pressure ultimately require drug therapy. The goals for BP lowering are SBP <140 mm Hg and DBP <90 mm Hg. The choice of drugs and their proper usage have been well detailed in JNC-VI. Pharmacological therapy could be considered for discontinuation for elderly patients with stage 1 hypertension in whom significant side effects persist despite attempts with a variety of pharmacological agents.

Basically, for older persons who have uncomplicated hypertension, generic low-dose diuretics or β-blockers are the first-line drugs of choice. Many older persons have one or more comorbid conditions that may alter the choice of the drug to be used to treat high blood pressure.

Complications or problems in the management of high blood pressure in older persons range from the subtle to the fatal. More subtle complications of antihypertensive medications include postural hypotension after meals, falls, depression, and mild-to-moderate clouding of the sensorium. On every visit, the clinician should include a formal evaluation of mental status and mood, should directly measure postural changes in blood pressure, and should question the patient about symptoms of dizziness. It is crucial also to obtain a history from family members with regard to the patient's relative vitality, cognition, and overall state of health. Older persons who experience side effects from prescription medications are more likely to attribute the cause of the side effect to the aging process than the drug itself. Therefore, both patients and their families must be cautioned with regard to subtle side effects of antihypertensive medications.

SUGGESTED READING

1. Applegate WB, Miller ST, Elam JT, Cushman W, el Derwi D, Brewer A, Graney MJ. Nonpharmacologic intervention to reduce blood pressure in older patients with mild hypertension. *Arch Intern Med.* 1992;152:1162–1166.
2. MRC Working Party. Medical Research Council Trial of Treatment of Hypertension in Older Adults: principal results. *Br Med J.* 1992;304:405–416.
3. National High Blood Pressure Education Program Working Group. Report on hypertension in the elderly. *Hypertension.* 1994;23:275–285.
4. Sixth Report of the Joint National Committee on Prevention, Detection, Evaluation, and Treatment of High Blood Pressure. *Arch Intern Med.* 1997;157:2413–2446.
5. Staessen JA, Fagard R, Thijs L, et al, for the Systolic Hypertension-Europe (Syst-Eur) Trial Investigators. Morbidity and mortality in the placebo-controlled European Trial on Isolated Systolic Hypertension in the Elderly. *Lancet.* 1997;360:757–764.
6. Stason WB. Cost and quality tradeoffs in treatment of hypertension. *Hypertension.* 1989;13(suppl I):I-145-I-148.
7. Systolic Hypertension in the Elderly Program (SHEP) Cooperative Research Group. Prevention of stroke by antihypertensive drug treatment in older persons with isolated systolic hypertension: final results of SHEP. *JAMA.* 1991;265:3255–3264.
8. Taylor JO, Cornoni-Huntley J, Curb JD, et al. Blood pressure and mortality risk in the elderly. *Am J Epidemiol.* 1991;134:489–501.

Chapter 87

Ethnicity and Socioeconomic Status in Hypertension

John M. Flack, MD, MPH; Beth A. Staffileno, DNSc; Carla Yunis, MD, MPH

KEY POINTS

- Epidemiological data consistently show a higher incidence and prevalence of hypertension in blacks than in whites, irrespective of age. The age-adjusted hypertension burden is similar among whites and Hispanics.

- Aggregate comparisons of various ethnic groups on mean blood pressure (BP) levels and hypertension risk are, to some degree, confounded by different average levels of socioeconomic status (SES) indicators and other lifestyle attributes.

- BP control rates are slightly higher in blacks than in whites and considerably higher in both these groups than in Hispanics. BP control rates within each ethnic group are usually higher in women than in men.

- Clinical outcomes from pressure-related target-organ damage are worse among those in low SES groups.

See also Chapters 88, 143

Rising blood pressure (BP), particularly systolic blood pressure (SBP), occurs commonly with advancing age in industrialized countries such as the United States. Although the lifetime risk of hypertension for most Americans probably exceeds 70%, specific ethnic patterns of hypertension onset, prevalence, and ultimately the occurrence of pressure-related sequelae have been noted. Hypertension risk and pressure-related clinical outcomes vary inversely with socioeconomic status (SES) indicators.

Ethnic Patterns of Hypertension

Epidemiological data consistently show a higher incidence of hypertension in blacks than in whites, irrespective of age. The hypertension excess in blacks is greatest at younger ages, particularly among women, and declines progressively with advancing age. Mean BP levels are higher in black men at all ages until 70 years of age. In women, mean BP levels are higher in blacks at all ages, although the differential narrows with advancing age. This ethnic differential in hypertension rates and premature hypertension onset probably results, in part, from a greater prevalence of obesity in blacks, particularly among women. Other factors possibly contributing to higher levels of hypertension in blacks include lower potassium and calcium intakes, lower levels of physical activity, high levels of psychosocial stressors, and, perhaps, greater salt sensitivity. Genetic factors have been proposed as having a role in the observed ethnic hypertension differentials. Nevertheless, there are virtually no confirmatory data to support this speculation.

Cross-sectional data from the first phase of National Health and Nutrition Examination Survey (NHANES) III, which evaluated 9901 participants (non-Hispanic whites, non-Hispanic blacks, and Mexican Americans), men and women, 18 years and older, from 1988 to 1991, indicate that 24% (or at least 43 million persons) of the noninstitutionalized, adult US population have hypertension. The overall prevalence of hypertension reported in the survey was slightly greater among men than among women (24.7% and 23.4%, respectively), and age-adjusted hypertension prevalence was higher in non-Hispanic blacks than in non-Hispanic whites and Mexican Americans (32.4%, 23.3%, and 22.6%, respectively). For both men and women, non-Hispanic blacks had the highest mean SBP until the end of the fifth decade. Between the sixth and seventh decades, Mexican American men had the highest mean SBP level. Among women, non-Hispanic blacks had the highest mean SBP until the end of the sixth decade; thereafter, all three ethnic groups had similar mean levels of SBP. In comparison, mean DBP levels in men and women of all three ethnic groups gradually increased from early adulthood through the fifth decade but plateaued and subsequently declined with advancing age. Over the last three decades, the average BP differential for black and white adults has narrowed considerably.

Hypertension-Related Morbidity and Mortality

BP correlates positively with risk for cardiovascular-renal disease for the broad range of BPs spanning from normal to hypertensive. The absolute level of risk for some BP-0related sequelae (eg, stroke and renal disease mortality) is usually higher in blacks than in whites at a given BP level, but across the broad range of BP, the fundamental association of BP with pressure-related clinical sequelae, including coronary heart disease, is similar in blacks and in whites. Blacks, Hispanics, and Native Americans all have higher rates of end-stage renal disease (ESRD) than whites. Because blacks develop hypertension at an earlier age than whites, at least some of the excess BP-related morbidity and mortality relates to a longer duration of hypertension rather than to race per se.

Geographic location appears to contribute to the expression of BP-related morbidity and mortality. A recent report form the Coronary Artery Risk development in Young Adults (CARDIA) study on a cohort of more than 5000 black and white men and women, aged 18 to 30 years, studied at four clinical centers located in different regions of the country, reported on hypertension prevalence and incidence over 7 years. Hypertension prevalence, sociodemographic characteristics, dietary habits, physical activity, weight, smoking, and alcohol consumption were similar at baseline in the four clinical centers. Nevertheless, over 7 years of follow-up, differences in hypertension incidence and prevalence emerged; at the 7-year follow-up visit, hypertension prevalence differed significantly by region (Birmingham, Ala, 14%; Oakland, Calif, 11.2%; Minneapolis, Minn, 7%; and Chicago, Ill, 6.6%). Also at the 7-year follow-up, hypertension prevalence in black and white men ranged from 9% to 5%, respectively, in Chicago and from 25% to 14%, respectively, in Birmingham. Among women, elevated BP did not differ significantly by regional center, but hypertension prevalence was highest in black and white women in the Birmingham cohort.

The observed regional disparities in hypertension incidence and prevalence are not fully understood. Regional dietary intake habits may contribute, at least in part, to these regional differences in hypertension. Accordingly, CARDIA participants in the Birmingham clinic had the highest level of dietary sodium intake, as well as the lowest consumption of potassium and magnesium, a trend that was present in both black and white participants. These dietary differences, as well perhaps as other unmeasured environmental factors, may contribute to the greater incidence and prevalence of hypertension, as well as to the high burden of pressure-related target-organ damage, in blacks and other low SES groups in the United States.

Ethnic Patterns of BP Control

Over the past two decades, the number of Americans aware of their hypertensive condition has increased, while the age-adjusted mortality from coronary heart disease and stroke has declined by almost 53% and 60%, respectively. Data from NHANES III indicate that overall hypertension awareness was greatest among non-Hispanic blacks (74%) and non-Hispanic whites (70%) compared with Mexican Americans (54%). Nevertheless, BP is not adequately controlled in the large majority of hypertensives. Hypertension control rates ($<$140/90 mm Hg) are highest among non-Hispanic blacks, non-Hispanic whites, and Mexican Americans (25%, 24%, and 14%, respectively). Non-Hispanic black women have the highest levels of hypertension awareness, treatment, and control (79%, 65%, and 29%, respectively). On the other hand, when only drug-treated hypertensives are considered, non-Hispanic white women have the highest BP control rates. The percentage of drug-treated, hypertensive adults with controlled hypertension ($<$140/90 mm Hg) has increased from 11% in the NHANES II (1976 to 1980) to 24% in the NHANES III (1988 to 1991). Moreover, in NHANES III, when individuals with BP $<$140/90 mm Hg following nonpharmacological therapy are included in the definition of controlled hypertension, the percentage increases to 35%.

Poor BP control appears to be an important factor in the excessive rate of pressure-related complications among blacks in the southeastern United States. Accordingly, Svetkey and colleagues reported a cross-sectional population survey of 4162 men and women, aged 65 years and older, who resided in mostly rural areas of North Carolina. They noted that among treated hypertensives, women were 52% more likely than men to have adequate BP control (DBP $\leq$90 mm

Hg) and that blacks were 40% less likely than whites to have adequate BP control. This black/white difference is in stark contrast to the previously mentioned national survey data on ethnic patterns of BP control.

SES and Hypertension

SES indicators (eg, education and income) function as surrogate markers of a constellation of lifestyle characteristics, including diet, physical activity, psychosocial and environmental stressors, social support, coping mechanisms, and health-seeking behaviors, as well as access to health-related information and medical care. The Treatment of Mild Hypertension Study (TOMHS) was a multicenter, randomized, double-blind, placebo-controlled clinical trial evaluating the efficacy of different classes of antihypertensive agents in 902 men and women, aged 45 to 69 years, with stage I diastolic hypertension. Recent analyses of baseline TOMHS data showed discrepant levels of urinary Na^+ and Na^+:K^+ ratio in blacks and whites that correlated to socioeconomic differences. Higher levels of urinary Na^+ and Na^+:K^+ ratio ($P<$.001 and $P<$.05, respectively) were documented for individuals of lower income and educational attainment among blacks, but not among whites. The higher urinary Na^+ levels and Na^+:K^+ ratio in lower SES TOMHS blacks represent a pattern of dietary electrolyte intake that if present in the black population at large would be a contributing factor to the excessive incidence and prevalence of hypertension and pressure-related target-organ damage (eg, stroke, left ventricular hypertrophy, and proteinuria) among blacks. Dietary intake of cations appears to be a quantitative difference in dietary intake between ethnic groups and in turn also relates to SES level, though dissimilarly in blacks and whites.

Aggregate comparisons of various ethnic groups on mean BP levels and hypertension, risk are to some, degree confounded by different average levels of SES indicators, such as income and education. Moreover, anthropometric measures, such as obesity, which correlate with low SES, especially in women, can also influence biological systems that are involved in BP regulation and the expression of pressure-related target-organ damage. For example, Cooper and coworkers reported data documenting positive association between obesity and both serum angiotensin-converting enzyme and angiotensinogen levels. This observation represents a potential mechanism through which obesity might contribute to elevated BP as well as to pressure-related target-organ damage. These data also highlight the complex interrelationships of ethnicity, SES, and body size with biological mechanisms likely to be involved in BP regulation.

Psychosocial factors correlated with lower SES may also contribute to the excess risk of developing elevated BP and to the disparity of hypertension incidence and prevalence among blacks and whites. Strogatz and colleagues examined the relationship between social support and perceived stress with BP in a cross-sectional, community-based sample of 1784 black women and women, aged 25 to 50 years, living in the southeastern United States. After adjustment for age, obesity, and waist/hip ratio, separate analyses of emotional support, instrumental support, and perceived stress revealed an inverse association for support and a direct association for stress with BP. The association was stronger for SBP than DBP. Differences in SBP associated with low support and high stress ranged from +5.2 to +3.6 mm Hg in women and +3.5 to +2.5 mm Hg in men. These data suggest that chronic and increased low SES, low social support, and high stress may contribute to the development of hypertension among blacks.

Aggregate measures of an individual's attainment of durable goods also appear to have a role in the relationship between education and BP. A recent study by Kaufman and colleagues suggests interactions between possession of material goods and level of education among populations of African origin in the United States, Africa, and the Caribbean. Unlikely previously reported associations between education and hypertension in the United States, in this report education was actually associated with a greater, not lesser, risk of hypertension among Caribbean women (odds ration 1.69, confidence interval [CI], 1.15–2.48).

SES and Hypertension-Related Disease Outcomes

SES not only influences risk for hypertension and other cardiovascular diseases, but lower SES also appears to predict a less desirable outcome from hypertension-related sequelae. Blacks have a higher incidence of ESRD compared with their white counterparts. It has been postulated that SES may be a significant factor contributing to the racial disparity of all-cause and hypertension-induced disease. Sixteen-year follow-up data from the prospective Multiple Risk Factor Intervention Trial (MRFIT) involving 332 544 black and white men, aged 35 to 57 years, estimated the risk of incident ESRD relative to BP and income. In both racial groups, higher BP and lower income was associated with an increased incidence of ESRD. The magnitude of risk, however, was greater among black men. After adjustment for covariates using a proportional hazards model, the relative risk (RR) of all-cause ESRD among black men was 1.87 (95% CI, 1.47–2.39) and the RR for hypertensive ESRD was even greater, 2.42 (95% CI, 1.52–3.84). These findings suggest that black men may be more susceptible to the deleterious effects of elevated BP than white men.

Overall, ethnic patterns of hypertensive-disease burden, BP control, and ultimately pressure-related clinical complications are influenced by geography, SES, secular trends, lifestyle attributes, dietary practices, psychosocial stressors, and, almost assuredly, other unknown factors. In turn, hypertension contrasts across SES strata are influenced by the same, and perhaps other, factors. Though genetic factors undoubtedly influence hypertension risk, the role of genetics in explaining racial/ethnic differentials in hypertension and its sequelae remains to be elucidated. Future research that focuses more on the understanding of intraethnic group disease variation will be fruitful. Such research will be the logical sequel to the increasingly greater recognition of the substantial within-group variation in the determinants of hypertension (including genetic susceptibility), overall hypertension risk, and the expression of adverse pressure-related clinical sequelae.

SUGGESTED READING

1. Burt VL, Whelton P, Roccella EJ, Brown C, Cutler JA, Higgins M, Horan MJ, Labarthe D. Prevalence of hypertension in the US adult population: results from the Third National Health and Nutrition Examination Survey, 1988–1991. *Hypertension.* 1995;25:305–313.
2. Cooper RS, McFarlane-Anderson N, Bennett FI, Wilks R, Tewsbury D, Ward R, Forrester T. ACE, angiotensinogen and obesity: a potential pathway leading to hypertension. *J Hum Hypertens.* 1997;11:107–111.
3. Flack JM, Neaton JD, Daniels B, Esunge P. Ethnicity and renal disease: lessons from the Multiple Risk Factor Intervention trial and the Treatment of Mild Hypertension Study. *Am J Kidney Dis.* 1993;21(suppl 1):31–40.
4. Ganguli MC, Grimm RH Jr, Svendsen KH, Flack JM, Grandits GA, Elmer PJ. Higher education and income are related to a better Na:K ratio in blacks. Baseline results of the Treatment of Mild Hypertension Study (TOMHS) data. *Am J Hypertens.* 1997;10:979–984.
5. Hall WD, Ferrario CM, Moore MA, Hall JE, Flack JM, Cooper W, Simmons JD, Egan BM, Lackland DT, Perry M Jr, Roccella EJ. Hypertension-related morbidity and mortality in the southeastern United States. *Am J Med Sci.* 1997;313:195–209.
6. Kaufman JS< Tracy JA, Durazo-Arvizu RA, Cooper RS. Lifestyle, education, and prevalence of hypertension in populations of African origin: results from the International Collaborative Study on Hypertension in Blacks. *Ann Epidemiol.* 1997;7:22–27.
7. Kiefe CI, Williams OD, Bild DE, Lewis CE, Hilner JE, Oberman A. Regional disparities in the incidence of elevated blood pressure among young adults: the CARDIA study. *Circulation.* 1997;96:1082–1088.
8. Klag MJ, Whelton PK, Randall BL, Neaton JD, Brancati FL, Stamler J. End-stage renal disease in African American and white men: 16-year MRFIT findings. *JAMA.* 1997;277:1293–1298.
9. Strogatz DS, Croft JB, James SA, Keenan NL, Browning SR, Garrett JM, Curtis AB. Social support, stress, and blood pressure in black adults. *Epidemiology.* 1997;8:482–487.
10. Svetkey LP, George LK, Tyroler HA, Timmons PZ, Burchett BM, Blazer DG. Effects of gender and ethnic group on blood pressure control in the elderly. *Am J Hypertens.* 1996;9:529–535.

Chapter 88

Socioeconomic Status and Blood Pressure

Daniel W. Jones, MD

KEY POINTS

- Socioeconomic status has an inverse relationship with blood pressure levels and hypertension prevalence in most populations.

- Low socioeconomic status predicts poor outcomes in hypertensive individuals.

- Most of the adverse effect of low socioeconomic status in hypertensives can be overcome by removal of social and economic barriers to health care and by adoption of healthier lifestyles.

See also Chapters 67, 96

The relationship between social status and health is generally inverse and is described for a large number of disease processes and diverse populations. The most commonly used markers of socioeconomic status are educational level and income. Most data regarding the relationship with blood pressure use arbitrary cutoffs for hypertension. The strength of the association is most likely underestimated by lower blood pressure cutoff points.

Socioeconomic Status and Hypertension Prevalence

An inverse relationship between socioeconomic status and blood pressure has been reported in a large number of observational studies. This relationship persists despite significant diversity in design, geography, race, and age in these studies. In the United States, the National Health and Nutrition Examination Surveys (NHANES I, II, and III) have all demonstrated this inverse relationship. NHANES II reported a mean diastolic blood pressure (DBP) 2 to 6 mm Hg lower for those with >13 years of education versus <9 years (depending on sex and race). Data from the INTERSALT Study showed that systolic blood pressure was 1.3 mm Hg higher in men and 4.5 mm Hg higher in women for each 10 fewer years of education.

Baseline data for the Hypertension Detection and Follow-up Program (HDFP) demonstrated a strong inverse relationship between educational status and hypertension prevalence. This study also showed that the effect on hypertension prevalence was strongest in blacks and at younger ages. In HDFP, blacks 30 to 49 years of age with a college education had a hypertension (DBP≥95 mm Hg or on medication) prevalence rate of 13.7% compared with 26.6% for those with <10 years of formal education.

Socioeconomic Status and Blood Pressure-Mechanisms

Few studies have attempted to explain the relationship between socioeconomic status and blood pressure. Proposed mechanisms include differences in diet (sodium, potassium, calories), physical activity, body mass, alcohol intake, exposure to trace metals (lead), psychosocial stress, and access to health care (including acceptance of and use of care). Obesity may be particularly important in this relationship in some groups. In HDFP, controlling for obesity reduced the association between socioeconomic status and hypertension prevalence among whites but not blacks. Other studies, including Intersalt, have demonstrated differences in sodium, potassium, and alcohol intake based on socioeconomic status. Attempts to demonstrate the importance of psychosocial factors are complicated by inadequate methodology and are confounded by race.

Socioeconomic Status and Hypertension-Related Target Organ Disease

End-stage renal disease (ESRD) is the hypertension-related target organ disease most studied. In a large ESRD incidence study, Whelton et al reported an odds ratio of 8.1 for blacks versus whites. Adjustment for socioeconomic factors reduced this ratio to 5.5, indicating a substantial socioeconomic effect. HDFP showed a higher prevalence of left ventricular hypertrophy at baseline in those in lower socioeconomic groups. Several studies have indicated an inverse relationship between socioeconomic status and cardiovascular disease mortality, including heart disease and stroke.

Socioeconomic Status and Treatment Effect

If individuals with a lower socioeconomic status as measured by income or education have a higher prevalence of hypertension, how much of this negative impact can be overcome by improving access to appropriate hypertension treatment? This was one of the central questions in the HDFP. In 14 communities in the United States, hypertensive patients identified through screening were randomly assigned to either a stepped-care program (the experimental group) or referred to their usual community sources of care (usual-care, the control group). The stepped-care program was designed to eliminate as many social and economic barriers to treatment as possible. In the usual-care group, lower socioeconomic status predicted lower clinic attendance, lower use of drugs, and lower achievement of goal blood pressure (DBP<90 mm Hg). Stepped-care eliminated much but not all of the influence of socioeconomic status on achievement of goal blood pressure. Also, all-cause mortality in the usual-care group was twice as high for those with less than a high school education as for high school graduates. The stepped-care program appeared to have eliminated much of this socioeconomic status gradient, and those at the lowest end of the scale appeared to have received the most benefit.

Socioeconomic Status and Health in Developing Societies

The relationship between hypertension (including its risk factors and target organ disease) and socioeconomic status is usually inverse as noted. Occasionally, though, it is absent or even direct in nature. In developing countries, markers of cardiovascular risk or disease sometimes initially show a positive relationship to socioeconomic status. Individuals with high socioeconomic status have the highest incidence of hypertension. Then, as countries become more developed, the risk factors move from those in the highest to the lowest socioeconomic groups. This phenomenon has been described in Great Britain and the United States. Recent studies from several Asian countries demonstrate a similar direct relationship for blood pressure and obesity.

Summary

In most populations, there is a strong inverse relationship between socioeconomic status and blood pressure (including hypertension prevalence, risk factors for hypertension, and hypertension-related target organ disease). Much of the adverse effect associated with lower socioeconomic status can be eliminated with systems that overcome social and economic barriers to health care and to adoption of healthier lifestyles.

SUGGESTED READING

1. Brogan DR, Lakatos E. Hypertension detection, treatment, and control in the United States: not as bad as it seems? *Am J Epidemiol.* 1986;124:738–745.
2. Daugherty SA. Hypertension Detection and Follow-up Program: description of the enumerated and screened population. *Hypertension.* 1983;5(suppl IV):IV 1-IV 43.
3. Holme I, Helgeland A, Hjermann I, Lund-Larsen PG, Leren P. Coronary risk factors and socioeconomic status: the Oslo study. *Lancet.* 1976;2:1396–1398.
4. Hypertension Detection and Follow-up Program Cooperative Group. Educational level and 5-year all-cause mortality in the hypertension detection and follow-up program. *Hypertension.* 1987;9:641–646.
5. Hypertension Detection and Follow-up Program Cooperative Group. Race, education, and prevalence of hypertension. *Am J Epidemiol.* 1977;106:351–361.
6. Liu K, Cedres LB, Stamler J, Dyer A, Stamler R, Nanas S, Berkson DM, Paul O, Lepper M, Lindberg HA, Marquardt J, Stevens E, Schoenberger JA, Shekelle RB, Collette P, Shekelle S, Garside D. Relationship of education to major risk factors and death from coronary heart disease, cardiovascular diseases, and all causes: findings of three Chicago epidemiologic studies. *Circulation.* 1982;66:1308–1314.
7. Marmot MG, Adelstein AM, Robinson N, Rose GA. Changing social-class distribution of heart disease. *Br Med J.* 1978;2:1109–1112.
8. Shulman N, Cutter G, Daugherty R, on behalf of the Hypertension Detection and Follow-up Program Cooperative Group. Correlates of attendance and compliance in the hypertension detection and follow-up program. *Control Clin Trials.* 1982;3:13–27.
9. Stamler R, Shipley M, Elliott P, Dyer A, Sans S, Stamler J. Higher blood pressure in adults with less education: Some explanations from INTERSALT. *Hypertension.* 1992;19:237–241.
10. Tyroler HA. Socioeconomic status, age, and sex in the prevalence and prognosis of hypertension in blacks and whites. In: Laragh JH, Brenner BM, eds. *Hypertension: Pathophysiology, Diagnosis, and Management.* 1st ed. New York, NY: Raven Press Ltd;1990:159–173.

Chapter 89

Overall Dietary Patterns and Blood Pressure

Frank M. Sacks, MD

KEY POINTS

- Populations eating mainly vegetarian diets have lower blood pressure levels, and their blood pressure increases less with age, than those eating omnivorous diets.

- Except for fish oil, which has a mild blood pressure–lowering effect, the type or amount of dietary fats does not affect blood pressure.

- A dietary pattern high in fruits and vegetables, high in low-fat dairy products, emphasizing fish and chicken rather than red meat, and low in saturated fat, cholesterol, sweets, and high-carbohydrate snacks lowered blood pressure.

- This diet lowered blood pressure in stage 1 hypertensive patients by amounts similar to drug monotherapy.

See also Chapters 90, 91, 92, 118

Dietary Patterns Associated With Low Blood Pressure

There are striking differences in the blood pressures of populations worldwide. Blood pressure is higher and rises more steeply with age in industrialized than in nonindustrialized societies. A predominantly vegetarian dietary pattern is often present in those cultures that have generally low blood pressure. In industrialized countries, vegetarians have lower average blood pressure levels than do comparable nearby nonvegetarian populations. The lowest average blood pressures in an industrialized country were found in strict vegetarians in Massachusetts ("macrobiotics") who consumed almost no animal products of any kind **(Figure 89.1)**. Their diet was very plentiful in whole grains, green leafy vegetables, squash, and root vegetables. The entire blood pressure distribution of the vegetarians was shifted to lower levels than the nonvegetarians who resided in the same area. This indicates that diet could have a population-wide effect on blood pressure. In clinical trials, less extreme vegetarian diets lowered blood pressure, although not to the levels of the strict vegetarian group. A dietary pattern that was high in potassium and polyunsaturated fats and low in starch, saturated fat, and cholesterol was inversely associated with blood pressure in a large population of US men. Prospective studies in the United States, one in women (Nurses Health Study) and the other in men (Health Professionals Follow-up Study), found that a high intake of fruits and vegetables was associated with lower blood pressure and less change in blood pressure with age, although dietary fat was not associated with blood pressure levels. These and other studies demonstrated the need to test dietary patterns and blood pressure by clinical trials.

The Dietary Approaches to Stop Hypertension (DASH) Trial

Epidemiological findings support several possible dietary changes to reduce blood pressure. The strongest evidence is for fruits and vegetables. Other hypotheses include increasing calcium intake, increasing vegetable oils or decreasing animal fats, increasing n-3 fatty acids as in fish oils, and increasing total or vegetable protein. DASH, a multicenter trial, tested two dietary patterns compared with a control dietary pattern that resembled average US intake: (1) a "combination" diet high in fruits, vegetables, whole-grain cereal products, low-fat dairy products, fish, chicken, and lean meats designed to be reduced in saturated fat, total fat, and cholesterol, moderately high in protein, and high in minerals and fiber, and (2) a "fruits-and-vegetables" diet that tested the effect of fruits and vegetables alone and was similar in other nutrients to the control dietary pattern. All food for the experimental diets was provided to the participants. The experimental diets were eaten for 8 weeks. The dietary patterns were constructed with commonly consumed food items, so that the results could be conveniently implemented in dietary recommendations to the general public. The study population consisted of 459 healthy men and women, mean age 44 years, with systolic blood pressure <160 mm Hg and diastolic blood pressure 80 to 95 mm Hg. The blood pressures of the population would be classified as either stage 1 hypertension, high-normal, or normal. Blacks composed 60% of the population. It is important to emphasize that sodium intakes were the same in all diets and that the participants maintained their prestudy body weights during the trial.

The combination diet reduced blood pressure significantly, by 5.5 mm Hg systolic and 3.0 mm Hg diastolic, according to measurements made in the clinics, and 4.5 mm Hg systolic and 2.7 mm Hg diastolic for 24-hour ambulatory measurements **(Figure 89.2)**. In contrast, the fruits-and-vegetables diet reduced blood pressure by about half this amount, −2.8/−1.1 mm Hg for clinic and −3.1/−2.1 mm Hg for ambulatory readings. The effects of the dietary patterns were similar in men and women. The blood pressure reductions in black participants were greater than those in whites. The diets were more effective in hypertensives than in those with high-normal or normal blood pressure. In hypertensives, who composed 29% of the group, the reductions in blood pressure were −11.4/−5.5 mm Hg for the combination diet and −7.2/−2.8 mm Hg for the fruits-and-vegetables diet. The therapeutic effects of the combination diet in the hy-

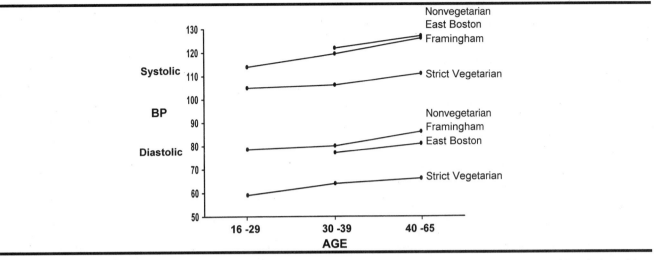

Figure 89.1. Blood pressure in a strict vegetarian population in Boston and in nonvegetarian populations in East Boston and Framingham, Mass. Adapted from Sacks FM, Kass EH. Low blood pressure in vegetarians: effects of specific foods and nutrients. *Am J Clin Nutr.* 1988;48:795–800.

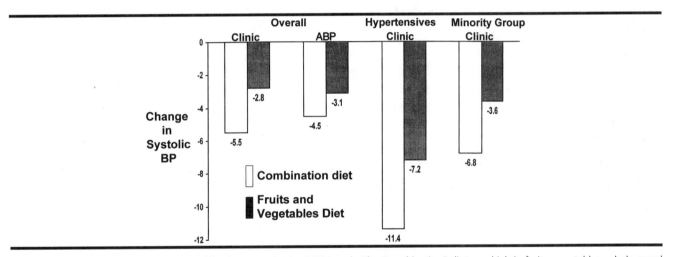

Figure 89.2. Effect of dietary patterns on blood pressure in the DASH study. The "combination" diet was high in fruits, vegetables, whole-cereal products, low-fat dairy products, fish, chicken, and lean meats and was designed to be reduced in saturated fat, total fat, and cholesterol, reduced in sweets and high-carbohydrate snacks, and high in minerals and fiber. The "fruits-and-vegetables" diet was high in fruits and vegetables but was similar in other nutrients to the control dietary pattern resembling average intake in the United States. ABP: Ambulatory Blood Pressure.

pertensives approached the magnitude of pharmacological treatment with a single drug over the 8 weeks of the study.

Foods or Nutrients Responsible for the Effects of the DASH Diet

Fruits and Vegetables

If we compare the blood pressure lowering caused by the fruits-and-vegetables diet with that caused by the combination diet, it may be surmised that the high intake of fruits and vegetables was responsible for ≈50% of the effect of the combination diet. Fruits and vegetables are high in potassium, magnesium, fiber, and many other nutrients. Of these, potassium is the most well-established for lowering blood pressure, particularly in persons with low potassium intake or with hypertension and in blacks. The DASH population had these characteristics associated with potassium-sensitive blood pressure, and the magnitude of blood pressure lowering in the fruits-

and-vegetables group is similar to that in potassium trials in such populations. Thus, a plausible explanation is that raising potassium intake by fruits and vegetables from a low intake, 1700 mg (44 mmol), to a high level, 4100 mg (105 mmol), reduced blood pressure.

Other Foods and Nutrients

Aside from testing fruits and vegetables, the DASH study was not designed to determine which additional foods or nutrients were responsible for the overall blood pressure–lowering effect. Compared with the fruits-and-vegetables diet, the combination diet had somewhat more vegetables, low-fat dairy products, poultry, fish, calcium, magnesium, potassium, protein, and cereal grains and was lower in saturated, monounsaturated, and total fat, as well as cholesterol, red meat, sweets, and high-carbohydrate snacks. Overall, trials that tested certain of these nutrients individually, eg, fat, fiber, calcium, or magnesium, have not found effects on blood pressure that could account for the effects of the DASH combination diet. However, it could be that very small hypotensive effects of several nutrients, too small to be detected in a clinical trial or in a meta-analysis, eg, 0.5 to 1 mm Hg, could combine to reduce blood pressure. Alternative explanations include the possibility that a nutrient in the combination diet that has blood pressure–lowering properties has not yet been identified or that the combination dietary pattern itself has a unique effect.

Dietary Fats and Blood Pressure

In two large US populations, one in female nurses and the other in male health professionals, neither the type nor the amount of dietary fats was related to the emergence of hypertension or blood pressure changes during 4 years of follow-up. In another US population of men, blood pressure was positively associated with saturated fats and inversely with polyunsaturated fats. The effects of saturated, monounsaturated, and polyunsaturated (linoleic acid) fatty acids and carbohydrates have been studied in many clinical trials. In most trials, replacing animal fat with either carbohydrates or unsaturated vegetable oils did not lower blood pressure in either normotensive or hypertensive patients. In particular, the larger and better-designed trials found no significant effect.

Fish Oil

From a physiological viewpoint, it is attractive to propose that fish oil lowers blood pressure. Fish oil has highly unsaturated fatty acids that stimulate vasodilating prostaglandins and inhibit platelet aggregation and the consequent release of vasoconstrictors. Fish oil is often prescribed as capsules that contain 1 mL of purified oil or as crude cod liver oil. Large doses of fish oil, eg, 30 to 45 mL, clearly lower blood pressure levels in hypertensive patients. However, intervention trials of moderate, more practical amounts of fish oil were inconsistent. Meta-analysis of these trials found a small hypotensive effect (3/1.5 mm Hg) of 10 to 15 mL of fish oil, particularly in hypertensive patients. A smaller dose, eg, 6 capsules daily, had no effect in either hypertensive or normotensive persons. The unpleasant taste of the fish oil and belching interfere with compliance. Therefore, fish oil is not considered to be a practical therapy for hypertension.

Dietary Protein, Carbohydrate, and Fiber

Vegetarians have relatively low protein intake, although in almost all cases it is above the Recommended Dietary Allowance. In Japan, in contrast, a high protein intake is associated with a low incidence of hypertension. Several small trials did not find that the type or amount of protein affects blood pressure, although the possibility of modest effects, eg, 2 to 3 mm Hg, cannot be ruled out. When substituted for fat, carbohydrate has not lowered blood pressure in most trials. However, the type of carbohydrate has not been studied adequately. It is possible that complex or unrefined carbohydrate that produces a low glucose and insulin response affects blood pressure differently than does sugar or refined carbohydrate, eg, white bread. Dietary fiber includes a variety of nonabsorbable biochemicals found mainly in plants. In two large epidemiological studies, a high dietary fiber intake was associated with low blood pressure and a decreased incidence of hypertension. Fruit fiber but not vegetable fiber was apparently protective; but because fruits, as a group, were protective, it is difficult to definitively identify the fiber as the cause as opposed to another nutrient in fruits, such as potassium. Controlled trials failed to confirm a hypotensive effect of various fibers, although the study populations were relatively small.

Applications to Public Health and Clinical Practice

The DASH trial proved that an overall dietary pattern that is high in fruits and vegetables, is high in low-fat dairy products, emphasizes fish and chicken rather than red meat, and is low in red meat, saturated fat and cholesterol, sweets, and high-carbohydrate snacks lowered blood pressure and is likely to protect against the development of hypertension and its complications. DASH also proved that fruits and vegetables lower blood pressure. If the population shifted to this type of diet, the blood pressure distribution would shift to lower levels, reducing the incidence of cardiovascular disease. For clinicians, the blood pressure reductions demonstrate an alternative to drug therapy as initial therapy for stage 1 hypertension. The Sixth Joint National Committee on the Prevention, Detection, Evaluation, and Treatment of Hypertension endorsed the results of DASH and recommended the DASH diet for the population and clinical practice.

SUGGESTED READING

1. Appel LJ, Moore TJ, Obarzanek E, Vollmer WM, Svetkey LP, Sacks FM, Bray GA, Vogt TM, Cutler JA, Windhauser MM, Lin PH, Karanja N. A clinical trial of the effects of dietary patterns on blood pressure: DASH Collaborative Research Group. *N Engl J Med.* 1997;336:1117–1124.

2. Ascherio A, Hennekens CH, Willett WC, Sacks FM, Rosner B, Manson J, Witteman J, Stampfer MJ. Prospective study of nutritional factors, blood pressure, and hypertension among US women. *Hypertension.* 1996;27:1065–1072.

3. Ascherio A, Rimm EB, Giovannucci EL, Colditz GA, Rosner B, Willett WC, Sacks FM, Stampfer MJ. A prospective study of nutritional factors and hypertension among US men. *Circulation.* 1992;86:1475–1484.

4. Morris MC, Sacks FM. Dietary fats and blood pressure. In: Swales JD, ed. *Textbook of Hypertension.* Oxford, UK: Blackwell; 1994:605–618.

5. Morris MC, Sacks FM, Rosner B. Does fish oil lower blood pressure: a meta-analysis of controlled trials. *Circulation.* 1993;88:523–533.

6. Obarzanek E, Velletri PA, Cutler JA. Dietary protein and blood pressure. *JAMA.* 1996;275:1598–1603.

7. Sacks FM, Kass EH. Low blood pressure in vegetarians: effects of specific foods and nutrients. *Am J Clin Nutr.* 1988;48:795–800.

8. Stamler J, Caggiula A, Grandits GA, Kjelsberg M, Cutler JA, for the MRFIT Research Group. Relationship to blood pressure of combinations of dietary macronutrients: findings of the Multiple Risk Factor Intervention Trial (MRFIT). *Circulation.* 1996;94:2417–2423.

Chapter 90

Salt and Blood Pressure

Norman M. Kaplan, MD

KEY POINTS

- For hypertension to develop, sodium intake beyond a certain threshold level is probably essential, but other genetic and environmental factors may modify its effect.

- In multiple population studies, the slope of blood pressure rise with age is significantly related to the level of sodium intake.

- Moderate sodium reduction to a level of 100 mmol/d is reasonably easy to achieve, and there are no dangers or discomfort in doing so. In properly controlled randomized trials, sodium reduction lowered blood pressure significantly.

- With the ability to identify hidden salt by the provision of improved labeling and the provision of more processed foods with less sodium in them, more people will be able to achieve a moderate degree of sodium reduction.

See also Chapters 48, 89, 91, 116

The epidemiological evidence for the involvement of sodium in the pathogenesis of essential hypertension is in keeping with an essential role for this element. The evidence is and will continue to be indirect, because direct proof of the role of any ubiquitous environmental factor in the pathogenesis of a slowly developing disorder that follows polygenic inheritance presents formidable difficulties. Experimental data from animals can support the epidemiological evidence, as can observations on relatively short-term manipulations of dietary intake. But to demand complete understanding of the role of sodium or any other factor before we can embark on either preventive or therapeutic maneuvers would paralyze all rational action.

The most convincing experimental study is that of Denton et al on free-living chimpanzees, the species closest to humans, with >98% genetic identity. Ten chimpanzees were given progressively increasing amounts of dietary sodium over the range ingested by humans; the others remained on their usual low-sodium diet. Over the 89 weeks of the study, the blood pressure (BP) rose an average of 33/10 mm Hg, only to return to baseline after 20 weeks without added sodium. A response was seen in 7 of the 10 animals on extra sodium.

Sodium or Chloride

Considerable animal data and increasing human evidence support a parallel need for both sodium and chloride in the pathogenesis of hypertension. Other salts of sodium do not induce changes in BP, nor does chloride given with other cations. The issue is largely academic, because chloride is the major anion accompanying sodium in the diet and in body fluids.

Population Studies

In most populations, a correlation exists between the levels of usual dietary sodium intake (almost always estimated from 24-hour urine sodium excretion) and the average BP (**Figure 90.1**). Elliott plotted the data from 28 populations around the world for 50-year-old men, showing a significantly positive association that has a slope of 10 mm Hg for systolic blood pressure per 100 mmol of dietary sodium. The relation between mean sodium intake and the change of slope of blood pressure with age, as estimated from pressures taken among subjects 20 and 50 years old, is also significantly positive.

In their analysis of 24 studies involving 47 000 people, Law et al found that a difference in sodium intake of 100 mmol/d was associated with an average difference in systolic BP that increased progressively with the age of the population. This difference averaged 5 mm Hg at age 15 to 19 years and 10 mm Hg at age 60 to 69 years. The differences in diastolic BP were ≈50% of those for systolic pressure. The association was also related to the initial level of BP: the higher the pressure, the greater the difference with changes in sodium excretion.

These data, collected from numerous investigators using disparate techniques for measurements of BP and sodium excretion, are subject to various degrees of bias and confounding factors, such as body weight. The greatest source of error is the large day-to-day variation of sodium intake (and excretion) within individuals, so that individuals may be grossly misclassified regarding their habitual sodium intake. As a result of this large variation in individual BP and sodium intake, ie, within-population data, most studies of individuals fail to show an association between the two, whereas the association is readily shown by studies of average BP and sodium intake of different populations, ie, between-population data.

In addition to the problem of day-to-day variation, a number of confounding factors could alter the relation. Therefore, Elliott examined only the 14 published studies in which appropriate safeguards for data collection and analysis were available, using a coefficient of reliability for sodium estimated from repeated measures to be 0.46. The overview of these population-based studies reveals statistically significant (all with probability values <0.001) positive relations, but with lesser values than shown in the plot of all 28 studies (**Table 90.1**).

Many of the methodological problems were addressed in the massive Intersalt study, in which 200 people from each of 52 centers worldwide had BP and 24-hour urine measurements according to a strict, uniform protocol. Among the entire 10 079 men and women 20 to 59 years old, sodium excretion in individual subjects within

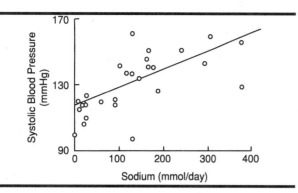

Figure 90.1. Scatterplot showing across-population association between mean systolic blood pressure and mean 24-hour sodium excretion for 28 populations in men 50 years old (slope *b,* 9.97 mm Hg/100 mmol sodium; *P*<.001; SE, 1.99). Reproduced with permission from Elliott P. Observational studies of salt and blood pressure. *Hypertension.* 1991;17(suppl I):I-3-I-8.

Table 90.1. Overview of Population-Based Studies of 24-Hour Urinary Sodium Excretion and Blood Pressure: Pooled Regression Slopes *b* (SE) (mm Hg/100 mmol Sodium) by Sex and for Men and Women Combined

	N	SYSTOLIC BP *b* (SE)*	DIASTOLIC BP *b* (SE)*
Men	7099	1.78 (0.66)	1.55 (0.42)
Women	6136	4.80 (0.98)	2.02 (0.59)
Men and Women Combined	12 503	3.65 (0.62)	1.98 (0.37)

BP indicates blood pressure.
*Corrected for reliability by use of Intersalt estimate of 0.46.
Reproduced with permission from Elliott P. Observational studies of salt and blood pressure. *Hypertension.* 1991;17(suppl I): I-3-I-8.

separate centers was significantly related to BP. In four remote, rural, unacculturated populations, sodium excretion was <50 mmol/d and BPs were very low, with virtually none in the hypertensive range, and there was no upward slope of BP with age. In the other 48 centers with sodium excretion >100 mmol/d, sodium was significantly related to the slope of BP with age **(Figure 90.2)**. Over a 30-year period, 100 mmol/d lower sodium intake was associated with 9 to 11 mm Hg lower systolic and 5 to 6 mm Hg lower diastolic pressure.

Threshold Effect

These data suggest a threshold relation between sodium intake and hypertension: Those who ingest less than the amount required for a hypertensinogenic effect of sodium do not develop hypertension. Those who ingest more than the amount required will develop hypertension if they have the requisite genetic makeup and unless they are exposed to such other interacting environmental cofactors as high potassium intake. Once above the threshold level, the relationship tends to be linear.

The lower limit below which hypertension does not develop is probably ≈50 mmol/d sodium, and intakes >100 mmol/d are enough to induce hypertension. Unfortunately, neither Elliott's nor Intersalt's multiple populations had any groups within the range of 50 to 100 mmol/d, so the exact threshold is uncertain.

Preventive Studies

In the Trials of Hypertension Prevention phase 2 study, a moderate reduction of dietary sodium intake has been shown to significantly reduce the incidence of hypertension in people with high-normal BP, in the 83 to 89 mm Hg diastolic range. Although the <2 mm Hg fall in BP overall may not seem like much in an individual patient, a population-wide reduction of even such a small degree would have a major impact on reducing the incidence of hypertension and, presumably, of cardiovascular complications.

The potential for prevention was demonstrated by Hofman et al in a study on 486 newborn infants, half of whom were assigned to a usual-sodium diet, the other half to a low-sodium diet for the first 6 months of life. At 6 months, the sodium intake of the low-sodium group was only one third that of the normal-sodium group, and their mean systolic BP was 2.1 mm Hg lower. Among the 35% of the participants who could be traced 15 years later, those originally on the low-sodium diet had 3.6/2.2 mm Hg lower blood pressure despite the absence of any demonstrated difference in current sodium intake.

Therapeutic Studies

A much larger number of controlled studies have been performed on hypertensive subjects to determine whether sodium reduction will reduce established high BP. Cutler et al analyzed 22 trials of reduced sodium intake that met their rigid inclusion criteria, involving 1043 hypertensive subjects. Weighted linear-regression analyses across the trials showed an overall decrease of 5.8/2.5 mm Hg for a 100-mmol/d reduction in sodium excretion. Midgley et al analyzed

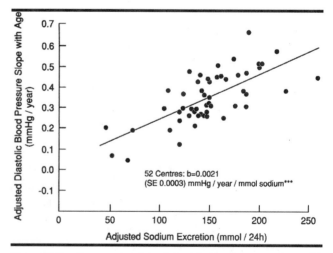

Figure 90.2. Cross-center plots of diastolic blood pressure slope with age and median sodium excretion and fitted regression lines for 52 centers, also adjusted for body mass index and alcohol intake. ***P*<.001. Reproduced with permission from Intersalt Cooperative Research Group. Intersalt: an international study of electrolyte excretion and blood pressure: results from 24-hour urinary sodium and potassium excretion. *BMJ.* 1988;297:319–328.

23 trials with 1131 hypertensive subjects who met their inclusion criteria of randomized allocation to control and sodium-reduction groups; monitored, timed sodium excretion; and outcome measures of both systolic and diastolic BP. The overall decrease in BP for a 100-mmol/d reduction in urinary sodium excretion was 3.9/0.9 mm Hg; in the 17 trials involving subjects ≥45 years (as the overwhelming majority of hypertensive patients would be), the decrease was a highly significant 6.3/2.2 mm Hg.

Hypertensive individuals vary in their sensitivity to sodium intake. In none of the studies analyzed by Cutler et al or Midgley et al were the subjects tested for sodium sensitivity. Clearly, some hypertensive persons who are more sodium-sensitive will achieve greater falls in BP from moderate sodium restriction than others who are less sodium-sensitive. However, there seems little reason to test patients for sodium sensitivity before prescribing moderately reduced dietary intake.

Putative Dangers of Sodium Reduction

Testing for sodium sensitivity appears to be unnecessary, for two simple reasons: Moderate sodium reduction to a level of 100 mmol/d is reasonably easy to achieve, and there are no dangers or discomfort in doing so. Critics of universal moderate sodium reduction have raised the specter of multiple potential hazards from this practice **(Table 90.2)**. A number of hazards have been seen in severely sodium-restricted experimental animals that were exposed to major stresses at sodium levels comparable to <10 mmol/d in humans. However, such hazards have rarely if ever been documented in humans, and certainly not in those whose dietary sodium intake is moderately reduced.

In a 3-year follow-up of almost 3000 treated hypertensive patients, Alderman et al noted that among the 483 men whose initial urinary sodium excretion in a single specimen collected after 4 days of reduced sodium intake was in the lowest quintile (averaging 65 mmol/d), myocardial infarctions occurred in 22. Among the 475 men in the highest sodium quintile, only 4 myocardial infarctions were seen. There were, however, no increases in infarctions among the women with lower sodium excretion or of strokes in men or women. Moreover, there was no ascertainment of sodium intake after the single urine collection, and a number of possible confounding factors were not controlled for.

Concern over these data led Kumanyika and Cutler to evaluate the adverse effects noted in all 20 randomized trials of sodium reduction with at least 6 months' follow-up published between 1984 and 1996. They found "no adverse effects of moderate reductions in sodium intake in controlled trials conducted in diverse settings and involving frequent monitoring of more than 3000 individuals for as long as 5 years."

Lest there be concern that people asked to lower sodium moderately may go overboard and restrict their intake down to the very low levels at which potential hazards might arise, remember that the average percentage of decrease in sodium intake achieved in multiple clinical trials was only about one third of baseline intake despite intensive counseling and careful follow-up. In routine clinical practice, most patients may be hard put to achieve even that degree of dietary reduction. With the ability to identify hidden salt by the provision of improved labeling and the provision of more processed foods with less sodium in them, more people will be able to achieve the moderate degree of sodium reduction that will provide significant decreases of established high BP and a meaningful protection against the development of hypertension.

Table 90.2. Putative Dangers of Sodium Restriction

| | LEVELS OF SODIUM RESTRICTION | |
DANGER	VERY LOW (0–20 MMOL/D)	MODERATE (70–120 MMOL/D)
Less cardiovascular reserve with Na+ depletion (exercising in hot weather)	+	−
Inability to reconstitute losses (acute gastrointestinal)	+	−
Danger to susceptible patients (Addisonian, Na-wasting nephritis)	+	−
Activation of renin-angiotensin and other deleterious responses	+	−
Decreased intake of other nutrients	?	−
Diminished enjoyment of food	+	−

SUGGESTED READING

1. Alderman MH, Madhavan S, Cohen H, Sealey JE, Laragh JH. Low urinary sodium is associated with greater risk of myocardial infarction among treated hypertensive men. *Hypertension.* 1995;25:1144–1152.
2. Cutler JA, Follmann D, Allender PS. Randomized trials of sodium reduction: an overview. *Am J Clin Nutr.* 1997;65(suppl):643S–651S.
3. Denton D, Weisinger R, Mundy NI, Wickings EJ, Dixson A, Moisson P, Pingard AM, Shade R, Carey D, Ardaillou R, et al. The effect of increased salt intake on blood pressure of chimpanzees. *Nat Med.* 1995;1:1009–1016.
4. Elliott P. Observational studies of salt and blood pressure. *Hypertension.* 1991;17(suppl I):I-3-I-8.
5. Elliott P, Stamler J, Nichols R, Dyer AR, Stamler R, Kesteloot H, Marmot M, for the Intersalt Cooperative Research Group. Intersalt revisited: further analyses of 24-hour sodium excretion and blood pressure within and across populations. *BMJ.* 1996;312:1249–1253.
6. Hofman A, Hazebroek A, Valkenburg HA. A randomized trial of sodium intake and blood pressure in newborn infants. *JAMA.* 1983;250:370–373.
7. Kumanyika SK, Cutler JA. Dietary sodium reduction: is there cause for concern? *J Am Coll Nutr.* 1997;16:192–203.
8. Law MR, Frost CD, Wald NJ. By how much does dietary salt reduction lower blood pressure? I: analysis of observational data among populations. *BMJ.* 1991;302:811–815.
9. Midgley JP, Matthew AG, Greenwood CM, Logan AG. Effect of reduced dietary sodium on blood pressure: a meta-analysis of randomized controlled trials. *JAMA.* 1996;275:1590–1597.
10. The Trials of Hypertension Prevention Collaborative Research Group. Effects of weight loss and sodium reduction intervention on blood pressure and hypertension incidence in overweight people with high-normal blood pressure: the Trials of Hypertension Prevention, phase II. *Arch Intern Med.* 1997;157:657–667.

Chapter 91

Potassium and Blood Pressure

Paul K. Whelton, MD, MSc

KEY POINTS

- Many studies suggest that potassium intake is inversely related to systolic and diastolic blood pressure. Potassium deficiency may play a special role in the strikingly high incidence and prevalence of hypertension in American blacks.

- Increased potassium intake reduces both systolic and diastolic blood pressure. This effect is more pronounced in hypertensives than in normotensives, in blacks than in whites, and in those consuming a high intake of sodium. Increased potassium intake, in combination with weight loss, sodium restriction, moderation in alcohol consumption, and increased physical activity, may provide the optimal means for prevention and treatment of hypertension.

- Increased potassium intake may provide cardioprotective benefits that are independent of its effects on blood pressure.

See also Chapters 24, 89, 90, 118

High blood pressure is among the most important of the modifiable risk factors for cardiovascular disease. With the exception of relatively isolated societies, there is a tendency for blood pressure levels to rise progressively with increasing age. Evidence from a variety of sources, including interpopulation and migrant studies, suggests that poor nutrition habits and physical inactivity play an important role in the genesis of age-related increases in blood pressure and in the occurrence of hypertension. Weight gain, alcohol consumption, excessive intake of sodium, and insufficient dietary potassium are the leading possibilities for nutritional causes of hypertension. Interest in the potassium–blood pressure relationship dates back to the early part of the 20th century, when increased potassium intake was advocated as a treatment for hypertension. Recent publications, including numerous cross-sectional studies in economically developed and economically developing countries as well as two meta-analyses of clinical trial results, have rekindled interest in the role of potassium as a means to prevent and treat hypertension.

Epidemiology

Cross-sectional studies conducted in the United States, Japan, England, Scotland, Sweden, Belgium, St Lucia, Kenya, Zaire, and China have identified an inverse relationship between blood pressure and various measures of serum, urine, and total body and dietary potassium. The most precise estimates come from the Intersalt study, a cross-sectional investigation conducted in 10 079 men and women 20 to 59 years old from 52 populations around the world. In this study, a 60 mmol/d higher level of urinary potassium excretion was associated with a 3.4 mm Hg (95% CI, 1.5 to 5.2 mm Hg) lower level of systolic and 1.9 mm Hg (95% CI, 0.7 to 3.0 mm Hg) lower level of diastolic blood pressure after adjustment for the potentially confounding influences of age, sex, body mass index, alcohol consumption, and urinary sodium excretion and correction for regression dilution bias. Epidemiological studies are also consistent with the suggestion that potassium deficiency may play a special role in the

strikingly high incidence and prevalence of hypertension in blacks and the elderly.

Isolated populations with a low prevalence of hypertension and a blunted age-related increase in blood pressure almost uniformly consume a diet that is relatively high in potassium and low in sodium content (**Table 91.1**). Potassium intake is often lower in economically developed countries than in isolated societies because commercially prepared foods are an important part of the diet, and potassium is frequently removed during the manufacturing process. Migration studies have identified a relationship between progressive diminution in potassium intake and increasing levels of blood pressure and hypertension. Typically, these changes have been noted in a setting in which there is a concurrent increase in sodium, calorie, and alcohol consumption and a decrease in physical activity. It has been hard to separate the independent contributions of each of these changes to the concurrent change in blood pressure. It is conceivable that they all play a role in the age-related increase in blood pressure that is so common in the United States and most other societies.

Clinical Trials

A critically important question is whether the previously mentioned inverse association between potassium intake and blood pressure is causal or merely reflects the presence of a confounding relationship between potassium and another variable that is causal. Clinical trials provide the most satisfactory study design for resolution of this question. Potassium was widely advocated as a means to lower blood pressure during the 1920s and 1930s. The rice/fruit diet of Kempner, which achieved great notoriety during the 1950s, was characterized by a relatively high content of potassium and a low sodium/potassium ratio. Kempner's diet, however, also resulted in weight loss and a variety of metabolic changes. During the 1960s and 1970s, Menelly, Dahl, and others conducted a series of animal experiments that suggested that potassium administration could blunt the rise in blood pressure after sodium loading in a variety of salt-sensitive rat models. Luft and colleagues reported similar findings in a series of metabolic studies during which humans were exposed to extremely high and extremely low intakes of dietary sodium. The first controlled trial of the efficacy of increased potassium intake in essential hypertension, however, was not reported until 1981. Since that time, a large number of randomized, controlled trials as well as many uncontrolled experimental studies have reported on the effect of increased and decreased potassium intake on blood pressure in both hypertensive and normotensive persons.

In a recent review, Whelton et al identified 33 randomized, controlled trials (2609 participants) in which the effects of an increased intake of potassium on blood pressure were evaluated. Of these, 21 trials (1560 participants) were conducted in hypertensive and 12 trials (1005 participants) in normotensive persons. In all but two trials, the dose of potassium prescribed in the active intervention arm was ≥60 mmol/d. The weighted mean net change in urinary potassium excretion for the intervention versus the control group was 53 mmol/24 h in the 31 trials in which such information was available. Overall, increased potassium intake was associated with a significant

reduction in mean (95% CI) systolic and diastolic blood pressure of 4.4 (2.5 to 6.4) and 2.5 (0.7 to 4.2) mm Hg, respectively (**Table 91.2**). After exclusion of one trial in which there was an extreme effect on systolic (−41 mm Hg) and diastolic (−17 mm Hg) blood pressure, the overall mean (95% CI) reduction was 3.1 (1.9 to 4.3) for systolic and 2.0 (0.5 to 3.4) mm Hg for diastolic blood pressure. Subgroup analysis suggested that the treatment effect was enhanced in hypertensives, blacks, and those consuming a high intake of sodium. In trials in which the participants were consuming a diet high in sodium content, there was a significant ($P<0.001$) dose-response relationship between 24-hour urinary potassium excretion and treatment effect size.

Using randomized, crossover design trials, Krishna et al demonstrated that short-term potassium depletion produces an increase in blood pressure in both hypertensive and normotensive persons.

Two randomized, controlled trials have explored the efficacy of increased potassium intake in reducing the need for antihypertensive drug therapy in patients with well-controlled hypertension. In a dietary modification trial conducted by Siani et al, an increased intake of potassium significantly reduced the need for antihypertensive drug therapy. In contrast, in a large and rigorously controlled trial of potassium chloride pill supplementation, Grimm et al were unable to identify any apparent effect of potassium supplementation on blood pressure. The fact that the participants in Grimm's study were concurrently counseled to reduce their salt intake may have blunted the effect of the potassium supplements.

Mechanism of Action

Various mechanisms have been proposed to explain the purported influence of potassium on blood pressure. These include a direct natriuretic effect, suppression of the renin-angiotensin and sympathetic nervous systems, an effect on kallikreins and eicosanoids, improvement of baroreceptor function, antagonism of the effects of natriuretic hormone, and direct arterial vasodilatation, resulting in a reduction of peripheral vascular resistance. Many studies have demonstrated short-term changes in sodium excretion, but it re-

Table 91.1. Urinary Excretion of Potassium and Sodium/Potassium Ratio in Seven Low-Blood-Pressure Populations*

POPULATION	URINARY POTASSIUM, MMOL/24 H	URINARY SODIUM/ POTASSIUM RATIO
Yanomamo Indians, Brazil	152	0.01
Kung Bushman, Botswana	70–103	0.28–0.44
Xingu Indians, Brazil	78–96	0.19–0.20
Asaro Valley, Papua New Guinea	62–79	0.53–0.70
Luo tribesmen, Kenya	32–35	1.9
Yi farmers, China	48–59	1.4–3.4

*Data from Reference 2.

Table 91.2. Pooled Estimates of Change in Blood Pressure After Potassium Supplementation in 33 Randomized, Controlled Clinical Trials*

TRIALS IN ANALYSIS (N)	SYSTOLIC BLOOD PRESSURE		DIASTOLIC BLOOD PRESSURE	
	MEAN CHANGE	95% CI	MEAN CHANGE	95% CI
All trials (n=33)	−4.44	−2.53, −6.36	−2.45	−0.74, −4.16
Obel trial excluded (n=32)	−3.11	−1.91, −4.31	−1.97	−0.52, −3.42
Hypertensive trials† (n=20)	−4.4	−2.2, −6.6	−2.5	−0.1, −4.9
Normotensive trials (n=12)	−1.8	−0.6, −2.9	−1.0	−0.0, −2.1
Trials in blacks† (n=6)	−5.6	−2.4, −8.7	−3.0	−0.7, −5.3
Trials in whites (n=25)	−2.0	−0.9, −3.0	−1.1	−0.1, −2.1
Urinary Na, mmol /d‡				
<140 (n=10)	−1.2	0.0, −2.4	0.1	1.1, −1.0
140–164 (n=10)	−2.1	−0.3, −4.0	−1.4	0.0, −2.8
≥165 (n=10)	−7.3	−4.6, −10.1	−4.7	−1.1, −8.3

*Data from Reference 8.
†Excludes outlier trial by Obel AO.
‡Urinary sodium excretion during follow-up.

mains unclear whether any long-term effects on blood pressure can be ascribed to a decrease in intravascular volume resulting from this initial and transient natriuresis.

Vasculoprotective Effect

In addition to its hypotensive effects, increased potassium intake may have independent vasculoprotective properties. In a series of animal models, including both spontaneously hypertensive and Dahl salt-sensitive rats, Tobian reported that the addition of either potassium chloride or potassium citrate markedly reduced the probability of death from a stroke. Khaw and Barrett-Conner examined the relationship between 24-hour dietary potassium intake at baseline and subsequent stroke-associated mortality in a population-based cohort of 859 men and women 50 to 79 years old living in a retirement community in southern California. Over 12 years of follow-up, 24 stroke-associated deaths occurred, and the relative risk of death from a stroke in the lowest versus the two highest tertiles of potassium intake at baseline was 2.6 ($P=0.16$) for men and 4.8 ($P=0.01$) for women. In multivariate analysis, a 10 mmol higher intake of potassium at baseline was associated with a 40% reduction in stroke mortality ($P<0.001$), independent of age, sex, blood pressure, blood cholesterol level, obesity, fasting glucose level, and a number of dietary variables, including intake of calories, fat, protein, fiber, calcium, magnesium, and alcohol. An inverse relationship has also been noted between mean 24-hour urinary potassium excretion in Intersalt populations and corresponding national stroke mortality experience in 25 countries. In the World Health Organization Cardiovascular Diseases and Alimentary Comparison Study, age-adjusted stroke mortality in 19 centers in 14 countries was significantly ($P<0.05$) and positively related to the mean ratio of urinary sodium/potassium ratio in both sexes. Evidence from a number of epidemiological studies suggests that stroke mortality is inversely related to intake of vegetables and fruits. These reports are consistent with a vasculoprotective effect of increased potassium intake, albeit they provide only indirect evidence in favor of the hypothesis.

Summary

An increased intake of potassium tends to lower blood pressure in both hypertensive and normotensive persons. In combination with other nonpharmacological approaches, such as weight loss, reduced sodium intake, moderation in alcohol consumption, and enhanced physical activity, increased intake of potassium may provide the optimal means for prevention and treatment of hypertension, but it is unlikely to be as important as these other approaches. Increasing potassium intake may play an especially important role in lowering blood pressure among certain subgroups of the population, such as the elderly and blacks.

SUGGESTED READING

1. Cappuccio FP, MacGregor GA. Does potassium supplementation lower blood pressure? A meta-analysis of published trials. *J Hypertens.* 1991;9:465–473.
2. He J, Whelton PK. Potassium, blood pressure, and cardiovascular disease: an epidemiologic perspective. *Cardiol Rev.* 1997;5:255–260.
3. Intersalt Cooperative Research Group. Intersalt: an international study of electrolyte excretion and blood pressure: results for 24 hour urinary sodium and potassium excretion. *BMJ.* 1988;297:319–328.
4. Khaw KT, Barrett-Connor E. Dietary potassium and stroke-associated mortality: a 12-year prospective population study. *N Engl J Med.* 1987;316:235–240.
5. National High Blood Pressure Education Program Working Group report on primary prevention of hypertension. *Arch Intern Med.* 1993;153:186–208.
6. The sixth report of the Joint National Committee on Prevention, Detection, Evaluation, and Treatment of High Blood Pressure (JNC VI). *Arch Intern Med.* 1997;157:2413–2446.
7. Whelton PK. Epidemiology of hypertension. *Lancet.* 1994;344:101–106.
8. Whelton PK, He J, Cutler JA, Brancati FL, Appel LJ, Follmann D, Klag MJ. Effects of oral potassium on blood pressure: meta-analysis of randomized controlled clinical trials. *JAMA.* 1997;277:1624–1632.
9. Xie JX, Sasaki S, Joossens JV, Kesteloot H. The relationship between urinary cations obtained from the Intersalt study and cerebrovascular mortality. *J Hum Hypertens.* 1992;6:17–21.
10. Yamori Y, Nara Y, Mizushima S, Sawamura M, Horie R. Nutritional factors for stroke and major cardiovascular diseases: international epidemiological comparison of dietary prevention. *Health Rep.* 1994;6:22–27.

Chapter 92

Calcium, Magnesium, and Blood Pressure

Lawrence J. Appel, MD, MPH

KEY POINTS

- In observational studies, an increased intake of calcium and magnesium is often associated with lower blood pressure.

- In clinical trials, the effects of calcium and magnesium supplements on blood pressure are small and inconsistent.

- A diet that includes foods rich in magnesium and calcium may reduce blood pressure.

- Calcium supplements may be necessary for older persons to consume an adequate intake of calcium.

See also Chapters 49, 110

In addition to weight, salt, potassium, and alcohol, other aspects of nutrition may affect blood pressure and account in part for the high prevalence of hypertension in most societies. Calcium and magnesium are two such nutrients.

Calcium: Overview of Basic Physiology and Nutrition

The adult body contains ≈1200 g of calcium, of which 99% is present in the skeleton. The remaining 1%, found in intracellular space, cell membranes, and extracellular fluids, has an essential role in numerous body functions, including nerve conduction, muscle contraction, blood clotting, and membrane permeability. Blood levels are tightly regulated within narrow limits through the effects of several hormones (vitamin D, parathyroid hormone, calcitonin, estrogen, testosterone, and perhaps others). These hormones control calcium absorption and excretion, as well as bone metabolism.

Calcium absorption occurs through active transport and passive diffusion across the intestinal mucosa. Active transport, which accounts for the absorption of calcium at low to moderate levels, is dependent on vitamin D. Passive diffusion becomes more important at higher levels of calcium intake. Fractional absorption depends on several factors including age (greater in infants and during puberty), pregnancy status (greater during the last two trimesters), and race (greater in blacks).

Calcium is lost through the body in feces, urine, and sweat. Urinary calcium excretion is typically 100 to 250 mg/d and varies as a function of the filtered load and the efficiency of reabsorption, which is regulated by parathyroid hormone levels. Increased intake of sodium, protein, and caffeine may increase calcium excretion. Other than a direct association between sodium intake and nephrolithiasis, the clinical relevance of these effects is unclear.

According to the US Department of Agriculture 1994 Continuing Survey of Food Intakes, the median dietary intake of calcium is less in women than in men and tends to decrease throughout adult ages (857 mg/d in men 31 to 50 years old and 702 mg/d in men ≥70 years old; 606 and 517 mg/d in women at corresponding ages). Also, in both sexes and across all age groups, blacks consume less calcium than whites. In terms of food sources, 73% of calcium in the food supply is from milk, 9% from fruits and vegetables, 5% from grain products, and the remaining 12% from all other sources. Milk products contain ≈300 mg of calcium per serving (for example, 8 oz of milk, 1.5 oz of cheddar cheese). Other calcium-rich foods include kale, calcium-fortified orange juice, and broccoli. Use of calcium supplements is high among adult women (25% in 1986) and is probably rising as a result of efforts to prevent osteoporosis through increased calcium intake.

In recent nutrition guidelines issued by the Institute of Medicine, an adequate intake of calcium for adults (men and women) is 1 g/d at 19 to 50 years old and 1.2 g/d at older ages. Few people meet this guideline. For instance, among persons ≥70 years old, <1% of women and <5% of men meet this dietary guideline.

Relationship Between Calcium and Blood Pressure

Reports from ecological studies of an inverse association between drinking water hardness and mortality from atherosclerotic diseases stimulated interest in the roles of calcium and magnesium intake on blood pressure. Evidence of an effect of calcium on blood pressure comes from a variety of sources including animal studies, observational studies, clinical trials, and most recently, meta-analyses of observational studies and controlled trials. In a meta-analysis of 23 observational studies, Cappuccio et al documented an inverse association between blood pressure and dietary calcium intake (as measured by 24-hour dietary recalls or food frequency questionnaires). However, the size of the effect was relatively small, and there was evidence of publication bias and of heterogeneity across studies. Subsequently, two meta-analyses of randomized trials documented that calcium supplementation significantly reduced systolic blood pressure (by 0.89 mm Hg in one analysis and 1.27 mm Hg in the other) but not diastolic blood pressure (**Figure 92.1**). Typical calcium doses in the trials were 1 to 1.5 g/d.

The unimpressive results of pill supplementation trials in the setting of inverse relationships in observational studies have several possible explanations. First, calcium may have an effect but only in combination with a high intake of other nutrients. However, in one trial of combinations of cation supplements (calcium, magnesium, and potassium) in hypertensive patients, none of the combinations

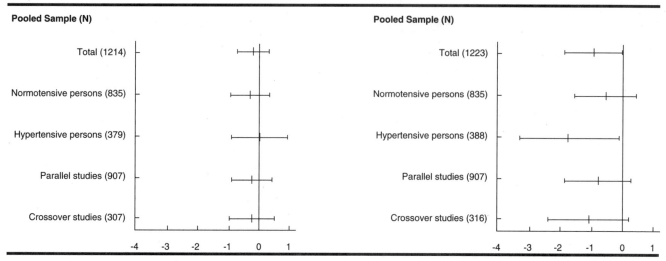

Figure 92.1. Mean change (95% CI) in systolic and diastolic blood pressure, overall and by subgroups, from a meta-analysis of 22 randomized trials (Allender et al, 1996).

reduced blood pressure. Alternatively, some nutrient closely associated with calcium (eg, protein, phosphorus, vitamin D, or an unknown nutrient) may be responsible for the blood pressure–lowering effect attributed to calcium. One small trial demonstrated that milk consumption in the context of a low calcium diet reduced systolic blood pressure. A recent clinical trial demonstrated that a healthy dietary pattern rich in low-fat dairy products, fruits, and vegetables, and reduced in saturated fat, total fat, and cholesterol lowered both systolic and diastolic blood pressure.

One issue still unanswered is whether certain subgroups of the population are particularly sensitive to the effects of calcium. Such groups may include pregnant women at risk for preeclampsia and persons with a low dietary intake of calcium or sodium. In the large and well-controlled Trials of Hypertension Prevention, calcium supplementation did not reduce blood pressure overall in the trial but may have reduced diastolic blood pressure in white women, particularly those with low urinary sodium excretion, calcium excretion, or low body mass index. In contrast, in another trial conducted in 300 female nurses with low dietary intakes of calcium, magnesium, and potassium, calcium supplementation did not lower blood pressure. Likewise, in one trial of 4589 pregnant women, calcium supplements had no effect on hypertension, blood pressure, or preeclampsia. Surprisingly, the effects of calcium supplementation on blood pressure in blacks has not been well studied, even though they consume much less calcium than their white counterparts. Although the effects of calcium supplementation on blood pressure have been small and inconsistent, clinical trials have demonstrated that calcium supplementation in combination with vitamin D can reduce the risk of bone fractures in older persons.

Magnesium: Overview of Basic Physiology and Nutrition

The adult body contains ≈25 g of magnesium, of which 40% is in soft tissues, 60% in the skeleton, and only 1% in extracellular fluids. Magnesium is a cofactor in >300 enzyme systems and is required for aerobic and anaerobic energy production, glycolysis, membrane function, and DNA and RNA synthesis. It has been called "nature's physiological calcium channel blocker." In magnesium depletion states, intracellular calcium rises and leads to contraction of smooth muscle and skeletal muscle along with a rise in blood pressure. Such findings raise the possibility that magnesium may be involved in blood pressure homeostasis in healthy populations.

The mechanisms controlling blood levels and intestinal absorption of magnesium are poorly understood. The kidney has a predominant role in magnesium homeostasis, reabsorbing most filtered magnesium, particularly in magnesium deficiency states. As with calcium, fractional absorption is inversely proportional to the amount of magnesium ingested.

According to data from the 1994 Continuing Survey of Food Intake, the median dietary intake of magnesium is nearly 300 mg/d in adult men and ≈225 mg/d in women. Magnesium intake decreases to a minor extent with age. Approximately 45% of dietary magnesium comes from fruits, vegetables, grains, and nuts and ≈30% from milk, meat, and eggs. According to recent guidelines, the estimated average daily requirement of magnesium is 350 mg for adult men (≥30 years old) and ≈265 mg for adult women.

Relationship Between Magnesium and Blood Pressure

The body of evidence implicating magnesium as a major determinant of blood pressure is limited and inconsistent. In observational studies, often cross-sectional in design, dietary magnesium is often inversely associated with blood pressure. This relationship was seen in cross-sectional analyses of 15 248 participants in the Atherosclerosis Risk in Communities study, in which hypertensive participants also had lower serum magnesium levels than did normotensives. In one prospective observational study, dietary magnesium intake was inversely related to systolic and diastolic blood pressure and change in blood pressure; however, these relationships did not persist after adjustment for fiber.

In the aggregate, clinical trials do not support a prominent role of magnesium in blood pressure homeostasis, at least in nondeficient general populations. Such was the opinion expressed by Whelton and Klag in their overview of eight small trials. Since then, several large, well-designed trials have been conducted. In Phase 1 of the Trials of Hypertension Prevention, supplemental magnesium had no effect on blood pressure in 461 persons with high normal blood pressure. Magnesium in combination with either potassium or calcium had no effect on blood pressure in a trial of 125 hypertensives. Most recently, in a trial of 300 female nurses with low dietary intake of magnesium, potassium, and calcium, magnesium had no effect on blood pressure. In contrast, in a crossover, dose-response trial of only 17 hypertensive patients, oral magnesium resulted in a significant dose-dependent reduction in blood pressure. Overall, it appears that magnesium supplementation in nondeficient general populations has little impact on blood pressure. However, a healthy diet rich in low-fat dairy products, fruits, and vegetables, and reduced in fat and cholesterol and that provided >400 mg/d of magnesium lowered both systolic and diastolic blood pressure.

Summary

Available evidence does not support pill supplementation with either calcium or magnesium as a means to reduce blood pressure in the general population. However, a healthy diet rich in fruit, vegetables, and low-fat dairy products and reduced in saturated fat, total fat, and cholesterol (and thereby rich in calcium and magnesium) can reduce blood pressure. In older persons, pill supplementation with calcium may be appropriate as a means to increase calcium intake and thereby prevent bone fractures related to osteoporosis.

SUGGESTED READING

1. Allender PS, Cutler JA, Follmann D, Cappuccio FP, Pryer J, Elliott P. Dietary calcium and blood pressure: a meta-analysis of randomized clinical trials. *Ann Intern Med.* 1996;124:825–831.

2. Appel LJ, Moore TJ, Obarzanek E, Vollmer WM, Svetkey LP, Sacks FM, Bray GA, Vogt TM, Cutler JA, Windhauser MM, Lin PH, Karanja N, for the DASH Collaborative Research Group. A clinical trial of the effects of dietary patterns on blood pressure. *N Engl J Med.* 1997;336:1117–1124.

3. Cappuccio FP, Elliott P, Allender PS, Pryer J, Follman DA, Cutler JA. Epidemiologic association between dietary calcium intake and blood pressure: a meta-analysis of published data. *Am J Epidemiol.* 1995;142:935–945.

4. Institute of Medicine. *Dietary Reference Intakes: Calcium, Phosphorus, Magnesium, Vitamin D, and Fluoride.* Washington, DC: National Academy Press; 1997.

5. Levine RJ, Hauth JC, Curet LB, Sibai BM, Catalano PM, Morris CD, DerSimonian R, Esterlitz JR, Raymond EG, Bild DE, Clemens JD, Cutler JA. Trial of calcium to prevent preeclampsia. *N Engl J Med.* 1997;337:69–76.

6. Ma J, Folsom AR, Melnick SL, Eckfeldt JH, Sharrett AR, Nabulsi AA, Hutchinson RG, Metcalf PA. Associations of serum and dietary magnesium with cardiovascular disease, hypertension, diabetes, insulin, and carotid arterial wall thickness: the ARIC Study. *J Clin Epidemiol.* 1995;48:927–940.

7. Sacks FM, Brown LE, Appel L, Borhani NO, Evans D, Whelton P. Combinations of potassium, calcium, and magnesium supplements in hypertension. *Hypertension.* 1995;26:950–956.

8. Sacks FM, Willett WC, Smith A, Brown LE, Rosner B, Moore TJ. Effect on blood pressure of potassium, calcium, and magnesium in women with low habitual intake. *Hypertension.* 1998;31:131–138.

9. Whelton PK, Klag MJ. Magnesium and blood pressure: review of the epidemiologic and clinical trial experience. *Am J Cardiol.* 1989;63:26G–30G.

10. Yamamoto ME, Applegate WB, Klag MJ, Borhani NO, Cohen JD, Kirchner KA, Lakatos E, Sacks FM, Taylor JO, Hennekens CH. Lack of blood pressure effect with calcium and magnesium supplementation in adults with high-normal blood pressure: results from Phase I of the Trials of Hypertension Prevention (TOHP). *Ann Epidemiol.* 1995;5:96–107.

Chapter 93

Obesity, Body Fat Distribution, and Insulin Resistance

Clinical Relevance

Steven M. Haffner, MD

KEY POINTS

- Obesity is widely recognized as a risk factor for the development of hypertension.

- The association between body fat distribution and blood pressure has been shown to be independent of obesity in a number of studies.

- An adverse body fat distribution has been associated with insulin resistance, and insulin resistance may be an important cause of hypertension.

- Persons who develop hypertension at an early age have an increased frequency of lipid disorders ("familial dyslipidemic hypertension"); a subset of these patients have increased glucose and insulin concentrations.

See also Chapters 46, 47, 94, 144

Obesity and Body Fat Distribution in Relation to Hypertension

Obesity in clinical and epidemiological studies is most often assessed by body mass index (BMI: weight divided by the square of height). Obesity is widely recognized as a risk factor for the development of hypertension. In the follow-up of the first National Health and Nutrition Examination Survey, overall adiposity measured by BMI strongly predicted the incidence of hypertension in both blacks and whites. Conversely, weight loss has been shown to be associated with decreases in blood pressure in many studies.

Recently, the pattern of body fat distribution has been recognized as a major risk factor, with upper-body obesity being associated with dyslipidemia, type II diabetes, and hypertension. The most common clinical and epidemiological assessments of body fat distribution have been made from measures of central or upper-body adiposity, such as subscapular skinfolds, the ratio of subscapular to triceps skinfolds, or the ratio of waist to hip circumferences (WHR). Unfortunately, there are no agreements on landmarks for the measurement of circumferences. Often the waist circumference is measured at the umbilicus or, alternatively, at the minimum diameter between the thorax and the hips. The hip circumference can be measured at the maximum diameter of the hips or, alternatively, at the level of the greater trochanter. There are also no internationally recognized standards as to what constitutes upper-body adiposity, although some authors have suggested a WHR >0.95 in men or >0.85 in women. The WHR and ratio of skinfolds are related to the general degree of adiposity.

Central adiposity, as assessed by skinfolds, has been related to blood pressure cross-sectionally in whites, blacks, and Hispanics. WHR has also been related to blood pressure in Hispanics and whites. The association between body fat distribution and blood pressure has been shown to be independent of obesity in a number of studies.

Recently, interest has focused on the possible role of visceral fat, measured by computerized tomography, compared with the less metabolically active central subcutaneous fat. The ratio of visceral fat to subcutaneous fat is more closely correlated with the risk of type II diabetes than are assessments of fat distribution using circumferences or skinfolds. Fewer data are available on the possible role of visceral fat in hypertension, although a recent report has suggested very high correlations between both visceral and retroperitoneal adipose tissue mass and blood pressure in normoglycemic humans. Pouliot et al believe that waist circumference may be a better indicator of visceral fat than WHR.

The mechanisms relating obesity and body fat distribution to an increased risk of hypertension are not well understood. An adverse body fat distribution has been associated with insulin resistance, and Reaven suggested that insulin resistance may be an important cause of hypertension.

Is Insulin Resistance Related to the Pathogenesis of Hypertension?

The clustering of cardiovascular risk factors, including dyslipidemia, diabetes, hypertension, obesity, and central adiposity, has long been recognized. A number of groups have shown that lean, normoglycemic untreated hypertensive subjects are more insulin-resistant than comparable normotensive subjects. Furthermore, subjects who develop hypertension at an early age had an increased frequency of lipid disorders ("familial dyslipidemic hypertension"); a subset of these patients have increased glucose and insulin concentrations. Insulin resistance may underlie this cluster of atherogenic changes. Multiple mechanisms have been proposed to explain a possible relationship between insulin resistance and hypertension, including increased sympathetic nervous system activity, proliferation of vascular smooth muscle cells, altered cation transport, and increased sodium retention. However, the association between insulin and hypertension is still controversial.

The reason for the discrepancy between studies is not clear, but one factor may be that the etiology of hypertension is different among ethnic groups. Saad et al, in a cross-sectional study, suggested a relationship between insulin resistance and blood pressure in whites but not in blacks or Pima Indians. However, Falkner et al found an association between insulin resistance and mild hypertension in young, lean black males. A relationship between insulin resistance and hypertension has been shown in lean type I diabetic subjects but not in obese type II diabetic subjects. Because the blacks in the report by Falkner et al were much leaner than those in the report by Saad et al (BMI, 24 versus 31 kg/m^2, respectively), the discrepancy of whether insulin resistance is associated with hypertension may have been due to differences in adiposity. Ferrannini et al showed that decreased insulin sensitivity (by the hyperinsulinemic euglycemic clamp) is associated with blood pressure in a large number of nonobese nondiabetic Europeans.

Other studies have disputed some of the proposed mechanisms that might underlie the relationship of insulin resistance and hypertension. Anderson et al showed that short-term insulin infusions (2 hours) raise catecholamines but not blood pressure in normotensive men. Similarly, short-term infusion leading to vasodilation rather than vasoconstriction has also been shown in men and in dogs. However, the effect of chronic hyperinsulinemia (ie, lasting months or years) is not known. Ecological data also do not support a strong relationship between insulin and blood pressure. Pima Indians and Mexican Americans have high rates of type II diabetes, hyperinsulinemia, and insulin resistance and yet have a lower prevalence of hypertension.

One problem in examining the relationship between insulin resistance and blood pressure has been the lack of prospective data. This limitation is important in subjects with preexisting hypertension. Certain antihypertensive agents have been reported to increase insulin resistance and induce dyslipidemia. Many studies have avoided this problem by studying hypertensive subjects not currently on medications. However, another potential problem with cross-sectional studies is that the clustering of risk factors (including insulin resistance) could result from compensatory mechanisms that induce secondary metabolic changes such as increased catecholamines.

A prospective study examined the role of obesity, body fat distribution, and insulin concentrations in relation to the development of hypertension in 1440 nonhypertensive Mexican American and non-Hispanic white subjects over 8 years. Obesity, glucose intolerance, and fasting insulin were each significantly related to the incidence of hypertension in univariate analyses. Subjects in the highest category of BMI ($\geq$30 kg/m^2) had an increased incidence of hypertension relative to subjects with lower BMIs (13.8% versus 6.3%, respectively; relative risk [RR]=2.00; $P<$.001). Similarly, subjects in the highest tertile of insulin concentrations ($>$95 pmol/L) had an increased incidence of hypertension relative to subjects with lower insulin concentrations (13.4% versus 6.9%, respectively; RR=1.93; $P=$.001).

Subjects with type II diabetes had an increased incidence of hypertension relative to subjects with normal glucose tolerance (17.1% versus 7.8%, respectively; RR=2.18; $P=$.04). None of the interactions of ethnicity with BMI, insulin, and glucose tolerance status were statistically significant ($P>$.50), suggesting that the effects of BMI, insulinemia, and glucose intolerance category on hypertension incidence were similar in each ethnic group.

In this population, subjects had dyslipidemia (increased triglyceride and decreased high-density lipoprotein cholesterol levels) before the onset of hypertension. This observation supports the general concept of the clustering of the cardiovascular risk factors with hypertensive subjects, as has been proposed in the "familial dyslipidemia hypertension syndrome"; furthermore, the lipid disorder may precede the development of hypertension. Because the relative impact of insulin resistance may be greater in lean than in obese subjects, the incidence of hypertension was examined stratified simultaneously by BMI and fasting insulin concentrations. In nonobese subjects (BMI $<$25 kg/m^2), the incidence of hypertension increased with baseline fasting insulin concentrations in a stepwise fashion. This relation was not consistently observed in more obese subjects. In lean subjects, the incidence of hypertension for those in the highest tertile of insulin concentration compared with those in the lowest two tertiles was 10.1% versus 4.5%, respectively (RR=2.24; $P=$.0032), in subjects with BMI between 25 and 30 kg/m^2, and the incidence in the corresponding insulin categories was 11.5% versus 15.0%, respectively (RR=0.70; $P=$NS). Thus, the effect of fasting insulin on the incidence of hypertension decreased with increasing obesity.

Relationship Between Hypertension, Antihypertensive Agents, and the Development of Type II Diabetes

A number of studies have suggested that thiazides and β-blockers might worsen glucose tolerance and insulin resistance. In contrast, calcium antagonists (with the possible exception of nifedipine) are believed not to affect insulin sensitivity, and certain ACE inhibitors and α-blockers might even improve insulin sensitivity. Antihypertensive agents that worsen insulin sensitivity might be expected to increase the risk of diabetes because hyperinsulinemia and insulin resistance are strongly related to the incidence of type II diabetes. This is important because hypertensive persons appear to be at increased risk of diabetes, as evidenced by the clustering of diabetes and hypertension. In a longitudinal study of Swedish women, it was observed that hypertensive women taking diuretics have a significant, 3.4-fold-higher risk of developing diabetes than hypertensive women not on therapy. Relative to hypertensive subjects not on therapy, the risk of developing diabetes was even higher in hypertensive subjects taking β-blockers and hypertensive subjects taking both thiazides and β-blockers. In a 10-year follow-up study, 12.7% of hypertensive men developed diabetes, as opposed to 3.6% of nonhypertensive men ($P<$.001). Others have found that whereas the use of antihypertensive agents is associated with an increased risk of diabetes, the risk of diabetes with thiazide diuretics is not different from that with other antihypertensive agents.

In another prospective study, subjects who were hypertensive at baseline had a higher 8-year incidence of type II diabetes (8.9%

versus 4.9%, $P=.041$) and impaired glucose tolerance (25.2% versus 10.0%, $P<.001$) than subjects who were normotensive at baseline. After adjustment for age, sex, ethnicity, obesity, body fat distribution, fasting glucose, and insulin, this excess was present only for impaired glucose intolerance. Thus, the excess risk of type II diabetes in hypertensive patients can be explained by their greater age, obesity, more unfavorable body fat distribution, and hyperinsulinemia, whereas their excess risk of impaired glucose intolerance is independent of these factors. The odds of developing type II diabetes for hypertensive subjects on β-blockers and thiazides versus other hypertensives were not greater than with other agents, contrary to the Swedish studies. In the Systolic Hypertension in the Elderly Program (SHEP), a clinical trial evaluating the effect of low-dose diuretics on the risk of coronary heart disease in the elderly, subjects randomized to the active treatment groups had significantly higher glucose levels (but the difference was quite small in magnitude).

Insulin resistance is moderately associated with the risk of development of hypertension in people of European ancestry and in Mexican Americans; the relationship of insulin resistance to hypertension may be weaker in blacks. Hypertensive subjects have an increased risk of developing diabetes; certain antihypertensive agents (ie, thiazides and β-blockers) may further increase the risk of developing diabetes by increasing insulin resistance, but this effect may depend on the dose of the antihypertensive drug.

SUGGESTED READING

1. Blair D, Habicht JP, Sims EA, Sylwester D, Abraham S. Evidence for an increased risk for hypertension with centrally located body fat and the effect of race and sex on this risk. *Am J Epidemiol.* 1984;119:526–540.

2. Falkner B, Hulman S, Tannenbaum J, Kushner H. Insulin resistance and blood pressure in young black men. *Hypertension.* 1990;16:706–711.

3. Ferrannini E, Natali A, Capaldo B, Lehtovirt M, Jacob S, Yki-Järvinen H. Insulin resistance, hyperinsulinemia, and blood pressure. *Hypertension.* 1997;30:1144–1149.

4. Haffner SM, Ferrannini E, Hazuda HP, Stern MP. Clustering of cardiovascular risk factors in confirmed prehypertensive individuals. *Hypertension.* 1992;20:38–45.

5. Haffner SM, Fong D, Hazuda HP, Pugh JA, Patterson JK. Hyperinsulinemia, upper body adiposity and cardiovascular risk factors in non-diabetics. *Metabolism.* 1988;37:338–345.

6. Hunt SC, Wu LL, Hopkins PN, et al. Apolipoprotein, low density lipoprotein subfraction, and insulin associations with familial combined hyperlipidemia: study of Utah patients with familial dyslipidemic hypertension. *Arteriosclerosis.* 1989;9:335–344.

7. Lithell HOL. Effect of antihypertensive drugs on insulin, glucose and lipid metabolism. *Diabetes Care.* 1991;14:203–209.

8. Morales PA, Mitchell BD, Valdez RA, Hazuda HP, Stern MP, Haffner SM. Incidence of NIDDM and impaired glucose tolerance in hypertensive subjects: the San Antonio Heart Study. *Diabetes.* 1993;42:154–161.

9. Pouliot MC, Després JP, Lemieux S, Moorjani S, Bouchard C, Tremblay A, Nadeau A, Lupien PJ. Waist circumference and abdominal sagittal diameter: best simple anthropometric indexes of abdominal visceral adipose tissue accumulation and related cardiovascular risk in men and women. *Am J Cardiol.* 1994;73: 460–468.

10. Saad MF, Lillioja S, Nyomba BL, et al. Racial differences in the relation between blood pressure and insulin resistance. *N Engl J Med.* 1991;324:733–739.

Chapter 94

Physical Activity, Fitness, and Blood Pressure

Denise G. Simons-Morton, MD, PhD

KEY POINTS

- Physical activity should be recommended to all sedentary individuals to prevent hypertension and to all patients with hypertension.

- Aerobic activity that increases heart and respiration rates, engaged in at least three times a week for 40 minutes, has been shown to lower BP.

- A formal screening examination and testing are recommended for individuals with cardiovascular symptoms or disease and for older individuals and those with two or more cardiovascular disease risk factors who wish to engage in vigorous exercise.

- Advice and counseling to increase physical activity should include information about recommended physical activity regimens, attention to behavioral issues, and follow-up.

See also Chapters 46, 47, 93, 144

Evidence has accumulated over the past several decades that physical activity and cardiorespiratory fitness are important influences on blood pressure (BP) as well as on overall cardiovascular disease (CVD) risk. Physical activity, which is a behavior that results in energy expenditure, and cardiorespiratory fitness, which is a physiological attribute of the body's ability to utilize oxygen, have been seen to be inversely associated with BP level and hypertension incidence. Randomized controlled trials have demonstrated that increasing exercise (a structured form of physical activity) can lower BP. The body of evidence strongly supports the assertion that engaging in a physically active lifestyle has the potential to decrease, delay, or prevent the development of hypertension or the need for antihypertensive medication.

In addition to effects on BP, physical activity increases cardiorespiratory fitness, which is most likely an independent protective factor for coronary heart disease, as well as provides other benefits that reduce risk of CVD, including favorable effects on blood lipids, weight, and insulin sensitivity. Physical activity and cardiorespiratory fitness are inversely associated with CVD incidence and mortality as well as with total mortality. In addition, physical activity has favorable effects on other conditions, such as osteoporosis, risk of some cancers, depression, and physical functioning in the elderly. Therefore, physical activity should be promoted for a variety of benefits, of which a favorable effect on BP is only one.

Observational Evidence That Physical Inactivity Is a Risk Factor for Hypertension

Numerous epidemiological studies, both cross-sectional and longitudinal, have observed inverse relationships between amount of physical activity and BP level. Prospective cohort studies have found that the incidence of hypertension is higher in those with lower activity levels or lower levels of cardiorespiratory fitness. The associations generally have held while age, sex, smoking, weight, body mass index, blood lipids, and/or other potentially confounding or mediating factors are controlled for. Most of the studies have examined self-reported leisure-time physical activity or have used an estimate of total amount of activity. This includes, for example, stair climbing and walking as well as exercise and sports. Some studies of physical activity and CVD have also measured activity at work, and some have examined cardiorespiratory fitness as measured by treadmill or bicycle tests. The general body of evidence from observational studies is very strong for an inverse relationship between physical activity level and BP level. Observational studies, however, are limited in their design by the inability to ensure that all other factors that may affect BP are the same between active and nonactive groups.

Interventional Evidence That Increasing Activity Reduces BP

Randomized, controlled trials provide additional strong evidence that physical activity favorably influences BP. The randomized trial can determine whether changing physical activity changes BP by using a study design that controls for other factors that affect BP, including both known and unknown factors. Some 45 controlled trials have been conducted that have examined the effects on BP of physical activity regimens. Both normotensive and hypertensive individuals have been studied.

Most of the tested physical activity interventions have been aerobic exercise, which is rhythmic exercise that involves large muscle movements such as running, walking, cycling, or swimming and that causes increases in heart and respiration rates (which results in increased oxygen consumption). The exercise regimens tested in most studies used a frequency, intensity, and duration based on the American College of Sports Medicine (ACSM) exercise prescription for improving cardiorespiratory fitness, which is summarized in **Table 94.1**. Several studies have examined the effects of dynamic resistance exercise, ie, weight training.

Five quantitative meta-analyses have summarized the results of the controlled trials. The results of one meta-analysis are shown in the **Figure 94.1**. All of the meta-analyses have concluded that physical activity significantly decreases both systolic and diastolic BP. Significant decreases have been found in normotensive as well as hypertensive participants with aerobic exercise and, more recently, with dynamic resistance exercise. The average magnitude of effect ranges from a net decrease of 2/3 mm Hg in normotensives to a net decrease of 10/8 mm Hg in hypertensives. The latter magnitude of effect is comparable to that seen in studies of single-drug treatment of hypertension. The better-designed studies (ie, randomized assignment, regular contacts in the control group) have resulted in an average reduction of 7 mm Hg for systolic BP and of 5 mm Hg for diastolic BP in hypertensives. The BP effects have been independent of weight changes.

Although some reviewers have concluded that moderate-intensity activity, such as walking, has BP-lowering effects as great as or greater than those of vigorous-intensity activity, such as running, few studies have directly compared the effects on BP of differing exercise intensities. Making comparisons across studies is problematic because of differences in populations, measurement protocols, length of follow-up, and other characteristics. A recent randomized study examined the effects of incorporating physical activity into daily activities, such as walking up stairs instead of taking the elevator or being more active in home and yard endeavors, compared with a more traditional exercise regimen based on the ACSM prescription for cardiorespiratory fitness. Both groups lowered BP, with no significant difference in effect between the groups, although the traditional exercise group increased cardiovascular fitness significantly more. More evidence is still needed about the relative biological effects of moderate- and vigorous-intensity activity, but behavioral intervention studies provide evidence that people may be more able to achieve moderate- than vigorous-intensity activity. The implication is that at least initial changes in sedentary or irregularly active people should target moderate-intensity activities, such as walking.

National Recommendations

Physical inactivity has been identified as an important modifiable risk factor for CVD by the American Heart Association and the National Institutes of Health. The National High Blood Pressure Education Program recommends physical activity as an adjunctive treatment for patients with stages 2 and 3 hypertension and in those with stage 1 or high normal BP who are diabetic or have demonstrable target-organ damage. It should be used as a first-line intervention for patients with high normal and stage 1 hypertension who are free

Table 94.1. Exercise Prescription to Control Blood Pressure and to Develop and Maintain Cardiorespiratory Fitness

PARAMETER	DESCRIPTION
Mode of activity	Large-muscle activity that is rhythmical and aerobic (eg, walking, running, cycling)
Frequency	3 to 5 days per week
Duration	20 to 60 minutes
Intensity	60% to 90% of maximum heart rate (50% to 85% of maximum oxygen uptake)

Source: American College of Sports Medicine.

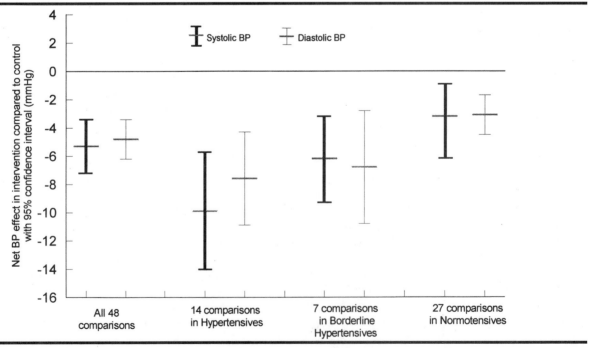

Figure 94.1.   Results of a meta-analysis of controlled trials testing aerobic exercise and blood pressure published through 1991; 36 studies with 48 intervention-control comparisons. Median characteristics of exercise programs: 3 times per week for 40 minutes at 65% maximum oxygen update over 16 weeks. Adapted from Fagard RH. Physical fitness and blood pressure. *J Hypertens.* 1993;11(suppl 5):S47–S52 and Fagard RH. Prescription and results of physical activity. *J Cardiovasc Pharmacol.* 1995;25(suppl 1):S20–S27.

of target-organ damage and as a population-wide behavior for preventing the increase in BP that occurs with age. The American Heart Association, the National Heart, Lung, and Blood Institute, the US Preventive Services Task Force, and the National Health Promotion and Disease Prevention Objectives in *Healthy People 2000* all recommend that physicians and other healthcare providers advise and counsel their patients to be physically active.

For controlling BP, the ACSM recommends the same exercise regimen as for developing and maintaining cardiorespiratory fitness **(Table 94.1)**. More recently, the focus has been on health in general, rather than on cardiorespiratory fitness. The ACSM and the Centers for Disease Control and Prevention as well as the *Surgeon General's Report on Physical Activity and Health* recommend a minimum of 30 minutes of moderate-intensity physical activity on most days to achieve health benefits. These recommendations also state that additional activity, which can be achieved by increasing frequency, duration, and/or intensity, can result in additional health benefits. An intensity of 50% to 69% of maximum heart rate is considered to be moderate, and an intensity of ≥70% of maximum heart rate is considered to be vigorous. Moderate-intensity activity for most people is comparable to a relatively brisk walking pace of 3 to 4 miles per hour, and vigorous-intensity activity is comparable to jogging or running.

All of the recommendations focus on aerobic exercise as the primary activity. Some of the recommendations include weight training as part of an overall fitness regimen, but none recommend weight training as a sole mode of exercise. The role of weight training in hypertension treatment or prevention needs further study, but it is recommended for overall fitness.

Physical Activity Advice and Counseling

Patients should be advised to engage in moderate-to-vigorous aerobic-type activity on a regular basis, at least three times per week, to prevent or treat hypertension. A physician's advice to increase physical activity can be a very strong motivator to patients. However, because behavior change is very difficult, advice alone is not sufficient. Advice should be accompanied by education about the recommended physical activity regimens and attention to behavioral issues, such as selecting an enjoyable activity, identifying and overcoming barriers, setting realistic goals, providing positive reinforcement, and enhancing social support. Advice by a physician followed by behavioral counseling by other members of the healthcare team is a reasonable approach.

Sedentary patients should start out slowly at a more moderate intensity and shorter duration than the ultimate goal. They should, for example, start with 10-minute walks two times a week and gradually increase over several weeks or months to 30 minutes of moderate- to vigorous-intensity activity three or more times a week. Achieving the ACSM exercise prescription, or achieving 30 minutes daily of moderate-intensity activity, is to be considered a long-term, not short-term, goal of physical activity counseling. The ultimate goal of counseling is for physical activity to be a permanent lifestyle behavior.

Determining the intensity of activity can be done in a variety of ways. The traditional method is self-monitoring of heart rate during exercise. To use this method, patients must be taught how to take their pulse, either radial or carotid, or to use a heart rate monitor. To identify the heart rate range that corresponds to the ACSM exercise

prescription for moderate to vigorous activity of 60% to 90% of maximum heart rate, one can estimate maximum heart rate by subtracting age from the constant 220 and then multiplying by 60% or by 90%, respectively, to obtain the lower and upper values for the range. Thus, for a 50-year-old person, the target heart rate range during exercise is from 102 to 153 beats per minute, calculated as follows:

Lower limit: $(220-50)\times0.60 = 102$ bpm

Upper limit: $(220-50)\times0.90 = 153$ bpm

The recent focus on moderate-intensity activity brings the lower limit of the target heart rate range down to 50% of maximum, which for the example given is 85 beats per minute. A heart rate anywhere within the heart rate range during activity is acceptable for achieving health benefits and improving fitness. Individuals who are not used to physical activity should start at the lower end of the range, which will be more comfortable; with increasing experience and fitness, values higher in the range can be targeted.

An alternative to pulse monitoring is to achieve a relative perceived exertion of "moderate to very hard." Perceived exertion or heart rate monitoring is preferred to providing an absolute pace in an exercise prescription, such as walking 4 miles per hour, because an individual's age and physical condition affect both the actual and perceived intensity of the activity. The phrase "brisk walking" should adequately convey a moderate intensity to most patients.

Two of the most important concepts of providing recommendations for increasing physical activity is that the activity must be regular (ie, at least several times a week to daily) and that the activity must be continued, because health benefits decline after activity is discontinued. Another important concept is that if a person relapses (ie, becomes sedentary again), it should be considered a temporary setback, not a failure. Achievements should be reinforced, and short-term goals should be selected that are realistic. Follow-up visits should incorporate attention to physical activity, either by the physician or by other medical staff, because it is known from behavioral intervention studies that after follow-up intervention ceases, health behaviors degrade.

Safety Issues and Screening Recommendations Before Exercise

Although a person with hypertension may have a greater BP increase during exercise than a person without hypertension, there is no evidence that the risks of exercise outweigh the benefits in hypertensives. General recommendations for screening before one engages in an exercise program have been provided by the ACSM, which are applicable to the hypertensive patient **(Table 94.2)**. For people who wish to engage in moderate-intensity activity, no medical screening is needed unless the person has CVD symptoms or known disease. For older people or people with two or more CVD risk factors (older age, family history of early heart disease, cigarette smoking, hypercholesterolemia, diabetes mellitus, hypertension) but no symptoms, screening is recommended only if they wish to engage in vigorous exercise. People with CVD symptoms or known CVD need a medical history and examination and, if not contraindicated, an exercise test no matter what intensity of activity they wish to engage in.

The goals of the medical history and examination are to determine whether there are any contraindications to exercise testing and to identify any medical conditions that would be a contraindication

Table 94.2. Recommendations for Medical Examination and Exercise Testing Before Exercise Participation, by Patient Characteristics

| | APPARENTLY HEALTHY | | ≥2 CVD RISK FACTORS | | |
EXERCISE INTENSITY	YOUNGER*	OLDER	NO SYMPTOMS	SYMPTOM(S)	KNOWN DISEASE†
Moderate	Not necessary	Not necessary	Not necessary	Recommended	Recommended
Vigorous	Not necessary	Recommended	Recommended	Recommended	Recommended

Source: American College of Sports Medicine.
* ≤ 40 years for men, ≤ 50 years for women.
†Persons with known cardiac, pulmonary, or metabolic disease.

to exercise. Absolute contraindications include acute ischemia, arrhythmias, congestive heart failure, and acute infections. Relative contraindications should take into account a physician's clinical judgment. Diastolic BP >115 mm Hg or systolic BP >200 mm Hg are considered relative contraindications; other relative contraindications include some cardiac conditions, such as valvular heart disease and ventricular aneurysm; electrolyte abnormalities; chronic infectious diseases; and pregnancy. The goals of an exercise test are to determine what intensity of exercise is safe and to determine whether exercise under supervision is necessary. In addition, the exercise test can determine the individual's maximum heart rate, which is much more accurate than using the constant 220 minus age and which can be used to develop an individualized exercise prescription.

Exercise and Antihypertensive Medications

Use of antihypertensive medication is not a contraindication to exercise participation of either moderate or vigorous intensity. β-Blockers diminish or eliminate the heart rate response to exercise, so for patients taking β-blockers, a perceived exertion of "moderate to very hard" is a preferable recommendation to a target heart rate range. An individual on antihypertensive medication who begins a regular physical activity regimen may be able to maintain BP control on a lower level of medication, or possibly without medication, as long as the physical activity is continued.

SUGGESTED READING

1. American College of Sports Medicine. *ACSM's Guidelines for Exercise Testing and Prescription.* 5th ed. Philadelphia, Pa: Williams & Wilkins; 1995.
2. American College of Sports Medicine. Position stand: physical activity, physical fitness, and hypertension. *Med Sci Sports Exerc.* 1993;25:i–x.
3. Fagard RH. Physical fitness and blood pressure. *J Hypertens.* 1993;11(suppl 5):S47–S52.
4. Fagard RH. Prescription and results of physical activity. *J Cardiovasc Pharmacol.* 1995;25(suppl 1):S20–S27.
5. Fletcher GF, Blair SN, Blumenthal J, Caspersen C, Chaitman B, Epstein S, Falls H, Sivarajan ES, Froelicher VF, Pina IL. Statement on exercise: benefits and recommendations for physical activity programs for all Americans: a statement for health professionals by the Committee on Exercise and Cardiac Rehabilitation of the Council on Clinical Cardiology, American Heart Association. *Circulation.* 1992;86:340–344.
6. Kelley G. Dynamic resistance exercise and resting blood pressure in adults: a meta-analysis. *J Appl Physiol.* 1997;82:1559–1565.
7. NIH Consensus Development Panel on Physical Activity and Cardiovascular Health. Physical activity and cardiovascular health. *JAMA.* 1996;276:241–246.
8. Pate RR, Pratt M, Blair SN, Haskell WL, Macera CA, Bouchard C, Buchner D, Ettinger W, Heath GW, King AC, Kriska A, Leon AS, Marcus BH, Morris J, Paffenbarger RS Jr, Patrick K, Pollock ML, Rippe JM, Sallis J, Wilmore JH. Physical activity and public health: a recommendation from the Centers for Disease Control and Prevention and the American College of Sports Medicine. *JAMA.* 1995;273:402–407.
9. US Department of Health and Human Services. *Physical Activity and Health: A Report of the Surgeon General.* Atlanta, Ga: US Department of Health and Human Services, Centers for Disease Control and Prevention, National Center for Chronic Disease Prevention and Health Promotion; 1996.

Chapter 95

Alcohol Use and Blood Pressure

William C. Cushman, MD

KEY POINTS

- More than 50 epidemiological studies have shown a direct relationship between ≥3 daily drinks of alcoholic beverages and hypertension.

- Reduction in alcohol intake is associated with lowering of blood pressure in randomized clinical trials: each reduction by 1 drink per day lowers systolic and diastolic blood pressure ≈1 mm Hg.

- Although regular alcohol intake is associated with lower risk for atherothrombotic cardiovascular events, excessive intake increases the risk of many medical and psychosocial problems, including hypertension.

- For persons with hypertension who drink excessively, average maximum alcohol intakes of 1 drink per day in women and 2 drinks per day in men are reasonable goals, if drinking is not otherwise contraindicated.

See also Chapter 118

Ethyl alcohol has been made and consumed by mankind throughout recorded history. Many serious adverse health and psychosocial consequences result from excessive alcohol intake, but there are what is considered by many cultures positive psychosocial effects of drinking, as well as potential health benefits of regular alcohol intake. One of the detrimental effects attributed to alcohol is its association with hypertension. What are the epidemiological associations, clinical trial evidence, and potential mechanisms of the alcohol-hypertension relationship, and what are reasonable public health recommendations based on this evidence?

Epidemiology

Alcohol consumption has one of the most consistently observed epidemiological associations with blood pressure (BP) among the known potentially modifiable risk factors for hypertension. More than 50 cross-sectional epidemiological studies from a variety of cultures have reported increasing average BP or a higher prevalence of hypertension with increasing levels of alcohol intake. Above an average intake of 2 drinks per day (a standard drink is defined as ≈14 g ethanol, which is contained in a 12-oz glass of beer, a 5-oz glass of table wine, or 1.5 oz of distilled spirits), the higher the alcohol intake, the higher the BP. This relationship usually persists as an independent effect even when age, body mass, sodium and potassium excretion or intake, cigarette smoking, and education are controlled for and has been demonstrated in whites, blacks, and Asians.

The **Figure 95.1** is from a classic early epidemiological study in the northern California Kaiser Permanente population that is illustrative of population studies. As in the women in the Kaiser Permanente study, sometimes a J-shaped relationship is apparent, with lower BP levels seen with low levels of alcohol intake compared with no drinking or compared with ≥3 drinks per day average. Sometimes low levels of alcohol have been associated with higher BP levels than no alcohol intake. Often, as in the men in the Kaiser Permanente study, there is no BP difference between the nondrinking group and those consuming ≤2 drinks per day. However, the BP differences between these two groups, when they are found, are usually small.

A reduction in alcohol consumption is also associated with a decrease in BP in prospective observational studies and in patient studies of alcohol cessation in alcoholics. When it has been examined, the hypertensive effect of alcohol appears to abate within several days of abstention, and the relationship between intake and BP is highest for alcohol consumed within the previous 24 hours. Sometimes a particular type of alcoholic beverage is more strongly associated with BP, but no beverage type has been consistently incriminated or absolved. It is possible that any differential effects are related to differences in accuracy of reporting between types. Overall, it appears that the relationship is dependent on the amount of absolute alcohol ingested.

Excess alcohol intake has also been associated with resistance to antihypertensive therapy. Although it is reasonable to assume that medication noncompliance in heavy drinkers contributes to this resistance, compelling data suggest a true interference with the BP-lowering effects of medications taken appropriately.

Alcohol intake of ≥3 drinks per day is associated with approximately a doubling of the prevalence of hypertension and has been estimated to account for 5% to 30% of hypertension, depending on the prevalence of heavy drinking in a population.

Randomized Controlled Trials

Randomized controlled trials provide a high level of evidence for the efficacy of an intervention. At least 11 randomized studies have been conducted to examine the effect of a reduction in alcohol intake on BP (**Table 95.1**). Although most of these studies included relatively few subjects, were of short duration, and were not designed as effectiveness trials, the results are consistent with the epidemiological evidence. Average differences in alcohol intake between intervention and control groups ranged from 1.0 to 5.7 drinks per day and resulted in significant reductions in systolic BP, diastolic BP, or both in all but two studies.

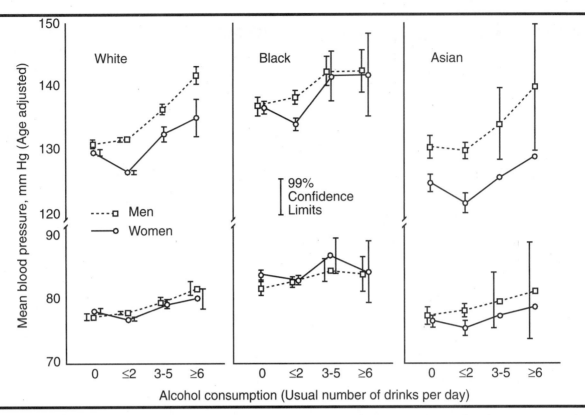

Figure 95.1.   Mean systolic blood pressures (upper half) and mean diastolic blood pressures (lower half) for white, black, or Asian men and women with known drinking habits. Small circles represent data based on fewer than 30 persons. (From Klatsky AL, Friedman GD, Siegelaub AB, Gerard MJ. Alcohol consumption and blood pressure. *N Engl J Med.* 1977;296:1194–1200. Used by permission.)

Table 95.1. Randomized Controlled Trials of the Effects of Alcohol Reduction on Blood Pressure

| | STUDY POPULATION | | | STUDY RESULTS | | | |
STUDY, YEAR	N	AGE, Y (MEAN ± SD OR RANGE)	DURATION, WK	BASELINE BP, MM HG	ALCOHOL INTAKE DIFFERENCE, DRINKS*/DAY	BP DIFFERENCE, MM HG	P
Puddey, 1985	46	35±8	6	133/76	3.7	3.8/1.4	<0.001/<0.05
Howes, 1985	10	25–41	0.6	120/66	5.7	8/6	<0.025/<0.001
Puddey, 1987	44	53±16	6	142/84	4.0	5/3	<0.001/<0.001
Ueshima, 1987	50	46±7	2	148/93	2.6	5.2/2.2	<0.005/NS
Wallace, 1988	641	42±20	52	136/82	1.0	2.1/?	<0.05/NS
Parker, 1990	59	52±11	4	138/85	3.8	5.4/3.2	<0.01/0.01
Cox, 1990	72	20–45	4	132/73	3.4	4.1/1.6	<0.05/<0.05
Maheswaran, 1992	41	40s	8	144/90	3.1	Not reported	NS
Puddey, 1992	86	44	18	137/85	3.0	4.8/3.3	<0.01/<0.01
Ueshima, 1993	54	44±8	3	144/96	1.7	3.6/1.9	<0.05/NS
PATHS, 1998	641	57±11	104	140/86	1.3	0.9/0.6	0.16/0.10

*A standard drink is defined as 14 g ethanol and is contained in a 12-oz glass of beer, a 5-oz glass of table wine, or 1.5 oz of distilled spirits.

The largest and longest of the intervention studies is the recently published Prevention and Treatment of Hypertension Study (PATHS). The National Heart, Lung, and Blood Institute, the National Institute on Alcohol Abuse and Alcoholism, and the Veterans Affairs Cooperative Studies Program collaborated in this randomized, controlled, multicenter effectiveness trial. The trial included both short- and long-term follow-up to determine whether BP was lowered by sus-tained reductions in alcohol intake in 641 moderate to heavy drinkers with above-optimal to slightly hypertensive levels of dias-tolic BP. Candidates for the trial with evidence of alcoholism, includ-ing any medical complications of excess alcohol intake, were ex-cluded. Although the difference in alcohol intake between the intervention and control groups was highly significant and sustained over the 2 years of follow-up, it averaged only 1.3 drinks per day rather than the projected 2.0 drinks per day. This happened in part because the control group lowered reported alcohol intake more than anticipated. The average difference in reduction in BP of 0.9/0.6 mm Hg was not significantly different between the intervention and control groups. However, the BP differences and the development or recurrence of hypertension were generally in the expected direction.

In the other, mostly short-term, efficacy studies, baseline levels of alcohol intake and changes in alcohol intake were generally larger than those observed in PATHS. The net reductions in BP were usually significant, averaging up to 8 mm Hg systolic and up to 6 mm Hg diastolic, for differences in alcohol intake of ≈6 drinks per day. Among these studies, two studies by Puddey et al in normotensives and hypertensives, respectively, are probably the best from which to derive a crude prediction for BP change: averaging over the two studies, a 3-drink-per-day net reduction was associated with a 4.4/2.2 mm Hg reduction in BP. Among all the studies, for every 1-drink-per-day reduction in alcohol intake in the intervention groups compared with the control groups, an ≈1 mm Hg decrease in either systolic or diastolic BP, or both, was observed. Overall, the randomized controlled trials give solid evidence that a reduction in alcohol intake in individuals who drink, on average, ≥3 drinks per day results in a significant lowering of BP.

Potential Mechanisms of Effect on BP and Cardiovascular Protection

There are a number of possibilities for the mechanism or mechanisms by which chronic alcohol consumption results in elevated BP. Proposed mechanisms include a chronic state of alcohol withdrawal in frequent drinkers, but there appears to be more evidence for a direct effect of alcohol. Suggested mediators of this effect have included (1) stimulation of the sympathetic nervous system, endothelin, the renin-angiotensin-aldosterone system, insulin (or insulin resistance), or cortisol; (2) inhibition of vascular relaxing substances; (3) calcium or magnesium depletion; (4) increased intracellular calcium in vascular smooth muscle; and (5) increased acetaldehyde.

Compared with abstention, even low levels of alcohol intake are associated with reduced incidence of atherothrombotic events, such as myocardial infarction and atherothrombotic stroke. These beneficial effects of alcohol appear to be at least in part because of increases in HDL and apolipoproteins A1 and A2, antioxidant effects, and reduced platelet aggregability. However, higher intake levels are associated with increased risk for hypertension, cardiomyopathy, and other cardiac complications, including hemorrhagic strokes, certain kinds of cancer, liver damage and other gastrointestinal disease, suicides, accidents, violence, and alcohol abuse and dependence.

Recommendations

In light of the association between heavy drinking and hypertension, other detrimental health consequences, and adverse psychosocial effects, as well as the potential benefits of alcohol, current public health recommendations in the United States are as follows: For those who drink, average alcohol intake should not exceed 2 drinks per day in men and 1 drink per day in women, because women are generally smaller and have markedly lower gastric alcohol dehydrogenase than men. Many persons should not drink at all, including those with a history of or who appear to be at risk for a drinking problem or serious medical complications from alcohol, and pregnant women. For those who are not in one of these high-risk categories and who drink within the limits outlined above, the risk of developing hypertension is probably not increased and beneficial effects of alcohol may predominate. However, anyone drinking an average of >1 or 2 drinks per day should be encouraged to reduce intake to reduce BP, the risk of developing hypertension, and the risk of other alcohol-related problems.

SUGGESTED READING

1. Cushman WC, Cutler JA, Hanna E, Bingham SF, Follmann D, Harford T, Dubbert P, Allender PS, Dufour M, Collins JF, Walsh SM, Kirk GF, Burg M, Felicetta JV, Hamilton BP, Katz LA, Perry HM, Willenbring ML, Lakshman R, Hamburger RJ, for the PATHS Group. The Prevention and Treatment of Hypertension Study (PATHS): effects of an alcohol treatment program on blood pressure. *Arch Intern Med.* 1998; 152:1197–1207.

2. Klatsky AL, Friedman GD, Siegelaub AB, Gérard MJ. Alcohol consumption and blood pressure: Kaiser-Permanente Multiphasic Health Examination Data. *N Engl J Med.* 1977;296:1194–1200.

3. MacMahon S. Alcohol consumption and hypertension. *Hypertension.* 1987;9: 111–121.

4. Marmot MG, Elliott P, Shipley MJ, Dyer AR, Ueshima H, Beevers DG, Stamler R, Kesteloot H, Rose G, Stamler J. Alcohol and blood pressure: the INTERSALT study. *BMJ.* 1994;308:1263–1267.

5. *Nutrition and Your Health: Dietary Guidelines for Americans, 4th Edition, 1995.* Washington, DC: US Department of Agriculture, US Department of Health and Human Services; 40–41.

6. Puddey IB, Beilin LJ, Vandongen R, Rouse IL, Rogers P. Evidence for a direct effect of alcohol consumption on blood pressure in normotensive men: a randomized controlled trial. *Hypertension.* 1985;7:707–713.

7. Puddey IB, Beilin LJ, Vandongen R. Regular alcohol use raises blood pressure in treated hypertensive subjects: a randomized controlled trial. *Lancet.* 1987;1:647–651.

8. Saunders JB, Beevers DG, Paton A. Alcohol induced hypertension. *Lancet.* 1981;2: 653–656.

9. Suh I, Shaten BJ, Cutler JA, Kuller LH. Alcohol use and mortality from coronary heart disease: the role of high-density lipoprotein cholesterol: the Multiple Risk Factor Intervention Trial Research Group. *Ann Intern Med.* 1992;116:881–887.

10. Thun MJ, Peto R, Lopez AD, Monaco JH, Henley SJ, Heath CW Jr, Doll R. Alcohol consumption and mortality among middle-aged and elderly US adults. *N Engl J Med.* 1997;337:1705–1714.

Chapter 96

Psychosocial Stress and Blood Pressure

Thomas G Pickering, MD, PhD

KEY POINTS

- There are important social and cultural determinants of blood pressure (BP).

- People working in stressful (or "high-strain") jobs have higher BP than people in less stressful jobs.

- Increased reactivity of BP to stressful stimuli is seen in hypertensive patients, but its ecological significance is unclear.

See also Chapters 45, 75, 87, 88

It is generally accepted that human essential hypertension derives from a number of causes and that both genetic and environmental factors contribute. Estimates based on twin studies suggest that about 50% of blood pressure (BP) variance is genetic, but exactly what is inherited and how it operates remains obscure. The leading candidates for environmental causes are dietary and psychosocial factors.

Evidence for a Role for Psychosocial Factors in Hypertension

There are three ways in which the roles of environmental stress on BP can be evaluated: animal experiments, laboratory studies, and field studies. Animal studies using mice housed in population cages, where there is social interaction, have indicated that dominant animals develop higher BPs than subordinates. The highest BPs are seen in subdominants attempting to achieve control. A human situation analogous to the social interaction of mice has been reported in prisoners. The systolic BP of men who had lived for several months in a dormitory was 131 mm Hg, whereas in men living in single-occupancy cells it was only 115 mm Hg. Furthermore, transfer from a cell to a dormitory caused the BP to increase and vice versa. These changes could not be attributed to diet, because all the prisoners ate the same food.

There is a large body of epidemiological evidence suggesting that the increase in BP with age is determined culturally and environmentally, rather than genetically. A good example is provided by a 30-year observational study of Italian nuns living in a secluded order, reported by Timio. The nuns were compared with a control group both at entry and after 30 years. BPs were the same at entry, but by the end of the study the systolic BP was approximately 30 mm Hg higher in the controls than in the nuns, who failed to show the usual increase of BP associated with aging. Cardiovascular morbidity and urine catecholamine secretion were also lower in the nuns. The differences could not be explained by changes in body weight, by diet, or by childbearing. The authors inferred that the differences were due to the nuns' monastic and relatively stress-free environment. Similar observations have been made in people who migrate from a stable traditional society to a westernized one, but the primary problem with nearly all of them is that it is difficult to know exactly what factors were responsible for the rise of BP. While stress may be a crucial factor, there are also

major dietary and other lifestyle changes associated with the transition between cultures. Nonetheless, these studies suggest that there is something about modern society that tends to elevate BP.

Another factor that has been associated with increased BP in several studies is "lifestyle incongruity," defined as the extent to which a high-status style of life exceeds the norm for an individual's occupational class. Its evaluation is relatively objective and is based on a comparison between occupation and income on the one hand and the possession of material goods on the other. Its effects on BP may be most noticeable when it is combined with a lack of social support.

A similar concept is John Henryism, a scale used to investigate the effects of socioecological stress in blacks. An individual who scores high on the John Henryism scale is one who believes that he can control environmental stressors through a combination of hard work and determination. Men who score below the sample mean on education but above the mean on John Henryism have higher BPs than men who score above the mean on both measures.

The effects of socioecological stress on BP in blacks have also been documented in a population survey of BP in different neighborhoods of Detroit, which were defined as either "high stress" or "low stress" according to the socioeconomic status of the inhabitants (defined by variables such as income, home ownership, and education) and instability variables (eg, crime rate and marital instability). The highest BPs were seen in black men under the age of 40 living in high-stress neighborhoods; black and white men living in low-stress neighborhoods had similar pressures.

Some of the most persuasive evidence for a role of chronic stress in the development of hypertension comes from studies of "job strain," defined as jobs that combine high demands and low control or decision latitude, which are typically blue-collar jobs. Men employed in such jobs have a threefold increased risk of hypertension, and those who stay in high-strain jobs over a 3-year period have BP that is 11/7 mm Hg higher than men who were in persistently low-strain jobs. Exposure to job strain is also associated with increased left ventricular mass and risk of coronary heart disease.

A common feature of all these observations is an element of discord between the individual and his or her social setting. Most of the models used to describe these phenomena rely on an interaction of two or more factors to produce hypertension, rather than one factor acting alone.

Individual Psychological Factors and the Perception of Stress

The concept of a "hypertensive personality" has been debated for many years but is still unresolved. The idea is that the hypertensive individual harbors repressed hostility, or "anger-in," which is channeled into increased activity of the sympathetic nervous system, resulting in an increased BP. Although many studies have reported varying degrees of association between inhibited aggression and BP, others have reported negative or inconsistent results.

Individual Differences in Susceptibility to Psychological Factors

The effects that a given level of perceived stress will have on the cardiovascular system will depend to some extent on the physiological susceptibility of the individual. It has been suggested that individuals who show increased reactivity to stressful stimuli are at increased risk of developing hypertension. It must be admitted, however, that direct evidence in support of this mechanism is limited. It has been demonstrated that neurogenically mediated pressor episodes do not by themselves lead to any sustained increase of BP, although they can cause left ventricular hypertrophy. Another problem is that BP reactivity measured in the laboratory does not provide good prediction of BP changes during daily life.

Hypertensive subjects tend to show an enhanced response to mental challenges, such as mental arithmetic, compared with normotensives. These findings would be consistent with increased reactivity being at least in part a consequence rather than a cause of the hypertension. The only population-based study (conducted in Tecumseh, Michigan) did not find any correlation between reactivity and BP. One reason for the discrepancy between the Tecumseh findings and those of other studies was that the Tecumseh subjects were not necessarily aware that their BP was high, while in most other studies they were. This finding relates to other observations demonstrating that simply labeling people as hypertensive increases their BP reactivity to stress.

SUGGESTED READING

1. D'Atri DA, Fitzgerald EF, Kasl SV, Ostfeld AM. Crowding in prison: the relationship between changes in housing mode and blood pressure. *Psychosom Med.* 1981;43: 95–105.
2. Dressler WW. Social support, lifestyle incongruity, and arterial blood pressure in a southern black community. *Psychosom Med.* 1991;53:608–620.
3. Harburg E, Erfurt JC, Chape C, Hauenstein LS, Schull WJ, Schork MA. Socioecological stressor areas and black-white blood pressure: Detroit. *J Chronic Dis.* 1973;26:595–611.
4. Henry JP, Stephens PM, Ely DL. Psychosocial hypertension and the defense and defeat reactions. *J Hypertens.* 1986;4:687–697.
5. Julius S, Jones K, Schork N, Johnson E, Krause L, Nazzaro P, Zemva A. Independence of pressure reactivity from pressure levels in Tecumseh, Michigan. *Hypertension.* 1991;17(suppl III):III-12-III-21.
6. Pickering TG, Devereux RB, James GD, Gerin W, Landsbergis P, Schnall PL, Schwartz JE. Environmental influences on blood pressure and the role of job strain. *J Hypertens Suppl.* 1996;14:S179–S186.
7. Poulter NR, Khaw KT, Hopwood BE, Mugambi M, Peart WS, Rose G, Sever PS. The Kenyan Luo migration study: observations on the initiation of a rise in blood pressure. *BMJ.* 1990;300:967–972.
8. Rostrup M, Kjeldsen S, Eide IK. Awareness of hypertension increases blood pressure and sympathetic responses to cold pressor test. *Am J Hypertens.* 1990;3:912–917.
9. Timio M. Blood pressure trend and psychosocial factors: the case of the nuns in a secluded order. *Acta Physiol Scand Suppl.* 1997;640:137–139.

Chapter 97

Trends in Blood Pressure Control and Mortality

Thomas J. Thom, BA; Edward J. Roccella, PhD, MPH

KEY POINTS

- Approximately 50 million Americans have hypertension.

- National surveys show that among persons 18 to 74 years of age, average systolic blood pressures have decreased since the 1960s.

- There were marked increases in the percentage of hypertensive persons who are aware of their condition, are being treated, and have their blood pressure under control after the 1971–1974 survey, but there was lack of improvement in the 1990s.

- The sharp acceleration in the rate of decline in stroke mortality since 1972, which resulted in the United States' having one of the lowest death rates from stroke in the world, has apparently ended in the 1990s, and the rate may possibly be increasing.

See also Chapters 98, 99, 100

Estimates extrapolated from the 1988–1991 National Health and Nutrition Examination Survey (NHANES III) indicate that ≈50 million Americans have hypertension, which is one of the major risk factors for stroke, coronary heart disease (CHD), heart failure, and other cardiovascular-renal diseases. The effectiveness of the detection, treatment, and control of hypertension plays a major role in the primary and secondary prevention of these diseases. This seems to be especially true for stroke, possibly because the relationship between blood pressure and risk of stroke is even stronger than the relationship between blood pressure and CHD. The marked acceleration of the downward trend in age-adjusted stroke mortality in the United States after 1972 coincided with the major national health education effort to detect, treat, and control hypertension.

Definitions and Data Sources

Data from the 1960–1962 National Health Examination Survey, from the NHANES studies of 1971–1974 (NHANES I), 1976–1980 (NHANES II), and 1988–1994 (NHANES III), and from national vital (mortality) statistics from the National Center for Health Statistics are the primary sources of information for this review. Methodology and limitations of the survey design and procedures for blood pressure measurements used in the national surveys are described elsewhere. Hypertension is defined as a systolic blood pressure of ≥140 mm Hg, a diastolic pressure of ≥90 mm Hg, or use of antihypertensive medication (treated hypertensive patients). To examine long-term trends, the formerly accepted definition of 160 mm Hg for systolic and 95 mm Hg for diastolic blood pressure or on treatment has been used. In the health interviews, respondents are asked whether a physician has ever told them that they have hypertension or whether they are taking antihypertensive medication. On the basis of the two interview questions plus actual blood pressure measurements, the hypertensive person's awareness of his or her condition and treatment and control status can be ascertained. Mortality data in this chapter are for stroke (cerebrovascular diseases), CHD, and major cardiovascular diseases based on tabulation of US death

certificates as coded to the International Classification of Diseases of the World Health Organization.

Trends

Average Blood Pressure and Prevalence of Hypertension

The national surveys show that among persons 18 to 74 years of age, average systolic and diastolic blood pressures have generally decreased since the 1960s **(Table 97.1)**. Decreases were observed in men and women and in the white and black populations. Declines were greater among older than among younger age groups (data not shown). Both mean systolic and diastolic pressures were significantly higher in the black than in the white population, and mean blood pressures were higher in men than women overall. Men had higher mean blood pressures than women at younger ages, but later in life the reverse is true.

The prevalence of hypertension for persons 20 to 74 years of age was essentially unchanged during the 1960s and 1970s for white and black men and women, but data from NHANES III (1988–1994) indicate a substantial decline in prevalence **(Table 97.2)**.

Hypertension Awareness, Therapy, and Control

For age 18 to 74 years, **Figure 97.1** shows the marked improvement since 1971–1974 in the proportion of persons with hypertension (≥160/95 mm Hg or those with lower pressures but taking antihypertensive medication) who are aware of their condition, are being treated, and have their blood pressure under control. In 1971–1974, only 54% of the hypertensive population knew of their condition, 37% were being treated with drugs, and 16% of the hypertensive population (42% of those treated) had their blood pressure under control. By 1988–1991, 89% of persons with hypertension were aware of their condition, 79% were being treated with medication, and 64% of the hypertensive population (82% of those treated) had their high blood pressure under control. In general, those favorable trends are observed in all race/sex groups. Comparable percent-

Table 97.1. Average Blood Pressure in Persons 18 to 74 Years of Age by Sex and Race, United States, 1960–1962 to 1988–1994 National Health Examination Surveys

	WHITE		BLACK	
	M	F	M	F
Systolic blood pressure, mm Hg				
1960–1962	130	127	135	137
1971–1974	133	129	138	136
1976–1980	129	121	130	127
1988–1994	123	116	127	122
Diastolic blood pressure, mm Hg				
1960–1962	78	77	83	83
1971–1974	85	81	89	86
1976–1980	82	77	84	81
1988–1994	75	69	77	71

Values are age-adjusted. Blood pressures are based on 1, 2, or (usually) 3 seated measurments on one occasion.

Table 97.2. Percent Prevalence of Hypertension* in Persons 20 to 74 Years of Age by Sex and Race, United States, 1960–1962 to 1988–1994 National Health Examination Surveys

	WHITE		BLACK	
	M	F	M	F
1960–1962	39.3	31.7	48.1	50.8
1971–1974	41.7	32.4	51.8	50.3
1976–1980	43.5	32.3	48.7	47.5
1988–1994	24.3	19.3	34.9	33.8

*Either systolic blood pressure ≥140 mm Hg or diastolic ≥90 mm Hg or taking antihypertensive medication. Values are age-adjusted.

ages (numbers inside the bars in Figure 97.1) are available only for the 1976–1980 and 1988–1991 periods for the hypertensive population at the blood pressure threshold ≥140 mm Hg systolic or ≥90 mm Hg diastolic or taking antihypertensive medication.

During the NHANES III survey, which was conducted in two phases (1988–1991 and 1991–1994), there were small declines in awareness (73% to 68%), therapy (55% to 54%), and control (29% to 27%) of hypertension based on 140/90 mm Hg cut points in persons 18 to 74 years of age. These changes indicate that no further progress has been made in the 1990s. Recent reports have shown decreases in awareness, treatment, and control of hypertension in Minnesota and increases in age-adjusted average blood pressure levels of a cohort in Iowa.

The long-term data demonstrate the progress made during the two decades of national and community hypertension control efforts. These programs alerted the public to the dangers of uncontrolled hypertension and its sequelae and encouraged the public to visit their physicians, have their blood pressure measured, follow their doctors' advice, and stay on therapy. Data from the National Disease and Therapeutic Index, a survey of US physicians in private practice conducted by IMS America Limited of Ambler, Pa, show that the population received the message to visit their physicians for high blood pressure. IMS America reported a doubling from 1970 to 1990 in the number of visits to physicians for hypertension, to 89 million in 1990. In contrast, visits for all causes remained relatively stable.

Mortality

Stroke is the third leading cause of death, accounting for ≈150 000 deaths each year. **Figure 97.2** shows that the age-adjusted death rates for stroke declined at a modest rate during the 22 years from 1950 to 1972, a decrease of 28%. After that year, there was a sharp acceleration of the rate of decline for 18 years, followed by a flat trend since 1992. Between 1972 and 1991, the decline was 59%. The annual decline was ≈2% per year before 1972 and as much as 6% per year after that. Acceleration of the rate of decline occurred in all age/race/sex groups. Figure 97.2 also shows the reduction in mortal-

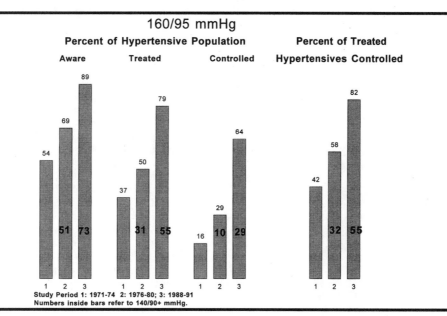

Figure 97.1. Hypertension awareness, treatment, and control rates reported in NHANES; age 18 to 74 years.

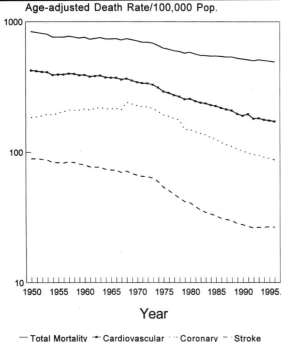

Age-adjusted Death Rate/100,000 Pop.

Year

─ Total Mortality ─•─ Cardiovascular ⋯ Coronary ─ ─ Stroke

Rates adjusted to U.S. population, 1940.
No correction made for changes caused by revision
in the International Classification of Diseases.

Figure 97.2. Death rates for total mortality and cardiovascular diseases in the United States, 1950 to 1996.

ity from CHD and demonstrates that the trend for total cardiovascular disease improved considerably more than did the trend for all causes of death combined.

Evidence of declining trends in incidence and immediate or long-term survival after stroke is not available on a national scale. Hospital discharge statistics for broad age groups do show very modest increases in rates of hospitalization for stroke between 1970 and ≈1985, followed by very modest declines to 1994. They also show steady and significant increases in the percentage of stroke patients discharged alive from hospitals and decreases in the length of stay since 1970. These trends are also apparent for CHD. These statistics, however, are an incomplete measure of incidence and case-fatality, and they are affected by repeat admissions and changes in hospital admission practices.

In addition, community-based studies conducted during the 1970s and 1980s (the Minnesota Heart Survey, the Honolulu Heart Program, the Framingham Study, and the study in Rochester, Minn) also report substantial declines in stroke incidence and rates of hospitalizations for stroke as well as improved survival.

The modest decline in mortality from stroke from 1950 to 1972 remains largely unexplained. During that time, there were few effective and pervasive means to control blood pressure. Data are not available from before 1960 on trends regarding population blood pressure. In the 1970s and 1980s, population average systolic and diastolic blood pressures and prevalence of hypertension declined.

Role of Education

The sharp acceleration in the rate of decline in stroke mortality that began after 1972 continued until recently. It resulted in the United States' having one of the lowest death rates from stroke in the world. Many factors contributed to the decline in mortality from stroke and from CHD. These include the introduction of well-tolerated oral antihypertensive drugs and heightened efforts to treat hypertension with these agents and with changes in lifestyle as both adjunctive and definitive care. Clinicians have become motivated to manage hypertension more effectively when clinical trial evidence demonstrated reductions in the risks of nonfatal and fatal cardiovascular diseases from lowering blood pressure. In 1972, a large national effort commenced, the National High Blood Pressure Education Program, designed to educate the public, health professionals, and hypertensive patients about the health risks posed by hypertension and the health benefits of its detection, treatment, and control. This program also developed a national infrastructure that supported and disseminated blood pressure management guidelines such as the six periodic reports of the Joint National Committee on Detection, Evaluation, and Treatment of High Blood Pressure.

It is widely believed that part of the mortality decline for stroke and CHD was the result of the massive and successful national campaign to detect, treat, and control hypertension. Simultaneous reductions in the prevalence of smoking and high blood cholesterol and improvements in the treatment of other cardiovascular diseases undoubtedly also contributed to the decline in cardiovascular mortality. It should be noted that many countries have also adopted the US guidelines and procedures for national efforts to control blood pressure and have experienced long-term declines in stroke mortality and, in some cases, acceleration of the rate of decline over the past 20 years.

SUGGESTED READING

1. Burt VL, Cutler JA, Higgins M, Horan MJ, Labarthe D, Brown C, Roccella EJ. Trends in prevalence, awareness, treatment, and control of hypertension in the adult US population: data from the Health Examination Surveys, 1960 to 1991 [published correction appears in *Hypertension.* 1996;27:1192]. *Hypertension.* 1995;26:60–69.
2. Burt VL, Whelton P, Roccella EJ, Brown C, Cutler JA, Higgins M, Horan MJ, Labarthe D. Prevalence of hypertension in the US adult population: results from the third National Health and Nutrition Examination Survey, 1988–1991. *Hypertension.* 1995;25:305–313.
3. *Health US, 1996–97 and Injury Chartbook.* Hyattsville, Md: National Center for Health Statistics; 1997.
4. Lenfant C, Roccella EJ. Trends in hypertension control in the United States. *Chest.* 1984;86:459–462.
5. National Heart, Lung, and Blood Institute. *Morbidity and Mortality Chartbook on Cardiovascular, Lung, and Blood Diseases, 1996.* Bethesda, Md: US Department of Health and Human Services, Public Health Service, National Institutes of Health; 1996.
6. Proceedings of the National Heart, Lung, and Blood Institute Conference on the Decline in Stroke Mortality, Bethesda, Maryland, November 30–December 1, 1992.. *Ann Epidemiol.* 1993;3:453–575.
7. *The Sixth Report of the Joint National Committee on Prevention, Detection, Evaluation, and Treatment of High Blood Pressure.* Bethesda, Md: NIH publication 98–4080; November 1987.
8. Stamler J, Stamler R, Neaton JD. Blood pressure, systolic and diastolic, and cardiovascular risks: US population data. *Arch Intern Med.* 1993;153:598–615.
9. Veterans Administration Cooperative Study Group on Antihypertensive Agents. Effects of treatment on morbidity in hypertension, II: results in patients with diastolic blood pressure averaging 90 through 114 mm Hg. *JAMA.* 1970;213:1143–1152.

Chapter 98

Hypertension

A Worldwide Epidemic

Patrick J. Mulrow

KEY POINTS

- Hypertension is a worldwide epidemic with an estimated 690 million people being hypertensive.

- Hypertension is recognized worldwide as a major cardiovascular risk factor. Cardiovascular disease accounts for 30% of the world's deaths.

- Hypertension is poorly controlled, with less than 25% controlled in developed countries and less than 10% in developing countries.

- Socioeconomic conditions in the world suggest that prevention through lifestyle modifications is the universal "vaccine" against hypertension.

See also Chapters 75, 97, 99, 100

Hypertension is a worldwide epidemic that can affect all ages but primarily occurs in adults. The prevalence increases dramatically with age, and in many populations 50% of the people more than 60 years of age have hypertension. It is estimated that there are 3.45 billion adults in the world (20 years and older), and on the basis of a 20% prevalence, approximately 690 million people would have hypertension. In China alone the estimated prevalence is 90 million.

Hypertension is one of the major risk factors for stroke, coronary heart disease, and heart and kidney failure. About 30% of worldwide deaths, or 15 million, are due to cardiovascular diseases. The World Health Organization (WHO) estimates there are 5 million deaths per year worldwide due to strokes, with another 30 million suffering from its disabling effects. In the United States and other countries, even inadequate hypertension treatment programs have significantly decreased the occurrence of strokes. Management of hypertension can significantly reduce the suffering from stroke around the world.

Approximately 135 million people suffer from diabetes mellitus worldwide. Hypertension significantly increases the already high incidence of stroke, heart attacks, and renal failure in diabetic patients.

Epidemiology of Hypertension Worldwide

Estimates of the prevalence of hypertension in various parts of the world may only be compared with caution because of differences in cut points, quality of the blood pressure measurements and surveys, age and ethnic groups studied, and socioeconomic conditions. Moreover, equal blood pressure levels may have different cardiovascular effects, depending upon associated risk factors, such as smoking, obesity, diabetes mellitus, and dyslipidemia.

Despite the differences in the quality of the epidemiological studies carried out throughout the world, several factors seem to be consistent. The adult population has approximately 20% prevalence of hypertension if the cut point is 140/90 mm Hg. The prevalence increases with age and more than 50% in the population >60 years of age. In earlier years, before the age of 40, men have a greater prevalence than women, but in the elderly, women have a greater prevalence. Fewer hypertensive men than women are aware of their hypertension or are treated or controlled. The urban population has a higher prevalence than the rural population. In some countries, different ethnic groups have different prevalence; for example, in Chinese males, Tibetans have a prevalence of 11.4% compared with only 5.85% in the Man ethnic group. Whites and Mexican-Americans in the United States have significantly lower prevalence than blacks.

Four rigorous national health surveys have been reported in the nineties, two in developed countries, United States, and Canada, and two in developing countries, Egypt and China (**Table 98.1**). Even in Canada, where access to the National Health Care System is easy and mostly free, the prevalence is high and the control rate is low. Egypt's control rate of less than 10% probably reflects the situation in many developing countries.

A Survey of the Status of Hypertension by the Members of the World Hypertension League

Thirty-five hypertension societies/leagues from 36 different countries submitted abstracts for the 17th World Hypertension League (WHL) Council Conference held in Montreal, Canada, on June 28, 1997.

Twenty-seven of the abstracts contained answers for all or part of the questionnaire that was sent to all league presidents. These data were collated and reviewed.

The information requested on the questionnaire was as follows:

- Blood pressure level used to define hypertension
- Prevalence of hypertension
- Percent of hypertensives who were aware of their diagnosis

Table 98.1. Comparison of Hypertension Surveys in Four Countries

COUNTRY	PREVALENCE	AWARE	TREATED	CONTROLLED
United States	20.4	73	55	21
Canada	22	58	39	16
Egypt	26.3	37	24	8
China	13.6	25	13	3

Values are percentages. These studies were performed following standardized protocols using trained personnel. Nationwide cross-sectional studies of randomly selected subjects were carried out. The results were adjusted for age and gender. Aware indicates the percentage of hypertensive subjects who knew they had hypertension; Treated indicates the percentage of hypertensive subjects on hypertension treatment; and Controlled indicates the percentage of hypertensive subjects whose blood pressure on treatment was below 140/90 mm Hg.

- Percent of hypertensive patients on treatment
- Percent of hypertensives controlled
- Drugs used for treatment

The answers were based primarily on national epidemiological surveys. Two surveys were of specific regions. A number of abstracts indicated that the Monitoring Trends and Determinants in Cardiovascular Disease (MONICA) study standards were followed, but the precise methodology of the surveys could not be ascertained from all of the abstracts.

The source of the data on drug usage in treatment was not clearly defined in most abstracts, but when stated, the source was the result of either hospital or physician surveys or government statistics.

The blood pressure cut point varied among countries. The European countries tended to use the WHO/International Society of Hypertension (ISH) recommendation of 160/95 mm Hg, while other countries used 140/90 mm Hg. Of the 27 countries reporting, 14 used 140/90 mm Hg, with a prevalence range from 11% to 43% and a median of 24%, and 13 used 160/95 mm Hg, with a prevalence from 5% to 34% and a median of 23%. However, even when countries used 160/95 mm Hg as a cut point for the diagnosis, 140/90 mm Hg was used by some as an index of control.

The prevalence of hypertension varied considerably and was influenced by a number of factors. By far, the most important influence was age. Most countries reported a >50% prevalence of hypertension in the population >60 years of age. Obviously, the blood pressure cut point has a significant influence on the prevalence of hypertension. In many countries, the rural population had a lower prevalence than the urban population. The rural population had less awareness of their hypertension, and there was a lower rate of treatment and hence control. The ethnic groups within a country had an influence on the prevalence of hypertension. The influence of gender on prevalence varied among countries, but consistently fewer men were on treatment than women. Far Eastern countries reported a lower prevalence than European countries.

The percent of patients aware of their hypertension and those on treatment have increased considerably in those countries that have reported recurrent surveys over several years. Of the 16 countries presenting data, the number controlled at below 140/90 mm Hg is de-pressingly small. The range was between 3% and 31%, a median of 16% being controlled.

The antihypertensive drugs used varied among countries and were influenced, to some extent, by the wealth of the countries. The richer countries tended to use more calcium antagonists and ACE inhibitors, while the poorer countries used diuretics, β-blockers, or other older drugs. When comparison with earlier years was shown, the trend was for more calcium antagonists and ACE inhibitors. The average use reported by 11 countries for diuretics was 26%, β-blockers 29%, calcium antagonists 28%, and ACE inhibitors 23%.

In summary, these preliminary and somewhat imprecise data point out the considerable variation among the countries in the results of the survey. Some of this variation is due to the different criteria used for defining hypertension prevalence and control. Obviously, different countries have different questions to be answered by a survey, but certain criteria need to be standardized, such as age, cut points, and definition of control.

Prevention of Hypertension

Despite the imprecise data on hypertension prevalence and control around the world, it is clear that hypertension is a worldwide epidemic and a major risk factor for cardiovascular disease. The main approaches to controlling adverse health effects on populations should be to prevent the development of hypertension as well as to modify the risk factors that accentuate the cardiovascular damage of hypertension. Small changes in the blood pressure of populations have marked effects on cardiovascular disease. It has been estimated that a downward shift of 2 mm Hg in the systolic blood pressure of a population will reduce annual stroke rates by 6% and coronary artery disease by 4%. Effecting lifestyle changes in communities will require collaboration among professionals, government, industry, media, and the public. Some of the factors that are possible to be modified on a community-wide basis are summarized below.

Reduction in Sodium Intake

Epidemiological surveys, clinical trials, and animal experiments show a relationship between salt intake and blood pressure. Individuals vary in their response to changes in sodium intake. Black and elderly subjects seem to be more sensitive to sodium intake. In one meta-analysis of 22 clinical trials in hypertensive subjects, a reduction in sodium intake of 56 to 105 mmol reduced SBP/DBP 4.8/2.5. The Intersalt multicenter international cooperative study indicated that over a 30-year age span, 100 mmol/d lower sodium intake would be associated with a 9–mm Hg less rise in blood pressure with age. To change sodium intake requires food industry involvement, particularly in industrial countries, and education of those who control food preparation, usually a wife or mother, in developing countries.

Weight Reduction

In many countries, elevated blood pressure is attributable to a considerable degree to increased body weight. Weight reduction lowers blood pressure and lipid levels. A report on the primary prevention of hypertension in individuals with high-to-normal blood pressure showed that weight reduction caused a significant decrease in blood pressure and hypertension incidence over 3 to 4 years. Prevention of obesity also reduces prevalence of diabetes mellitus.

Smoking

Cigarette smoking substantially increases the cardiovascular risk from hypertension. A major effort to reduce smoking in populations will have an impact on cardiovascular effects of hypertension.

SUGGESTED READING

1. Burt VL, Cutler JA, Higgins M, Horan MJ, Labarthe D, Whelton P, Brown C, Roccella EJ. Trends in the prevalence, awareness, treatment, and control of hypertension in the adult US population: data from the health examination surveys, 1960–1991 [published correction appears in *Hypertension.* 1996;27:1192]. *Hypertension* 1995;26:60–69.

2. Cutler JA, Follmann D, Allender PS. Randomized trials of sodium reduction: an overview. *Am J Clin Nutr.* 1997;65(suppl 2):643S–651S.

3. Elliott P, Stamler J, Nichols R, Dyer AR, Stamler R, Kesteloot H, Marmot M, for the Intersalt Cooperative Research Group. Intersalt revisited: further analyses of 24 hour sodium excretion and blood pressure within and across populations. *BMJ.* 1996;312:1249–1253.

4. Ibrahim MM, Rizk H, Appel LJ, el Aroussy W, Helmy S, Sharaf Y, Ashour Z, Kandil H, Roccella E, Whelton PK, for the NHP Investigative Team. Hypertension prevalence, awareness, treatment, and control in Egypt: results from the Egyptian National Hypertension Project (NHP). *Hypertension.* 1995;26:886–890.

5. Joffres MR, Ghadirian P, Fodor JG, Petrasovits A, Chockalingam A, Hamet P. Awareness, treatment, and control of hypertension in Canada. *Am J Hypertens.* 1997;10: 1097–1102.

6. Joint World Health Organization/International Society of Hypertension Meeting. 1991 guidelines for the prevention of hypertension and associated cardiovascular disease. *J Hypertens.* 1992;10:97–99.

7. Mulrow PJ, Pötzsch J, Sleight P, eds. *WHL—Yearbook 1997.* Toledo, Ohio: World Hypertension League; 1997.

8. Tao S, Wu X, Duan X, Fang W, Hao J, Fan D, Wang W, Li Y. Hypertension prevalence and status of awareness, treatment and control in China. *Chin Med J* (*Engl*). 1995; 108:483–489.

9. World Health Organization. *Hypertension Control: Report of a WHO Expert Committee.* Geneva, Switzerland: World Health Organization; 1996.

10. World Health Organization. *The World Health Report 1997: Conquering Suffering, Enriching Humanity.* Geneva, Switzerland: World Health Organization; 1997.

Chapter 99

Prevention of Hypertension

Jeffrey A. Cutler, MD, MPH; Jeremiah Stamler, MD

KEY POINTS

- A wide variety of evidence supports the potential for hypertension prevention through weight control, increased physical activity, moderation of sodium and alcohol intake, increased potassium intake, and a dietary pattern rich in fruits, vegetables, and low-fat meat, fish, and dairy products.

- Clinical trials evaluating blood pressure changes in response to nutritional and behavioral interventions provide key evidence for hypertension prevention.

- Both targeted (including clinical) and population-wide (public health) strategies are important approaches to hypertension prevention.

See also Chapters 97, 98, 118

Background: The Strategic Challenge

The prevalence of hypertension in US adults is estimated as ≈1 in 4, or 50 million persons; incidence, ≈1 million new cases per year. Tens of millions of others have blood pressure (BP) levels above optimal, although not hypertensive, and they are at increased risk of major cardiovascular and renal diseases **(Figure 99.1)**.

Until the 1990s, the approach to coping with this mass BP problem was primarily a "high-risk" strategy: detect, evaluate, and treat people with definite hypertension. This emphasis has accomplished much during the past three decades: it ended therapeutic nihilism in regard to hypertension and has resulted in control of hypertension for millions of Americans. It is a reasonable inference that this effort has been one of the most important factors contributing to the decades-long, substantial declines in mortality rates from coronary heart disease and stroke and consequent increases in life expectancy for adult men and women. But this high-risk strategy has serious limitations: it is defensive rather than proactive, and it relies primarily on drug treatment, with its mix of favorable and unfavorable effects and costs. In addition, despite great progress, it still leaves millions of Americans with hypertension treated inadequately or not at all, and it neglects the tens of millions of people with BP elevations that are associated with increased risk although not yet at levels considered to be hypertensive. Above all, this approach is never-ending; it offers no possibility of terminating the epidemic of high BP. Only the primary prevention of this major risk factor offers this possibility **(Figure 99.2)**.

In this regard, a pivotal fact is that the adverse BP levels rampant among adults result from a rise in systolic and diastolic pressure experienced by most people during the decades from youth through middle age, with a continuing rise in systolic pressure through later years. Maintenance of young-adult favorable BP levels throughout life would therefore end high BP as a mass problem. Recent research advances make it possible to set this as a strategic goal.

Key Evidence Supporting Ability to Prevent BP Rise During Adulthood and High BP

Evidence is now available on the relationship to BP of lifestyle, particularly nutritional traits, common in the population. These in-

clude caloric imbalance with consequent overweight, habitual high salt (NaCl) intake, inadequate potassium intake, excess alcohol consumption, and sedentary habits. By the early 1990s, the extensive data on these traits served as a scientific foundation for the first international and US expert group reports on the prevention of high BP. During the mid-1990s, new findings also indicated relationships of several other dietary factors to BP. These data are from both observational studies and randomized controlled trials, as well as from animal experiments.

Observational Studies

Methodological problems. Aside from overweight, all other candidate risk factors are difficult to measure reliably. Most are dietary components, regarding which this problem is especially great. Self-report methods suffer from limitations in reporting, recording, and analysis; objective methods, principally collection of 24-hour urine for sodium and potassium excretion, are inconvenient and, given inevitable intermittence with free-living people, give only an estimate of usual intake. Importantly, intakes vary considerably from day to day, so that accurate characterization of an individual's usual intake requires repeated observations over time. Because of BP variability, the outcome variable is also more accurately assessed with repeated measurements. Finally, there must be sufficient variation among members of the study population to detect associations of lifestyle factors with BP level or change (and hypertension prevalence/incidence). Large study groups help to accomplish this.

Few prospective cohort studies examine associations of multiple factors, singly and in combination, with BP change or hypertension incidence. Such studies are faced with formidable methodological challenges, related primarily to the need for repeated measurements in large samples of individuals over a lengthy follow-up period.

Findings from cross-sectional epidemiological studies. One epidemiological strategy that has been successfully used to examine relationships to BP of a broad range of factors is the international comparative study. Although such studies have used only cross-sectional designs thus far, they have been informative. For example, the Intersalt Study involved >10 000 men and women 20 to 59 years old, sam-

CLASSIFICATION OF BLOOD PRESSURE FOR ADULTS AGE 18 YEARS OR OLDER

Average DBP mm Hg	Average SBP mm Hg			
	< 120	120-129	130-139	≥ 140
< 80	Optimal†	Normal	High Normal	High
80-84	Normal	Normal	High Normal	High
85-89	High Normal	High Normal	High Normal	High
≥ 90	High	High	High	High

† Optimal blood pressure, with regard to cardiovascular risk, is SBP <120 mm Hg and DBP <80 mm Hg. However, unusually low readings should be evaluated for clinical significance.

Figure 99.1. Systolic and diastolic BP criteria for classification of BP as optimal, normal (not optimal), high-normal, and high. The recommendation is to classify on the basis of average BP for an individual from ≥2 readings at each of ≥2 visits after an initial screening, with the individual not taking drugs and not acutely ill. Optimal BP, with regard to cardiovascular risk, is systolic BP <120 mm Hg and diastolic BP <80 mm Hg; however, unusually low readings should be evaluated for clinical significance. When systolic and diastolic BPs fall into different categories, the higher category should be selected to classify the individual's BP status, eg, 138/82 should be classified as high-normal BP. Reproduced with permission from the Fifth Report of the Joint National Committee on Detection, Evaluation, and Treatment of High Blood Pressure, National High Blood Pressure Education Program, National Institutes of Health, National Heart, Lung, and Blood Institute, NIH publication 93–1088, January 1993.

pled at 52 centers in 32 countries. It tested both cross-population (ecological) (N=52) and within-population (N>10 000) prior hypotheses. To deal with the methodological problem in assessing individual intake, it used a large sample size and a single carefully collected 24-hour urine per person to assess intake of sodium, potassium, and other variables. Also, the study used repeat urine collection in a random 8% of participants to estimate measurement reliability and correct for it. Its cross-population and within-population analyses gave concordant results, substantiating the relationships of sodium and potassium excretion (direct and inverse, respectively) and the direct associations of body mass index and alcohol intake with BP levels, hypertension prevalence, and slope of BP on age. Subsequent analyses from Intersalt, based on measurement of urinary nitrogen

excretion as a marker of dietary protein, provided evidence for an inverse association of protein intake with systolic and diastolic BP. Additional support for this intriguing relationship has come from other observational studies, including analyses of data collected over 6 years from 11 342 middle-aged men in the Multiple Risk Factor Intervention Trial (MRFIT). The MRFIT results support the concept that multiple dietary factors influence BP, including direct associations with saturated fat and dietary cholesterol, overweight, and dietary sodium and alcohol intake and an inverse association with potassium intake in addition to protein.

Findings from prospective observational epidemiological studies. In the Chicago Western Electric Study of 1560 middle-aged men examined annually for 9 years, usual dietary intake during the previous

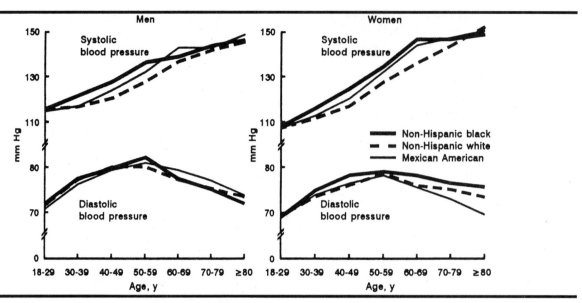

Figure 99.2.   Mean systolic and diastolic BPs by age and race/ethnicity for men and women, US population ≥18 years old. Reproduced with permission from Burt VL, Whelton P, Roccella EJ, et al. Prevalence of hypertension in the US adult population: results from the Third National Health and Nutrition Examination Survey, 1998–1991. *Hypertension.* 1995;25:305–313.

month was assessed by in-depth interview at years 0 and 1. Baseline dietary cholesterol and alcohol intake were directly related to BP change over time; dietary vegetable protein and antioxidant intake (vitamin C and β-carotene), inversely related. Change in weight over the years was also directly related to BP change. (Sodium and potassium intake were not measured.)

Two large cohort studies of health professionals, conducted entirely by questionnaire, relied on self-report of usual postbaseline BP or diagnosis of incident hypertension, with the assumption that this would be sufficiently accurate in these well-informed individuals. Usual intake of foods and nutrients was determined at baseline by the Willett food frequency questionnaire. Several of the expected variables—weight (body mass index) and alcohol intake—were found to be strong BP predictors. Dietary potassium, magnesium, and fiber were inversely related to BP change over time and incidence of high BP. Sodium intake was not, but salt intake is particularly difficult to measure by questionnaire, and those health professionals with originally higher intake and high-normal BPs may have reduced dietary salt, with resultant confounding of the analysis.

These findings from large epidemiological studies, cross-sectional and prospective, on relationships of several dietary variables (macronutrients and micronutrients) to BP and BP change, along with previous reports on inverse relationships of vegetarian diets with BP and hypertension, gave impetus to the conduct of the Dietary Approaches to Stop Hypertension (DASH) trial.

Intervention Trials

Four large, randomized clinical trials conducted in adults with high-normal BPs have reported findings on the effects of nutritional and other lifestyle changes on BP levels and hypertension incidence. The 5-year Primary Prevention of Hypertension (PPH) Study found that a multifactor intervention (weight loss, reduction of sodium and alcohol intake, increased physical activity) significantly lowered av-

erage follow-up BP by 1 to 2 mm Hg and hypertension incidence by 54% (8.8% versus 19.2% for intervention and control participants, respectively). This outcome was attributable to the modest weight loss (average of ≈3 kg) and, to a lesser extent, sodium reduction (average of ≈20%). The Hypertension Prevention Trial (HPT) studied these two intervention approaches both separately and combined and tested increased dietary potassium as well. Again, weight loss lowered BP throughout the 3 years of the trial, with the effect waning as weight was partially regained. Nevertheless, the data trended toward a lower incidence of hypertension, by 27%. Sodium reduction was very modest (10% at 3 years) and did not significantly lower mean BP, although here, too, the incidence of hypertension was apparently reduced. The combined intervention encountered diminished effectiveness in weight reduction, perhaps because too much was being asked of participants at once, and consequently, BP results were not better than with single interventions. Only a modest increase of 8% in potassium intake was maintained through most of the follow-up, and evidence for a BP effect was minimal.

The Trials of Hypertension Prevention (TOHP) phase I tested a broad range of interventions aimed at factors thought to be related to BP levels. In addition to counseling overweight participants for weight reduction (with inclusion of an exercise component) or sodium reduction, a third lifestyle approach (stress management) was evaluated; also, four nutritional supplements (calcium, magnesium, potassium, and fish oil) were tested in placebo-controlled, double-blind designs. During the first 6 months of intervention, only weight loss and sodium reduction produced significant BP reductions, by 2 to 4 mm Hg systolic and 1 to 3 mm Hg diastolic BP. By design, lifestyle groups were also followed up for a period of 18 months to assess maintenance of behavioral change. During this relatively short period, weight and sodium reduction each demonstrated tendencies to decrease hypertension incidence, by 51% and 24%, respectively. Stress management showed no such trend.

TOHP phase II, a longer trial, further evaluated benefits of weight loss and sodium reduction, singly and in combination. The most important additional finding of TOHP-II was that each of the interventions lowered the incidence of hypertension significantly, by ≈20% over the 3- to 4-year duration of the trial. In addition, during the initial 6-month follow-up period, the effects of weight loss and sodium reduction on hypertension incidence were additive. A combination of the two interventions was also more effective than either one alone in the Trial on Nonpharmacological Intervention in the Elderly (TONE), which studied hypertensive participants for 2.5 years. At the other extreme of age, a group of Dutch investigators showed that consumption of infant formula with decreased sodium content starting in the neonatal period resulted in lower systolic BP at 6 months of age. Of potentially great significance, reexamination of 35% of these infants after 15 years showed maintenance of a 3.6/2.2 mm Hg advantage in BP levels for the initially lower sodium cohort, despite little evidence of difference in current sodium intake or any other BP determinants at the follow-up examination.

Participants in clinical trials (including those just described) are volunteers and thus are apt to be more highly motivated toward lifestyle change and enjoy socioeconomic circumstances more conducive to modifying behavior than other social groups. To achieve broad public health benefits, efficacious methods to prevent hypertension should be shown to be effective in broadly representative populations. Over a 5.5-year period in the Stanford Five-City Project, there was some evidence for lesser weight gain and somewhat stronger indication of improved physical fitness among adults 25 to 74 years old in intervention cities compared with control cities.

Reducing dietary salt should be one approach that is particularly amenable to a population approach, because upward of 85% of dietary sodium comes from processed foods. Two community-intervention salt-reduction trials have been completed in Europe using "quasi experimental" designs (one intervention, one control community). In the Portuguese Salt Trial, two rural communities were compared, with random samples of residents 15 to 69 years old examined before intervention, then annually for 2 years. The health education program in the intervention community was facilitated by the fact that 50% of the very high salt consumption (360 mmol/d sodium) came from that added in cooking at home, and another 33% was derived from one food item, salt-dried codfish. There was also a focus on reducing salt used in commercial bread-baking. Results of this trial showed sodium excretion to be 42% lower in the intervention community at 1 year, and there were significant reductions of mean BPs of 4 to 5 mm Hg at both 1 and 2 years.

In contrast, the Belgian salt trial was much less successful in its intervention; there were no net changes in sodium excretion or BP for men, sodium changes for women were modest (20%), and differences in mean BP reductions (2.9 mm Hg systolic and 1.6 mm Hg diastolic BP) were not significant. In contrast to the Portuguese trial, the same individuals were not examined at baseline and follow-up, leading to less precise estimation of BP change.

Another community intervention experiment studied adolescents at two boarding schools. In a crossover design with each phase lasting 1 academic year, sodium intake was reduced 15% to 20% merely by changes in food purchasing and preparation, with a significant effect on systolic and diastolic BP of ≈2 mm Hg. This study is encouraging because of the simplicity of the intervention and because prevention is theoretically most attractive when begun in childhood. A recent 3-year community trial in urban north China also reported significant reductions of systolic BP (5 mm Hg in men and 6 mm Hg in women 15 to 64 years old) associated with net reductions in sodium intake of only 14% in men and 6% in women.

Current Recommendations and Future Directions

Consistent recommendations for preventive medicine and public health have emerged from the World Health Organization/International Society of Hypertension Guidelines Committee and the comprehensive US Working Group Report on the Primary Prevention of Hypertension. The reports emphasize (1) weight control and increased physical activity (for effects on BP and other risk factors), (2) no more than moderate alcohol intake (daily average of ≤2 standard drinks, ie, no more than 1 oz or 26 g of ethanol), (3) limitation of dietary sodium to ≤2.4 g/d (equivalent to 6 g of sodium chloride), and (4) increased dietary potassium.

Regarding reduction of psychosocial stress, more study is required, and no specific roles for supplementing calcium or magnesium intake were noted.

In addition to the foregoing reports, the 1997 Sixth Report of the Joint National Committee on Prevention, Detection, Evaluation, and Treatment of High Blood Pressure gave special emphasis to the very encouraging results of the DASH trial. In this 8-week outpatient feeding trial, DASH found that a diet rich in fruits, vegetables, and fat-free and low-fat dairy foods, with reduced total and saturated fat and dietary cholesterol, plus modestly increased protein, lowered BP in adults by 5.5/3.0 mm Hg. Importantly, body weight and sodium intake were maintained at constant levels in all participants, who consumed little or no alcohol. Also, in nonhypertensives separately, the diet reduced BP by 3.5/2.1 mm Hg.

Thus, the results of DASH add to the extensive evidence on established lifestyle causes of rise in BP with age and resultant high incidence of hypertension. This evidence leads to the reasonable inference that most of the knowledge is in hand for the primary prevention of high BP. While ongoing or needed research pursues such issues as (1) the full potential of combined lifestyle approaches, (2) the effects in special population groups, (3) better methods for estimation of food and nutrient intake, and (4) potential for incorporation of hypertension prevention into primary medical care, it is possible to apply existing knowledge in pursuit of making the rise in BP with age rare and optimal BP levels common, thereby ending the epidemic.

SUGGESTED READING

1. Ellison RC, Capper AL, Stephenson WP, Goldberg RJ, Hasmer DW Jr, Humphrey KF, Ockene JK, Gamble WJ, Witschi JC, Stare FJ. Effects on blood pressure of a decrease in sodium use in institutional food preparation: the Exeter-Andover project. *J Clin Epidemiol.* 1989;42:201–208.

2. Farquhar JW, Fortmann SP, Flora JA, Taylor CB, Haskell WL, Williams PT, Maccoby N, Wood PD. Effects of communitywide education on cardiovascular disease risk factors: the Stanford Five-City Project. *JAMA.* 1990;264:359–365.

3. Forte JG, Miguel JM, Miguel MJ, de Pádua F, Rose G. Salt and blood pressure: a community trial. *J Hum Hypertens.* 1989;3:179–184.

4. Geleijnse JM, Hofman A, Witteman JC, Hazebroek AA, Valkenburg HA, Grobbee DE. Long-term effects of neonatal sodium restriction on blood pressure [published erratum appears in *Hypertension.* 1997;29:1211]. *Hypertension.* 1996;29:913–917.

5. Stamler J, Caggiula A, Grandits GA, Kjelsberg M, Cutler JA. Relationship to blood pressure of combinations of dietary macronutrients: findings of the Multiple Risk Factor Intervention Trial (MRFIT). *Circulation.* 1996;94:2417–2423.

6. Stamler J, Stamler R, Neaton JD. Blood pressure, systolic and diastolic, and cardiovascular risks: US population data. *Arch Intern Med.* 1993;153:598–615.

7. Stamler R, Stamler J, Gosch FC, Civinelli J, Fishman J, McKeever P, McDonald A, Dyer AR. Primary prevention of hypertension by nutritional-hygienic means: final report of a randomized, controlled trial [published erratum appears in *JAMA.* 1989;262:3132]. *JAMA.* 1989;262:1801–1807.

8. The Hypertension Prevention Trial Research Group. The Hypertension Prevention Trial: three-year effects of dietary changes on blood pressure. *Arch Intern Med.* 1990;150:153–162.

9. The Trials of Hypertension Prevention Collaborative Research Group. The effects of nonpharmacologic interventions on blood pressure of persons with high normal levels: results of the Trials of Hypertension Prevention, phase I [published erratum appears in *JAMA.* 1992;267:2330]. *JAMA.* 1992;267:1213–1220.

10. The Trials of Hypertension Prevention Collaborative Research Group. Effects of weight loss and sodium reduction intervention on blood pressure and hypertension incidence in overweight people with high-normal blood pressure: the Trials of Hypertension Prevention, phase II. *Arch Intern Med.* 1997;157:657–667.

Chapter 100

Treatment Trials: Morbidity and Mortality

Bruce M. Psaty, MD, PhD; Curt D. Furberg, MD, PhD

KEY POINTS

- Control of elevated systolic or diastolic blood pressure reduces the risk of stroke, myocardial infarction, congestive heart failure, and death.

- High-risk patients, such as the elderly, are prime candidates for antihypertensive therapy.

- Diuretics in low doses are effective, economical, and safe, especially in the elderly.

- Only 60% to 70% of patients respond to single-drug therapy.

See also Chapters 97, 98, 101

With rare exceptions, high blood pressure is an asymptomatic risk factor for cardiovascular disease. Pharmacological treatment is initiated to prevent the complications of untreated hypertension: major disease end points such as stroke, acute myocardial infarction, and congestive heart failure. This chapter focuses on the evidence from the completed randomized trials of antihypertensive therapy that specified cardiovascular morbidity and mortality as their primary outcomes. Several key issues in the design of studies that evaluate a therapy are reviewed; two major randomized trials, the Hypertension Detection and Follow-up Program (HDFP) and the Medical Research Council (MRC) trials, are described; and the results of several recent meta-analyses are summarized.

Issues in Study Design

In 1958, Dustan and colleagues reported that the long-term treatment of patients who presented with malignant hypertension was associated with a 1-year survival rate of 70%, far better than the rate of 20% among untreated patients with malignant hypertension in previous studies. The design used by Dustan was a cohort study that relied on historical controls. In addition to cohort studies, case-control studies are also available to evaluate the risks and benefits of a therapy. Observational studies, however, are subject to a variety of potential biases that may threaten the validity of the treatment-control comparison.

The preferred design to evaluate a therapy is the randomized controlled clinical trial. On average, randomization produces groups that are similar at baseline with respect to their expected response to therapy, their propensity for compliance, and their risk for the outcome of interest. With randomization, the study becomes an unbiased test of the therapy. Complete follow-up of subjects, careful ascertainment of events, and blinded classification of outcomes ensure the validity of the comparison between the treatment and the control groups. Even if some participants are noncompliant with therapy or cross over to the other therapy, the analysis should follow the intention-to-treat principle, which compares the treatment and the control groups exactly as they were initially randomized.

Randomized controlled clinical trials can assess a therapy in terms of a variety of outcomes. For antihypertensive therapy, examples include physiological measures, such as level of blood pressure; measures of subclinical disease, such as angiographically assessed coronary atherosclerosis; or major disease end points, such as stroke and myocardial infarction. In the absence of evidence from trials that include major disease end points, it is common to consider evidence concerning other intermediate or surrogate end points. The underlying assumption is that the effect of the therapy on coronary atherosclerosis, for instance, is an adequate surrogate for its effect on major disease end points. In practice, this assumption has not always turned out to be true. In one randomized clinical trial of patients with coronary disease, nifedipine suppressed the development of new coronary lesions but unexpectedly and significantly increased total mortality. Thus, the randomized trials that specify major disease end points as their primary outcomes provide the best evidence regarding the key risks or benefits associated with specific forms of antihypertensive therapy.

Randomized trials are also important to evaluate adverse drug reactions, including symptoms that may influence quality of life or general well-being. Because high blood pressure is asymptomatic, it is important that treatment is associated with as few symptoms as possible. A comparison of side effects among various drugs is of interest, however, primarily when the drugs are known to be equally effective in terms of preventing the major disease end points associated with hypertension.

Two Major Randomized Trials

Once early studies had shown a benefit from treating participants with diastolic blood pressures >115 mm Hg, it was no longer ethical to randomize subjects with high diastolic pressures to receive a placebo. The HDFP and MRC investigators responded in different ways **(Table 100.1)**. In the HDFP trial, researchers recruited subjects with elevated levels of diastolic blood pressure and randomized them to either diuretic-based stepped care or referred (usual) care. Referred-care participants had an opportunity to be evaluated by their own physicians for some form of therapy, and the stepped-care group received systematic care. Conversely, the MRC investigators limited eligibility to those with mild hypertension, and participants

Table 100.1. Two Major Randomized Trials of the Treatment of Hypertension: the HDFP and MRC Trials

SAMPLING	HDFP (1979)	MRC (1985)
Sampling	Population-based	General practice clinic
Centers, n	14	176
Eligibility		
Age, years	30–69	35–64
Blood pressure		
Systolic, mm Hg		< 200
Diastolic, mm Hg	> 90	90–109
Subjects excluded	Bedfast and Institutionalized	Those with secondary or treated hypertension, congestive heart failure, angina, recent myocardial infarction diabetes, gout, asthma
Subject		
Screened, n	178,009	515,000
Randomized, n	10,940	17,354
Blinding	Neither subjects nor physicians	Subjects only
Treatment	Offered free standardized program of stepped care anti-hypertensive therapy	Thiazide diuretic (bendrofluazide) or beta-blocker (propranolol)
Control	Referred to personal sources of medical care	Matching thiazide placebo or matching beta-blocker placebo
Target diastolic blood pressure (DBP)	< 90 mm Hg if entry DBP > 100 mm Hg 10 mmHg reduction if entry DBP was 90–99 mm HG	< 90 mm Hg
Trial duration, yrs	5	5.5
Primary endpoint	Total mortality	Fatal and non-fatal stroke

	HDFP		MRC	
	STEPPED CARE	REFEREED CARE	ACTIVE	PLACEBO
Baseline DBP, mm Hg	101.1	101.2	98.5	98.0
Subjects with DBP at or below target at the end of trial	64.9%	43.6%	74.1%	46.3%
Total mortality				
Randomized	5485	5455	8700	8654
Deaths, n	349	419	248	253
Cumulative mortality, %	6.4	7.7	2.9	2.9
Relative risk	0.83		0.98	
(95%CI)	(0.72–0.95)		(0.82–1.16)	
Total strokes				
Events, n	102	158	60	109
Cumulative incidence, %	1.9	2.9	0.7	1.3
Relative risk	0.64		0.55	
(95% CI)	(0.50–0.82)		(0.40–0.75)	

DBP indicates diastolic blood pressure; CI, confidence interval.

were randomized to one of two active drugs or matching placebos. In both studies, the intervention reduced mean diastolic blood pressure by about 5 mm Hg more than it was reduced in the control groups.

These initial choices affected other aspects of the design. In the HDFP, the use of referral of participants to their personal sources of medical care as the "control" therapy precluded the possibility of blinding; and to avoid any potential bias in ascertaining morbid events, the investigators defined total mortality as the outcome of primary interest. In the MRC trial, the use of a matching placebo allowed blinding, and the investigators defined their primary end point as fatal or nonfatal stroke.

Table 100.1 also summarizes the primary results of the two trials. The typical measure of the intervention effect is the "relative risk," which is the event rate in the intervention group divided by the event rate in the control group; for total mortality in the HDFP, for instance, $0.83 = (349/5485)/(419/5455)$. Values <1.0 indicate a benefit from therapy, and values >1.0 indicate an adverse effect from therapy. The 95% confidence interval (CI) uses the observed data to estimate the likely range of the true underlying relative risk. A 95% CI that excludes 1.0 corresponds to a value of $P<.05$.

On occasion, the benefits of therapy are expressed in terms of the "relative risk reduction," which is calculated as 1 minus the relative risk. An alternative measure is "the number requiring treatment to prevent one event," which is calculated as 1 divided by the difference in event rates between the treatment and comparison groups. In the HDFP trial, stepped care was associated with a percent relative risk reduction of 17% for total mortality $(1-0.83)$, and 76 hypertensive subjects received stepped care for 5 years to prevent 1 death $[1/(0.077-0.064)]$. Because this form of expression maybe used to

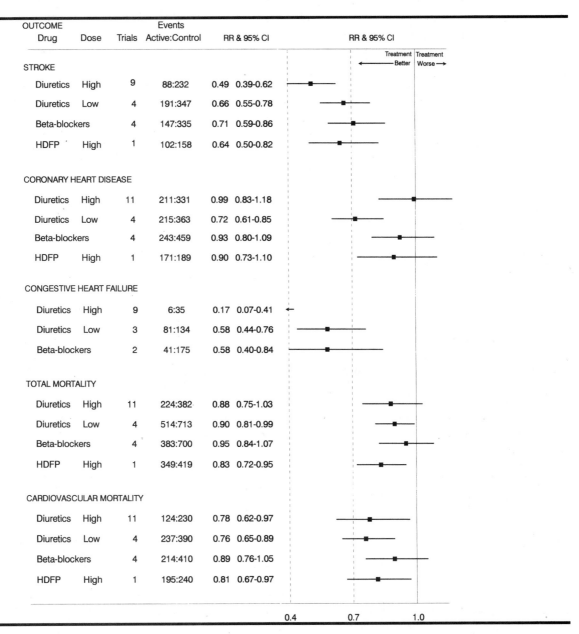

Figure 100.1. Meta-analysis of randomized, controlled clinical trials in hypertension according to first-line treatment strategy. Trials indicates number of trials with at least 1 end point of interest; RR, relative risk; CI, confidence interval; and HDFP, Hypertension Detection and Follow-up Program Study (5484 in stepped care and 5455 in referred care). For these comparisons, the numbers of participants randomized to active therapy and control were 7768 and 12 075 for high-dose diuretic therapy, 4305 and 5116 for low-dose diuretic therapy, and 6736 and 12 147 for β-blocker therapy. Because the MRC trials included two active arms, the control group is included twice in these totals, once for a diuretic comparison and again for a β-blocker comparison. The total numbers of participants randomized to active therapy and control therapy were 24 294 and 23 926, respectively. Reprinted with permission from JAMA.

guide treatment decisions, it is important to recognize the possibility that benefit may be underestimated in clinical trials, especially when a high proportion of the comparison group, such as the placebo group in the MRC trial, receives drug treatment.

Meta-analyses of the Randomized Trials

In 1986, the term "meta-analysis" first appeared in the Medline database of the National Library of Medicine; in the same year, MacMahon and colleagues published the first meta-analysis of the randomized trials to estimate the overall effect of the treatment of hypertension on morbidity and mortality. The technique of meta-

analysis is commonly used to combine data from studies to gain statistical power. As new trials have been completed, additional meta-analyses have been published.

Compared with control groups, active treatment generally produces a long-term difference of 5 to 6 mm Hg in diastolic blood pressure. The reduction in stroke incidence is quite close to the estimate of 35% to 40% derived from the association of blood pressure with event rates in epidemiological studies. For coronary heart disease, the risk reduction of 8% to 14% is less than the 20% to 25% predicted from the epidemiological studies.

In a meta-analysis that included the results of recent trials in older adults, such as SHEP, we analyzed the findings of 18 trials according to the first-line treatment strategy **(Figure 100.1)**. Compared with the control group, β-blocker therapy was effective in preventing stroke (RR, 0.71; 95% CI, 0.59 to 0.86) and congestive heart failure (0.58; 0.40 to 0.84). The findings were similar for high-dose diuretic therapy (for stroke: 0.49; 0.39 to 0.62, and for congestive heart failure: 0.17; 0.07 to 0.41). Low-dose diuretic therapy prevented not only stroke (0.66; 0.55 to 0.78) and congestive heart failure (0.58; 0.44 to 0.76) but also coronary disease (0.72; 0.61 to 0.85) and total mortality (0.90; 0.81 to 0.99). These data indicate clearly that the use of low-dose diuretic therapy is effective in preventing many of the major disease complications of untreated high blood pressure. Another recent meta-analysis of the treatment trials suggests that the benefits of treatment are similar in men and women. **(Table 100.2)**

Calcium Channel Blockers and ACE Inhibitors

With one recent exception, calcium channel blockers and ACE inhibitors have not been evaluated in large, long-term trials in patients with hypertension. The reports of increased risks of myocardial infarction, total mortality, gastrointestinal hemorrhage, and cancer associated with the use of short-acting calcium channel blockers have raised questions about the safety of some of the calcium channel blockers. In Syst-Eur, the use of nitrendipine compared with placebo was associated with a reduced risk of stroke in older adults with isolated systolic hypertension. Several recent studies comparing ACE inhibitors and calcium channel blockers in patients with diabetes or glucose intolerance suggest that there may be a higher rate of cardiovascular events in subjects randomized to calcium channel blockers. Low-dose diuretics are effective in patients with diabetes. Large, long-term trials, such as ALLHAT, which compares 4 major classes of drugs in terms of their effects on fatal and nonfatal coronary disease, will be important in helping to guide clinical practice in the future.

Summary

The randomized trials that examined major disease end points as an outcome have generally used diuretics or β-blockers as first-line therapy for high blood pressure. Antihypertensive therapy, both β-blocker and high-dose diuretic therapy, results in significant reductions in incidence of stroke and congestive heart failure. The use of low-dose diuretic therapy also reduces the incidence of coronary disease and total mortality (Figure 1). The findings are consistent across a number of meta-analyses, and the health benefits of the treatment of hypertension are similar in men and women (Table 100.2).

Despite the wealth of information from a score of trials, a number of questions remain unanswered. Although calcium channel blockers and ACE inhibitors are commonly used to treat high blood pressure in the United States, we still lack the results of large, long-term studies that directly compare these newer agents with standard therapy, such as low-dose diuretic therapy. The newer agents also tend to be much more costly than diuretics and β-blockers. The recently published recommendations of the Joint National Committee on the Detection, Evaluation, and Treatment of High Blood Pressure are to use low-dose diuretics and β-blockers as first-line treatment of hypertension under most circumstances. These recommendations are well supported by the available data on major disease end points from the randomized clinical trials.

Table 100.2. **Estimate of Treatment Effect by Sex**

OUTCOME	WOMEN		MEN	
	OR	95% CI	OR	95% CI
Total mortality	0.91	0.81–1.01	0.88	0.81–1.01
CVD-related death	0.86	0.74–1.01	0.80	0.70–0.91
Fatal strokes	0.71	0.53–0.96	0.57	0.41–0.78
All strokes	0.62	0.52–0.73	0.66	0.56–0.78
Fatal coronary events	0.92	0.74–1.16	0.83	0.71–0.97
All major coronary events	0.85	0.72–1.01	0.82	0.73–0.92
Main CVD events	0.74	0.66–0.83	0.78	0.71–0.86

OR indicates odds ration; CI, confidence interval; and CVD, cardiovascular. None of the differences in the ORs between men and women were statistically significant (all interaction values of $P \geq 0.31$).

Acknowledgments

The research reported in this article was supported by grants HL-40628 and HL-43201 from the National Heart, Lung, and Blood Institute and AG-09556 from the National Institute on Aging. Dr Psaty is a Merck/SER Clinical Epidemiology Fellow (sponsored by the Merck Co Foundation, Rahway, NJ, and the Society for Epidemiological Research, Baltimore, Md).

SUGGESTED READING

1. Collins R, Peto R, MacMahon S, Hebert P, Fiebach NH, Eberlein KA, Godwin J, Qizilbash N, Taylor JO, Hennekens CH. Blood pressure, stroke, and coronary heart disease, II: short-term reductions in blood pressure: overview of randomised drug trials in their epidemiologic context. *Lancet.* 1990;335:827–838.

2. Curb JD, Pressel SL, Cutler JA, Savage PJ, Applegate WB, Black H, Camel G, Davis BR, Frost PH, Gonzalez N, Guthrie G, Oberman A, Rutan GH, Stamler J, for the Systolic Hypertension in the Elderly Program Cooperative Research Group. Effect of diuretic-based antihypertensive treatment on cardiovascular disease risk in older diabetic patients with isolated systolic hypertension. *JAMA.* 1996;276:1886–1892.

3. Davis BR, Cutler JA, Gordon DJ, Furberg CD, Wright JT Jr, Cushman WC, Grimm RH, LaRosa J, Whelton PK, Perry HM, Alderman MH, Ford CE, Oparil S, Francis C, Proschan M, Pressel S, Black HR, Hawkins CM, for the ALLHAT Research Group. Rationale and design for the Antihypertensive and Lipid Lowering Treatment to Prevent Heart Attack Trial (ALLHAT). *Am J Hypertens.* 1996;9:342–360.

4. Gueyffier F, Boutitie F, Boissel JP, Pocock S, Coope J, Cutler J, Ekbom T, Fagard R, Friedman L, Perry M, Prineas R, Schron E. Effect of antihypertensive drug treatment on cardiovascular outcomes in women and men: a meta-analysis of individual patient data from randomized, controlled trials. The INDANA Investigators. *Ann Intern Med.* 1997;126:761–767.

5. MacMahon SW, Cutler JA, Furberg CD, Payne GH. The effects of drug treatment for hypertension on morbidity and mortality from cardiovascular disease: a review of randomized controlled trials. *Prog Cardiovasc Dis.* 1986;29(suppl 1):99–118.

6. Psaty BM, Heckbert SR, Koepsell TD, Siscovick DS, Raghunathan TE, Weiss NS, Rosendaal FR, Lemaitre RN, Smith NL, Wahl PW, et al. The risk of myocardial infarction associated with antihypertensive drug therapies. *JAMA.* 1995;274:620–625.

7. Psaty BM, Smith NL, Siscovick DS, Koepsell TD, Weiss NS, Heckbert SR, Lemaitre RN, Wagner EH, Furberg CD. Health outcomes associated with antihypertensive therapies used as first-line agents: a systematic review and meta-analysis. *JAMA.* 1997;277:739–745.

8. SHEP Cooperative Research Group. Prevention of stroke by antihypertensive drug treatment in older persons with isolated systolic hypertension: final results of the Systolic Hypertension in the Elderly Program (SHEP). *JAMA.* 1991;265:3255–3264.

9. Estacio RO, Jeffers BW, Hiatt MR, Biggerstaff SL, Gifford N, Schrier RW. The effect of nisolidipine as compared with enalapril on cardiovascular outcomes in patients with non-insulin-dependent diabetes and hypertension. *N Engl J Med* 1998;338:645-652.

Antihypertensive Treatment Trials: Quality of Life

R.H. Grimm, Jr, MD, PhD

KEY POINTS

- Quality of life is the patient's ability to function well in daily living, including psychological and physical well-being, social and leisure activity, and satisfaction with life.

- In placebo-controlled studies, incidence rates of adverse events in patients on placebo are frequently the same as or sometimes even greater than in active drug–treated patients.

- Quality of life is usually not impaired and may even improve with use of modern treatments, including drugs and/or lifestyle advice.

- Quality of life and drug side effects are important concerns but should not be major obstacles to effectively managing and controlling high blood pressure.

See also Chapters 58, 100

Background

Lowering blood pressure (BP) with drugs (particularly diuretics and β-blockers) has now been clearly shown to reduce incidence of cardiovascular disease. Quality of life is an important concern with management of hypertension. Roughly 60 million Americans have BP high enough (systolic BP >140 mm Hg and/or diastolic BP >90 mm Hg) to need lifestyle changes and/or drug treatment to lower their BP. The majority of these patients will require treatment for life. The prospect of millions of Americans being treated for decades with drugs to lower BP is sobering; quality of life is therefore an important concern. Surprisingly, despite clear evidence demonstrating the benefit of lowering BP, only 54% of hypertensives are treated with drugs, and just 27% have controlled BPs. This poor performance is at least in part due to concerns about the effects of treatment on the patient's quality of life and drug side effects.

Drug Treatment of Hypertension: Historical Paradigm

Historically, the dominant paradigm has been that treating hypertension and lowering BP with drugs will impair quality of life. This view has been shared by patients and physicians alike and no doubt evolved from the early years of experience treating hypertension.

In the 1930s and 1940s, hypertension was clearly established as the major factor associated with severe cardiovascular morbidity and mortality. The term "malignant hypertension" was used to describe the pathological entity of renal arterial hyperplasia with classic "onion-skinning" of the renal arterioles. This condition was associated with extreme elevation of BP and a near certainty of serious cardiovascular events occurring within a relatively short period of time (dissecting aneurysms, myocardial infarctions, stroke, congestive heart failure, renal failure, etc). At that time, however, there were no safe and effective treatments for lowering BP. In the late 1940s, BP could be lowered by extreme reduction in dietary sodium and weight loss with the "Kempner rice diet," but this required months of residential treatment during which diet and activity were rigidly controlled. Obviously, this was not conducive to quality of life, and once back into the community, the group tended to resume their pretreatment lifestyle and BPs went up. Other treatments used in the early 1950s for hypertension include (1) surgical sympathectomy, (2) injection of pyrogens, and (3) rauwolfia plant extract. These treatments were accompanied by severe side effects and poor quality of life. Because of these limitations, the practical effect of these treatments for lowering BP was nil to minimal. In the mid 1950s, a few oral drugs became available, such as ganglionic blocking agents and the nonselective α-blockers phenoxybenzamine and phentolamine, but these drugs were also associated with severe, life-limiting side effects, including orthostatic hypotension and syncopy, which severely impaired the patient's quality of life. In the late 1950s and early 1960s, high-dose thiazide diuretics, high-dose reserpine, nonselective α-blockers, and centrally acting α_2-agonists such as methyldopa were commonly used but, relative to today, were grossly overdosed and also associated with a high rate of side effects, intolerance, and poor quality of life. Given this history, it is not difficult to understand how antihypertensive drug treatment and poor quality of life were strongly linked in the physician's and patient's minds.

Adverse Events

All drug treatments have the potential to produce unwanted side effects. It is important, however, to make the distinction between a drug side effect and an adverse event. Side effects are causally related to the drugs given, whereas an adverse event is a symptom or complaint that occurs in a patient taking drugs but is not necessarily causally related to the drug.

In placebo-controlled studies, incidence rates of adverse events in patients on placebo are frequently the same or sometimes even greater than in active drug–treated patients.

The **Table 101.1** illustrates this point in data from the 1-year results from the Treatment of Mild Hypertension Study (TOMHS).

Antihypertensive drugs do cause side effects that occasionally can be life-threatening (ie, ACE inhibitors and angioneurotic edema); more commonly, however, such symptoms are mild, do not interfere with daily activities, and are not necessarily directly caused by the drugs.

Factors that aid in assessing whether or not an adverse event is a drug side effect are whether the symptom is persistent, whether discontinuing the drug eliminates the symptom, and whether it returns after the patient is rechallenged with the suspect drug.

Quality of Life: Definition

Although the context of quality of life has not been well defined, it now generally is thought to be the patient's ability to function well in daily living, including psychological and physical well-being, social and leisure activity, and satisfaction with life. It has also been defined as the capacity to function well, enjoy a sense of well-being, and experience with satisfaction the social, emotional, physical, and intellectual aspects of life.

Over the past 25 years, there has been an explosion of new classes of antihypertensive drugs. There has also been more rigorous scientific evaluation of lifestyle treatments for lowering BP, mainly weight loss, reduction of dietary sodium and alcohol, and increased physical activity. These classes of drugs include β-blockers, selective α_1-antagonists, ACE inhibitors, calcium channel blockers (1980s), and recently, angiotensin receptor blockers. All these types of drugs are very effective in lowering BP and are well tolerated. Results are now available on the quality-of-life effects with different types of drugs and lifestyle treatments for hypertension.

Effects of Lifestyle Changes on Quality of Life

Weight loss has been clearly shown to improve quality of life; in fact, the greater the weight loss in the Treatment of Mild Hypertension Study and the Trial of Antihypertensive Interventions and Management (TAIM), the greater the improvement in quality of life.

The above-mentioned studies also observed that reducing dietary sodium by 20% to 30% will not impair quality of life (TOMHS/TAIM). In the TOMHS study, increased leisure physical activity was also associated in graded fashion with improvements in quality of life, independent of weight loss.

Antihypertensive Drugs and Quality of Life

In 1986, Croog et al reported the first study that examined antihypertensive drugs and quality of life. This study of 626 hypertensive men randomly allocated to either methyldopa, propranolol, or captopril observed that there were between-drug differences in changes of quality of life.

Other groups have examined between–drug group differences in change of quality of life. However, these studies are frequently limited by short study duration and lack of a placebo comparison.

Two large placebo-controlled studies, TAIM and TOMHS, have reported on the effects of different antihypertensive drugs on quality of life. Both these studies also included lifestyle interventions involving weight loss and sodium reduction. The drugs studied in TAIM were the diuretic chlorthalidone and the β-blocker atenolol. TAIM observed general improvements in quality-of-life measures in all groups but no differences between placebo and active drugs. Improvements were more striking with weight reduction.

TOMHS has also reported on quality-of-life changes with placebo versus five active drugs: (1) the β-blocker acebutolol, (2) the calcium antagonist amlodipine, (3) the diuretic chlorthalidone, (4) the α-blocker doxazosin, and (5) the ACE inhibitor enalapril. All these groups also received lifestyle intervention involving weight loss, sodium and alcohol reduction, and increased leisure physical activity. TOMHS recruited 902 men and women with stage 1 diastolic hypertension who were treated for an average of 4.4 years. Quality of life was measured by a questionnaire adapted from the Medical Outcomes Study, modified for hypertension. The results were consistent with the TAIM study in that quality of life improved in all treated groups. It was of interest that the active drug group combined had significantly better improvements in most aspects of improved quality of life compared with placebo. Quality-of-life improvements were also related to the degree of weight loss and BP lowering. TOMHS also demonstrated statistically significant differences between drugs, in-

Table 101.1. Selected Adverse Events in TOMHS Participants Attending the 12-Month Visit*

CONDITION	β-BLOCKER ACEBUTOLOL, N (%)	CALCIUM BLOCKER AMLODIPINE, N (%)	DIURETIC CHLORTHALIDONE, N (%)	α-BLOCKER DOXAZOSIN, N (%)	ACE INHIBITOR ENALAPRIL, N (%)	PLACEBO, N (%)
Tiredness/fatige	35 (36)	36 (31)	43 (35)	38 (31)	33 (26)	72 (34)
Waking up early	28 (22)	24 (21)	30 (24)	36 (30)	34 (28)	70 (33)
Feeling depressed	23 (18)	21 (18)	19 (15)	20 (16)	24 (20)	41 (19)
Faintness/dizziness	23 (18)	22 (19)	24 (19)	28 (23)	28 (23)	44 (21)
Blacking out	1 (1)	1 (1)	0 (0)	1 (1)	2 (2)	8 (4)
Lightheadedness on standing	21 (17)	19 (16)	23 (19)	35 (29)	36 (29)	31 (15)
Headaches	27 (22)	27 (23)	26 (22)	38 (31)	31 (25)	72 (34)
Swelling of feet	14 (11)	16 (14)	11 (9)	13 (11)	14 (11)	22 (10)
Joint pain	34 (27)	32 (28)	38 (31)	46 (38)	42 (34)	65 (31)
Dry mouth	23 (18)	28 (24)	24 (19)	28 (24)	19 (15)	34 (16)

*Adverse event data are selected from a more complete list.

dependent of the weight loss, with the largest improvements noted in the chlorthalidone (diuretic) and acebutolol (β-blocker) groups.

Overall, the weight of the evidence is that quality of life is usually not impaired and may even improve with use of modern treatments, including drugs and/or lifestyle advice. This improvement is enhanced by the degree of weight loss and BP lowering. Most antihypertensive drugs studied thus far also tend to improve quality-of-life measures. Evaluation of the effects on quality of life should be routine for the introduction of new drugs. It now appears that effective management of hypertension with lifestyle and drugs can enhance rather than impair quality of life. Quality of life and drug side effects are important concerns but should not be major obstacles to effectively managing and controlling high BP.

Hypertension can be readily diagnosed, and numerous safe and effective treatments are available that work well to lower the BP, which will significantly prevent cardiovascular disease. However, only 50% of hypertensives are treated with drugs, and only 27% of hypertensives in America have their BP at goal (<140/90 mm Hg). Appreciating that properly prescribed antihypertensive agents will not adversely affect quality of life and may actually improve it is very valuable information and should help improve these alarming statistics.

SUGGESTED READING

1. Burt VI, Cutler JA, Higgins M et al. Trends in prevalence, awareness, treatments, and control of hypertension in the adult US population: data from the Health Examination Surveys. *Hypertension.* 1995;26:60–69.

2. Croog SH, Levine S, Testa MA, et al. The effects of antihypertensive therapy on quality of life. *N Engl J Med.* 1986;314:1657–1664.

3. Grimm RH, Grandits GA, Cutlet JA, Stewart AL, McDonald RH, Svendsen K, Prineas RJ, Liebson PR, for the TOMHS Research Group. Relationships of quality of life measures to long-term lifestyle and drug treatment in the Treatment of Mild Hypertension Study (TOMHS). *Arch Intern Med.* 1997;157:638–648.

4. Grimm RH, Grandits GA, Prineas RJ, et al. Long-term effects on sexual function of five antihypertensive drugs and nutritional hygienic treatment in hypertensive men and women: the Treatment of Mild Hypertension Study (TOMHS). *Hypertension.* 1997;29:8–14.

5. Neaton JD, Grimm RH, Prineas RJ, et al. Treatment of Mild Hypertension Study: final results. *JAMA.* 1993;270:713–724.

6. Tarlov AR, Ware JE, Greenfield S, et al. The Medical Outcomes Study: an application of methods for monitoring the results of medical care. *JAMA.* 1989;262:925–930.

7. The Treatment of Mild Hypertension Study: A randomized, placebo-controlled trial of a nutritional-hygienic regimen along with various drug monotherapies. *Arch Intern Med.* 1991;151:1413–1423.

8. Wassertheil-Smoller A, Blaufox MD, Oberman A, et al. Effect of antihypertensives on sexual function and quality of life: the TAIM Study. *Ann Intern Med.* 1991;114:613–620.

Chapter 102

Economic Impact of Blood Pressure

William B. Stason, MD, MSc

KEY POINTS

- Cost-effectiveness analysis adds an economic perspective that allows priorities for health care to be set according to the relationship of costs to benefits.

- The cost-effectiveness of treatment for hypertension depends most importantly on the magnitude of cardiovascular risk from untreated blood pressure elevation, the success of treatment in reducing blood pressure and reducing risk, and the net cost of so doing.

- The risk from elevated blood pressure and the benefits of treatment have been shown to be directly, if imperfectly, related to pretreatment blood pressure levels.

- Opportunities to reduce the costs of hypertension care without loss of benefits include starting treatment with lower-cost medications, limiting office visits to those that are clinically necessary, and selective use of laboratory tests.

See also Chapter 103

Current emphasis on cost containment in health care creates the need for healthcare professionals to examine their practice patterns in an effort to identify opportunities to reduce costs while maintaining or improving health outcomes.

This chapter will discuss the role of cost-effectiveness analysis in the management of hypertension and identify promising opportunities for increasing the cost-effectiveness of treating hypertension. The essence of cost-effectiveness analysis is the assessment of health benefits. The incorporation of costs per unit of benefit adds the economic perspective and allows the possibility of setting priorities for health care according to the relationship of costs to benefits.

Global Cost-Effectiveness of Hypertension Treatment

The cost-effectiveness of treatment for hypertension depends most importantly on the magnitude of cardiovascular risk from untreated blood pressure elevation, the success of treatment in reducing blood pressure and reducing risk, and the net costs of so doing. Net costs reflect the balance of the costs of treatment and any cost savings that may result from the prevention of hypertension-related complications. Especially important considerations for the cost-effectiveness of treatment from a clinical perspective are (1) the need for accurate determination of pretreatment blood pressure and other measures of risk, (2) the adverse impact of failures in adherence, (3) the importance of the patient's quality of life on treatment, and (4) the fact that antihypertensive medications account for a sizable proportion of out-of-pocket costs of treatment for those with health insurance who do not need hospitalization or extensive evaluation.

Our study of the cost-effectiveness of hypertension treatment serves to highlight some of these issues. The basic results of this study are summarized in the **Figure 102.1**. The cost-effectiveness ratio is expressed in dollars per quality-adjusted life-year (QALY), which reflects the extent to which a year of life with medication side effects or clinical symp-

tomatology is worth less than a year of full health. This study showed, first, that hypertension treatment does not pay for itself. Only 22% of the cost of treating those with a diastolic blood pressure of ≥105 mm Hg and 15% of the cost of treating diastolic blood pressures of 90 to 104 mm Hg are recovered. The value of treating hypertension, therefore, must be measured in lives saved and morbidity prevented. Second, the cost-effectiveness of treatment is directly related to the level of pretreatment blood pressure. Assuming full adherence to medical regimens, the cost-effectiveness ratios are ≈$45 000, $22 000, and $9000 per QALY (1984 dollars) for diastolic blood pressures of 90 to 94, 95 to 104, and ≥105 mm Hg, respectively. Problems with adherence to medications and dropouts from care reduce the cost-effectiveness by one-third.

Concepts of Cost-Effectiveness Analysis for Clinical Practice

This cost-effectiveness analysis compares treatment of hypertension with no treatment, taking a societal perspective that required consideration of all medical care costs over the lifetime of individuals and all health benefits summarized as QALYS. Discounting of future costs and benefits became extremely important because the stream of the costs of treating hypertension and the adverse effects of medications on the quality of life begin immediately, whereas cost savings and benefits from cardiovascular events prevented are commonly many years in the future.

The realities of clinical practice require a somewhat different approach to cost-effectiveness analyses if they are to be maximally useful in assessing cost and quality-of-care trade-offs and guiding practice decisions. Especially important will be the perspective from which the analysis is performed, the treatments that are compared, the time frame of analysis, and the measures of health benefits and costs that are included.

Cost-effectiveness may be assessed from the point of view of the patient, the physician, or the health maintenance organization

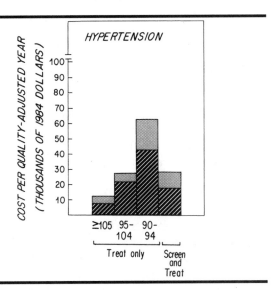

Figure 102.1.   Cost-effectiveness of hypertension treatment in 1984 dollars for sustained diastolic hypertension and screening plus treatment of persons with diastolic blood pressures of 95 mm Hg or greater. Full adherence (dark cross-hatched areas) and expected adherence (stippled plus cross-hatched areas) are shown. Adapted and reproduced with permission from the *Annu Rev Public Health*. 2985;6:41–63.

clinical decisions and to health system changes and increasing the benefits of hypertension treatment, reducing costs, or both (**Table 102.2**).

Accurate Classification of Blood Pressure

Maximal benefits of treatment will be achieved only if each patient's blood pressure is accurately classified before a diagnosis of hypertension is made or treatment is begun. Accurate blood pressure measurements are needed to avoid the deleterious effects of falsely labeling a patient with the diagnosis and to prevent unnecessary treatment in patients for whom the risks of medications outweigh the benefits.

Benefits Versus Risks of Treatment

The risk from elevated blood pressure and the benefits of treatment have been shown to be directly, if imperfectly, related to pretreatment blood pressure levels. Prudence suggests a conservative approach to initiating pharmacological treatment in patients with stage 1 hypertension in the lowest ranges and suggests that a trial of nonpharmacological treatment may be the better decision on net-benefits grounds as well as cost-effectiveness grounds.

(HMO) or insurer, as well as from that of society at large. The patient is likely to be most concerned about out-of-pocket costs not covered by health insurance and near-term effects of the disease or its treatment on the quality of life. The longer-term effects on the risk of cardiovascular events are usually not as much of a concern. The physician is guided by the interests of the patient but also by professional and financial self-interests. The HMO or insurer is inevitably influenced by costs of care, patient satisfaction, and other factors that may influence its competitive position in the healthcare marketplace.

The person performing the assessment must choose the perspective that best serves the needs of relevant decision makers. Most commonly, the goal will be to compare treatment with no treatment, one type of treatment with another (for example, two types of drugs as monotherapy or nonpharmacological therapy with monotherapy), or one practice setting or organizational scheme with another. A relatively short time frame will be preferable. This does not mitigate the importance of long-term costs and benefits but rather reflects the realities of clinical practice that focus, by necessity, on proximate outcomes such as blood pressure control, end-organ damage, and patient quality of life. Measures of ambulatory care cost, in order of importance, include medications, office visits and consultations, laboratory examinations, and the indirect costs borne by the patient because of the time off work and travel connected with receiving medical care (**Table 102.1**). The costs of hospitalizations for the treatment of cardiovascular events or treatment complications are large but, fortunately, occur in a relatively small number of patients each year.

Opportunities to Improve the Cost-Effectiveness of Hypertension Management

A range of opportunities exist for improving the cost-effectiveness of hypertension management. These relate both to individual

---

Table 102.1.   Measures of Costs and Health Benefits for Assessing the Cost-Effectiveness of Hypertension Management

Measures of cost
  Medication
  Office visits
  Consultations (eg, physician specialist, dietitian)
  Laboratory tests (eg, blood tests, electrocardiogram, echocardiogram)
  Hospitalizations (for hypertension, medication side effects, cardiovascular events)
Measures on health benefits
  Blood pressure control
  Quality of life
  Avoidance of end organ damage (eg, left ventricular hypertrophy)
  Control of risk factors (eg, cholesterol, weight, smoking, alcohol)
  Prevention of cardiovascular events (eg, strokes, myocardial infarction, congestive heart failure)

Table 102.2.   Opportunities to Improve the Cost-Effectiveness of Hypertension Management

Improve effectiveness of treatment
  Accurate classification of blood pressure
  Balance benefits versus risks of treatment
  Maximize quality of life on treatment
  Adherence to treatment regimens
  Control of other cardiovascular risk factors
Reduce costs
  Start treatment with lower-cost medications
  Limit office visits to those with a clear clinical objective
  Limit laboratory tests to those that are medically necessary

Quality of Life

Increasing emphasis is being placed on the importance of the patient's quality of life on treatment. From a cost-effectiveness perspective, maintaining or improving quality of life on treatment may be as important as or more important than normalizing blood pressure.

Many studies have compared the effects of different medication regimens on the overall quality of life, vitality, perceived health, sleep patterns, sexual function, mood, and emotional control. Although early studies in this area have suggested advantages of ACE inhibitors, the Treatment of Mild Hypertension Study found the best quality of life in the diuretic and β-blocker groups, even compared with placebo.

Patient Adherence

Failures in adherence to prescribed medication regimens and in the continuity of follow-up may dramatically reduce both the effectiveness and cost-effectiveness of hypertension treatment. Medications that are purchased but not consumed add costs without corresponding benefits. Partial or intermittent adherence cannot achieve the full benefits of treatment.

Reducing the Costs of Treatment

Opportunities to reduce the costs of treatment should be pursued vigorously to the extent that cost reductions can be achieved without clinically significant sacrifice in blood pressure control, quality of life, or the incidence of metabolic side effects.

The medication cost/efficacy dilemma has been intensified in recent years by the introduction and widespread acceptance of calcium channel blockers and ACE inhibitors. There is no question that these agents have attractive pharmacological properties, but they are also very expensive.

In brief, available studies report that all major drug groups are equivalent in their blood pressure–lowering abilities. Except for one trial in Systolic Hypertension in the Elderly that found a reduction in stroke with a long-acting dihydropyridine calcium channel blocker, only thiazides and β-blockers have been shown to reduce cardiovascular mortality and morbidity. Arguments supporting the newer agents relate to the favorable quality-of-life profile of the ACE inhibitors, favorable metabolic profiles for both ACE inhibitors and calcium channel blockers, and the attractive potential for the newer agents to prevent the progression of vascular and cardiac disease processes. The Sixth Report of The Joint National Committee on the Prevention, Detection, Evaluation, and Treatment of High Blood Pressure recommended diuretics and β-blockers for uncomplicated hypotensives but recognized that there were many possible indications that could affect the choice of therapy.

A reasonable approach to treatment, therefore, that would also meet cost-effectiveness objectives would be to initiate antihypertensive treatment with generic hydrochlorothiazide or propranolol in patients with no indication for another agent. The more expensive medications could then be reserved for situations in which they really do "add value."

Cost reductions can also be achieved by avoiding routine follow-up visits and laboratory tests. In both cases, there should be a clear clinical justification. Selective use of laboratory tests to monitor metabolic effects of medications or end-organ damage can reduce costs without loss of benefit.

Concern about the cost-effectiveness of hypertension management is a highly germane policy issue with important implications for medical practice. Healthcare facilities will be under ever-increasing pressure to confront cost-quality trade-offs in delivering services. Fortunately, several attractive opportunities exist in hypertension management for achieving economies with little loss, or even gain, in health benefits.

SUGGESTED READING

1. Appel LJ, Stason WB. Ambulatory blood pressure monitoring and blood pressure self-measurement in the diagnosis and management of hypertension. *Ann Intern Med.* 1993;118:867–892.
2. Beto JA, Bansal VK. Quality of life in treatment of hypertension: a meta-analysis of clinical trials. *Am J Hypertens.* 1992;5:125–133.
3. Croog SH, Levine S, Testa MA, et al. The effects of antihypertensive therapy on the quality of life. *N Engl J Med.* 1986;314:1657–1664.
4. Edelson JT, Weinstein MC, Tosteson AN, Williams L, Lee TH, Goldman L. Long-term cost-effectiveness of various initial monotherapies for mild to moderate hypertension. *JAMA.* 1990;263:407–413.
5. Johannesson M, Borquist L, Jonsson B. The costs of treating hypertension in Sweden: an empirical investigation in primary health care. *Scand J Prim Health Care.* 1991;9:155–160.
6. The Treatment of Mild Hypertension Research Group. The Treatment of Mild Hypertension Study: a randomized, placebo-controlled trial of a nutritional-hygienic regimen along with various drug monotherapies. *Arch Intern Med.* 1991;151: 1413–1423.
7. Weinstein MC, Stason WB. Cost-effectiveness of interventions to prevent or treat coronary heart disease. *Annu Rev Public Health.* 1985;6:41–63.

Chapter 103

Economic Considerations in the Management of Hypertension

William J. Elliott, MD, PhD

KEY POINTS

- Cost-effectiveness calculations compute the cost per year of life saved by an intervention, balancing the overall cost of treatment against its effectiveness in avoiding future adverse events. Cost-utility analyses incorporate quality-of-life data and "correct" for disabilities from both adverse side effects of treatment and nonfatal adverse events.

- Beneficial cost-effectiveness ratios result from lower-cost treatments for patients at higher baseline risk (eg, older patients with higher initial blood pressures).

- The cost-benefit ratio for treating hypertension may be improved by selecting treatments that minimize the total cost of care while not adversely affecting quality of life; by enhancing compliance; and by avoiding unnecessary office visits and laboratory testing.

See also Chapter 102

Cost-effectiveness calculations are a formalized method of comparing the cost of an intervention with the (discounted) benefits that presumably accrue to a population to whom it is administered. Perhaps because hypertension is the most common chronic condition for which healthcare services are provided in the United States, much effort has been focused on understanding the relationship between costs and benefits of treatment for this medical problem. The difficulties inherent in these considerations (eg, regional and temporal variation in the cost of medicines and medical services, lack of morbidity and mortality data with newer medications) have limited the impact on public policy of this important issue, but more attention is being paid to economic considerations for hypertension treatment, both nationally (as in JNC VI) and locally (by managed-care organizations).

The cost-effectiveness ratio (cost per year of life saved) for hypertension treatment depends largely on four factors: (1) the absolute risk for cardiovascular events for a given patient group (which depends on age, blood pressure stage, and concomitant comorbidities); (2) the success of treatment in reducing the future risk of stroke, myocardial infarction, heart failure, dialysis, or renal transplantation; (3) the (discounted) future cost of these adverse events; and (4) the total cost of treatment. In cost-utility analyses (cost per quality-adjusted life-year saved), discounts are incorporated from quality-of-life data for discomfort or disability due to (1) side effects of treatment and (2) nonfatal adverse events (stroke, heart failure, angina pectoris, dialysis).

Early cost-effectiveness calculations were based on theoretical and computer models (eg, Coronary Heart Disease Policy Model, Framingham Heart Study), but more recently, data from large outcome studies in actual patients have provided "real-world" estimates of both costs and benefits. The most recent results from a large, single-country experience come from Sweden, where the government pays for nearly all of the medical care and therefore has solid data on both costs and morbid events; these are summarized in **Table 103.1.**

Table 103.1 shows, as have previous studies, that higher-risk patients (older people with higher untreated blood pressures) have more beneficial cost-effectiveness ratios and that there are some subgroups for whom antihypertensive drug therapy actually saves money in the long term. These results have also been seen in secondary prevention (for people who have survived an initial myocardial infarction or stroke).

Cost-effectiveness calculations for hypertension treatment have consistently shown that pharmacological treatment for all patients with elevated office blood pressures actually costs money overall. Nonetheless, there are several simple steps that can be easily incorporated into medical practice that would improve the cost-effectiveness ratio of treating hypertension. These include (1) accurate diagnosis and classification of hypertension, (2) baseline risk assessment to guide prescribing of costly medications, (3) drug therapy choice that leads to the lowest overall cost, (4) maximization of compliance with medications, and (5) reduction of unnecessary office visits and laboratory testing.

It has been estimated that ≈20% of individuals with elevated blood pressure in the medical office setting do not have sustained hypertension and may not benefit from therapy to the same extent as people with sustained hypertension. Cost-effectiveness analyses of ambulatory blood pressure monitoring as an initial diagnostic tool have shown that its selective use may lead to an overall reduction in costs, but these analyses have not yet convinced many payers to reimburse for the procedure. Home blood pressure monitoring and even repeated office visits to document the presence of sustained hypertension are recommended to avoid "wasting" treatment on patients with labile blood pressures who are at low cardiovascular risk.

Perhaps the most important change in the recent JNC VI report is risk stratification before initiation of drug therapy. For patients with low baseline risk (no other risk factors, no target-organ damage, and

Table 103.1. Cost for 1 Additional Year of Life for Swedish Hypertensives Treated With Diuretics or β-Blockers, Translated Into 1992 US Dollars

DIASTOLIC BP, mm Hg	AGE <45 YEARS		AGE 45–69 YEARS		AGE ≥ 70 YEARS	
	MEN	WOMEN	MEN	WOMEN	MEN	WOMEN
90–94	$118 375	$313 250	$8500	$26 875	$3125	$2625
95–99	$97 500	$236 750	$4250	$16 625	$1750	$875
100–104	$79 500	$173 500	$8500	$7375	$375	. . .*
≥105	$55 000	$93 250	. . .	. . .	. . .	. . .

* For this subgroup, antihypertensive drug therapy saves money.
Adaped with permission from Jönsson.

no cardiovascular disease), even with blood pressures as high as 159/99 mm Hg, JNC VI recommends a year of lifestyle modification before initiation of drug therapy. This is expected to improve the cost-effectiveness ratio, because it delays starting costly drug therapy for patients with a very low risk of cardiovascular events. At the other extreme, JNC VI recommends aggressive drug therapy for patients with diabetes or chronic renal impairment until the blood pressure is <130/85 mm Hg. This strategy has recently been suggested to be cost-effective as long as the marginal annual cost of such treatment does not exceed $260 for a 50 year old cohort.

Although lower-cost medications are easy to recommend over higher-cost drugs, the cost of medications is a complex subject. The American Heart Association estimates that medications account for 24% of the total cost of care for hypertension in 1998 in the United States. Pricing of medications is quite variable, particularly at the retail pharmacy. Even generic medications, which typically have much lower average wholesale prices than their branded counterparts, have a markup of up to 10 times higher than the traditional 7% for branded drugs, which sometimes makes the retail costs similar. Much effort is currently being expended by pharmacies and their managers to reduce pharmaceutical expenditures. Although some of these efforts are likely to be beneficial, enforced reduction in pharmaceutical benefits by administrative means led to worsened blood pressure control and increased morbid events in several previous studies. Some "innovations" (eg, monthly bidding for an exclusive contract to use a single ACE inhibitor in a large HMO) reduce the pharmacy budget but incur more office visits and lead to a higher total cost of care. Despite large differences in average wholesale prices between the least expensive diuretic and the most expensive calcium antagonist, after considering the cost of other needed medications, office visits, laboratory studies, and evaluation of adverse experiences, one large clinic in Omaha was unable to demonstrate a significant difference in the total cost of the first year of treatment among five different classes of antihypertensive drugs used as initial therapy for hypertension. When more than one medication is needed to control blood pressure, some pharmacy programs vigorously pursue prescribing economically advantageous fixed-dose combination products, which often cost less than two separate prescriptions for the components.

The choice of initial antihypertensive drug therapy has been based on cost-effectiveness calculations in several countries, including South Africa and Belgium, where all patients must take 12.5 mg of a diuretic for at least the first month. Such mandates have been recommended by some for patients in the United States but have not yet become popular. Initial reports of the better long-term tolerability and lack of side effects of some of the newer medications (eg, angiotensin II receptor antagonists) may eventually prove important in cost-utility analyses, which factor in not only "extra" visits to healthcare providers for evaluation of perceived side effects but also the subjective annoyance caused by antihypertensive drugs in some patients.

Compliance with medications is seldom thought of when cost-effectiveness calculations are performed but may have the most important effect of all factors that can be assessed in everyday medical practice. Patients who are prescribed antihypertensive medications but who do not take them properly clearly incur all the costs attendant to obtaining such therapy but derive no benefit from these transactions. Compliance may be enhanced by educating the patient about the disease and the medication, prescribing once-daily pills that do not adversely affect quality of life, and minimizing "out-of-pocket" costs.

In 1998 the United States spends $31.7 billion on hypertension treatment. Current estimates suggest that 26% goes for "indirect costs" (transportation, time off work, and "lost opportunity"), 21% pays healthcare providers, and an equal amount pays for hospital and nursing home services. If patients were able to monitor home blood pressures and receive healthcare advice by telephone rather than making unnecessary office visits, these costs could presumably be reduced. Similarly, laboratory testing can often be minimized by choosing low doses of drug therapy having few adverse metabolic effects and not often escalating into dose ranges that have been associated with hypokalemia, altered cholesterol levels, and the like.

The issue of how to enhance cost-effectiveness of hypertension treatment is expected to intensify in the next several years, as newer studies are completed that compare the effectiveness of some of the newer and currently more expensive drug classes with the traditional (and generically available) diuretics and β-blockers. How these clinical results are incorporated by healthcare policymakers in their approved "critical pathways" for treatment will likely be guided by future cost-effectiveness considerations.

SUGGESTED READING

1. Hilleman DE, Mohiuddin SM, Lucas BD Jr, Stading JA, Stoysich AM, Ryschon K. Cost-minimization analysis of initial antihypertensive therapy in patients with mild-to-moderate essential diastolic hypertension. *Clin Ther.* 1994;16:88–102.

2. Johannesson M. The cost-effectiveness of hypertension treatment in Sweden. *Pharmacoeconomics.* 1995;7:242–250.

3. Jönsson BG. Cost-benefit of treating hypertension. *J Hypertens.* 1994;12(suppl): S65–S75.

4. Kaplan NM, Gifford RW Jr. Choice of initial therapy for hypertension. *JAMA.* 1996;275:1577–1580.

5. Littenberg B. A practice guideline revisited: screening for hypertension. *Ann Intern Med.* 1995;122:937–939.

6. Reif MC, Carter VL. The retail cost of antihypertensive therapy: physician and patient as educated consumers. *Am J Hypertens.* 1994;7:571–575.

7. Roccella EJ, Lenfant C. Considerations regarding the cost and effectiveness of public and patient education programmes. *J Hum Hypertens.* 1992;6:463–467.

8. Siegel D, Lopez J. Trends in antihypertensive drug use in the United States: do the JNC V recommendations affect prescribing? *JAMA.* 1997;278:1745–1748.

9. Weinstein MC, Seigel JE, Gold MR, Kamlet MS, Russell LB. Recommendations of the Panel on Cost-effectiveness in Health and Medicine. *JAMA.* 1996;276: 1253–1258.

10. Yarows SA, Khoury S, Sowers JR. Cost effectiveness of 24-hour ambulatory blood pressure monitoring in evaluation and treatment of essential hypertension. *Am J Hypertens.* 1994;7:464–468.

Part C

CLINICAL MANAGEMENT

Section Editors: *Sheldon G. Sheps, MD*
Dominic A. Sica, MD
Donald G. Vidt, MD

General Diagnostic Aspects
Evaluation of Target Organs
Principles of Management
Antihypertensive Drugs
Managing Hypertension (Target Organ Damage)
Management of Special Populations
Management of Secondary Hypertension

Chapter 104

Blood Pressure Measurement

Carlene M. Grim, RN, MSN, SpDN; Clarence E. Grim, MS, MD

KEY POINTS

- Indirect blood pressure measurement is one of the most frequently and, in so many cases, most poorly performed healthcare procedure.

- Blood pressure should be measured in both arms at the first visit; the higher arm should then be used as the reference blood pressure.

- Virtually all epidemiological data used to determine hypertension detection, referral, and treatment guidelines are based on blood pressures taken by trained observers using the standardized blood pressure technique recommended by the American heart Association.

- A mercury manometer, the "gold standard" for indirect blood pressure measurement, is the most accurate and reliable instrument available.

See also Chapters 105, 106

Indirect BP Measurement

Indirect blood pressure (BP) measurement is safe, is relatively painless, and provides reliable information when performed accurately. Virtually all the epidemiological data used to determine hypertension detection, referral, and treatment guidelines are based on BPs obtained by the American Heart Association (AHA) standardized indirect measurement method.

Because high BP is almost always "silent" (without symptoms), diagnosis and treatment hinge on accurate BP measurement. The proven benefits of treating high BP can be accomplished only if health professionals are measuring BP accurately. Crucial clinical decisions are based on these measurements. Accurate BP measurement requires the ability to hear, interpret, and record Korotkoff (K) sounds; good eye-to-hand coordination for equipment operation; and the ability to perform the steps outlined below. Failure to practice correct technique and the use of inaccurate equipment are the major reasons for inaccurate BP determinations. Standardized curricula have been developed to ensure mastery of this critical healthcare skill.

Selecting and Caring for BP Measurement Equipment

The manometer is either a mercury or an aneroid instrument calibrated to the nearest 2 mm Hg. The mercury manometer is read at the top edge (the meniscus) of the mercury column. It is considered the "gold standard" measurement device because it is the most accurate device available. The aneroid manometer consists of a metal bellows that expands as the pressure in the cuff increases and is read at the point indicated by a needle on its dial. It is fragile and easily damaged. Users cannot be certain that it is accurate even when the needle is positioned at zero. Therefore, it is necessary to use a "Y" connector to compare the aneroid device to an accurate mercury

manometer at least every 6 months (**Figure 104.1**). Calibration is required when the readings differ from the standard mercury manometer by 3 mm Hg.

The stethoscope head should have a low-frequency detector or bell for listening to the low-pitched sounds. Earpieces should fit comfortably forward in the direction of the ear canal and block out external noise. For best sound transmission, the tubing should be no longer than 15 in.

Automated BP Measurement Devices

Before using any automated BP instrument, you must document the accuracy of its pressure-registering system (Y tube to mercury device). Then, simultaneously compare digital and mercury readings on the patient, because automated devices fail to give accurate readings on many individuals. The use of automated devices is discouraged in most clinical settings.

Steps Needed to Obtain Accurate and Reliable Readings

Step 1. Environment

The setting should be private and quiet, with a comfortable room temperature.

Rationale. To get the best estimate of the patient's usual BP, you must control for environmental factors that may cause BP variation or interfere with hearing Korotkoff sounds.

The manometer must be positioned so the observer can view it at eye level.

Rationale. Viewing the manometer above or below the observer's eye level results in inaccurate readings.

The room should have a straight-backed chair next to a table for the patient, a seat for the BP observer, and an adjustable surface to support the arm at heart level during standing measurements. The height of the table should be such that the midpoint of the cuff when in place on the patient's right arm is supported at heart level, that is, approximately at the level of the fourth intercostal space (at the sternum) in the seated position or at the level of the midaxillary line in the supine position. Achieving heart level may require using a cushion to increase the height of the patient in the chair or using an object (such as a book) to support the arm at the correct level.

Rationale. Avoids errors induced by differences in hydrostatic pressure between the point of artery compression by the cuff and the heart. If the center of the cuff on the arm or leg is above the heart level, the reading will be falsely low by 0.8 mm Hg for each 1 cm above the heart

Table 104.1. Phases of the Korotkoff Sounds

Phase I
  The pressure level at which the first faint, consistent tapping sounds are heard. The sounds gradually increase in intensity as the cuff is deflated. The first of at least two of these sounds is defined as the systolic pressure.
Phase II
  The time during cuff deflation when a murmur of swishing sounds are heard.
Phase III
  The period during which sounds are crisper and increase in intensity.
Phase IV
  The time when a distinct, abrupt, muffling of sound (usually of a soft blowing quality) is heard. This is defined as the diastolic pressure in anyone in whom sounds continue to zero.
Phase V
  The pressure level when the last regular BP sound is heard and after which all sound disappears. This is defined as the diastolic pressure unless sounds are heard to zero.

To avoid error, the observer must be prepared to recognize two normal Korotkoff sound variations associated with BP readings. (1) The auscultatory gap is a period of silence occurring during Korotkoff phases I and II. This disappearance of sound is temporary and is usually short, but the gap can occur over a period of 40 mm Hg. It seems to be associated with higher BP readings. (2) An absent Korotkoff phase V occurs when sounds are heard to "0." When this is the case, phase IV should be recorded along with phase V. In this case phase IV is the best reference for diastolic pressure.

level. If below heart level, it will be falsely high by a similar amount. Supporting the back in the seated position and the arm in any position avoids increases in BP due to isometric muscle contraction.

Step 2. Preparation and Rest Period

Inquire about biological factors that may affect the reading at this time, including the time and dose of medications. If not wearing short, loose sleeves, patients should bare their arm(s). Explain the procedure and that you will take at least two readings.

Rationale. To get the best estimate of the patient's usual BP, you must control for biological factors that may cause BP variation at this time: pain, stress, full urinary bladder, recent meal; prescription, over-the-counter, and street drugs, as well as caffeine and nicotine. Clothing interferes with cuff placement, pressure, and sound transmission. Prepares patient and avoids elevated readings due to anxiety about the procedure and repeated readings.

Instruct patients to sit up straight with legs uncrossed, back resting against the chair, and feet flat on the floor, and to remain silent until you finish taking the BP readings, after which you will answer their questions. Allow a 5-minute rest period before the first reading.

Rationale. The lack of back and foot support, such as occurs when the patient is seated on an examination table, causes BP elevation averaging 5 mm Hg diastolic. Talking or active listening during measurement causes BP elevation.

Step 3. Proper Cuff (Bladder) Size

To get an accurate reading, the width of the cuff bladder should encircle at least 40% of the arm circumference and the length at least 80%. At the first visit, measure circumference at the midpoint of the upper arm, between the olecranon and acromion processes. Arms >53 cm in circumference should have the BP measured with a cuff of the appropriate size on the forearm. When arm circumference measurement is not practical, as during screening situations, it is acceptable to estimate the proper cuff size by comparing the bladder width and length to arm circumference.

When BP is not measured in both arms, the reading should be taken in the right arm unless it is known that BP in the left arm is higher. Note the appropriate cuff/bladder size on each chart.

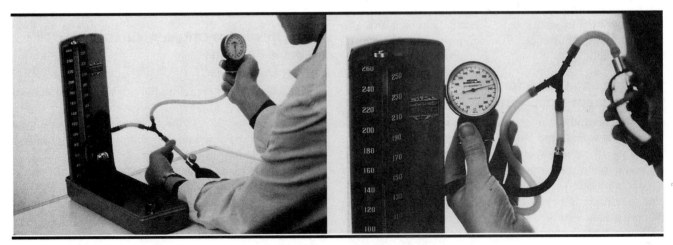

Figure 104.1.   Aneroid instrument being tested by inserting a Y-tube connector or stopcock to create a communicating system with one pressure source. Allows simultaneous pressure application to both instruments. Courtesy of Shared Care Research and Education Consulting, Inc, Torrance, Calif.

Rationale. Using a bladder that is too narrow or short for the limb is a common error that is serious because it yields false high readings. Diseases that cause BP differences between the arms are much more likely to cause a falsely low BP in the left arm.

Step 4. Cuff Placement

Locate the patient's brachial artery at the midpoint of the upper arm by palpating between the biceps and triceps muscles on its inner surface. Wrap the cuff smoothly and snugly around the arm with its bladder center directly over the palpated artery and the lower edge of the cuff 2.5 cm above the antecubital fossa.

Rationale. Avoids false high readings that occur when cuff pressure is not equally distributed over the artery. Avoids errors that result from extra sounds when the stethoscope comes in contact with cuff or tubing.

Step 5. Determine the Maximum Inflation Level

Before listening for the BP, determine the inflation level necessary to obtain an accurate systolic reading, the maximum inflation level (MIL).

(1) Locate the radial pulse and note the heart rate and rhythm.

Rationale. When the heart rate is irregular, systolic BP may vary beat to beat. Then additional readings are needed to get the best estimate of the systolic BP.

(2) Continue feeling the pulse and rapidly inflate the cuff to 60 mm Hg and then by 10-mm increments until the pulse is no longer palpable. This is the first estimate of the palpated pressure. Stop inflating the cuff.

(3) Begin deflation at 2 mm Hg/s. Note the pressure at which the pulse reappears.

This is the palpated systolic pressure and will usually be within 10 mm Hg of the level at which the pulse disappeared. Additional readings are needed for accurate estimation of the palpated systolic BP when the pulse is irregular.

(4) Immediately release all pressure. Add 30 mm Hg to the palpated systolic reading to determine the MIL.

Rationale. Determines the minimum pressure needed to get an accurate systolic BP on a patient and decreases patient discomfort. Avoids errors that result from failure to inflate above systolic BP reading, including an inaccurately low systolic BP reading, which occurs when the observer begins listening during an auscultatory gap.

Step 6. Stethoscope Placement

Position the stethoscope earpieces pointing forward in your ears.

Rationale. Sound is not transmitted well when the eartips fail to point into the ear canal.

Find the point at which the brachial artery pulse is the strongest, usually just above the antecubital fossa on the inner aspect of the arm. Using light pressure, position the chestpiece over this point with all edges gently touching the skin surface. The stethoscope bell or a low-frequency detector is recommended.

Rationale. The loudest sounds will be heard over this pulse. Avoids errors due to difficulty hearing and interpreting Korotkoff sounds. Errors result when too much stethoscope pressure causes additional artery occlusion and distorts BP sounds. Korotkoff sounds are of low frequency.

Do not allow the stethoscope head to touch the cuff or tubing.

Rationale. Extraneous sounds mask and confuse Korotkoff sounds.

Step 7. Inflation/Deflation

Rapidly inflate the cuff to the MIL. If sounds are heard immediately, completely release all pressure and repeat step 5 to repeat the palpated pressure.

Rationale. Rapid inflation to correct level ensures listening above systolic BP. Slow inflation traps venous blood in the arm and may result in pain and diminished or distorted sounds.

Release the air from the cuff so that the mercury falls at a rate of 2 mm Hg/s until Korotkoff sounds are heard. Continue deflation at the rate of 2 mm Hg per beat. If unable to hear sounds clearly, quickly release all pressure, and check position of eartips and stethoscope. Repeat the procedure.

Rationale. Slow deflation is necessary to allow the observer to hear the systolic and diastolic pressures at the point of onset. A reading can be no more accurate than the rate of deflation, ie, a deflation rate of 10 mm Hg/s will result in a pressure accurate to only 10 mm Hg, and if one beat is missed, to only 20 mm Hg.

Step 8. Systolic BP

Reading to the nearest 2 mm Hg mark, remember the systolic pressure at the onset of Korotkoff phase 1, the first of at least two regular "tapping" sounds **(Table 104.1).** When the reading falls between two 2 mm Hg marks, round to the higher of the two. Concentrate and remember the reading by silently repeating the systolic number with every heart beat until you confirm disappearance. Immediately record both systolic and diastolic BPs.

Rationale. Observers must learn to rule out sound artifacts. Single sounds inconsistent with heart rate are insignificant artifacts unless the pulse was irregular during palpation. In the case of arrhythmia, additional readings are needed to get the best estimate of the systolic BP.

Forgetting the reading is a common source of errors of 8 to 10 mm Hg, especially in the presence of a wide pulse pressure (difference between the systolic and diastolic pressures).

Step 9. Diastolic BP

Remember the pint at which the last regular Korotkoff sound is heard. When the sounds continue to very low diastolic levels or 0, remember the reading at the onset of KIV, the point at which sounds begin to muffle, as well as the last sound heard. This is best determined on a second reading if the pressure is heard to zero.

Rationale. The onset of KV (disappearance) is more reliably interpreted when observers listen for the last sound heard. The absence of KV occurs often in children, during pregnancy, and in other high-cardiac-output states. In these cases, the onset of KIV is the most accurate diastolic indicator.

If the diastolic BP is heard above 90 mm Hg, listen for an additional 40 mm Hg. Otherwise, listen for 10 to 20 mm Hg below the last sound to confirm disappearance.

Rationale. Avoids inaccurately high diastolic BP due to failure to listen until sounds reappear after a period of silence when an auscultatory gap is present.

Step 10. Recording

Record the reading, the arm used, the position of the patient, and the cuff size used. Immediately record the reading as KI/KV. If KIV is recorded, write the three numbers as KI/KIV/KV. If sounds do not cease, record KV as 0.

Rationale. Standardized recording methods are necessary to correctly interpret and compare readings by different observers. When phase V is absent, Korotkoff phase IV is the best indication of diastolic pressure.

Step 11. Repeat the Reading

Make certain all air is out of cuff. Wait 1 to 2 minutes and repeat steps 6 through 10.

Rationale. BP normally changes from minute to minute, especially during clinical measurements. The average of two or more BP readings in a single arm is more reliable and a better indicator of usual readings than is a single reading or one reading in each arm.

Step 12. Repeat the Process

Repeat the measurements in the other arm during initial workup and standing or supine as dictated by the patient's situation. Postural changes in BP are measured after 1 and 3 minutes of standing. Note the arm with the higher reading for future comparisons.

Rationale. BP can differ by >10 mm Hg between arms. The higher pressure more accurately reflects intra-arterial pressure.

Special Techniques and Populations
Absence of Korotkoff Phase V

When cardiac output is high, as in some children, in thyrotoxicosis, during fever, and in pregnant women, KV is often absent. In this event, Korotkoff sounds are heard until the mercury column falls to zero. BP should be recorded as three numbers (KV/KIV/0).

BP Measurement in Children

The principles of measurement are the same in newborns, infants, and children. A most important consideration is the selection of a cuff that is appropriate for the arm circumference, as described above.

BP Measurement in the Elderly

In the elderly, the brachial arteries occasionally become very thickened and stiff. When this happens, the indirect cuff pressure may overestimate intra-arterial pressure, because higher cuff pressure is required to compress such a rigid vessel. The presence of a radial artery that is still palpable after the cuff is inflated above the systolic BP should be a warning of this error. If the artery feels excessively thick when rolled back and forth under the finger, the BP reading measured with indirect techniques may be falsely high. Recheck the pressure by palpation in the forearm. If the palpated systolic pressure differs by >15 mm Hg, then a direct arterial puncture may be needed to be certain of the true pressure. The patient should be informed and the problem noted on the patient's record to alert others who measure BP in that individual.

Very Large, Cone-Shaped, and Muscular Arms

If the patient's arm is >41 cm in circumference or if it is shaped so that a cuff will not fit on it well, then accurate pressure measurement may be impossible. In this case, palpated and auscultated readings should be attempted, with a cuff of the appropriate size, in both the upper arm and forearm. If these differ by >15 mm Hg, then a better estimate of true pressure will be the palpated systolic pressure with the cuff on the forearm.

SUGGESTED READING

1. Bailey RH, Knaus VL, Bauer JH. Aneroid sphygmomanometers: an assessment of accuracy at a university hospital and clinics. *Arch Intern Med.* 1991;151: 1409–1412.
2. Blood-pressure monitors: convenience doesn't equal accuracy. *Consumer Reports.* 1996;61:53–55.
3. Cushman WC, Cooper KM, Horne RA, Meydrech EF. Effect of back support and stethoscope head on seated blood pressure determinations. *Am J Hypertens.* 1990;3:240–241.
4. Grim CM, Grim CE. A curriculum for the training and certification of blood pressure measurement for health care providers. *Can J Cardiol.* 1005;11(suppl H): 38H–42H.
5. Hayes MV. Managing mercury: simple, effective methods for cleaning up small spills. *Medical Waste.* 1993;1:3–7.
6. McKay DW, Campbell NR, Parab LS, Chockalingam A, Fodor JG. Clinical assessment of blood pressure. *J Hum Hypertens.* 1990;4:639–645.
7. National High Blood Pressure Education Program Working Group Update on the 1987 Task Force Report on High Blood Pressure in Children and Adolescents: a working group report from the National High Blood Pressure Education Program. *Pediatrics.* 1996;90:649–658.
8. Perloff D, Grim CM, Flack J, Frohlich ED, Hill M, McDonald M. Morgenstern BZ. Human blood pressure determination by sphygmomanometry. *Circulation.* 1993;88:2460–2470.
9. Prisant LM, Alpert BS, Robbins CB, Berson AS, Hayes M, Cohen ML, Sheps SG. American national standard for nonautomated sphygmomanometers: summary report. *Am H Hypertens.* 1995;8:210–213.
10. Sixth Report of the Joint National Committee on Prevention, Detection, Evaluation, and Treatment of High Blood Pressure (JNC VI). *Arch Intern Med.* 1997;157: 2413–2446.

Chapter 105

Initial Workup of the Hypertensive Patient

Marvin Moser, MD

KEY POINTS

- A history, physical examination, basic serum chemistries, urinalysis, total and HDL cholesterol, and an ECG are recommended for the initial evaluation of a hypertensive patient.

- Goals of initial evaluation are (1) estimation of the severity of the hypertension, (2) evaluation of other cardiovascular risk factors, and (3) evaluation of secondary hypertension.

- An echocardiogram, 24-hour ambulatory blood pressure monitoring, and renin determinations are not recommended unless there are specific indications for these procedures.

- Particular attention should be paid to systolic blood pressure, which more closely predicts morbidity and mortality than diastolic pressure.

See also Chapters 104, 106

The initial diagnostic evaluation of the hypertensive patient should have three major objectives: (1) to define the severity of the hypertension, (2) to determine the presence or absence of other risk factors for cardiovascular disease, and (3) to search for clues of secondary causes for hypertension.

The Sixth Joint National Committee on the Prevention, Detection, Evaluation, and Treatment of High Blood Pressure (JNC VI) recommends a careful history, a complete physical examination, several basic laboratory tests, and an ECG for the diagnostic evaluation. It is recognized from epidemiological studies that hypertension, in conjunction with any one of several other cardiovascular risk factors, such as a smoking history, elevated serum lipid levels, hyperglycemia, an increased intake of alcohol, and obesity, puts a person at greater risk than when hypertension is the only risk factor. The presence of target organ involvement, such as left ventricular hypertrophy (LVH), indicates that treatment should be undertaken more readily than in subjects without evidence of target organ involvement. Even though only about 5% of all cases of hypertension in a general population are secondary to an identifiable specific cause, patients with these diseases should be identified, if possible, because they may be curable and may be treated differently from patients with essential hypertension.

Establishing the Diagnosis of Hypertension

The initial step in the evaluation of a patient with newly discovered hypertension is to decide whether or not he or she actually has a sustained blood pressure elevation. Before a diagnosis of hypertension is established, blood pressure should be measured on at least two occasions after the original determination unless initial levels are >160–170/105–110 mm Hg (stage 3 hypertension). In this case, the diagnosis is probably established, and therapy may be initiated without additional recordings. Follow-up readings will often be lower than the first reading, and fewer people will be categorized as hypertensive if these subsequent pressures are considered. Individuals with initially

elevated blood pressures who become normotensive on further evaluation should not be ignored, however, because they have a tendency to develop more consistently elevated blood pressures in the future. They should be carefully followed up at regular intervals of between 6 months and 1 year. Careful attention should be paid to measurement techniques to ensure that blood pressure readings are accurate.

Risk increases as pressure rises—the higher the level of blood pressure, the greater the incidence of cardiovascular complications at all ages and in both sexes. Recent data from more than 300 000 men screened in the Multiple Risk Factor Intervention Trial (MRFIT) determined that elevation of systolic blood pressure may be a more reliable and important prognostic factor than an elevated diastolic blood pressure, at least in men. This finding confirms data from Framingham and other studies, but the perception persists that the diastolic blood pressure is of more importance than systolic blood pressure as a predictor of events. An increased pulse pressure (systolic-diastolic), which reflects decreased arterial compliance in older persons, may be an even better indicator of cardiovascular risk. Risk is related to pressure; although risk increases linearly with levels of blood pressure >110/80 mm Hg, it does not become significant to an individual until pressure reaches 135 to 140/85 to 90 mm Hg.

White Coat Hypertension?

Routine use of ambulatory blood pressure monitoring to diagnose "white coat hypertension," defined as persistently elevated blood pressures in a doctor's office with normal blood pressures at home or at work, is rarely necessary and has not been recommended by the JNC VI. This opinion and recommendation are based on the following: (1) All of the major epidemiological studies have based their estimations of risk on casual pressures taken on one or two occasions in a doctor's office or clinic, not on home or worksite pressures. If the office blood pressure is high, the risk of a future cardiovascular event is increased compared with someone with a normal casual blood pressure. (2) In all of the long-term clinical trials, patients were treated on the basis of blood pressures measured in a clinic or doctor's office. The lower the office blood pressure, the better the outcome. (3) Recent data from the Tecumseh study have established that patients with slightly elevated blood pressures in doctors' offices but with normal pressures at home are different physiologically from those who are normotensive (<135/85 mm Hg) both at home and in a medical office. Peripheral resistance is increased, and changes in left ventricular diastolic function and in certain metabolic parameters such as insulin resistance, levels of serum cholesterol, and serum glucose have already occurred.

Clues for Secondary Hypertension

If an elevated blood pressure is discovered, efforts should be made to rule out, if possible, the presence of secondary hypertension **(Table 105.1)**. Although a number of very rare causes exist, most fall into a few diagnostic groups:

Chronic renal insufficiency can usually be ruled out by the absence of proteinuria and the presence of a normal serum creatinine level.

Renovascular hypertension can be suspected if there is (1) new-onset hypertension over the age of 55 to 60 years, particularly in smokers; (2) hypertension in a child <10 to 12 years of age; (3) sudden increase in blood pressure in patients who were previously controlled by medication; (4) failure of triple-drug therapy; and (5) a periumbilical bruit with radiation to the flanks, especially in younger women, which is characteristically holosystolic and high-pitched with a short diastolic component.

Primary hyperaldosteronism can be suspected if the serum potassium level is <3.5 mEq/L in the absence of diuretic therapy or <3.0 mEq/L on diuretic.

Coarctation of the aorta can be identified by the presence of a short, rough systolic murmur in the second left interspace, the palpation or auscultation of bruits over the back, the absence of or marked decrease in the amplitude of the femoral pulses or blood pressures in the legs, a chest radiograph demonstrating notching of the posterior ribs, or an imaging test.

Table 105.1. Some Symptoms or Findings That May Suggest Further Studies For Causes of Hypertension

Obesity, unusual truncal distribution of fat and abdominal striae, and excessive body or facial hair (hyperadrenalism)

Anxiety, tremor, headaches, sweating, or rapid pulse (hyperthyroidism or pheochromocytoma)

Pallor and diaphoresis (pheochromocytoma)

Skin lesions (pheochromocytoma is associated with several neurocutaneous syndromes; pigmented striae are consistent with hyperadrenalism)

Muscle weakness, cramps (primary aldosteronism)

Periods of impaired consciousness (cerebrovascular disease or hypersomnolence due to sleep apnea, also associated with hypertension)

Absent or diminished femoral pulses (coarctation or aorta)

Periumbilical holosystolic bruit with diastolic component (renovascular disease)

Pheochromocytoma or thyroid crisis may be suspected with a history of palpitations, sweating, headaches, weight loss, and the presence of orthostatic hypotension.

Cushing's disease, a rare form of hypertension, can be suspected in an obese person with purple abdominal striae and abnormal chemistries.

Every case of accelerated or malignant hypertension should be evaluated for secondary hypertension after the blood pressure is lowered.

Specific Aspects of the History

In the determination of urgency in treatment, it is often helpful to establish whether there is a strong family history of hypertension, stroke, or coronary disease, especially if any of these events had occurred in close relatives <60 years old. The history should specifically include information regarding symptoms and any prior cardiovascular disease.

Although stages 1 and 2 hypertension (blood pressures of 140–159/90–99 and 160–179/100–109 mm Hg) are generally asymptomatic, there is one symptom, an early morning occipital headache that clears as the patient moves about, that we have found to be correlated with an elevated blood pressure. Although most people cannot accurately predict their blood pressures, some get a sense of fullness in the head, redness in the face, or a "general unease" when their blood pressures are high. Recent data demonstrating improvement in general well-being when blood pressure is lowered with antihypertensive agents suggest that hypertensive individuals may not be as free of symptoms as has been commonly believed.

A history of the use of other medications (prescribed or over-the-counter) or street drugs (cocaine, amphetamines, etc) should be obtained, because these may cause an elevation of pressure or aggravate existing hypertension. Among drugs that may increase blood pressure are high-dose estrogens, adrenal steroids, nonsteroidal anti-inflammatory agents, nasal decongestants, some other cold remedies, appetite suppressants, cyclosporine, and tricyclic antidepressants. The number of patients, however, who experience an elevated blood pressure from these agents is small. The average blood pressure of women on low-dose oral contraceptives is only slightly increased. If blood pressure is well controlled in treated subjects, there is little reason to totally interdict the use of any of these medications if they are indicated for medical reasons.

Physical Examination

On the first visit, it is useful to measure blood pressure in both arms. These should be similar, although if there is a time lapse between the two measurements, there may be a difference of ≈5 to 10 mm Hg. If the difference is much more than 15 to 20 mm Hg of systolic blood pressure, an atherosclerotic plaque may be present in the circulation of the arm with the lower pressure. Always use the blood pressure measured in the arm with the higher reading to determine therapy. Specific symptoms or signs may present clues as to the presence of a variety of other diseases.

Funduscopic examination is not very helpful in the majority of subjects with stages 1 and 2 hypertension, but the presence of significant arteriolar narrowing or arteriovenous nicking indicates that blood pressure has been elevated for a considerable length of time or has been higher at other times. Flame-shaped hemorrhages,

Table 105.2. Initial Laboratory Evaluation

TEST	IMPLICATIONS
Urine examination	Helpful in ruling out parenchymal renal disease
Urea nitrogen or serum creatinine determination	Can rule out kidney failure; provides an index of baseline kidney function
Serum potassium: hypokalemia (<3.5 mEq/L) in patients not taking medication*	Strongly suggests a search for primary hyperaldosteronism
Serum glucose elevation*	Assists in diagnosis of diabetes mellitus and can be seen in pheochromocytoma, hyperthyroidism, and hyperadrenal states
Uric acid measurements*	Provides baseline; may be predictor of future gout
Serum cholesterol with HDL, LDL, and triglycerides if indicated*	Provides information about another risk factor for heart disease
Calcium level*	Excludes hypercalcemia as a primary cause of hypertension
ECG	Helpful in determining the presence of LVH, ischemia, heart block, etc

*An automated blood chemistry may be less expensive than individual determinations.

exudates, or papilledema with an elevated blood pressure suggest severe target-organ damage and a poor prognosis unless therapy is instituted quickly.

Physical examination of the heart includes an evaluation of rate and rhythm. Ectopic beats are not uncommon in persons with hypertension, especially if LVH is present. Atrial fibrillation, however, is not a common finding unless there are other complicating factors. Physical signs of cardiomegaly, especially of LVH, may be present, with a forceful apical impulse and palpation of cardiac dullness to the left of the midaxillary line. An accentuated aortic second sound is frequently present, especially if the diastolic blood pressure is >100 mm Hg. A fourth heart sound is common in adults with hypertension and atrial enlargement, but a third heart sound suggests decreased ventricular function. Specific valvular murmurs are not usually related to hypertension, but marked elevations of diastolic pressures cause dilatation of the aortic ring, and an aortic diastolic murmur will occasionally be heard.

Examination of the peripheral pulses helps both to rule out peripheral arterial disease and to confirm the diagnosis of aortic coarctation. The carotid arteries should be palpated and auscultated for the presence of bruits, which might indicate narrowing or plaques.

During examination of the abdomen, special efforts should be made to listen for a periumbilical bruit (renovascular disease) and to palpate for a spongy mass that might suggest polycystic kidneys (this entity is obviously quite rare). Active, forceful pulsations along the aorta might be a normal finding in young, thin people but might suggest an abdominal aortic aneurysm in older individuals. Palpation of the abdomen, especially laterally, may trigger a typical attack in individuals with a pheochromocytoma.

Laboratory Evaluation

The JNC VI report again stressed that the laboratory evaluation of hypertensive patients need not be extensive or costly (**Table 105.2**). If proteinuria is absent, a renal cause of the hypertension is rarely found. Patients with renovascular disease, however, may present with a normal urinalysis. White and red blood cells with proteinuria and/or casts suggest the presence of accelerated or malignant hypertension or chronic glomerulitis or pyelonephritis. Certain blood chemistries are suggested as baseline data (Table 105.2). An automated blood chemistry is recommended to include those tests to

provide baseline information for the treatment of hypertension as well as other risk factors, such as diabetes and hyperlipidemia. A complete blood count is also advised.

An ECG is suggested to determine the presence or absence of arrhythmias, myocardial ischemia, and/or LVH. The presence of a heart block would indicate caution in the use of a β-blocker or one of the nondihydropyridine calcium antagonists. Although an echocardiogram is a more sensitive indicator of LVH than an ECG, a full echocardiogram is expensive, and the information other than ventricular mass is probably not of great importance for the average hypertensive patient. This procedure has not been recommended in the routine evaluation of a hypertensive subject.

Chest radiograph, intravenous pyelogram, and plasma renin are also not currently recommended as routine procedures in the evaluation of the hypertensive patient and are rarely indicated. These are relatively insensitive indicators of secondary hypertension and should be reserved for use in individuals in whom there is a high suspicion of a specific disease.

SUGGESTED READING

1. Gifford RW Jr, Kirkendall W, O'Connor DT, Weideman W. Office evaluation of hypertension: a statement for health professionals by a writing group of the Council for High Blood Pressure Research, American Heart Association. *Circulation.* 1989; 79:721–731.
2. Grimm RH Jr, Grandits GA, Cutler JA, Stewart AL, McDonald RH, Svendsen K, Prineas RJ, Liebson PR, for the TOMHS Research Group. Relationships of quality-of-life measures to long-term lifestyle and drug treatment in the Treatment of Mild Hypertension Study. *Arch Intern Med.* 1997;157:638–648.
3. Julius S, Mejia A, Jones K, Krause L, Schork N, van de Ven C, Johnson E, Petrin J, Sekkarie MA, Kjeldsen SE, et al. "White coat" versus "sustained" borderline hypertension in Tecumseh, Michigan. *Hypertension.* 1990;16:617–623.
4. Moser M. Can the cost of care be contained and quality of care maintained in the management of hypertension? *Arch Intern Med.* 1994;154:1665–1671.
5. Moser M. Hypertension. In: Rakel RE, ed. *Conn's Current Therapy 1995.* Philadelphia, Pa: WB Saunders Co; 1995:263–280.
6. Moser M. Hypertension can be treated effectively without increasing the cost of care. *J Hum Hypertens.* 1996;10(suppl 2):533–538.
7. Neaton JD, Wentworth D, for the Multiple Risk Factor Intervention Trial Research Group. Serum cholesterol, blood pressure, cigarette smoking, and death from coronary heart disease: overall findings and differences by age for 316 099 white men. *Arch Intern Med.* 1992;152:56–64.
8. The Sixth Report of the Joint National Committee on Prevention, Detection, Evaluation, and Treatment of High Blood Pressure. *Arch Intern Med.* 1997;157: 2413–2446.

Chapter 106

Out-of-Office Blood Pressure Monitoring

William B. White, MD

KEY POINTS

- One important advantage of self-monitoring of the blood pressure (BP) is that multiple readings during different times of the day may be taken and recorded by patients.

- A useful feature of self-monitoring of the BP is that it usually avoids the pressor response ("white-coat" effect) seen in 15% to 20% of stage I and II hypertensive patients in the doctor's office.

- Several cross-sectional studies have shown that out-of-office BPs correlate better with echocardiographically determined left ventricular mass than clinic pressures.

- While more costly than self-monitoring, ambulatory BP monitoring can often be useful because it may lead to more accurate identification of those who truly require antihypertensive therapy as well as those who may be best managed with nonpharmacological therapy.

See also Chapters 104, 105

Out-of-Office Blood Pressure Monitoring

Monitoring of the blood pressure (BP) outside of the medical care environment has become an important part of clinical hypertension assessment and management. There are two main forms of out-of-office BP monitoring: self-monitoring, usually performed by the patient (or a relative) with an aneroid manometer or portable semiautomated device, and ambulatory BP monitoring, which uses automated devices for repeated determinations during an extended time period, typically 24 hours. Both techniques can greatly enhance the clinician's understanding of BP behavior in patients and aid in diagnosis and therapeutic decision-making.

Self-Monitoring of the BP

There are a number of advantages of self-monitoring, or home measurement of the BP **(Table 106.1)**. One important advantage of self-monitoring of the BP is that multiple readings during different times of the day may be taken and recorded by patients. These values can be reviewed by the physician as adjunct information to the office pressures for therapeutic decision-making. A second useful feature of self-monitoring of the BP is that it usually avoids the pressor response ("white-coat" effect) seen in 15% to 20% of stage I and II hypertensive patients in the doctor's office.

Techniques for Self-Monitoring

Several types of BP monitors are available for use at home, including aneroid (dial-type) manometers, semiautomated electronic sphygmomanometers (generally using an oscillometric method of BP measurement), and mercury-column sphygmomanometers. Aneroid manometers with a stethoscope are relatively simple to use and generally are the most economical type of self-monitoring units available. However, in older patients lacking manual dexterity or when hearing loss is an issue, an electronic device may be preferable to a nonautomated sphygmomanometer. Electronic devices are convenient, but before they are used in practice by patients, they should be validated according to a rigorous standard, such as the American Association for Medical Instrumentation (AAMI) guidelines. In addition, clinical calibration against a mercury-column sphygmomanometer should be performed on a regular basis. Patients are usually fairly accurate when recording their own pressures but may tend to underreport high BP levels and monitor the BP at home, while relaxed, rather than during work or other stressful situations.

Usefulness of Self-Monitored BPs for Hypertension Management

Although the theoretical advantages of self-monitoring are obvious, there are still no definitive prognostic data comparing the prediction of cardiovascular risk by home BP versus doctor's office BP. Conversely, several cross-sectional studies have shown that self-monitored BPs correlate better with echocardiographically determined left ventricular mass than clinic pressures. One population study based in Japan has suggested that home BP is a better predictor of cardiovascular risk than office BP in older patients. The self-monitored BP has the potential for reducing the bias and error in assessing the "true" pressure in a patient (which may be quite large if a small number of readings in the doctor's office are used). In some studies, the self-monitored pressure has been shown to be similar to the attenuated BP seen with repeated measurements over time (ie, weeks and months) in the clinic.

Table 106.1. Usefulness of Self or Home Bound Pressure Monitoring

Distinguishes sustained hypertension from white-coat hypertension
Assesses response to antihypertensive therapy
Improves patient adherence to treatment
Potentially reduces management costs

Note: Only validated electronic devices or aneroid sphygmomanometers with appropriately sized cuffs are recommended.

Because the self-monitored BP may be more representative of the true BP for an individual, it can be useful in therapeutic decision-making. Once antihypertensive therapy has been initiated, self-monitoring of the BP is an excellent way to evaluate the effectiveness of the therapy and avoid multiple doctor or nurse visits. Furthermore, the relationship between time of dosing of antihypertensive therapy and BP levels may be easier to assess with self-monitoring patients. As a final tribute, adherence to therapy and BP control have been shown to improve when patients (even previously noncompliant ones) self-monitor their BP.

Table 106.2. Values of Clinic and Ambulatory Blood Pressures in Normal and Untreated Hypertensive Patients (Based on Clinic Pressures)

	NORMOTENSIVES	HYPERTENSIVES
Clinic systolic BP	120±9	151±10
Clinic diastolic BP	79±6	101±6
24-hour systolic BP	113±9	139±12
24-hour diastolic BP	72±5	87±8
Awake systolic BP	118±9	149±12
Awake diastolic BP	76±5	93±9
Sleep systolic BP	98±9	117±9
Sleep diastolic BP	60±5	77±7

Reproduced with permission from White WB, Morganroth J. Usefulness of ambulatory blood pressure monitoring in assessing antihypertensive therapy. *Am J Cardiol.* 1989;63:94–98.

Ambulatory Monitoring of the BP
The Recorders

Over the past 20 years, noninvasive automated devices have been developed for hypertension management and clinical research. In recent years, the ambulatory BP monitors have become much more practical to use in patient care, because the devices are quite small (<1 lb in most instances), simple to apply by a nurse or technician, and precise. These fully automated, programmable recorders are capable of 100 to 200 BP and pulse measurements from an energy source of two to four small batteries. The devices measure BP either by oscillometry or auscultation of Korotkoff sounds. Oscillometric measurement is derived from oscillations emanating from the brachial artery into the BP cuff; the amplitudes of the oscillations are related to a standard form of BP (usually mercury column measurements by auscultation), and an algorithm is then developed. The oscillometric methodology is fairly accurate in patients who have midrange BPs and hold their arms still during cuff inflation and deflation. Some recent data suggest that oscillometric BP determination is less accurate in older patients or in those with extremely low or high pressures. Auscultatory measurements mimic those of clinicians and use a microphone for detection of the Korotkoff sounds. Auscultatory devices are also subject to noise artifact when the patient has excessive arm motion during the actual BP measurement.

Comparison of Ambulatory BP With Office or Clinic Measurements

Full clinical utility of ambulatory BP recordings depends on the frame of reference for the values derived. There is a reproducible diurnal/nocturnal pattern to BP during a 24-hour period of measure-

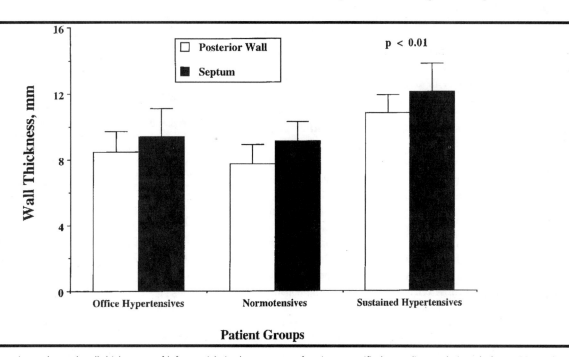

Figure 106.1. Posterior and septal wall thicknesses of left ventricle in three groups of patients stratified according to their ambulatory BP monitoring results. Office hypertensive patients had an office BP >140/90 mm Hg and an awake BP <130/80 mm Hg; normotensives had an office BP <140/90 mm Hg and an awake BP <130/80 mm Hg; sustained hypertensives had an office BP and awake BP >140/90 mm Hg. Wall thicknesses were significantly greater in sustained hypertensive patients ($P<0.01$) vs two other groups. Reproduced with permission from White WB, Schulman P, McCabe EJ, Dey HM. Average daily blood pressure, not office blood pressure, determines cardiac function in patients with hypertension. *JAMA.* 1989;261:873–877.

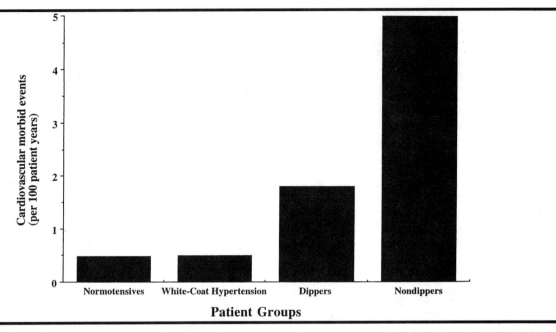

Figure 106.2. Cardiovascular event rates (per 100 patient-years of follow-up) according to ambulatory BP profiles (normotensives and white-coat hypertensives had awake BP <136/86 and 131/86 mm Hg for men and women, respectively; dipper hypertensives had awake BP >136/86 and 131/86 mm Hg in men and women, respectively, with >10% decline in BP during the night, whereas nondippers had <10% decline in BP during the night compared with daytime BP values. Reproduced with permission from Verdecchia P, Porcellati C, Schillaci G, Borgioni C, Ciucci A, Battistelli M, et al. Ambulatory blood pressure: an independent predictor of prognosis in essential hypertension. *Hypertension*. 1994;24:790–798.

ment in ≈80% of patients. Typically, the pressure is highest while the patient is awake (especially during work) and lowest during sleep. The data are expressed as 24-hour mean BP and often as the values during wakefulness and sleep. BP during sleep is quite low compared with the office or clinic pressure, whereas BP during the awake state is similar to the values obtained in the office **(Table 106.2)**. One must keep these differences in mind when trying to interpret ambulatory BP recordings. A major effort has been made to publish normative data for ambulatory BP during the past several years, but none have been linked to cardiovascular events.

Relationship Between the Ambulatory BP and Hypertensive Disease

One of the most important findings with regard to the ambulatory BP has been its relationship to hypertensive target organ disease. The majority of cross-sectional studies published to date have shown the ambulatory BP to be superior to office BP in predicting target organ involvement. The most striking evidence has come from assessment of the relations among office BP, ambulatory BP, and indexes of left ventricular hypertrophy **(Figure 106.1)**. More recent data have also demonstrated that ambulatory BP is superior to office BP in predicting hypertensive cerebrovascular disease, retinopathy, renal abnormalities, and alterations in vascular compliance. Certain studies using intra-arterial pressure measurements (where beat-to-beat BP values are obtained) also show that variability of BP is a predictor of morbidity. Two studies have also shown ambulatory BP to be an independent predictor of cardiovascular risk. One of these has also demonstrated that a loss of nocturnal decline in BP (as in so-called nondippers) conveys excessive risk for stroke and myocardial infarction **(Figure 106.2)**.

Table 106.3. Clinical Diagnosis or Problems in Which Noninvasive Ambulatory Blood Pressure Monitoring Is Useful

Borderline hypertension with or without target organ involvement
Office of white-coat hypertension
Evaluation of patients refractory to antihypertensive therapy
Episodic hypertension
Hypotensive symptoms associated with antihypertensive medications
Autonomic dysfunction/nocturnal hypertension
Exclusion of placebo reactors when determining efficacy of antihypertensive drug therapy in controlled clinical trial

Adapted with permission from National High Blood Pressure Education Program Working Group Report on Ambulatory Blood Pressure Monitoring. *Arch Intern Med.* 1990;150:2270–2280.

Clinical Usefulness of Ambulatory BP

Several clinical diagnoses have actually been discovered as a result of ambulatory BP monitoring **(Table 106.3)**. Clinical problems appropriate for ambulatory BP monitoring that are seen most often by practicing physicians include borderline hypertension (with and without evidence for target organ damage), possible "white-coat" hypertension, and evaluation of refractory hypertension in patients on complex antihypertensive regimens. Not uncommonly, refractory patients (regardless of age) on antihypertensive drugs have a hypertensive response in the medical care environment, yet their out-of-office values are normal. Conversely, it is not unusual to find acceptable office pressures that increase to hypertensive levels late in the dosing period of the medication **(Figure 106.3)**.

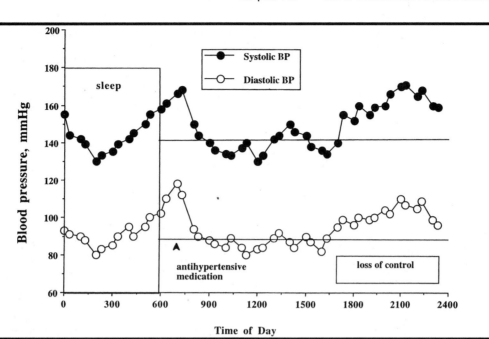

Figure 106.3. Twenty-four-hour profile obtained by noninvasive ambulatory BP monitoring in a stage III hypertensive patient. After antihypertensive medication, BP is relatively well controlled. At ≈5 PM (1700 hours), BP control is lost as antihypertensive effect of medication is attenuated. Early morning BP is also high before drug administration. Patient's office BP was 135 to 140/85 mm Hg on three long-acting medications. However, self-monitoring showed BPs to be variably high and low, leading to this ambulatory BP study.

Ambulatory BP monitoring is usually well tolerated by patients, especially as the technology has improved. A few problems do exist, however. An important minority of patients do not sleep well with the recorders, but unless they get out of bed and move about, the BP values will not be much higher than in patients who sleep well. Rarely, patients may develop erythema, ecchymoses, petechiae, or superficial phlebitis in the area distal to cuff placement. These soft-tissue injuries are typically mild and self-limiting.

Cost Considerations

The cost of self-monitoring to the patient using a nonautomated recording device is relatively low (≈$30 to $100 for the instrumentation and $0 to $30 for a nurse training session), and the data that it yields can be helpful in hypertension management. In contrast, ambulatory BP monitoring may cost the physician, hospital, or heart station several thousand dollars to provide one or two adequate recorders and software for data analysis and report generation. Individual studies generally charged to patients range from $60 for short daytime studies to $75 to $300 for 24-hour studies. Although it is more costly than self-monitoring, ambulatory BP monitoring can often be useful because it may lead to more accurate identification of those who truly require antihypertensive

therapy as well as those who may be best managed with nonpharmacological therapy.

SUGGESTED READING

1. Mansoor GA, White WB. Ambulatory blood pressure is a useful clinical tool in nephrology. *Am J Kidney Dis.* 1997;30:591–605.
2. National High Blood Pressure Education Coordinating Committee. National High Blood Pressure Education Program Working Group report on ambulatory blood pressure monitoring. *Arch Intern Med.* 1990;150:2270–2280.
3. Pickering TG, Kaplan NM, Krakoff L, Prisant LM, Sheps S, Weber MA, White WB. American Society of Hypertension Expert Panel: conclusions and recommendations on the clinical use of home (self) and ambulatory blood pressure monitoring. *Am J Hypertens.* 1996;9:1–11.
4. Soghikian K, Casper SM, Fireman BH, Hunkeler EM, Hurley LB, Tekawa IS. Home blood pressure monitoring: effect on use of medical services and medical costs. *Med Care.* 1992;30:855–865.
5. Staessen JA, Bienaszewski L, O'Brien E, Imai Y, Fagard RH. An epidemiological approach to ambulatory blood pressure monitoring: the Belgian population study. *Blood Press Monitoring.* 1996;1:13–26.
6. Tsuji I, Imai Y, Nagai K, Ohkubo T, Watanabe N, Minami N, et al. Proposal of reference values for home blood pressure measurement: prognostic criteria based on a prospective observation of the general population in Ohasama, Japan. *Am J Hypertens.* 1997;10:409–418.
7. White WB, Daragjati C, Mansoor GA, McCabe EJ. The management and follow-up of patients with white-coat hypertension. *Blood Press Monitoring.* 1996;1(suppl 2):S33–S36.

Chapter 107

Genetic Profiling in Hypertension

Haralambos Gavras, MD

KEY POINTS

- Essential hypertension is associated with genetic variants or polymorphisms in several candidate genes, but the findings are inconsistent in different racial or ethnic groups.

- Rare disorders with distinct phenotypes and Mendelian inheritance due to a single abnormal gene have been described for mineralocorticoid hypertension.

- Essential hypertension is a polygenic multifactorial disorder attributed to interplay of multiple causative or modifier genes with the environment, limiting the usefulness of genetic profiling in essential hypertension.

See also Chapters 39, 40, 41, 80, 81

Candidate Genes

The absence of a bimodal distribution of blood pressure that separates the population into clear-cut normal and abnormal groups indicates that hypertension is a polygenic or "complex" trait. The hypertensive phenotype thus does not follow the classic Mendelian rules of dominant or recessive inheritance attributable to a single gene locus. Approximately 30% to 50% of the variation in blood pressure between individuals is attributed to genetic factors.

Genes encoding for various hormones, hormone precursors, enzymes, receptors, or other biological principles relevant to the pathophysiology of blood pressure regulation are reasonable candidates for analysis. Such "candidate genes" include those encoding for various components of the renin-angiotensin-aldosterone system, the kallikrein-kinin system, the cation-transport systems regulating flux across cell membranes, the sympathetic system, vasoactive autacoids, and neurotransmitters. Genetic variants or polymorphisms in these genes have been proposed to confer susceptibility to hypertension or to specific target-organ complications, such as cardiac hypertrophy, coronary disease, renal failure, and stroke.

Several linkage and association studies have implicated a number of candidate gene variants in the etiology of essential hypertension, but the results differ, depending on the ethnic and racial background of the population studied. Examples include variants of the angiotensinogen gene that are associated with hypertension in French and North American but not in British or Mexican-American subjects. An association between the SA gene and hypertension has been found in Japanese but not white hypertensives. A renin gene restriction fragment length polymorphism has been associated with hypertension in blacks but not in whites. α_2-Adrenoceptor or β_2-adrenoceptor variants have been associated with hypertension in selected racial groups. In some cases when an association was found between a gene polymorphism and hypertension (eg, the angiotensin II receptor AT_1 gene), no linkage could be demonstrated by sib-pair analysis.

Within the large essential hypertensive population, there are rare families with particular phenotypical characteristics and quasi-Mendelian inheritance of hypertension, suggesting a single abnormal gene. Such hypertensive syndromes include glucocorticoid-remediable aldosteronism, the syndrome of apparent mineralocorticoid excess, Liddle's syndrome (pseudoaldosteronism), Gordon's syndrome (pseudohypoaldosteronism), and a syndrome characterized by severe hypertension, short stature, and brachydactyly. Some of these syndromes are associated with specific hypertensive complications. For example, subjects affected by the syndrome of glucocorticoid-remediable aldosteronism, which was found to be due to a chimeric gene involving the aldosterone synthase and 11-β-hydroxylase genes, appear to be particularly prone to hemorrhagic strokes. Members of the brachydactyly/ hypertension kindred are also prone to neurovascular malformation and early strokes.

Current Status of Genetic Profiling in Hypertension

Genetic profiling is not part of the routine diagnostic work-up of the hypertensive patient at this time. Exceptions are the rare cases of secondary hypertension in which clinical data, family history, and biochemical profiling point to anatomic or functional aberrations, such as abnormal production of hormones or abnormal receptor responses. Other rare sporadic or familial hypertensive disorders with distinct clinical and biochemical characteristics are also likely to be discovered in the future and found to be caused by specific gene mutations. In such cases, genotyping may confirm the diagnosis and dictate specific treatment strategies for the affected individual or may help identify other family members at risk.

For the vast majority of hypertensives, ie, those who remain classified as having essential hypertension, genetic profiling is unlikely to contribute to diagnosis or treatment. Furthermore, polymorphisms in some of the candidate genes associated with hypertension in one population appear to be common variants unrelated to hypertension in other populations of different ethnic ancestry and genetic background. It is likely that the intense current research in the molecular genetics of hypertension, aided by the recent advances in positional cloning and genotyping technology, such as the development of high-throughput methods for mutation analysis and of "linking libraries," will eventually provide the means for identifying and localizing aberrant genes in a more efficient and practical manner. The diagnostic value of genotyping for a polygenic and multifactorial disorder such as hypertension is further diminished by the interplay of multiple causative or modifier genes with the environment.

Therapeutic Implications

With the exception of the rare monogenic Mendelian disorders, it is difficult at this point to contemplate gene treatment as a therapeutic option for hypertension. However, it is possible that discovery of specific genotypes potentially linked to defined pathogenic mechanisms might lead to selective application of preventive or therapeutic measures in appropriate subgroups of the hypertensive population. Such strategies might replace the current indiscriminate application of expensive and not innocuous lifelong pharmacotherapy to all hypertensives on an empirical basis and might improve the success rates and cost-effectiveness of treatment in reducing cardiac and renal complications.

SUGGESTED READING

1. Lander ES, Schork NJ. Genetic dissection of complex traits [published correction appears in *Science.* 1994;266:353]. *Science.* 1994;265:2037–2048.
2. Lifton RP, Dluhy RG, Powers M, Rich GM, Cook S, Ulick S, Lalouel JM. A chimaeric 11-β-hydroxylase/aldosterone synthase gene causes glucocorticoid-remediable aldosteronism and human hypertension. *Nature.* 1992;355:262–265.
3. Litchfield WR, Weiss RJ, Coolidge CR, Lifton RP, Dluhy RG. Glucocorticoid-remediable aldosteronism is associated with hemorrhagic stroke. *Hypertension.* 1997;30:479. Abstract.
4. Mansfield TA, Simon DB, Farfel Z, Bia M, Tucci JR, Lebel M, Gutkin M, Vialettes B, Christofilis MA, Kauppiunen-Makelin R, Mayan H, Risch N, Lifton RP. Linkage of familial hyperkalemia and hypertension, pseudohypoaldosteronism type II, to 1q3-42 and 17p11–q21. *Hypertension.* 1997;30:475. Abstract.
5. Mune T, Rogerson FM, Nikkilä H, Agarwal AK, White PC. Human hypertension caused by mutations in the kidney isozyme of 11β-hydoxysteroid dehydrogenase. *Nat Genet.* 1995;10:394–399.
6. Naraghi R, Schuster H, Toka HR, Bähring S, Toka O, Oztekin O, Bilginturan N, Knoblauch H, Wienker TF, Busjahn A, Haller, Fahlbusch R, Luft FC. Neurovascular compression at the ventrolateral medulla in autosomal dominant hypertension and brachydactyly. *Stroke.* 1997;28:1749–1754.
7. Schuster H, Wienker TE, Bähring S, Bilginturan N, Toka HR, Neitzel H, Jeschke E, Toka O, Gilbert D, Lowe A, Ott J, Haller H, Luft FC. Severe autosomal dominant hypertension and brachydactyly in a unique Turkish kindred maps to human chromosome 12. *Nat Genet.* 1996;13:98–100.
8. Shimkets RA, Warnock DG, Bositis CM, Nelson-Williams C, Hansson JH, Schambelan M, Gill JR Jr, Ulick S, Milora RV, Findling JW, Canessa CM, Rossier BC, Lifton RP. Liddle's syndrome: heritable human hypertension caused by mutations in the beta subunit of the epithelial sodium channel. *Cell.* 1994;79:407–414.
9. Shuber AP, Michalowsky LA, Nass GS, Skoletsky J, Hire LM, Kotsopoulos SK, Phipps MF, Barberio DM, Klinger KW. High throughput parallel analysis of hundreds of patient samples for more than 100 mutations in multiple disease genes. *Hum Mol Genet.* 1997;6:337–347.
10. Smith CL, Klco S, Zhang TY, et al. Analysis of megabase DNA using pulsed field gel electrophoresis. In: Adolph KW, ed. *Methods in Molecular Genetics.* San Diego, Calif: Academic Press; 1993:155–196.

Chapter 108

Neurological Evaluation in Hypertension

Stephen J. Phillips, MBBS, FRCPC; Irene Meissner, MD, FRCPC

KEY POINTS

- Neurovascular evaluation is indicated in all hypertensive patients with focal or global cerebral dysfunction or with painless monocular vision loss.

- In stroke, the clinical assessment is directed at localization, differentiation of infarct from hemorrhage, and determination of cause.

- Computerized tomography and MRI can be used to confirm localization and stroke type.

- Vascular imaging is a priority in patients with carotid-territory transient ischemic attack or minor ischemic stroke.

See also Chapters 70, 72, 76, 137

Among the principal aims of antihypertensive treatment is prevention of neurovascular complications such as hypertensive encephalopathy, transient retinal ischemia, retinal infarction, anterior ischemic optic neuropathy, transient focal cerebral ischemia, cerebral infarction, and intracerebral hemorrhage. Neurovascular evaluation is indicated if the hypertensive patient presents with clinical features of acute global cerebral dysfunction, acute painless monocular vision loss, or acute focal cerebral dysfunction. In each of these situations, precise diagnosis is necessary to optimize subsequent management of the patient. The most important part of the evaluation is a careful history and neurological examination.

Hypertensive Encephalopathy
Diagnosis

Although there is some disagreement as to how to diagnose and classify this syndrome, there is usually a marked elevation of blood pressure, typically $\approx$250/150 mm Hg, plus neurological target organ damage characterized by severe headache, impaired consciousness (confusion, drowsiness, stupor, or coma), nausea and vomiting, vision disturbances, fleeting focal neurological symptoms and signs, seizures, or retinopathy (papilledema, hemorrhages, and exudates). Rarely are all of these features present in the same patient, but usually three or more are noted.

Neurological Investigation

Computed x-ray tomography (CT) of the brain should be performed to exclude subarachnoid hemorrhage, cerebral infarction, and intracerebral hemorrhage. A magnetic resonance image (MRI) may show diffuse or multifocal cerebral edema or small focal ischemic infarcts. Neither is necessary for the emergency management of the patient, however, and appropriate treatment should not be delayed to obtain these tests.

Retinal Ischemia

The retina and optic nerve head are supplied by branches of the internal carotid artery. Thromboembolic disease of the eye is both an important cause of vision impairment and an indicator of increased risk of cerebral and myocardial infarction.

Clinicopathological Syndromes

Transient monocular blindness (amaurosis fugax) is the sudden loss ("like a curtain coming down" or "graying out") of vision in one eye, lasting minutes. This is highly correlated with carotid occlusive disease in patients >50 years old but is usually due to migraine in younger patients.

Retinal artery occlusion causes sudden, painless, permanent monocular vision loss associated with ophthalmoscopic evidence of retinal infarction. In cases of central retinal artery occlusion, the vision loss is complete, there is an afferent pupillary defect, and the entire retina (excluding the macula) loses its transparency and appears milky white. The macula remains red because its choroidal blood supply is preserved. In cases of branch retinal artery occlusion, the vision loss is incomplete, pupil reactions are usually normal, and only a segment of the retina is infarcted.

Anterior ischemic optic neuropathy (infarction of the optic nerve head) is sudden, painless, permanent, monocular vision loss, accompanied by a nerve fiber bundle–type (arcuate) visual field defect, an afferent pupillary defect, and edema of the optic disc. The underlying lesion has been described as a lacunar infarct of the optic nerve head. Giant cell arteritis, lupus, or polyarteritis nodosa must be excluded by appropriate blood tests, and for suspected giant cell arteritis, a temporal artery biopsy may be required.

Neurological Investigation

Brain imaging. A CT scan of the brain is useful to look for coexisting silent cerebral infarct(s). The presence of such a lesion indicates that the patient is at higher risk of subsequent cerebral reinfarction than a patient who has had an isolated retinal ischemic event.

Vascular imaging. The technique used depends on the clinical situation and the availability of resources and expertise. The main reason for imaging the carotid arteries is to look for a surgically correctable lesion. Therefore, there is little need to proceed if the patient is not a candidate for carotid endarterectomy. If the patient presents with a history of several recent episodes of amaurosis fugax and has an ipsilateral neck bruit, the clinician should proceed directly to the most definitive test because the probability of finding severe carotid occlusive disease is high. To date, the most definitive procedure to evaluate the extracranial and intracranial circulation remains cerebral angiography. Magnetic resonance angiography is fast becoming a widely used technique to provide high-resolution images without the risks of catheter angiography. However, as with carotid ultrasound, it is limited in its ability to distinguish carotid occlusion from preocclusive stenosis and in defining intracranial stenoses and collateral supply, factors important in the surgical decision-making process.

In other clinical situations, it is appropriate to first perform a noninvasive study, usually duplex ultrasound. If a technically adequate study shows a <50% diameter stenosis in the appropriate carotid artery, angiography usually need not be performed. Stenoses >50% should be generally confirmed by angiography, which will also provide information about the remainder of the cerebral circulation of importance to the physician and surgeon.

Transient Focal Cerebral Ischemia

A transient focal cerebral ischemic attack (TIA) is an episode of focal cerebral dysfunction of sudden onset and offset, of presumed vascular cause, that usually lasts for a few minutes and always <24 hours. Distinction must be made, almost always on the basis of the patient's history, from other causes of transient focal cerebral dysfunction, such as migraine and epilepsy. TIA is an indicator of increased risk of myocardial as well as cerebral infarction. The symptoms of an attack are variable and depend on the vascular territory involved (**Table 108.1**). Management of the patient also depends on the vascular territory involved, because surgical treatment may be indicated in patients with carotid-territory TIA but not vertebrobasilar-territory TIA. Carotid endarterectomy substantially reduces the risk of stroke in patients who present with a carotid-territory TIA and an ipsilateral internal carotid artery diameter stenosis of ≥70%. Therefore, vascular imaging is a priority in patients with carotid-territory TIA.

Brain imaging may be unrevealing in patients with TIA; CT scan or MRI shows evidence of acute cerebral infarction in only a small proportion of patients who present with early resolution of symptoms. Patients in whom the CT scan shows white matter rarefaction (leukoaraiosis) have a higher risk of subsequent stroke. However, neither of these two findings influences subsequent management of the patient. Rarely, the brain imaging study shows evidence of a "TIA mimic," such as a glioma, that requires different treatment. The mechanisms underlying TIA are the same as those for cerebral infarction; consequently, the hematological and cardiac investigation of the two conditions is similar.

Cerebral Infarction and Intracerebral Hemorrhage

These are considered together because they cannot be distinguished reliably on clinical grounds. They present as "stroke," ie, the sudden onset of a persistent focal neurological deficit, by definition lasting >24 hours unless death occurs. The clinical picture depends

Table 108.1. Differentiation of the Involved Vascular Territory in Patients With TIA or Stroke

VASCULAR TERRITORY	CLINICAL FEATURE
Carotid	1. Unilateral motor or sensory abnormalities (or both) 2. Aphasia 3. Combination of 1 and 2 4. Homonymous hemianopsia plus 1 or 2 5. Dysarthria with unilateral motor or sensory abnormalities
Vertebrobasilar	1. Bilateral motor or sensory abnormalities 2. Bilateral limb or gait ataxia 3. Bilateral homonymous hemianopsia 4. Any combination of 1 through 3 5. Dysarthria plus any combination of 1, 2, 3, 9 and 10 6. Homonymous hemianopsia alone 7. Homonymous hemianopsia plus any combination of 1, 2, 9, and 10 8. Unilateral motor or sensory abnormalities plus any combination of 2, 3, 9, and 10 9. Vertigo plus any combination of 1 through 8 10. Diplopia plus any combination of 1 through 9

on the part of the brain involved and the size of the infarct or hematoma. Diagnosis is a three-step process: (1) localization, (2) differentiation of infarction from hemorrhage, and (3) determination of the cause of the stroke.

Localization

The clinical evaluation and a brain imaging study will allow localization of the lesion in the majority of patients. The aim is to determine which part of the brain and which vascular territory is involved. Localization is important for the following three reasons. First, it may indicate the need for urgent intervention such as surgical decompression of the posterior fossa in cerebellar infarction or hemorrhage (clinical features of a cerebellar stroke are shown in **Table 108.2).** Second, it may indicate a potential for specific treatment, such as carotid endarterectomy, aimed at reducing the risk of stroke recurrence, which may be appropriate for a minor carotid-territory ischemic stroke. Endarterectomy is not usually indicated for patients with vertebrobasilar-territory infarcts. Third, it helps predict the functional difficulties likely to be encountered by the patient, which is important for planning rehabilitation treatment.

CT is the most useful brain imaging study because it is relatively fast, inexpensive, and accessible. The disadvantages of CT are that it may not show an infarct in the brain stem or any infarct within the first few hours of a stroke. However, determining whether an initial CT scan demonstrates hemorrhage, early edema, or subtle acute changes of infarction is crucial to the decision regarding the use of intravenous thrombolytic therapy. If localization is critical and the CT scan unhelpful, an MRI is indicated.

Table 108.2. The Presenting Clinical Features of Cerebellar Stroke

Symptoms
   Dizziness or vertigo
   Nausea or vomiting
   Slurred speech
   Loss of balance
Signs
   Dysarthria
   Small pupils
   Ocular movement disorder
   Facial weakness or sensory loss
   Truncal, limb, or gait ataxia

Table 108.3. Nonhypertensive Causes of Spontaneous Intracerebral Hemorrhage

Arteriovenous malformation
Intraparenchymal rupture of a saccular or mycotic aneurysm
Neoplasm
   Primary (eg, glioblastoma multiforme)
   Secondary (eg bronchogenic carcinoma, renal-cell carcinoma, melanoma, or choriocarcinoma)
Cerebral amyloid angiopathy
Bleeding diathesis
Anticoagulant therapy
Thrombolytic therapy
Sympathomimetic drugs (eg, cocaine)

Differentiation of Infarction From Hemorrhage

For acute stroke, differentiation of infarction from hemorrhage is best achieved by CT. If the stroke occurred more than a few weeks before, the distinction can be made only by MRI. In the setting of acute stroke, intracerebral hemorrhage should be excluded by CT if the neurological condition of the patient is deteriorating. In this setting, CT should be performed before thrombolytic or anticoagulant therapy is administered. Early CT is indicated also if a cerebellar stroke is suspected. In other situations, it is advantageous to delay the CT scan until ≈48 hours after stroke onset because if the underlying lesion is an infarct, it is more likely to be visible at this time than in the first few hours. If the lesion is a hematoma, the characteristic CT signs will still be present.

Determining Cause

Intracerebral hemorrhage. The clinical evaluation and CT scan may be sufficient to diagnose the likely cause of the stroke and guide subsequent management. For example, cerebral amyloid angiopathy would be the most likely cause of a hemorrhage located superficially in the cerebral hemisphere of an 85-year-old patient. Such a patient could be spared cerebral angiography, might not require neurosurgical intervention, and should not be treated with antithrombotic drugs. Hemorrhages located in the basal ganglia, thalamus, pons, and cerebellum are usually due to hypertension-induced rupture of small-diameter penetrating end arteries. If the patient is young or does not have a history of hypertension, an alternative explanation should be considered (**Table 108.3**) and the appropriate investigations performed.

Cerebral infarction. Ischemic strokes are due to either (1) thrombotic or embolic occlusion of precerebral or cerebral arteries or (2) hemodynamic compromise with relative or absolute hypotension. Emboli may arise from the heart or from arterial lesions between the heart and the brain. Rarely, emboli may arise from the venous side of the circulation and gain access to the arterial circulation via a pulmonary arteriovenous fistula or an atrial septal defect. Therefore, determining the etiology of a cerebral infarct involves investigation of the heart, the precerebral and cerebral arteries, and the blood.

The nature and extent of investigation should be guided by the patient's age, family history, timing of symptom onset, the severity of the stroke, the presence or absence of comorbid factors, and the paucity of data concerning the effects of treatment on subtypes of cerebral infarction. Young patients tend to be more extensively investigated than older patients because there is a greater likelihood of finding an unusual cause. A strong family history of stroke is suggestive of a hereditary disorder. Patients who have mild strokes tend to be more extensively investigated than patients with severe strokes, because the milder the stroke, the more the patient may lose if there is a recurrence. In mild strokes, there is typically a greater effort at secondary prevention, which, in turn, depends on an understanding of the cause of the first stroke. Certain comorbid factors may point to the cause of the stroke. For example, a recent large transmural anterior myocardial infarction makes a cardioembolic mechanism likely. Other comorbid factors, such as terminal cancer, may carry such a poor prognosis that they render moot the investigation of the stroke. The recent FDA approval of tissue plasminogen activator (t-PA) as an intravenously administered thrombolytic agent for acute stroke has led to a more proactive approach to acute stroke management. Careful control of blood pressure in the acute care setting, early timing of treatment after the onset of stroke symptoms, and negative CT scan appear to be critical factors in the safe and efficacious administration of t-PA.

SUGGESTED READING

1. Brown RD Jr, Evans BA, Wiebers DO, Perry GW, Meissner I, Dale AJ. Transient ischemic attack and minor ischemic stroke: an algorithm for evaluation and treatment. Mayo Clinic Division of Cerebrovascular Diseases. *Mayo Clin Proc.* 1994; 69:1027–1039.
2. Caplan LR. Diagnosis and treatment of ischemic stroke. *JAMA.* 1991;266: 2413–2418.
3. Donnan GA. Investigation of patients with stroke and transient ischaemic attacks. *Lancet.* 1992;339:473–477.
4. Dunbabin DW, Sandercock PA. Investigation of acute stroke: what is the most effective strategy? *Postgrad Med J.* 1991;67:259–270.
5. Landi G. Clinical diagnosis of transient ischaemic attacks. *Lancet.* 1992;339: 402–405.
6. National Institute of Neurologic Disorders and Stroke rt-PA Stroke Study Group. Tissue plasminogen activator for acute ischemic stroke. *N Engl J Med.* 1995; 333:1581–1587.
7. Practice advisory: thrombolytic therapy for acute ischemic stroke: summary statement. Report of the Quality Standards Subcommittee of the American Academy of Neurology. *Neurology.* 1996;47:835–839.
8. Special report from the National Institute of Neurological Disorders and Stroke. Classification of cerebrovascular diseases III. *Stroke.* 1990;21:637–676.
9. Stroke—1989. Recommendations on stroke prevention, diagnosis, and therapy. Report of the WHO Task Force on Stroke and Other Cerebrovascular Disorders. *Stroke.* 1989;20:1407–1431.

Basic Cardiac Evaluation

Physical Examination, Electrocardiogram, and Chest Radiograph

Clarence Shub, MD; John A. Rumberger, PhD, MD

KEY POINTS

- Hypertensive heart disease can be detected by clinical examination, ECG, and cardiac imaging.

- Left ventricular hypertrophy (LVH) is a manifestation of "target organ damage" and implies an adverse prognosis and the need for aggressive therapy in the hypertensive patient.

- ECG remains the traditional and standard method for detecting LVH despite its relative lack of sensitivity.

See also Chapters 67, 110, 111, 138

Because the heart is one of the major target organs adversely affected by high blood pressure, a careful and thorough evaluation of cardiac structure and function is an obligatory part of the examination of the hypertensive patient.

Physical Examination

The presence of abnormalities on the cardiac and vascular physical examination contributes significantly to the cardiac assessment of the hypertensive patient and to cardiovascular risk stratification as recommended by JNC VI. The presence of "target organ" damage or clinical cardiovascular diseases, eg, the detection of left ventricular hypertrophy (LVH) or peripheral vascular disease, prompts more aggressive antihypertensive therapy and risk factor modification.

Palpation of the Cardiac Apex

One of the most important physical signs of LVH is a localized, sustained, and forceful apical impulse. This is best appreciated with the patient in the left lateral decubitus position but may be more difficult to elicit in obese patients and in those with chronic obstructive pulmonary disease. If the apical impulse in the supine position is laterally displaced, left ventricular (LV) dilatation should be suspected. In patients with hypertensive heart disease, LV dilatation is frequently associated with impaired ventricular function.

Auscultation
Heart Sounds

A loud first heart sound (S_1) and brisk carotid upstroke in a hypertensive patient suggest a hyperdynamic circulatory state. The second heart sound (S_2) is usually narrowly split, and the aortic component may be accentuated. Although paradoxical splitting of S_2 may occur, it is uncommon and, in the absence of left bundle-branch block, suggests LV systolic dysfunction. A third heart sound (S_3) is unusual except when LV systolic failure occurs. In almost all patients, a fourth sound (S_4) develops before the S_3 is heard, and when the S_3 is heard, the S_4 is almost always present.

The incidence of an S_4 in hypertensive patients has been estimated to be between 50% and 70%, especially in the presence of LVH and in older patients. An S_4 is the auscultatory counterpart of a vigorous atrial contraction into a relatively noncompliant left ventricle. An S_4 may be associated with a palpable presystolic impulse or A wave, the S_4 best appreciated when the patient is in the left lateral decubitus position and the bell of the stethoscope is gently placed directly on the point of maximal apical impulse. Because of the difficulty in routine clinical assessment of an S_4, the presence of a palpable A wave appears to be more specific for the pathophysiological mechanisms described above. An aortic systolic ejection sound (or click) is occasionally heard in hypertensive patients and appears to be related to forceful expansion of a dilated aortic root.

Murmurs

A systolic murmur can frequently be heard in older hypertensive patients. This murmur is usually ejection in type, early in timing, and of low intensity (grade 1 or 2). It most often represents aortic outflow turbulence related to a sclerotic aortic valve. This murmur can be heard at both the apex and the base, but occasionally the murmur is localized to the apex alone and can be confused with mitral regurgitation.

Some hypertensive patients with systolic murmurs may have LV outflow tract obstruction, a condition that has been referred to as "hypertensive hypertrophic cardiomyopathy." Such patients often have a small LV cavity with hypertrophied walls and normal or hyperdynamic systolic function. Recognition of this disorder is important, because it may worsen with the administration of certain antihypertensive drugs, especially diuretics or direct-acting vasodilators. Bedside hemodynamic maneuvers, such as the Valsalva maneuver, that accentuate the systolic murmur, may provide an important clue to the presence of LV outflow tract obstruction.

An early diastolic murmur of aortic regurgitation, which may be variable in intensity and duration, may occasionally be found in hypertensive patients. Usually there is no anatomic defect of the aortic valve, but rather the aortic root is dilated and the aortic regurgitation represents a "functional" abnormality secondary to dilatation of the aortic ring. This abnormality is more common in older hypertensive patients and may lessen in severity or even disappear as blood pressure is lowered.

Examination of the carotid, femoral, and extremity arterial pulses is also important. Reduced volume of the femoral pulses and/or a delay in femoral pulse timing (especially in a young patient) compared with simultaneous palpation of the radial pulse suggests the possibility of coarctation of the aorta. The presence of femoral and/or carotid bruits and reduced arterial pulses in the lower extremities suggests vascular obstructive disease, which in older patients is most commonly due to atherosclerosis. This process of vascular damage is enhanced and accelerated in the presence of systemic hypertension.

Electrocardiogram

Compared with the chest radiograph, the routine scalar electrocardiogram (ECG) is more sensitive in detecting LVH in hypertensive patients. Various ECG diagnostic criteria exist, eg, the scoring system recommended by Estes, the criteria of McPhie (sum of tallest precordial R and S waves >45 mm), and the Minnesota code. ECG evidence of left atrial enlargement may occur in the early stages of hypertension, is associated with LV diastolic dysfunction, and may precede abnormalities in the QRS complex.

Improved diagnostic sensitivity with excellent specificity is provided by sex-specific Cornell voltage criteria ($S_{V3} + R_{V1} \geq 20$ mm in women or ≥ 28 mm in men). With regard to QRS amplitudes, considerable overlap exists in normal and hypertensive patients. Factors such as age, sex, race, and body weight affect the QRS amplitude and may influence the predictive value of QRS criteria for the diagnosis of LVH. In the presence of left bundle-branch block, LVH is difficult to diagnose. Thus, when precordial QRS voltages alone are used as criteria for LVH, significant numbers of false-positive and false-negative results may occur.

Vectorcardiographic analysis increases diagnostic sensitivity. The vectorcardiographic forces are shifted posteriorly and to the left. This is manifested in the scalar ECG as an increased R wave in leads I, aVL, V_5, and V_6. As anterior forces decrease (diminished R waves in precordial leads V_1 through V_3), the pattern of anterior infarction may be simulated. Left axis deviation in the frontal plane may occur.

With increasing severity of hypertension, T-wave amplitude decreases, and T-wave inversion may occur in leads I, aVL, V_5, and V_6. The addition of J-point and ST-segment depression constitutes the pattern that has been called "LV strain." Relative subendocardial ischemia may be responsible for these repolarization abnormalities. The ECG diagnosis of LVH is considerably strengthened in the presence of increased QRS voltages combined with typical repolarization abnormalities ("LV strain").

The QRS duration has been reported to widen with increasing severity of hypertension, and the finding of ventricular conduction delay on the ECG has been correlated with certain histological abnormalities, eg, myocardial fibrosis. The ECG abnormalities may improve or even revert to normal with successful antihypertensive therapy (decreased QRS voltages and resolution of ST-T–wave abnormalities).

In the late stages of hypertensive heart disease, typical signs of LVH are almost always seen on the ECG. Thus, when a patient presents with heart failure that is attributed to hypertension, in addition to other target organ involvement, he or she almost always will have some evidence of LVH on the ECG; if not, other causes for heart failure should be considered.

The ECG is the traditional and standard method for detecting LVH. However, it detects only 20% to 50% of instances of autopsy-proven LVH in patient populations and <10% of echocardiographic LVH in the general population. Despite this relative insensitivity, ECG LVH is a strong predictor of cardiovascular morbidity and mortality. The cost-effectiveness of the ECG may be questioned when detection of hypertensive LVH is the only goal and its prognostic value appears to be less than that of echocardiography. However, it does provide important information when other clinical abnormalities (myocardial ischemia or infarction, arrhythmias, or conduction defects) are sought.

24-Hour Ambulatory ECG Monitoring

Clinical investigations using 24-hour ambulatory ECG monitoring have shown a greater incidence of ventricular arrhythmias in hypertensive patients with LVH. Ventricular arrhythmias appear to worsen as the hypertrophy progresses. These patients have an increased risk of sudden cardiac death. Atrial fibrillation and other supraventricular tachycardias are more common in patients with hypertension than in the general population. Although it is not indicated for asymptomatic patients, 24-hour ambulatory ECG monitoring can be useful in assessing atrial and ventricular arrhythmias in patients with palpitations, near syncope, or syncope.

Chest Radiograph

The chest radiograph of patients with uncomplicated hypertension usually is normal, although occasionally an abnormal cardiac contour suggesting LV enlargement or LVH may be found. However, one cannot rely on the routine chest radiograph to diagnose LVH. Subtle dilation of the ascending aortic shadow can be found in many patients with hypertension and no evidence of cardiac disease. In young patients and sometimes in adults, the presence of aortic coarctation as a cause of hypertension can be suspected on the chest radiograph.

SUGGESTED READING

1. Frohlich ED, Apstein C, Chobanian AV, Devereux RB, Dustan HP, Dzau V, Fouad-Tarazi F, Horan MJ, Marcus M, Massie B, et al. The heart in hypertension [published correction appears in *N Engl J Med.* 1992;327:1768]. *N Engl J Med.* 1992;327:998–1008.

2. Levy D, Garrison RJ, Savage DD, Kannel WB, Castelli WP. Prognostic implications of echocardiographically determined left ventricular mass in the Framingham Heart Study. *N Engl J Med.* 1990;322:1561–1566.

3. Levy D, Labib SB, Anderson KM, Christiansen JC, Kannel WB, Castelli WP. Determinants of sensitivity and specificity of electrocardiographic criteria for left ventricular hypertrophy. *Circulation.* 1990;81:815–820.

4. McLenachan JM, Henderson E, Morris KI, Dargie HJ. Ventricular arrhythmias in patients with hypertensive left ventricular hypertrophy. *N Engl J Med.* 1987;317:787–792.

5. Topol EJ, Traill TA, Fortuin NJ. Hypertensive hypertrophic cardiomyopathy of the elderly. *N Engl J Med.* 1985;312:277–283.

Chapter 110

Cardiac Imaging

Clarence Shub, MD; John A. Rumberger, PhD, MD

KEY POINTS

- Determination of left ventricular (LV) mass by echocardiography is the most commonly used noninvasive clinical method of diagnosing LV hypertrophy.

- Radionuclide angiography can be used to assess the dynamic changes in the LV blood pool but cannot directly evaluate the myocardium or the great vessels.

- MRI is a precise method to image the heart and great vessels, generally without need for contrast.

- Choice of imaging modality depends on clinical presentation, availability, and local expertise.

See also Chapters 67, 109, 111, 138

Proper evaluation of the heart in hypertension often requires the use of imaging procedures.

Echocardiography

The type of overload to which the heart is subjected determines not only the specific chamber (or chambers) involved but also the pattern of left ventricular hypertrophy (LVH). These patterns can be determined by echocardiography **(Figure 110.1)**. In concentric hypertrophy, the ratio of ventricular wall thickness to radius (relative wall thickness) is increased to >0.45. The ratio is decreased in eccentric hypertrophy. Eccentric hypertrophy should not be confused with the term asymmetric hypertrophy, in which a portion of the ventricle, usually the ventricular septum, is thicker than the other wall segments. Eccentric (or volume-overload) hypertrophy refers to a ventricle with an expanded cavitary volume in proportion to wall thickness, whereas concentric hypertrophy refers to a ventricle with thick walls relative to cavity volume. The usefulness of assessing these specific geometric patterns in terms of prognosis is not yet clear.

Interventricular septal and posterior wall thicknesses and left ventricular internal dimensions can indicate LVH and chamber size, respectively, but are more sensitive for detection of LVH when used to determine LV muscle mass. LV muscle mass may be calculated by use of standard M-mode echocardiographic measurements of the left ventricle in necropsy-validated formulas. LV mass is directly related to body size and should be indexed to body surface area or body height with use of sex-specific normative values. In addition, age appears to have a small but significant independent effect on LV mass in women but not in men. In comparison with autopsy-validated LVH, echocardiography has a specificity of 97% and a sensitivity of 57% for mild, 92% for moderate, and 100% for severe LVH. In contrast, the sensitivity for the Romhilt-Estes electrocardiographic point score is only 7% in the general population and 54% in autopsied patients with relatively severe LVH.

LV dimensions, mass, and ejection fraction (EF) can also be measured by two-dimensional echocardiography, a technique that provides more complete global and regional information than M-mode echocardiography. Recent studies have shown that three-dimensional echocardiography is more accurate and reproducible than either M-mode or two-dimensional echocardiography in the diagnosis of LVH. However, technical and feasibility issues need to be overcome before this modality will become available for clinical purposes.

Partition values for detection of LVH by M-mode echocardiography, derived from apparently normal subjects in the primarily white Framingham population, were an LV mass index in men >131 and in women >100 g/m^2. The upper-normal limits derived in a racially mixed normotensive population were >134 and 110 g/m^2, respectively. In obese subjects, identification of LVH is enhanced without loss of prognostic power by indexing LV mass to height. LV mass is best viewed as a continuous variable, and current partition values should ultimately be replaced by upper-normal limits that identify subjects with a more adverse prognosis.

Echocardiographic LV mass is elevated in 20% to 50% of patients with stage 1 hypertension and up to 90% of hospitalized patients with stage 2 to 3 hypertension. Echocardiography and, in selected circumstances, comprehensive echocardiography and Doppler assessment would appear to be appropriate in the situations listed in **Table 110.1.** Limited, or focused, echocardiography has been proposed as a less costly screening method to detect LVH in hypertensive patients. Its clinical role in hypertensive patients needs to be further defined.

"Hypertensive hypertrophic cardiomyopathy" can be readily diagnosed by combined two-dimensional and Doppler echocardiography. Echocardiography also allows imaging of the aorta, which can be useful in the evaluation of suspected aortic coarctation. Transesophageal echocardiography is especially valuable for the rapid diagnosis of aortic dissection.

LV systolic function can be assessed by calculating systolic fractional shortening by M-mode echocardiography or EF or by two-dimensional echocardiography. The latter is preferable if LV shape or pattern of wall motion is abnormal.

Standard measurements of cardiac function in hypertensive patients show that EF is preserved but that diastolic filling, as assessed

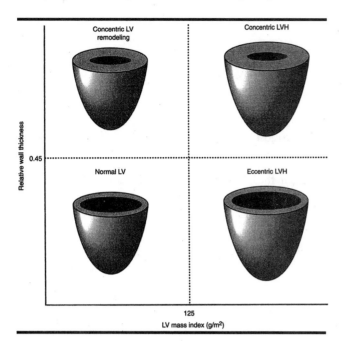

Figure 110.1.   Diagram depicting relation between LV mass index and relative wall thickness. An increase in LV mass index (defined as >125 g/m²) denotes development of LVH. If relative wall thickness (ratio of wall thickness/LV cavity radius) does not increase proportionately, chamber volume is increased and a more volume-dependent "eccentric" LVH occurs. However, if there is an increase in relative wall thickness along with LV mass index, a more "concentric" pressure-dependent LVH occurs. Conversely, if LV mass index does not increase but selective wall thickness increases, the more recently described "remodeling" phenomenon occurs. Adapted with permission from Frohlich ED, Apsten C, Chobanian AV, et al. The heart in hypertension. *N Engl J Med.* 1992;327:998–1008.

Table 110.1.   Indications for Use of Echocardiography, Comprehensive Echocardiography and Doppler Assessment

Possible cardiac involvement requires further confirmation (eg, ECG diagnosis of LVH based on voltage criteria alone)*
Patient has a coexisting cardiac condition (eg, valvular heart disease)
A child or adolescent has mild hypertension*
Etiology and significance of systolic murmurs need better definition
Hypertension occurs during exercise, but resting pressures are normal*
Dyspnea of unknown etiology (differentiate systolic vs diastolic dysfunction and assess pulmonary artery pressures by Doppler)

---

*Limited or focused echocardiography in order to assess LVH only may be appropriate under these circumstances.

---

by radionuclide angiography (RNA) or Doppler echocardiography, is often impaired. Studies using Doppler echocardiography have shown a high prevalence (≈30% to 45%) of impaired diastolic function in hypertensive patients, even in the absence of systolic dysfunction or LVH. These diastolic abnormalities reflect impaired ventricular relaxation but may also represent impaired chamber compliance due to LVH, deposition of increased or altered collagen tissue, and abnormalities of contractile proteins or intracellular calcium flux.

Doppler echocardiography allows separation of diastolic dys-

function into different patterns of LV filling abnormalities, eg, delayed relaxation or restrictive filling patterns. The latter reflect a more severe diastolic abnormality and are more likely to be associated with clinical symptoms, eg, dyspnea. The compliance curve of the stiff and poorly compliant ventricle is shifted to the left and is steeper than normal in patients with LVH. This implies that for an equivalent increase in diastolic volume, the diastolic pressure increases more in the hypertrophic than in the normal ventricle.

Radionuclide Angiography

RNA is a widely available and extensively used, validated method to assess cardiac size and function. RNA is used to assess dynamic changes in LV chamber volumes during the cardiac cycle by registering externally the dynamic changes in the ventricular "blood pool." RNA examines relative changes in total LV chamber blood pool "counts" during the cardiac cycle, and no assumptions regarding LV geometry are needed to quantify EF (as are necessary with echocardiography). As a result, RNA remains a very accurate clinical method to determine LVEF, although imaging is suboptimal in very obese subjects.

By defining dynamic changes in the LV during the cardiac cycle, we can graphically define the dynamics of contraction and relaxation **(Figure 110.2)**. Radionuclide LV "volume" curves can be analyzed to determine relative rates of systolic contraction (peak emptying rate) and early diastolic relaxation (peak filling rate). Abnormalities of early diastolic filling are frequently observed in patients with hypertension before there is evidence of systolic dysfunction. Because RNA examines the blood pool and not the myocardium directly, LV muscle mass cannot be quantified.

Electron Beam (Ultrafast) CT

Electron beam CT (EBCT), also known as ultrafast CT and cine CT, is a more recently developed x-ray imaging modality. This device uses an electron beam and stationary target/detector pairing to replace the physical rotation of the x-ray source/detector pair required by conventional CT. Ultrafast CT can acquire tomographic images very rapidly.

The methods for image display and analysis of cardiac (50-ms) images are derived from two-dimensional echocardiography to quantify regional myocardial motion, EF, and chamber volumes **(see Figure 110.3)** and from RNA to define the dynamics of LV volumes during the cardiac cycle. Unlike RNA and MRI, imaging by EBCT is "triggered" (as opposed to "gated") by the patient's ECG. Thus, dynamic imaging from the entire heart can be completed in seconds.

EBCT, like echocardiography and MRI, defines both the cardiac chambers and myocardium and can also be used to define great-vessel anatomy in hypertensive patients. Because of the speed at which imaging can be done, EBCT, if available, is extremely useful in assessing diseases of the aorta in severely ill patients and (because no sedation is necessary) in children.

Magnetic Resonance Imaging

MRI provides exquisite tomographic images of the heart and great vessels that can be displayed from virtually any plane or orientation. There is no radiation exposure to the patient. There is also no need for contrast injection, and patients can be imaged without concern as to their renal excretory function.

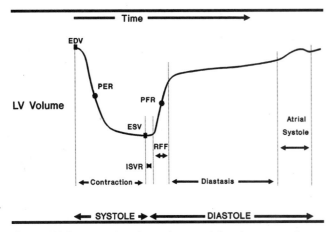

Figure 110.2. Dynamics of LV volume and function as may be assessed by RNA, ultrafast CT, and MRI. EF can be determined directly from the end-diastolic volume (EDV) and end-systolic volume (ESV). ISVR indicates isovolumetric relaxation phase; RFF, rapid (early) diastolic filling phase; PER, peak systolic emptying rate; and PFR, peak (early) diastolic filling rate.

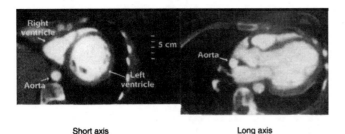

Short axis   Long axis

Figure 110.3. Ultrafast CT scans at end diastole in the cardiac short-axis (transverse cardiac) and horizontal long-axis planes from the mid left ventricle in a patient with congestive heart failure. Note that this well-known complication of hypertension results in a dilated left ventricle that has poor contractile performance. Similar images can be obtained with MRI.

MRI is useful to image the cardiac chambers and/or great vessels. Specific "cine" techniques have been developed to allow quantification of EF, LV volumes, and LV muscle mass. MRI is used extensively to define aortic dissection and coarctation and to follow such patients after surgical or pharmacological therapy.

The major disadvantages to MRI are the necessity of prolonged times for completion of the entire study (15 minutes to 1 hour) and the fact that the subject needs to remain still during image acquisition. Patients with claustrophobia or pacemakers or who are acutely ill cannot be imaged effectively with MRI. Although the method is safe for patients who have prosthetic (natural or metallic) valve replacements, MRI is contraindicated in patients who have metal plates anywhere in the body or metallic hip replacements. Although MRI technology is widely available, its application to cardiac imaging is not, mainly because of the need for additional software for analysis and proper image sequencing and limited experience in cardiac MRI.

Comparison of Imaging Modalities

Echocardiography, RNA, EBCT, and MRI are each imaging modalities that can be used to diagnose or quantify cardiovascular manifestations of hypertension (**Table 110.2**). Their relative utilization depends on their availability and the degree of local expertise with each technique. Each has a role in defining specific complications of hypertension, such as diastolic dysfunction, reduced EF, heart failure, aortic aneurysm, and dissection, or concomitant cardiac disease, eg, valve abnormality. In addition, each has distinct advantages and disadvantages in clinical practice (**Table 110.3**).

The clinician must choose which method to apply to a specific patient, largely guided by individual clinical circumstances, the objectives of the study, relative costs of the various techniques, and the expertise of the local or referral laboratory or imaging center. Mere availability of a particular technique to image the heart and great vessels does not absolve the clinician of first establishing the necessity and objectives of the study.

Table 110.2. Comparison of RNA, CT, and MRI Methods to Define Cardiac Function and Great Vessel Anatomy

IMAGING MODALITY	CARDIAC/VASCULAR APPLICATIONS					
	EF	LVM	LV VOLUME	DIASTOLIC FUNCTION	RWMA	GREAT VESSEL ANATOMY
RNA	Yes	No	Yes	Yes	Yes	No
Conventional CT	No	No	No	No	No	Yes
Ultrafast CT	Yes	Yes	Yes	Yes	Yes	Yes
MRI	Yes	Yes	Yes	Yes	Yes	Yes

RNA indicates radionuclide angiography; CT, computed tomography; MRI, magnetic resonance imaging; EF, ejection fraction; RWMA, regional wall motion (contraction) abnormalities; and LVM, left ventricular muscle mass.

Table 110.3. Advantages and Disadvantages of RNA, CT, and MRI in Assessing Patients With Hypertension

IMAGING MODALITY	ADVANTAGES	DISADVANTAGES
RNA	Widely available in major medical centers	Radiation, limitations in large patients
Conventional CT	Widely available in major medical centers	Radiation, contrast media
Ultrafast CT	Highly versatile and precise	Availability to only a few major medical centers, radiation, contrast
MRI	Versatile, precise, no radiation	Limited availability,* contrast,† prolonged imaging

*Although MRI is widely available, at present there are limited facilities that can perform dynamic cardiac studies.
†See section on "Magnetic Resonance Imaging."

SUGGESTED READING

1. Breen JF, Julsrud PR, Ehman RL. Cardiac magnetic resonance imaging. In: Giuliani ER, Fuster V, Gersh BJ, McGoon MD, McGoon DC, eds. *Cardiology: Fundamentals and Practice.* St Louis, Mo: Mosby Year-Book; 1991:chap 14.

2. Clements IP, Sinak LJ, Gibbons RJ, Brown ML, O'Connor MK. Determination of diastolic function by radionuclide ventriculography. *Mayo Clin Proc.* 1990;65:1007–1019.

3. Devereux RB, Alonso DR, Lutas EM, Gottlieb GJ, Campo E, Sachs I, Reichek N. Echocardiographic assessment of left ventricular hypertrophy: comparison to necropsy findings. *Am J Cardiol.* 1986;57:450–458.

4. Gibbons RJ. Equilibrium radionuclide angiography. In: Marcus ML, Skorton DJ, Schelbert HR, Wolf GL, eds. *Cardiac Imaging: A Companion to Braunwald's Heart Disease.* Philadelphia, Pa: WB Saunders Co; 1991:chap 57.

5. Gibbons RJ. Nuclear cardiology. In: Giuliani ER, Fuster V, Gersh BJ, McGoon MD, McGoon DC, eds. *Cardiology: Fundamentals and Practice.* St Louis, Mo: Mosby Year-Book; 1991:chap 13.

6. Gopal AS, Keller AM, Shen Z, Sapin PM, Schroeder KM, King DL Jr, King DL. Three-dimensional echocardiography: in vitro and in vivo validation of left ventricular mass and comparison with conventional echocardiographic methods. *J Am Coll Cardiol.* 1994;24:504–513.

7. Krumholz HM, Larson M, Levy D. Prognosis of left ventricular geometric patterns in the Framingham Heart Study. *J Am Coll Cardiol.* 1995;25:879–884.

8. Marcus ML, Weiss RL. Evaluation of cardiac structure and function with ultrafast computed tomography. In: Marcus ML, Skorton DJ, Schelbert HR, Wolf GL, eds. *Cardiac Imaging: A Companion to Braunwald's Heart Disease.* Philadelphia, Pa: WB Saunders Co; 1991:chap 33.

9. Park SH, Shub C, Nobrega TP, Bailey KR, Seward JB. Two-dimensional echocardiographic calculation of left ventricular mass as recommended by the American Society of Echocardiography: correlation with autopsy and M-mode echocardiography. *J Am Soc Echocardiogr.* 1996;9:119–128.

10. Spirito P, Maron BJ, Bonow RO. Noninvasive assessment of left ventricular diastolic function: comparative analysis of Doppler echocardiographic and radionuclide angiographic techniques. *J Am Coll Cardiol.* 1986;7:518–526.

Chapter 111

Exercise Stress Testing

Michael F. Wilson, MD; Mofid N. Khalil Ibrahim, MD, PhD

KEY POINTS

- Exercise stress testing provides useful information for cardiac diagnosis, prognosis, and management.

- An exaggerated blood pressure response to exercise stress testing is due in part to impaired vasodilation.

- Subjects who exhibit this exaggerated blood pressure response have increased risk of target organ damage.

- Added prognostic value is provided by stress myocardial perfusion imaging.

See also Chapters 67, 109, 110, 138

Stress testing, which is also known as exercise tolerance testing, is commonly performed by use of a programmed treadmill electrocardiographic (ECG) evaluation. The treadmill ECG protocol developed by Bruce is generally recognized as the standard. This protocol begins at 1.7 miles per hour and a 10% grade, then increases both speed and grade at 3-minute intervals to symptom-limited exercise capacity. Others believe that treadmill speed should be held constant while the grade is increased gradually (Balke test) or that speed and grade should be increased separately (Naughton test) to produce a linear progression of work load.

Bike exercise ergometry is a valuable method for stress testing that is especially useful in conjunction with radionuclide ventriculography. Both the first-pass and the multi-gated acquisition (MUGA) techniques measure ventricular contractile (ejection fraction) response to exercise. However, myocardial perfusion imaging in conjunction with treadmill stress testing or with a vasodilating agent (dipyridamole or adenosine) has largely replaced exercise ventriculography in many institutions. The MUGA scan at rest remains valuable to assess resting ventricular function through accurate ejection fraction and regional wall motion measurements. Nuclear cardiology myocardial perfusion imaging with exercise or pharmacological stress has increased sensitivity and specificity compared with exercise ECG testing and also increased precision in prognosis and management decisions.

Cardiovascular Responses to Exercise

With exercise, there is an increase in metabolic demand for oxygen, and the cardiac output (CO) responds through an increase primarily in heart rate (HR) but also in stroke volume (SV). Cardiac output is the product of heart rate and stroke volume ($CO = HR \times SV$). Systemic vascular resistance (SVR) decreases with exercise, but the increase of cardiac output is greater. Therefore, mean arterial blood pressure (MBP) increases according to the relationship $SVR \times CO = MBP$. With exercise, the normal pattern is for systolic blood pressure (SBP) to increase and diastolic blood pressure (DBP) to decrease. However, there may be an abnormal hypertensive response to exercise, defined as SBP ≥ 220 mm Hg and/or DBP ≥ 100 mm Hg. The maximum HR level in beats per minute (bpm) is a function of age and equals ≈ 220 minus age in years. Myocardial work, oxygen consumption ($M\dot{V}O_2$), coronary blood flow, CO, and HR all increase proportionately.

HR is a useful and practical index to record the level of stress placed on the heart. Optimum stress testing requires an HR $\geq 85\%$ of age-predicted maximum. Physical conditioning will decrease the HR response to a given work load, as will some cardiac medications, such as β-blockers. Rate-pressure product ($RPP = HR \times SBP$) is recorded as a clinical measure of $M\dot{V}O_2$. A value of $\geq 25\ 000$ (bpm $\times$ mm Hg) at peak exercise is considered to be an adequate response for stress testing purposes. See **Table 111.1** for indications for exercising or pharmaceutical stress testing.

If $\geq 85\%$ of optimum HR and RPP is reached and the exercise tolerance test is negative (normal by ECG criteria, with no defects in myocardial perfusion imaging), there is a high probability that no disease is present. However, the sensitivity is substantially lower if the HR and RPP maximal responses are less than optimal.

Contraindications for Stress Testing

There are both absolute and relative contraindications to stress testing. There is general agreement that in the presence of certain conditions, stress testing should not be done **(Table 111.2)**. For example, patients with left main coronary artery disease or left main equivalent, those with high-grade obstruction ($\geq 80\%$ diameter narrowing) in all proximal branches of the left main coronary artery, should not undergo stress testing. The danger is a large mass of myocardium at risk of ischemia and myocardial infarction, arrhythmia, and sudden cardiac death secondary to ventricular fibrillation. Left main coronary artery disease is best managed by surgical bypass of the obstructed artery.

Relative Contraindications
Severe Hypertension

There is a danger of further aggravating an unstable and progressive hypertensive state. In general, hypertension should be brought under control before the exercise stress test. However, stress testing in the presence of mild to moderate hypertension (DBP ≤ 105 mm Hg) does not present a significant additional risk. Sometimes the SBP and DBP are mildly or moderately elevated in the stress testing

Table 111.1. Indications for Stress Testing

Diagnosis
    Chest pain syndrome
    Screening for latent heart disease
    Evaluation of dysrhythmias
Prognosis and severity of disease
    Functional capacity and exercise prescription
    After myocardial infarction
    Before noncardiac surgery
Management
    Evaluating effects of medical and surgical treatment
    Stimulus to change lifestyle
Myocardial viability

Table 111.2. Contraindications to Stress Testing

Acute myocardial infarction
Acute myocarditis or pericarditis
Rapid ventricular or atrial arrhythmias
Severe aortic stenosis, hypertrophic obstructive cardiomyopathy
Second- or third-degree heart block without pacemaker
Stage 3 elevated blood pressure $\geq$ 180/110 mm Hg
Unstable progressive angina
Severe illness from infection or other processes (eg, hyperthyroidism, sever anemia, or liver, renal, pulmonary, or cardiac failure)

milieu before exercise, even when the blood pressure was previously normal with or without medication. This is considered a variant of white-coat hypertension secondary to augmented sympathoadrenal activity, usually associated with mental stress.

Aortic Stenosis

Patients with clinical signs of critical aortic stenosis and angina should not undergo a stress test. These patients should be referred directly to the cardiac catheterization laboratory for evaluation of the aortic valve and the coronary arteries. In adults with evidence of moderate aortic stenosis, stress testing has some increased risk but may be quite useful, especially when accompanied by myocardial perfusion imaging. In children, stress testing in the presence of aortic stenosis has been useful and safe.

Unstable Angina Syndrome

A progressive increase in the intensity, frequency, duration, or ease of onset of exertional angina or angina at rest heralds the potential to develop into an acute myocardial infarction. Stress testing could aggravate this situation by increasing platelet aggregability and triggering the coagulation cascade through augmented sympathoadrenal and neurohumoral pathways. However, after appropriate therapy to control stable angina, it is sometimes useful to perform a stress test, especially in association with myocardial perfusion imaging, to assist in management decisions.

Compensated Heart Failure

Patients who have heart failure with dependent edema and pulmonary rales by auscultation should not undergo exercise stress test-

ing until these signs have responded to therapy. Conversely, careful exercise tolerance testing that monitors symptoms, HR, and BP responses relating to work load (and measures of oxygen consumption and carbon dioxide elimination when available) is useful for determining the appropriate rehabilitation exercise schedule. The Naughton stress test and the Borg scale of perceived effort are commonly used.

Exaggerated Pressure Response to Exercise

In normotensive individuals, an exercise SBP >220 mm Hg or DBP >100 mm Hg is beyond the standards for normal and is considered to be an exaggerated response. Only a small percentage of the usual population exhibits an exaggerated BP response to exercise. Normotensive individuals with a parental history of hypertension are at greater risk for developing hypertension and more frequently display the exaggerated BP pattern. Borderline hypertensives and those with treated hypertension and adequate resting BP control may display an exaggerated pressure response to exercise. The exaggerated response pattern may also be observed during mental stress or other behavioral states requiring greater attentiveness and mental performance. Hemodynamic measurements demonstrate vasodilatory impairment in those with an exaggerated response to exercise (**Figure 111.1**). This blunted vasodilation is manifest even at submaximal exercise and is associated with a trend toward a reduced CO response.

In subpopulations at high risk for hypertension or treated hypertensive patients who exhibit this exaggerated BP response to exercise, there is the added risk of accelerated target organ damage. This BP response pattern needs to be evaluated and appropriate adjustments to the antihypertensive drug therapy instituted in the process of exercise prescriptions. Repeat exercise tests may be necessary to achieve optimal BP regulation.

Added Prognostic Value of Stress Myocardial Perfusion Imaging

Stress myocardial perfusion imaging has many advantages over exercise ECG testing alone for identifying high-risk coronary disease patients: (1) the sensitivity of reversible stress-induced perfusion defects for detection of ischemia is greater than that of ST-segment depression and is more apparent in patients who fail to achieve 85% of maximum predicted heart rate; (2) the superiority of perfusion in localizing ischemia and determining the extent of myocardium at risk; (3) its greater ability to identify patients with underlying left main or three-vessel disease compared with exercise ECG alone; and (4) its enhanced capability for detecting residual ischemia within an infarct zone, because resting ST- and T-wave changes in the ECG may preclude an accurate interpretation of ST response to exercise. The total extent of stress defects has been shown by Pollock et al to be the best independent predictor of future major events and provides additional prognostic information compared with clinical ECG exercise testing and cardiac catheterization variables.

Several reports have indicated that patients with chest pain who have a totally normal myocardial perfusion scan have an excellent prognosis (yearly mortality rate of 0.5% and nonfatal myocardial infarction rate of 0.6%) during follow-up. A large study using stress ^{201}Tl single photon emission computed tomography has also demonstrated that

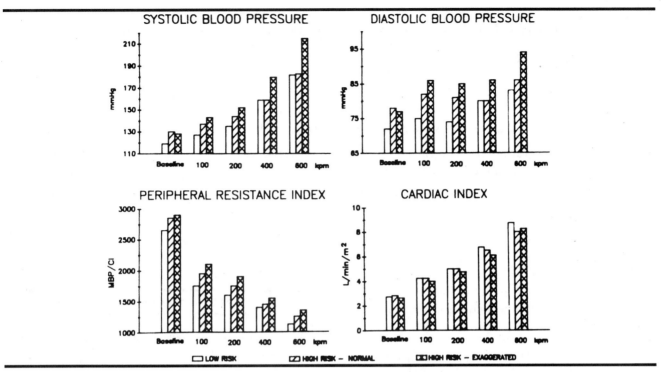

Figure 111.1.   Hemodynamic measurements of three groups at baseline control and during mild to moderate bicycle exercise (100 to 600 kpm). CI indicates cardiac index; DBP, diastolic blood pressure; PRI, peripheral resistance index; and SBP, systolic blood pressure.

cardiac mortality was 0.42% per year in patients with normal scans and 2.1% per year in those with abnormal scans. The cardiovascular mortality rose to 2.4% per year when three or more scan territories were involved and to 17% (over 32 months of follow-up) when four or more segments were abnormal. These data have extended the application of stress myocardial perfusion imaging using pharmacological agents (eg, dipyridamole or adenosine) beyond the diagnostic indications of the test and into risk stratification of patients after acute MI and before noncardiac (eg, vascular) surgery. In these patients, maximal exercise testing is either contraindicated or difficult for patients to perform.

SUGGESTED READING

1. Beller GA. New directions in myocardial perfusion imaging. *Clin Cardiol.* 1993;16: 86–94.

2. Borer JS, Brensike JF, Redwood DR, Itscoitz SB, Passamani ER, Stone NJ, Richardson JM, Levy RI, Epstein SE. Limitations of the electrocardiographic response to exercise in predicting coronary artery disease. *N Engl J Med.* 1975;293:367–371.

3. Bruce RA, Kusumi F, Hosmer D. Maximal oxygen intake and nomographic assessment of functional aerobic impairment in cardiovascular disease. *Am Heart J.* 1973;85:546–562.

4. Ellestad MH. Cardiovascular limits to exercise. In: Ellestad MH, ed. *Stress Testing: Principles and Practice.* 3rd ed. Philadelphia, Pa: FA Davis Co; 1975:177–195.

5. Esquivel L, Pollock SG, Beller GA, Gibson RS, Watson DD, Kaul S. Effect of the degree of effort on the sensitivity of the exercise thallium-201 stress test in symptomatic coronary artery disease. *Am J Cardiol.* 1989;63:160–165.

6. Iskandrian AS, Chae SC, Heo J, Stanberry CD, Wasserleben V, Cave V. Independent and incremental prognostic value of exercise single-photon emission computed tomographic (SPECT) thallium imaging in coronary artery disease. *J Am Coll Cardiol.* 1993;22:665–670.

7. Machecourt J, Longere P, Fagret D, Vanzetto G, Wolf JE, Polidori C, Comet M, Denis B. Prognostic value of thallium-201 single-photon emission computed tomographic myocardial perfusion imaging according to extent of myocardial defect: study in 1,926 patients with follow-up at 33 months. *J Am Coll Cardiol.* 1994;23:1096–1106.

8. Pamelia FX, Gibson RS, Watson DD, Craddock GB, Sirawatka J, Beller GA. Prognosis with chest pain and normal thallium-201 exercise scintigrams. *Am J Cardiol.* 1985;55:920–926.

9. Pollock SG, Abbott RD, Boucher CA, Beller GA, Kaul S. Independent and incremental prognostic value of tests performed in hierarchical order to evaluate patients with suspected coronary artery disease: validation of models based on these tests. *Circulation.* 1992;85:237–248.

10. Wilson MF, Sung BH, Pincomb GA, Lovallo WR. Exaggerated pressure response to exercise in men at risk for systemic hypertension. *Am J Cardiol.* 1990;66:731–736.

Chapter 112

Evaluation of Renal Parenchymal Disease

Michael A. Moore, MD

KEY POINTS

- Renal parenchymal diseases are almost always associated with impaired renal function.

- Glomerular disease can present as five clinical syndromes, including isolated proteinuria, idiopathic hematuria, nephrotic syndrome, nephritic syndrome, or renal insufficiency.

- Diabetic retinopathy and neuropathy usually establish the diagnosis of diabetic nephropathy in a nephrotic patient.

See also Chapters 73, 78, 141

Renal parenchymal diseases (RPDs)—cystic renal disease, glomerular disease, interstitial nephritis, nephrosclerosis, and end-stage kidney disease causing hypertension—are almost always associated with impaired renal function.

Patients with RPD present with renal insufficiency, proteinuria, or hematuria. Patients suspected of having RPD should initially have a urinalysis and renal function determination. Evaluation for RPD includes a history and physical examination seeking appropriate clues **(Table 112.1)**. Laboratory studies include a urinalysis, renal sonogram, blood urea nitrogen, serum creatinine, electrolytes and albumin, 24-hour urine for protein and creatinine content, and occasionally, renal biopsy. An algorithm for the laboratory evaluation of RPD is shown in **Figure 112.1.**

Evaluation of Proteinuria

Urinary reagent dipsticks detect albumin when it is present at concentrations >30 mg%. Urine should also be tested for protein with sulfosalicylic acid (one part sulfosalicylic acid to nine parts urine), which precipitates any protein, including light chains in dysproteinemic states. Proteinuria should be quantified with a 24-hour urinary protein collection. In nondiabetic patients, proteinuria is defined as >150 mg/24 h. An alternative method is determining the ratio of protein/creatinine (P/C) concentration in a randomly voided urine. The P/C ratio correlates closely with a 24-hour urine for protein (normal P/C <0.2; 1.0 to 3.5 ratio correlates with 1 to 3.5 g/24 h).

The earliest form of diabetic nephropathy is microalbuminuria (30 to 300 mg/24 h urinary albumin). Annual screening for microalbuminuria is important in all adult-onset and in postpuberty insulin-dependent diabetic patients. Microalbuminuria is not detected by standard urinary dipsticks for protein, and the urine must be sent to a laboratory for urinary albumin measurement in the microalbuminuria range.

RPD can have variable amounts of proteinuria. Proteinuria >3.5 g/d is considered to be in the nephrotic range. Patients with any amount of proteinuria should be followed up with an annual 24-hour urinary protein measurement to determine whether the glomerular disease is worsening.

A sample of the first voided urine of the day should be analyzed for protein content. "Orthostatic" proteinuria is present if protein is

Table 112.1. Clues to Renal Parenchymal Disease

Clinical clues

Recurrent urinary tract infections, particulary in young patient, suggest congenital bladder abnormalities and/or "reflux nephropathy."

A careful medication history, including proprietary analgesics to screen for any potential nephrotoxins (Table 112.2).

Locate previous renal function studies, such as blood urea nitrogen, serum creatinine, or urinalysis, because these can indicate preexisting chronic rather than acute renal failure.

A history of ingestion of moonshine or illicit alcohol suggests potential lead exposure.

Diabetic retinopathy establishes the diagnosis of diabetic nephrophathy in a nephrotic patient.

An abdominal bruit, particularly diastolic, suggests renal artery disease or an arteriovenous malformation.

Proteinuria always indicates glomerular disease.

Red cell casts always indicate glomerular inflammation.

A urine negative for protein by dipstick (albumin) but positive for protein by sulfosalicylic acid (any protein) suggests the presence of light chains with dysproteinemia

Physical examination clues

FINDINGS	SIGNIFICANCE
Periorbital edema	Expanded extracellular fluid volume
Edema in legs or lower back	
Rales	
Pallor	Anemia of chronic renal failure
Systolic murmur	Functional flow murmur
Diastolic murmur	Precedes pericarditis
Pericardial rub	Uremic pericarditis
Decreased tactile sensation/reflexes	Uremic neuropathy
Loss of muscle mass	Uremic myopathy

not present in a first voided urine but is present in subsequent urine during the day. Patients with persistent proteinuria (not orthostatic) should be screened for diabetes mellitus, connective tissue diseases, multiple myeloma, and measurement of the activity of the serum complement system.

ALGORITHM FOR EVALUATION OF RENAL PARENCHYMAL DISEASE

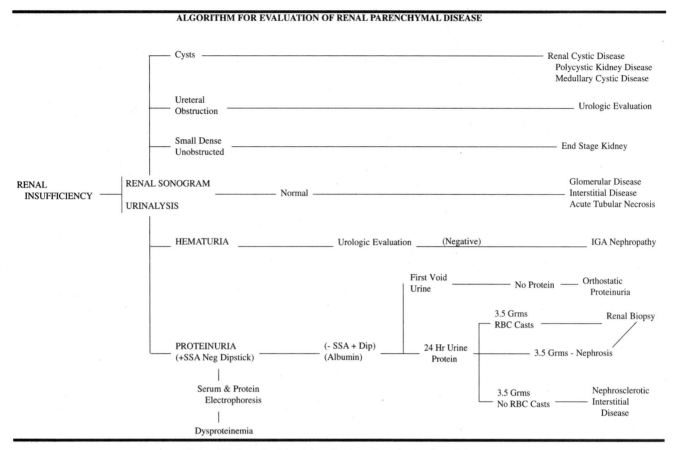

Figure 112.1. Algorithm for evaluation of renal parenchymal disease.

Glomerular Disease

Glomerular disease can present as five clinical syndromes, including isolated proteinuria, idiopathic hematuria, nephrotic syndrome, nephritic syndrome, or renal insufficiency. All treatable glomerular diseases except minimal change, membranous, and antineutrophil cytoplasmic antibody–mediated glomerulonephritis can be identified from blood studies. Renal biopsy is needed to diagnose these three treatable diseases. A specific pathological diagnosis of glomerular disease is particularly important in patients who may receive a renal transplant, because certain glomerular disease can recur in the transplanted kidney. These recurrent syndromes include membranoproliferative glomerulonephritis, focal glomerulosclerosis, and IgA nephropathy. Diabetic nephropathy and renal oxalosis also recur, but the rate of impairment is slow.

Hematuria usually requires urological evaluation. If no urological disease is found and kidney function is normal, IgA nephropathy is probably present. If kidney function is decreased or if proteinuria is also present, further workup may be necessary, including a renal biopsy.

Waxy or hyaline urinary casts represent the contents of renal tubules when protein condenses within them. These casts are always seen in patients with proteinuria but can be seen in normal urinalysis. Red blood cell (RBC) casts represent blood and protein derived from the glomerulus and indicate glomerular arteritis with bleeding into the renal tubule.

Patients with the nephritic syndrome have proteinuria to a lesser degree than those with the nephrotic syndrome ($<3.5/24\,h$), as well as variable hematuria and RBC casts in the urine. RBC casts are pathognomonic of the nephritic syndrome. Serum complement should be measured, because a low level of one or more components of the complement system is characteristic of several types of glomerulonephritis. Renal biopsy should be considered early in the course of the nephritic patient with renal insufficiency, because treatment information can be obtained from the pathological pattern found on biopsy.

Renal biopsy should be done only when the information will be necessary for the treatment of the patient. It is important to have an experienced renal pathologist available. Open renal biopsy is necessary only in severely obese or noncooperative patients and in patients with a solitary kidney. Some centers advocate treatment for isolated proteinuria with a 6- to 8-week course of steroids before further consideration of renal biopsy.

Interstitial Renal Disease

Chronic interstitial disease is diagnosed in patients with renal insufficiency (often nonoliguric), a history of a known cause of interstitial disease (usually a drug), and an essentially normal urinalysis. Chronic interstitial disease typically has $<1\,g$ of proteinuria and can reduce urinary concentrating capacities so that the urine specific gravity is low or fixed, but this is not a pathognomonic finding. The finding of eosinophils in the urine, although uncommon even in

Table 112.2. Normal Parameters of Renal Function

Normal values
  Blood urea nitrogen   5 to 22 mg/dL (1.8 to 7.9 mmol/L)
  Serum creatinine
    Men   0.5 to 1.3 mg/dL (40 to 110 μmol/L)
    Women   0.5 to 1.1 mg/dL (40 to 100 μmol/L)
  Creatinine clearance
    Men   110 to 150 mL/min (1.83 to 2.5 mL/s)
    Women   105 to 132 mL/min (1.75 to 2.2 mL/s)
Calculation of values
  Creatinine clearance = [urine creatinine (mg/dL) × urine volume (mL)]/
                         [plasma creatinine (mg/dL) × collection time (min)]
Formula for estimating creatinine clearance
  Men = [(140−age) × weight (kg)]/[72 × serum creatinine (mg/dL)]
  Women = [(140−age) × weight (kg)]/[72 × serum creatinine (mg/dL)] ×0.85

Reproduced by permission from Kassirer JP. Clinical evaluation of kidney function-glomerular function. *N Engl J Med.* 1971;285:385–389; and Rakel RE, ed. *Textbook of Family Practice.* 4th ed. Philadelphia, PA: WB Saunders; 1990.

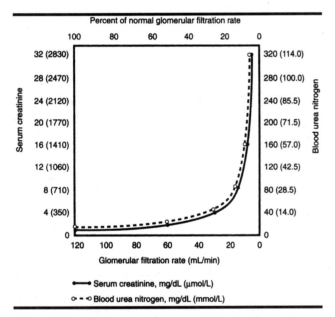

Figure 112.2. Relation among serum creatinine, blood urea nitrogen, and glomerular filtration rate. Adapted with permission from Kassirer JP. Clinical evaluation of kidney function-glomerular function. *N Engl J Med.* 1971;285:385–389.

proven cases of interstitial nephritis, is pathognomonic for "allergic" or drug-induced interstitial disease.

Nephrosclerosis

Nephrosclerosis is RPD secondary to chronic renal small-vessel disease. It occurs in hypertensive and older patients. All will have some degree of renal insufficiency, usually a history of hypertension, <2 g of proteinuria daily, and an otherwise unremarkable urinalysis. Renal sonography often demonstrates symmetrical normal to small kidneys with some increase in echogenicity.

End-Stage Kidney Disease

End-stage kidney disease is diagnosed by azotemia, elevated serum phosphorus (>5.5 mg/dL), anemia, urinalysis with variable amounts of proteinuria, broad casts, and small, dense, unobstructed kidneys on renal sonogram.

Recognizing and Defining Renal Insufficiency

Renal insufficiency can be recognized only by measurement of blood urea nitrogen, serum creatinine, or a creatinine clearance **(Table 112.2)**. Blood in the intestinal tract will raise the blood urea nitrogen level but not the serum creatinine; overhydration, decreased dietary protein, or malnutrition will lower the blood urea nitrogen. Creatinine is the product of daily muscle metabolism, and a fixed amount related to muscle mass is produced daily.

The creatinine clearance approximates the glomerular filtration rate. A creatinine clearance should be done if a more precise level of kidney function is needed. Because creatinine is also secreted by the renal tubules, the creatinine clearance overestimates the actual glomerular filtration rate, with the discrepancy increasing as renal function decreases. A timed collection (3 to 24 hours) is used. The creatinine clearance can be estimated by several methods; the one most commonly used is shown in Table 112.2.

There is an inverse relationship between the serum creatinine and creatinine clearance, in which an initial relatively large fall in creatinine clearance is reflected in only a small change in serum creatinine **(Figure 112.2)**. In an average-size patient <60 years of age, a serum creatinine level of ≥1.6 mg% usually reflects a 40% loss of glomerular filtration rate. In patients >60 years of age with a smaller muscle mass and, hence, a lower normal serum creatinine, a serum creatinine level of ≥1.4 mg% may reflect a similar loss of renal function.

SUGGESTED READING

1. American Diabetes Association. Diabetic nephropathy. *Diabetes Care.* 1997;20 (supp I):S24–S27.
2. Anderson S. Proteinuria. In: Greenberg A, ed. *Primer on Kidney Disease.* New York, NY: Academic Press Inc; 1990.
3. Bennett PH, Haffner S, Kasiske BL, Keane WF, Mogensen CE, Parving HH, Steffes MW, Striker GE. Screening and management of microalbuminuria in patients with diabetes mellitus: recommendation to the Scientific Advisory Board of the National Kidney Foundation from the ad hoc committee of the Council on Diabetes Mellitus of the National Kidney Foundation. *Am J Kidney Dis.* 1995;25:107–112.
4. Ginsberg JM, Chang BS, Matarese RA, Garella S. Use of single voided urine samples to estimate quantitative proteinuria. *N Engl J Med.* 1983;309:1543–1546.
5. Moore MA, Porush JG. Hypertension and renal insufficiency: recognition and management. *Am Fam Physician.* 1992;45:1248–1256.
6. National High Blood Pressure Education Program Working Group. 1995 update of the working group reports on chronic renal failure and renovascular hypertension. *Arch Intern Med.* 1996;156:1938–1947.

Chapter 113

Evaluation of the Peripheral Circulation

Jeffrey W. Olin, DO

KEY POINTS

- Evaluation of the entire vascular system is important because of the increased prevalence of peripheral arterial disease in patients with hypertension.

- The primary symptom of peripheral arterial disease is intermittent claudication.

- Blood pressure should be measured in both arms to detect the presence of innominate or subclavian artery stenosis due to atherosclerosis.

- A systolic and diastolic bruit heard over one carotid artery may be indicative of severe bilateral carotid artery disease.

- Evaluation of the peripheral circulation includes functional testing (ankle/brachial index, pulse volume recordings) and imaging (duplex ultrasound, CT scanning, magnetic resonance angiography, arteriography).

See also Chapters 65, 79, 142

Evaluation of the peripheral circulation is extremely important in the hypertensive patient because hypertension is a potent risk factor for the development of peripheral arterial disease (PAD), carotid atherosclerosis, and aneurysmal disease. The Framingham Study showed a significant relationship between systolic and diastolic blood pressure levels and the 26-year incidence of intermittent claudication.

Signs and Symptoms

There are several clues in the history that suggest the presence of carotid atherosclerosis, PAD, or aneurysmal disease. A history of transient ischemic attacks (focal neurological deficit that resolves within 24 hours), including amaurosis fugax (monocular blindness), aphasia, dysphagia, hemiparesis, hemiplegia, or focal sensory abnormalities or stroke, suggests the presence of cardiac disease, aortic arch atherosclerosis, or carotid artery atherosclerosis.

The primary symptom of PAD is intermittent claudication, which is characterized as discomfort, cramping, tightness, or tiredness in one of the muscle groups in the lower extremity. Most commonly, it occurs in the calf as a result of superficial femoral artery obstruction. However, thigh, hip, or buttock claudication occurs in patients with aortoiliac occlusive disease. As a general rule, the discomfort is brought on by exercise (usually walking) and is quickly relieved within 2 to 5 minutes after the individual stops walking. Intermittent claudication can usually be differentiated from pseudoclaudication (neurogenic claudication) caused by lumbar canal stenosis or disk disease on the basis of the history and physical examination (**Table 113.1**).

When the vascular disease becomes advanced, the patient may experience pain at rest, indicating that critical limb ischemia is present. It is not uncommon for individuals with rest pain to hang their leg over the side of the bed or sleep sitting in a chair so that gravity can improve the circulation to the lower extremity. This may lead to significant edema, which may falsely lead the clinician to suspect venous or lymphatic disease.

Cold hands and feet are poor clues to the presence of arterial insufficiency because they also occur in patients who are extremely tense, have overactivity of the sympathetic nervous system, or have some degree of vasospasm. Some patients have a condition called vasomotor instability, which prevents the blood vessel from reacting normally.

Physical Examination of the Circulation

At the initial physical examination, blood pressure should be measured in both arms. If the blood pressures are different, the

Table 113.1. Differentiating True Claudication From Pseudoclaudication

	INTERMITTENT CLAUDICATION	PSEUDOCLAUDICATION
Character of discomfort	Cramping, tightness, tiredness	Same, or tingling, weakness, clumsiness
Location of discomfort	Buttock, hip, thigh, calf, foot	Same
Exercise induced	Yes	Yes or no
Distance to claudication	Same each time	Variable
Occurs with standing	No	Yes
Relief	Stop walking	Often must sit or change body positions

From Krajewski LP, Olin JW. Atherosclerosis of the aorta and lower extremities. In: Young JR, Graor RA, Olin JW, Bartholomew JR, eds. *Peripheral Vascular Diseases*. St Louis, Mo: Mosby Yearbook; 1991:183. Used by permission.

higher value should be used for subsequent blood pressure readings. A discrepancy in blood pressure readings between arms is usually indicative of innominate or subclavian artery stenosis (commonly due to atherosclerosis) on the side of the lower blood pressure. Occasionally, both subclavian arteries are narrowed. Under these circumstances, the blood pressure will be higher in the legs than in the arms.

The carotid arteries should be palpated in every hypertensive patient. The carotid artery should be palpated low in the neck, generally at the level of the thyroid gland anterior to the sternocleidomastoid muscle. The carotid bifurcation (located at the angle of the jaw) should be avoided because palpation of this area may cause significant bradycardia or asystole in patients who have a hypersensitive carotid sinus or cause dislodgment of atheromatous material, producing a transient ischemic attack or a stroke. A fullness in the carotid pulsation in the elderly is most commonly due to a tortuous (kinked) carotid artery. Carotid artery aneurysms are quite uncommon. The subclavian artery pulse should be palpated in the supraclavicular fossa with the thumb while the fingers are placed behind the neck. The character of the pulsation as well as the presence or absence of an aneurysm should be noted. Next, the superficial temporal artery should be palpated. A decrease in the arterial pulsation may indicate stenosis of the common or external carotid artery.

After careful palpation, one should listen in the cervical and supraclavicular regions for the presence of bruits. Bruits can be heard best with the bell of the stethoscope with the patient in the sitting position. The location and quality of the bruit should be described and characterized as being a systolic bruit or a combined systolic and diastolic bruit. It is important to listen over the base of the heart to be certain that the bruit is not a transmitted murmur from the aortic or pulmonary valve. A bruit that is heard during both systole and diastole indicates that there may be severe bilateral carotid artery disease. In fact, the artery on the contralateral side to the continuous systolic/diastolic bruit is often more severely stenotic than the index vessel or totally occluded **(Figure 113.1)**. Other conditions that cause a systolic/diastolic bruit include arteriovenous malformation, arteriovenous fistula, or a venous hum. A venous hum is usually heard at the base of the neck and can easily be detected by its disappearance on light compression of the external jugular vein.

The axillary, brachial, radial, and ulnar pulses should be palpated. If there is evidence of ischemia of the hands or fingers or if there is any reason to believe that the arteries distal to the wrist are diseased, Allen's test should be performed. The patient is asked to make a tight fist, which will cause most of the blood to empty from the hands and fingers. The examiners' thumbs then swipe over the thenar and hypothenar eminences to occlude the radial and ulnar arteries. When the patient opens his hand, it should be blanched. When the radial or ulnar artery is released, prompt return of color to the hand indicates that the artery is open distal to the wrist. The maneuver is then repeated releasing the second artery. A positive test is failure of the hand to return to normal color promptly on release of the occluded artery.

The chest should be examined because occasionally, a large aneurysm in the ascending aorta may be visualized or palpated as a pulsation high in the chest near the suprasternal notch.

Careful auscultation of the abdomen for the presence of bruits (systolic, systolic/diastolic) in the epigastric region may reveal steno-

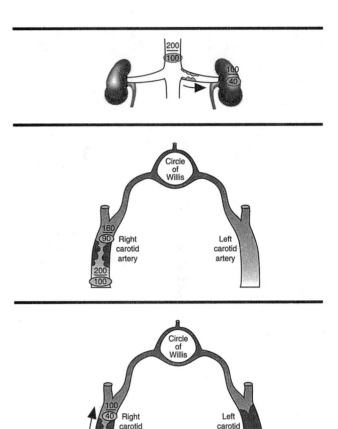

Figure 113.1. Top, Systolic/diastolic bruit in the renal artery. The kidney is an end organ, and when stenosis of a main renal artery becomes severe enough, a systolic/diastolic bruit may be present. During systole (left ventricular contraction), blood moves through a narrow arterial segment, turbulence is produced, and a bruit is heard. If the stenosis is severe enough, there is a significant pressure gradient during diastole as well (ie, 100 vs 40 mm Hg); therefore, blood continues to flow in a forward direction (arrow) from an area of high pressure to an area of low pressure. Middle, The right carotid artery is severely narrowed. When blood moves through this narrowed segment, turbulence is produced and a systolic bruit is heard. Because the left carotid artery is patent, there may be crossover from the left cerebral hemisphere to the right cerebral hemisphere through the circle of Willis. This keeps the pressure up in the distal right carotid artery, and no forward flow occurs during diastole; thus, a diastolic bruit is not heard. Bottom, The left carotid artery is occluded; therefore, there will be no crossover from the left cerebral hemisphere through the circle of Willis. Pressure in the distal right carotid artery will be very low. Since there is a substantial diastolic pressure difference (circled numbers), blood will flow forward (arrow) during diastole, producing a systolic/diastolic bruit. A systolic/diastolic carotid bruit indicates severe stenosis or occlusion of the contralateral carotid artery.

sis of the celiac artery, superior mesenteric artery, or renal arteries. A short systolic bruit is often heard in thin individuals and is generally not a cause of concern (Figure 113.1, top).

An attempt should be made to palpate the abdominal aorta in every individual. Infrarenal abdominal aortic aneurysms are not uncommon in the elderly hypertensive patient. By palpating the lateral border and the medial border of the aorta at the same time, the ex-

Sample Ankle-Brachial Index (ABI) Worksheet

Patient Name: _____

Date: _____   Patient Number: _____

Ankle-Brachial Index Interpretation
Above 0.90 – Normal
0.71 - 0.90 – Mild Obstruction
0.41 - 0.70 – Moderate Obstruction
0.00 - 0.40 – Severe Obstruction

Right Arm
Pressure:

_____

Left Arm
Pressure:

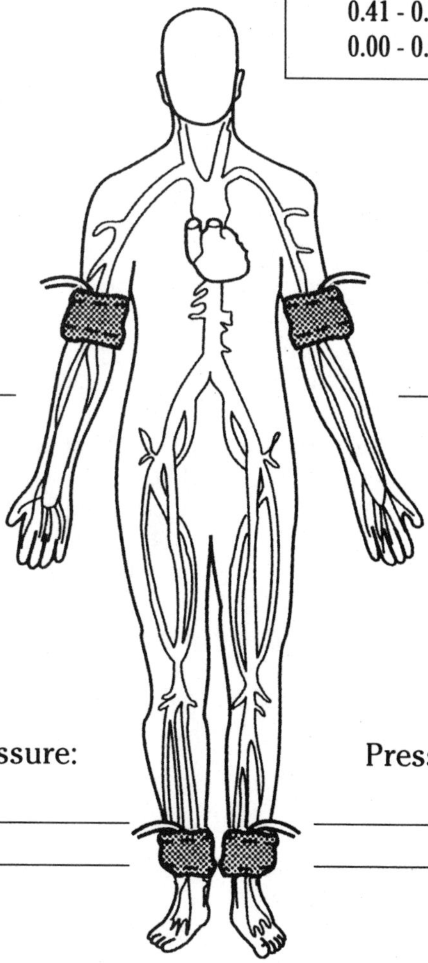

_____

Pressure:

PT _____
DP _____

Pressure:

_____ PT
_____ DP

Right ABI

$$\frac{\text{Right Ankle Pressure}}{\text{Highest Arm Pressure}} = \frac{\text{mm Hg}}{\text{mm Hg}} = \underline{\quad}$$

Left ABI

$$\frac{\text{Left Ankle Pressure}}{\text{Highest Arm Pressure}} = \frac{\text{mm Hg}}{\text{mm Hg}} = \underline{\quad}$$

Example
$$\frac{\text{Ankle Pressure}}{\text{Brachial Pressure}} = \frac{125 \text{ mm Hg}}{114 \text{ mm Hg}} = 1.09 \quad \textit{See ABI Chart}$$

Figure 113.2. Sample ABI worksheet. Reproduced with permission from the Society for Vascular Medicine and Biology, Peripheral arterial disease: marker of cardiovascular risk.

aminer can assess the size of the aorta. Gently rolling the aorta back and forth under the fingertips can help differentiate an aneurysm from a tortuous aorta.

Pulses in the lower extremities should be graded as normal, diminished, or absent. The femoral pulse should be palpated just below the inguinal ligament, with firm, constant pressure applied to feel the pulse, which is deep in most individuals. The size of the femoral artery should be noted, and an aneurysm should be considered if it is large. The amplitude and timing of the pulse should be compared with those of the radial artery, which may be diminished and delayed in coarctation of the aorta.

The popliteal pulse should be palpated in every individual. This pulse is often the most difficult for physicians to detect. Normally, the pulse should be palpated directly under the lateral aspect of the patella with the knee flexed $\approx 10°$. Firm pressure must be applied to allow the fingers to go deep into the popliteal space. The artery should be palpated with the pads of the fingers and not the fingertips. Popliteal artery aneurysms occur in 20% of patients with abdominal aortic aneurysms. The major complication of a popliteal aneurysm is thrombosis; when this occurs, the limb may become acutely ischemic, leading to limb loss in up to 50% of individuals.

Next, the posterior tibial, dorsalis pedis, and peroneal pulses should be palpated. The posterior tibial pulse can be felt posterior to the medial malleolus. The dorsalis pedis pulse is usually located over the second metatarsal bones. The dorsalis pedis pulse may not be detected in some normal individuals because the anterior tibial artery dives deep at the level of the ankle. If the dorsalis pedis pulse cannot be detected, one should attempt to find the anterior tibial artery. If neither can be felt, the peroneal artery can often be detected in the lateral aspect of the ankle.

Further Diagnostic Studies
Carotid Atherosclerosis

If carotid artery atherosclerosis is suspected, if a transient ischemic attack or a stroke has occurred, or if a carotid bruit is heard on physical examination, a duplex ultrasound examination of the carotid arteries is warranted. This study can estimate the degree of narrowing of the common carotid artery, the external carotid artery, and the internal carotid artery within several centimeters of the carotid bifurcation. The intracranial portion of the internal carotid artery cannot be adequately visualized with this technique. Although arteriography has been required in the past if carotid artery surgery was to be performed, many centers now perform carotid endarterectomy on the basis of the results of carotid ultrasound alone. Therefore, it is very important to be certain that the vascular laboratory is accredited and that appropriate quality control measures are followed.

Abdominal Aortic Aneurysm

An ultrasound, CT, or MRI scan can confirm the presence of an abdominal aortic aneurysm and give an accurate assessment of its size and location. An ultrasound examination is useful in determining the size of the femoral or popliteal arteries if aneurysms are suspected. Often the surgeon will operate on the basis of one of these

noninvasive imaging modalities. However, if clues that suggest the presence of renal artery stenosis or mesenteric ischemia are present, an arteriogram should be performed before surgical repair of the aneurysm.

Peripheral Arterial Disease

If the patient has intermittent claudication, ischemic rest pain, or digital ulcerations, the circulation can be assessed noninvasively with Doppler blood pressures or pulse volume recordings (pulse waveform analysis). The least expensive way to screen for the presence of PAD is to measure the ankle-brachial index (ABI). An ABI can easily be performed in any physician's office to accurately predict the severity of PAD and the risk of future cardiovascular events. With a hand-held Doppler (5 to 10 MHz), the systolic blood pressure should be measured in both arms, followed by the systolic blood pressure in the right and left posterior tibial and dorsalis pedis arteries. A sample worksheet for measuring the ABI is shown in **Figure 113.2.** Segmental pressures can be measured by placing blood pressure cuffs at the high thigh, calf, ankle, transmetatarsal region, and toe. Pressures and pulse volume waveforms are obtained at each level, and an ABI is obtained by comparing blood pressures in the ankle and in the arm. After this examination is performed in the resting position, the patient exercises on a treadmill, and repeat blood pressures and pulse waveforms are obtained. Segmental pressure measurements help determine the location of the arterial obstruction or predict the level at which an amputation should occur.

Although most patients with significant PAD demonstrate a decrease in the arterial pulsation, some have normal arterial pulses at rest. Therefore, it is important to perform pulse volume recordings and Doppler blood pressures not only at rest but after the patient has walked on a treadmill until symptoms are reproduced. When arterial obstruction is present, the pressures in the ankles decrease after exercise.

In severe arterial insufficiency (rest pain, ischemic ulcerations, or gangrene) or disabling claudication, the patient may require an arteriogram to determine whether surgical reconstruction or nonsurgical intervention, such a balloon angioplasty or stent placement, is feasible.

SUGGESTED READING

1. Ernst CB. Abdominal aortic aneurysm. *N Engl J Med.* 1993;328:1167–1172.
2. Graor RA, deWolfe VG, Elliot I. A clinical vignette: the clinical significance of systolic-diastolic bruits in the carotid arteries. *Cleve Clin Q.* 1984;51:155–158.
3. Kannel WB, McGee DL. Update on some epidemiologic features of intermittent claudication: the Framingham Study. *J Am Geriatr Soc.* 1985:33:13–18.
4. Krajewski LP, Olin JW. Atherosclerosis of the aorta and lower extremities. In: Young JR, Olin JW, Bartholomew JR, eds. *Peripheral Vascular Diseases.* 2nd ed. St Louis, Mo: CV Mosby Co; 1996:208–233.
5. Newman AB, Sutton-Tyrell K, Vogt M, Kuller LH. Morbidity and mortality in hypertensive adults with a low ankle/arm blood pressure index. *JAMA.* 1993;270:487–489.
6. Sumner DS. Volume plethysmography in vascular disease. In: Bernstein EF, ed. *Vascular Diagnosis.* 4th ed. St Louis, Mo: Mosby; 1993:181–193.
7. Yao JST. Pressure measurement in the extremity. In: Bernstein EF, ed. *Vascular Diagnosis.* 4th ed. St Louis, Mo: Mosby; 1993:169–175.
8. Young JR. Physical examination. In: Young JR, Olin JW, Bartholomew JR, eds. *Peripheral Vascular Diseases.* 2nd ed. St Louis, Mo: CV Mosby Co; 1996:18–32.

Chapter 114

Evaluation of Arterial Compliance

Gary E. McVeigh, MD, PhD

KEY POINTS

- Arterial compliance, defined as a change in volume for a given change in pressure, represents the best clinical measure of the buffering function of the aorta and its major branches.

- Reduced arterial compliance increases systolic blood pressure and pulse pressure, impairs coronary perfusion, and increases left ventricular afterload.

- Compliance changes may be inhomogeneous with respect to location within the arterial tree but pulse contour analysis allows consistent evaluation of the effects of aging, disease, and perhaps therapy.

See also Chapters 61, 62, 149

Structure of Blood Vessels

Arterial blood vessels are complex three-dimensional structures. The components of the arterial wall differ in mechanical, biochemical, and physiological characteristics. The endothelium represents a single monolayer of cells and possesses little tensile strength but can alter the mechanical behavior of arterial blood vessels through the production and release of vasoactive substances that influence vascular tone and structure. The arterial media bears most of the tensile strain of blood vessels. The relative proportions of its constituents—elastin, smooth muscle, and collagen—as well as the thickness of the media can vary considerably between blood vessels, according to their type, site, and physiological function. The tunica adventitia is the outermost layer of the arterial blood vessels; it contains a large number of collagen fibers and can also influence the mechanical properties of the vessels.

Resistance and Compliance

Traditionally, systemic vascular resistance has been used to estimate vascular adaptations in response to disease in arterial blood vessels and to monitor the hemodynamic effect of drug interventions. The resistance calculation reflects a reduction in capillary density and changes in the thickness:lumen ratio of the media in small arteries and arterioles. It ignores pressure fluctuations occurring in the aorta and its major branches, where the compliance characteristics provide the vital buffering function required to smooth pulsatile outflow from the heart.

Arterial compliance is defined as a change in area, diameter, or volume for a given change in pressure and is dependent on vessel geometry in addition to the mechanical properties of the vessel wall. Arterial wall properties are different in different vessels, in the same vessel at various distending pressures, and with the activation of smooth muscle in the vessel wall. Although no single descriptor of arterial physical characteristics can completely describe the mechanical behavior of the vasculature, arterial compliance represents the best clinical index of the buffering function of the arterial system. Changes in the mechanical behavior of blood vessels manifested by reduced arterial compliance can influence growth and remodeling of the left ventricle, large arteries, small arteries, and arterioles. The pathophysiological consequences of a reduced arterial compliance are outlined in **Figure 114.1**.

Estimation of Compliance in Humans

Unfortunately, no "gold standard" exists for estimating arterial compliance in human subjects, and each of the techniques has inherent limitations (**Table 114.1**). Although it is generally accepted that the structural and functional changes associated with arterial aging and disease impair the compliance characteristics of the circulation, recent studies have emphasized that changes in pulsatile arterial function do not progress in a uniform or consistent manner in all arteries. Previous studies using pulse-wave velocity to estimate the stiffness of arterial segments indicate that the aorta stiffens progressively at an accelerated rate compared with other arterial segments. Echo-tracking technology has revealed that age-related changes in pulsatile function are inhomogeneous within localized arterial segments of elastic and muscular arteries and that the compliance characteristics of the radial artery may paradoxically increase with age.

In contrast to the heterogeneity in the physical characteristics of localized arterial segments with aging and disease, consistent and predictable changes occur in the arterial pulse contour, regardless of the site of measurement. These measurements provide important information about the pulsatile arterial function. The changes in the arterial wave shape can be quantified by frequency-domain or time-domain analysis techniques. The former technique is invasive, making it unsuitable for clinical studies.

In hypertension, arterial compliance decreases as blood pressure increases because of the nonlinear mechanical behavior of arteries. Thus, a reduction in arterial compliance is a well-accepted finding in hypertension, whatever the site or method of measurement. Currently, considerable controversy exists as to whether abnormalities in compliance in hypertensive patients represent intrinsic change in the arterial wall (structural) or merely a reflection of pressure change (functional) and whether the changes in compliance are located

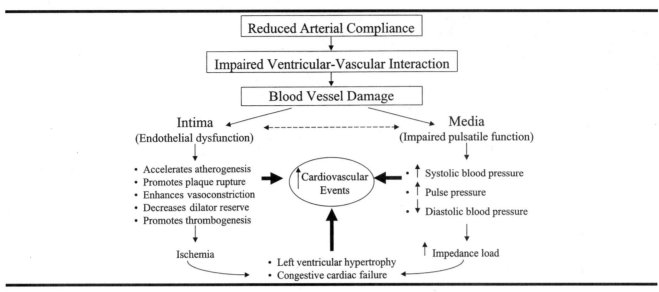

Figure 114.1. Schematic depiction showing how a reduced arterial compliance may promote blood vessel damage and predispose to premature clinical events.

Table 114.1. Methods Used to Estimate Arterial Compliance

METHODS	ADVANTAGES	LIMITATIONS	INFORMATION
Direct			
Angiography	Evaluation of different aortic segments	Expensive, invasive, limited clinical application	Regional aortic compliance
Magnetic resonance imaging	Noninvasive, not limited by acoustic window, able to examine multiple segments, not overly operator dependent	Claustrophobia, expensive, limited availability, remote site of BP measurement	Regional aortic compliance
TTE/TEE	TTE noninvasive, reasonable availability	Expensive, TTE limited by acoustic window, operator-dependent techniques; TEE invasive, remote site of BP measurement	Regional aortic compliance
Transcutaneous ET/IVUS techniques	Transcutaneous technique noninvasive; both techniques reproducible	Operator dependent, IVUS invasive, remote site of BP measurement with ET, clinical research application	Regional compliance of peripheral arteries
Venous occlusion plethysmography	Noninvasive, reasonable availability clinical research application	Remote site of BP measurement, Compliance of vascular bed under cuff	
Indirect			
Stroke volume/pulse pressure ratio	Noninvasive, reasonable availability	Noninvasive estimate of stroke volume required brachial sphygmomanometer BP measurement	Total arterial compliance
Pulse wave velocity	Noninvasive, reasonable availability reproducible	Limited to larger arteries, errors estimating path length and waveform distortion with pulse propagation	Segmental arterial compliance
Fourier analysis of pressure and flow waveforms	Standard technique, reproducible	Expensive, invasive, limited to the clinical research arena	Total arterial compliance
Pulse contour analysis	Can be noninvasive, reproducible, potential for widespread clinical application	Measurement of stroke volume	Total arterial compliance

BP indicates blood pressure; TTE, transthoracic echocardiography; TEE, transesophageal echocardiography; ET, echo-tracking; and IVUS, intravascular ultrasound.

primarily in the large or small vessels. The conflicting results reported in studies addressing the compliance characteristics of the arterial vasculature in human hypertension relate to confusion with the usage of terms describing vessel wall mechanical properties, diversity of the methods used, and heterogeneity of the patient populations and vascular regions studied.

An understanding of age- and disease-related physiological changes that occur in the arterial system is crucial to appreciate their influence on the occurrence of cardiovascular diseases and their response to treatment. By providing a direct assessment of abnormal structure or tone in the arterial vasculature, abnormalities in arterial compliance may improve risk stratification and identify individuals with early vascular damage who are predisposed to future vascular events **(Figure 114.1)**. It may also serve as a sensitive parameter to assess the effects of therapeutic interventions on pulsatile arterial function. Emerging data support the concept that the cardioprotective actions of drug interventions may depend, at least in part, on improvement in the compliance characteristics of the arterial circulation.

SUGGESTED READING

1. Boudoulas H, Toutouzas P, Wooley CF. *Functional Abnormalities of the Aorta.* Armonk, NY: Futura Publishing Co Inc; 1996.
2. Glasser SP, Arnett DK, McVeigh GE, Finkelstein SM, Bank AJ, Morgan DJ, Cohn JN. Vascular compliance and cardiovascular disease: a risk factor or a marker? *Am J Hypertens.* 1997;10:1175–1189.
3. Kelly R, Hayward C, Avolio A, O'Rourke M. Noninvasive determination of age-related changes in the human arterial pulse. *Circulation.* 1989;80:1652–1659.
4. Lee RT, Kamm RD. Vascular mechanics for the cardiologist. *J Am Coll Cardiol.* 1994;23:1289–1295.
5. McVeigh GE, Bank AJ, Cohn JM. Vascular compliance. In: Willerson JT, Cohn JN, eds. *Cardiovascular Medicine.* New York, NY: Churchill Livingstone; 1995: 1212–1227.
6. McVeigh GE, Burns DE, Finkelstein SM, McDonald KM, Mock JE, Feske W, Carlyle PF, Flack J, Grimm R, Cohn JN. Reduced vascular compliance as a marker for essential hypertension. *Am J Hypertens.* 1991;4:245–251.
7. Murgo JP, Westerhof N, Giolma JP, Altobelli SA. Aortic input impedance in normal man: relationship to pressure waveforms. *Circulation.* 1980;62:105–116.
8. Safar ME, Frohlich ED. The arterial system in hypertension: a prospective view. *Hypertension.* 1995;26:10–14.
9. Simon A, Megnien JL, Levenson J. Detection of preclinical atherosclerosis may optimize the management of hypertension. *Am J Hypertens.* 1997;10:813–824.

Chapter 115

Evaluation of Aortocarotid Baroreflexes

Addison Taylor, MD, PhD

KEY POINTS

- Hypertension leads to baroreceptor resetting, blunted baroreflex control of the blood pressure, and increased blood pressure variability.

- Autonomic failure is associated with wide fluctuations in blood pressure, usually manifest as supine hypertension and orthostatic hypotension.

- Exaggerated baroreflex responses in the carotid sinus hypersensitivity syndrome can cause bradycardia, excessive vasodilation, or syncope.

- Diagnosis of autonomic dysfunction in patients with hypertension or orthostatic hypotension and syncope can improve therapeutic management.

See also Chapters 34, 135, 136

The autonomic nervous system, through its sympathetic and parasympathetic divisions, modulates rapid adaptation of the cardiovascular system to changing conditions. This system is intimately involved in the maintenance of normal blood pressure during posture or temperature changes, metabolic alterations, or other environmental stresses. Precise cardiovascular regulation is achieved through a series of highly differentiated but closely integrated reflex arcs, including the aortocarotid, or high-pressure, and cardiopulmonary, or low-pressure, baroreflex arcs.

A number of factors modulate the cardiovascular response to baroreflex activation. These include the following: (1) origin and strength of the activating stimulus, (2) the "set point" of the reflex, (3) neuronal input from the hypothalamus and higher cortical centers as well as input from brainstem centers that modulate other autonomic functions such as respiration and gastrointestinal motility, (4) the state of responsiveness of the cardiovascular structures or their receptors that mediate the response to nerve stimulation, (5) the modulatory influence of neurohumoral and vasoactive substances (catecholamines, angiotensin, prostanoids, neuropeptides, etc), and (6) interactions of aortocarotid with baroreflex and chemoreflex arcs.

Assessment of Baroreflex Function

A variety of physiological and pharmacological maneuvers have been used to characterize the cardiovascular responses to autonomic reflex activation in normal subjects and to evaluate the integrity of the autonomic cardiovascular reflexes in patients with specific cardiovascular diseases. Some of the maneuvers and their effects on baroreflexes are summarized in **Table 115.1.**

Baroreceptor sensitivity is usually defined as a change in the R-R interval (reciprocal of the heart rate) on the ECG plotted as a function of the change in blood pressure during the preceding cardiac cycle. Although a quantitative assessment of baroreceptor sensitivity requires continuous monitoring of the ECG and intra-arterial pressure, a qualitative assessment of baroreflex arc integrity can be obtained at the bedside by measurement of the change in heart rate from baseline during the Valsalva maneuver for 15 seconds. The heart rate usually increases 10 to 30 bpm by the end of the 15-second Valsalva maneuver.

Blood pressure and heart rate are the hemodynamic parameters usually monitored at the bedside to assess the effects of autonomic reflex activation. However, a more comprehensive evaluation is obtained if one or more of the following hemodynamic measurements are also included: cardiac output, cardiac contractility, venous capacitance, peripheral and central venous pressure, or limb (forearm or leg) blood flow. Direct measurements of peripheral muscle sympathetic nerve firing rates in the arm or leg by microneurographic techniques provide a useful adjunct to these cardiovascular measures in the research laboratory but are limited to studies of sympathetic neural activity in specific vascular beds. Power spectral analysis of heart rate variability or arterial pressure signals provides an indirect assessment of changes in autonomic function, but there is significant controversy about which (if any) components of cardiovascular autonomic function are actually represented by low- versus high-frequency power spectra. Assessment of systemic and regional norepinephrine spillover rates, plasma norepinephrine and epinephrine concentrations, plasma renin activity, plasma angiotensin II concentrations, plasma arginine vasopressin, plasma atrial natriuretic peptides, and measurements of adrenergic receptor number or affinity offer additional although indirect information about the neurohormonal consequences of autonomic reflex activation.

Changes in arterial high-pressure baroreceptor activity can be induced by any physiological or pharmacological maneuver that produces an abrupt increase or decrease in blood pressure (**Table 115.1**). For example, the transient hypotension that occurs with standing or passive tilt results in a reflex increase in heart rate, whereas the post-Valsalva increase in blood pressure causes reflex slowing. Such drugs as α-adrenergic agonists or angiotensin II, which increase blood pressure by vasoconstriction, produce reflex slowing of the heart rate, whereas such agents as sodium nitroprusside or hydralazine that vasodilate augment sympathetic efferent nerve activity, heart rate, and cardiac contractility.

Because baroreceptor sensitivity decreases with age, the baroreceptor response obtained in a patient with suspected autonomic abnormalities should be compared with the response obtained in normal subjects of comparable age. Maneuvers, such as neck suction or neck pressure, that alter the transmural pressure or stretch in the carotid sinus can also be used to activate or deactivate arterial baroreceptor reflexes (**Table 115.1**).

Clinical Conditions Associated With Aortocarotid Baroreflex Abnormalities
Impaired Aortocarotid Baroreflex Function

Aortocarotid baroreflex abnormalities have been documented in a wide variety of clinical conditions in which autonomic neuronal control of blood pressure is altered. Some of the more common conditions are summarized in **Table 115.2.** Many of these conditions,

Table 115.1. Physiological and Pharmacological Maneuvers That Modulate Autonomic Cardiovascular Reflexes in Humans

ARTERIAL BAROREFLEXES	
ACTIVATE	**DEACTIVATE**
Neck Pressure	Neck Suction
Phenylephrine	Nitroglycerin
Angiotensin II	Amyl nitrite
Valsalva, phase IV	Nitroprusside

Table 115.2. Selected Clinical Conditions Associated With Autonomic Dysfunction

Neurological diseases	Drugs/toxins
Friedreich's ataxia	α-Adrenergic agonists
Guillain-Barré syndrome	β-Adrenergic agonists
Parkinson's disease	Cocaine
Central Nervous System	Amphetamines
Demyelinating Disease	Endotoxin shock
Syringomyelia	Certain snake venoms
Multiple-system atrophy	Familial dysautonomia
Endocrine/metabolic diseases	Cigarette smoking
Diabetes mellitus	**Neoplastic diseases**
Hyperthyroidism	Spinal meningiomas
Fabry's disease	Brainstem meningiomas
Cardiovascular conditions	Systemic mastocytosis
Hypertension	**Trauma**
Congestive Heart Failure	Spinal cord transection
Myocardial infarction	Neurocardiogenic syncope
Mitral valve prolapse	**Psychiatric diseases**
Genetic diseases	Panic disorder
Familial dysautonomia	Agoraphobia
Dopamine β-hydroxylase	**Environmental**
deficiency	Microgravity (space)
Primary/unknown	Prolonged bed rest
Carotid sinus hypersensitivity	
Idiopathic orthostatic hypotension	
Baroreceptor failure	

most notably idiopathic orthostatic hypotension, multiple-system atrophy, Shy-Drager syndrome, and diabetes mellitus, are characterized by orthostatic lightheadedness, weakness, or syncope due to interruption of the high-pressure baroreflex arc by the underlying disease.

If the disease affects primarily the postganglionic nerve, as in diabetes mellitus or amyloidosis, supine resting plasma norepinephrine concentrations are reduced and do not increase with standing (a stimulus that usually increases plasma norepinephrine by 50% to 100% above the supine value). Patients with autonomic insufficiency also demonstrate increased pressor sensitivity to α-adrenergic agonists (phenylephrine) due to vascular α-receptor upregulation.

When the disease affects primarily the preganglionic sympathetic nerve, as in multiple-system atrophy, supine values for plasma norepinephrine are normal but there is no increase with standing, because the aortocarotid baroreflex arc is interrupted within the central nervous system. Since there is normal basal release of norepinephrine from the intact postganglionic nerve, vascular α-receptors are normally sensitive to α-agonists.

Identification of the site of baroreflex dysfunction has therapeutic implications. For example, orthostatic hypotension in patients with preganglionic disease often improves with a high-tyramine diet. Monoamine oxidase inhibitors can increase norepinephrine release from the normal postganglionic nerve and decrease its metabolism in the synaptic cleft in these patients. Conversely, patients with diseases involving the postganglionic nerve may respond best to α-agonists, such as phenylpropylamine, clonidine, or midodrine. All patients, regardless of the site of baroreflex dysfunction, require fluid volume expansion with a high-salt diet, often combined with fludrocortisone.

Carotid Sinus Hypersensitivity

Orthostatic lightheadedness, weakness, or syncope may also occur in patients with exaggerated activity of the aortocarotid baroreflex. This condition, called carotid sinus hypersensitivity, is characterized by hypotension and syncope or near-syncope due to mechanical deformation of the carotid sinus located at the bifurcation of the common carotid artery. Symptoms may be produced by lateral rotation or hyperextension of the neck or by garments with tight-fitting collars that impinge on the carotid arteries. The condition has also been observed in patients with tumors of the neck that impinge on the carotid artery or encircle the glossopharyngeal or vagus nerves and in patients with extensive scarring in the neck secondary to radical neck dissection or radiation fibrosis. In the majority of these patients, however, there is no obvious cause for the condition, although it tends to occur more frequently in the elderly. It has recently been noted that a majority of patients with carotid sinus sensitivity have concomitant denervation of the sternocleidomastoid muscle, but the pathophysiological significance of this observation is not yet clear.

The diagnosis is established by demonstrating that massage of one carotid sinus for 5 to 10 seconds produces a fall of >50 mm Hg in the blood pressure or a sinus pause of >3 seconds accompanied by near-syncopal or syncopal symptoms. Three different types of carotid sinus syndrome have been noted and form the basis of the classification of this syndrome into the cardioinhibitory type (bradycardia only), the vasodepressor type (hypotension without bradycardia), and the mixed cardioinhibitory plus vasodepressor type. In patients who meet the criteria for cardioinhibitory carotid sinus syndrome, it is essential to repeat the carotid sinus massage after insertion of a temporary transvenous pacemaker to maintain the heart rate to exclude the possibility of a vasodepressor component that was undetected during the initial evaluation. If no significant vasodepressor component is demonstrated during carotid sinus massage with cardiac pacing, a permanent cardiac pacemaker of the dual-chamber type will usually prevent further symptoms. In the newest pacemakers, a rate-drop algorithm is incorporated into the firmware that activates the pacemaker impulse in response to a predetermined reduction in heart rate. A patient who has a significant vasodepressor component should be managed medically with elastic support garments, α-agonists, and fluid expansion in a fashion similar to that described above for orthostatic hypotension. Should this fail, surgical interruption of the carotid sinus reflex by stripping of the adventitia from the carotid artery or by transection of the glossopharyngeal nerve as it enters the brain could be considered; these procedures have been reported to prevent symptoms in a small series of patients.

SUGGESTED READING

1. Akselrod S, Oz O, Greenberg M, Keselbrener L. Autonomic response to change of posture among normal and mild-hypertensive adults: investigation by time-dependent spectral analysis. *J Auton Nerv Syst.* 1997;64:33–43.
2. Almquist A, Gornick C, Benson W Jr, Dunnigan A, Benditt DG. Carotid sinus hypersensitivity: evaluation of the vasodepressor component. *Circulation.* 1985;71: 927–936.
3. Bannister R. *Autonomic Failure: A Textbook of Clinical Disorders of the Autonomic Nervous System.* New York, NY: Oxford University Press; 1992.
4. Blanc J-J, L'Heveder GL, Mansourati J, Tea SH, Guillo P, Mabin D. Assessment of a newly recognized association: carotid sinus hypersensitivity and denervation of sternocleidomastoid muscles. *Circulation.* 1997;95:2548–2551.
5. Ewing DJ, Martyn CN, Young RJ, Clarke BF. The value of cardiovascular autonomic function tests: 10 years experience in diabetes. *Diabetes Care.* 1985;8:491–498.
6. Grubb BP, Olshansky B. *Syncope: Mechanisms and Management.* Armonk, NY: Futura Publishing; 1997.
7. Lye M, Vargas E, Faragher EB, Davies I, Goddard C. Haemodynamic and neurohumoral responses in elderly patients with postural hypotension. *Eur J Clin Invest.* 1990;20:90–96.
8. Manolis AS, Linzer M, Salem D, Estes NA III. Syncope: current diagnostic evaluation and management. *Ann Intern Med.* 1990;112:850–863.
9. Robertson D, Low PA, Polinsky RJ. *Primer on the Autonomic Nervous System.* San Diego, Calif: Academic Press; 1996.
10. Schellack J, Fulenwider JT, Olson RA, Smith RB III, Mansour K. The carotid sinus syndrome: a frequently overlooked cause of syncope in the elderly. *J Vasc Surg.* 1986;4:376–383.

Approach to Treatment of the Hypertensive Patient

Ray W. Gifford, Jr, MD

KEY POINTS

- The goal of antihypertensive therapy is to reduce cardiovascular morbidity and mortality and to prolong useful life by the least intrusive means possible.

- In selecting the initial drug, the sixth report of the Joint National Committee on Prevention, Detection, Evaluation, and Treatment of High Blood Pressure (JNC-VI) recommends that diuretics, β-adrenergic blockers, ACE inhibitors, calcium antagonists, selective α_1-adrenergic antagonists, α,β-blockers, or angiotensin II receptor blockers are appropriate choices.

- JNC-VI stated that preference be given to a diuretic or a β-blocker in uncomplicated cases because of their proven ability in randomized clinical trials to decrease cardiovascular morbidity and mortality.

- Other factors to be considered in selecting the appropriate drug for initial therapy include presence or absence of other risk factors or target-organ damage, demographics such as race and age, concomitant but unrelated symptoms or diseases, quality of life, and cost.

See also Chapters 117, 118, 121, 152

The goal of antihypertensive therapy is to reduce cardiovascular (CV) morbidity and mortality and to prolong useful life by the least intrusive means possible. There is abundant evidence from randomized, controlled trials that reduction of blood pressure (BP) by pharmacological therapy will reduce fatal and nonfatal CV events, including stroke, myocardial infarction, heart failure, and renal failure. No long-term trials have been designed to demonstrate similar benefits for lifestyle modifications (nonpharmacological therapy). Nevertheless, the sixth report of the Joint National Committee on Prevention, Detection, Evaluation, and Treatment of High Blood Pressure (JNC-VI, 1997) advocates lifestyle modifications as the first approach for most patients with uncomplicated stage 1 hypertension (systolic BP, 140 to 159 mm Hg; diastolic BP, 90 to 99 mm Hg). If target-organ damage (TOD) or diabetes is present (**Table 116.1**), however, pharmacological therapy is indicated.

Lifestyle Modifications (Nonpharmacological Therapy)

For many patients, the lifestyle modifications recommended to control high BP and concomitant risk factors can be intrusive and detract from quality and enjoyment of life to such an extent that adherence is often difficult to achieve. Conversely, these approaches are safe and relatively inexpensive, have been effective in reducing BP in short-term trials, and may obviate the need for drug therapy (**Table 116.2**).

Dietary modifications are more likely to succeed if patients are counseled initially and at regular intervals by a dietitian or nutritionist. Psychological counseling is often helpful for patients who must moderate their ethanol consumption or stop smoking. Nicotine chewing gum and patches often fail without simultaneous counseling.

When lifestyle modifications are prescribed as initial therapy, the patient should understand that drug treatment will be necessary if BP is not reduced to or toward a desirable range (usually <135/85 mm Hg) within 3 to 6 months. During this period, patients should be seen in the office at least every 2 months for the physician to monitor BP and adherence to the regimen and to reinforce the importance of the lifestyle modifications. If at the end of 6 months no progress has been made in reducing BP, drug therapy should be strongly advised. Too often, promises by nonadherent patients to do better in the future lead to indefinite postponement of drug therapy, to the detriment of the patient.

Appropriate lifestyle modifications should be advised for all hypertensive patients, even if drug treatment is also indicated. Adherence to hygienic measures will minimize the doses and numbers of drugs required to control BP and will ultimately enhance the chances for success of step-down therapy after the BP has been well controlled for ≥1 year. In the Trial of Mild Hypertension Study (TOMHS), lifestyle modifications alone reduced average BP from 141/91 to 134/82 mm Hg for 234 participants after 4 years.

Lifestyle modifications are also recommended for persons with high normal BP (diastolic BP, 85 to 89 mm Hg; systolic BP, 130 to 139 mm Hg) in an effort to keep the BP from rising into a definitely hypertensive range. The exception is some patients in risk category C, for whom drug treatment is also indicated (**Table 116.1**).

Pharmacological Therapy

For patients with stage 1 hypertension in risk group A, pharmacological therapy should be prescribed if BP is not normalized by lifestyle modifications within 12 months, or sooner if no progress has been made after 3 to 6 months. For patients with stage 1 hypertension

Table 116.1. Risk Stratification and Treatment

BP STAGES, MM HG	RISK GROUP		
	A: NO RISK FACTORS; NO TOD/CCD*	B: AT LEAST ONE RISK FACTOR, NOT INCLUDING DIABETES MELLITUS; NO TOD/CCD*	C: TOD/CCD* AND/OR DIABETES, WITH OR WITHOUT OTHER RISK FACTORS
High normal (130–139/85–89)	Lifestyle modification	Lifestyle modification	Drug therapy‡
Stage 1 (140–150/90–99)	Lifestyle modification (up to 12 months)	Lifestyle modification† (up to 6 months)	Drug therapy
Stages 2 and 3 (≥160/≥100)	Drug therapy	Drug therapy	Drug therapy

For example: A patient with diabetes and a BP of 142/94 mm Hg plus left ventricular hypertrophy (LVH) should be classified as having stage 1 hypertension with TOD (LVH) and with another major risk factor (diabetes). This patient would be categorized as stage 1, risk group C and recommended for immediate initiation of pharmacological treatment. Lifestyle modification should be adjunctive therapy for all patients recommended for pharmacological therapy.
* TOD/CCD indicates target-organ damage/clinical cardiovascular disease.
† For patients with multiple risk factors, clinicians should consider drugs as initial therapy plus lifestyle modifications.
‡ For those with heart failure or renal disease or diabetes.
Adapted from JNC-VI with permission.

Table 116.2. Lifestyle Modifications Advocated for Managing Hypertension as Either Definitive or Adjunctive Treatment

Effective in reducing BP (listed in approximate order of effectiveness)
1. Weight reduction by at least 10 lb (preferably more) for patients >10% above ideal body weight
2. Limitation of alcohol intake to 1 oz (30 mL) of ethanol daily (equivalent to 2 oz of 100-proof whiskey, 10 oz of wine, or 24 oz of beer; < 0.5 oz ethanol (15 mL) for women and lighter-weight men.
3. Limitation of dietary sodium to <2.4 g daily (equivalent to 6 g sodium chloride)
4. Aerobic exercise (brisk walking for 30 to 45 minutes 3 to 5 times a week has been shown to be beneficial in reducing blood pressure modestly)
5. Adequate potassium intake (≥ 90 mmol/d)
Not demonstrated to be effective in reducing BP
1. Supplements of calcium, magnesium, fish oil*
2. Stress management
3. Macronutrients
4. Garlic and onion
Effective for reducing cardiovascular risk but not for reducing BP
1. Tobacco avoidance
2. Reduction of dietary saturated fat and cholesterol

*Although dietary supplements of calcium and magnesium, have not been shown to reduce blood pressure for hypertensive patients, deficiency of these minerals might result in elevated blood pressure, so minimal daily requirements are recommended.

in risk group B, a trial of no more than 6 months of lifestyle modifications should be permitted before antihypertensive drug therapy is initiated. Drug treatment may be indicated initially, along with lifestyle modifications, for patients who have multiple risk factors. Pharmacological therapy should be prescribed from the outset (along with lifestyle modifications) for patients with stage 2 or 3 hypertension, and in risk group C, even for those who have high normal BP if they also have diabetes mellitus, heart failure, or renal disease.

Systolic Hypertension

The Systolic Hypertension in the Elderly Program (SHEP) showed that morbidity and mortality (including stroke, coronary events, and heart failure) are reduced when patients >60 years old with systolic BP ≥160 mm Hg and diastolic BP <90 mm Hg are effectively treated. In SHEP, a diuretic and a β-blocker, if necessary were compared with placebo in a double-blind trial. Benefit was equally evident for patients >80 years old and for those <80 years old. A comparable placebo-controlled trial in Europe (SYST-EUR) using nitrendipine, a dihydropyridine calcium antagonist not available in the United States, showed a statistically significant reduction in stroke events in elderly patients with isolated systolic hypertension.

Initial Therapy

The algorithm suggested in JNC-VI for managing hypertension is shown in the **Figure 116.1.** In selecting the initial drug, JNC-VI recommended that preference be given to a diuretic or a β-blocker because these were used in randomized, controlled trials demonstrating decreased CV morbidity and mortality with these agents. JNC-VI also stated that other classes of antihypertensive agents should be selected if there are special indications for them in a given patient (eg, ACE inhibitors in heart failure or diabetic nephropathy), if there is a contraindication to diuretics and β-blockers, or if these agents are ineffective or poorly tolerated.

Factors to be considered in selecting the appropriate drug for initial therapy include presence or absence of clinical CV disease or TOD, demographics such as race and age, concomitant but unrelated symptoms or diseases, quality of life, and cost. There is no evidence of gender differences in response to antihypertensive drugs.

The reliability of measurements of hemodynamic or biochemical parameters such as plasma catecholamines or plasma renin activity has not been great enough to justify their routine use in selection of the appropriate initial drug. Our desire to prospectively select the best drug for a given patient exceeds our ability to do so. At best, it is an educated guess. Guidelines are imprecise, are subject to revision as new data become available, and should not contravene the physi-

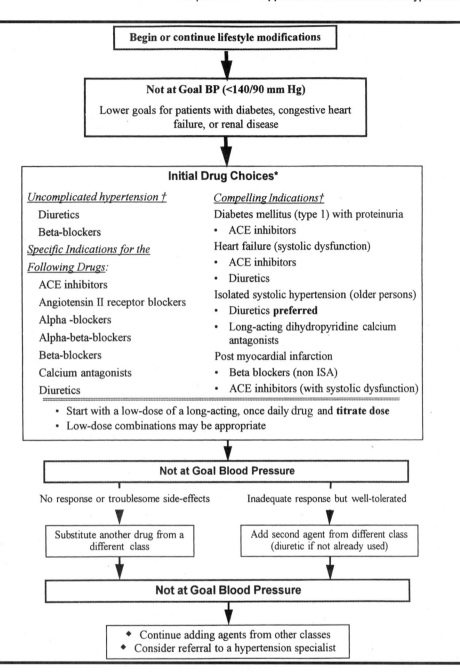

Figure 116.1. Algorithm for the treatment of hypertension. ISA indicates intrinsic sympathomimetic activity. *Unless contraindicated. †Based on randomized controlled trials. Adapted from Joint National Committee. The sixth report of the Joint National Committee on the Prevention, Detection, Evaluation and Treatment of High Blood Pressure (JNC-VI). *Arch Intern Med.* 1997;157:2413–2446.

cian's best judgment in selecting the appropriate agent to initiate therapy.

The "two-for-one" concept, in which a drug is selected not only for its effect on BP but also for its benefit on coexisting diseases or symptoms, should be given high priority. Examples include β-blockers or calcium antagonists for hypertensive patients with angina pectoris, β-blockers for hypertensive patients with migraine headache or senile tremor, ACE inhibitors for hypertensive patients with heart failure, β-blockers or nondihydropyridine calcium antagonists for hypertensive patients with atrial fibrillation (to slow ventricular rate),

thiazide diuretics for patients with osteoporosis, and selective α_1-adrenergic blocking agents for hypertensive men with symptomatic benign prostatic hypertrophy.

The algorithm **(Figure 116.1)** provides two options if the initial drug in optimal doses is suboptimally effective or poorly tolerated: (1) Substitute another agent for the first drug (sequential monotherapy). This would be particularly appropriate if the initial drug was ineffective or caused adverse effects. (2) Add a second agent from a different class (stepped care). This option might be selected if the first drug was partially effective but well tolerated.

Usually it is preferable to start treatment with a single agent or low-dose combination and to change the regimen as described above only if BP is not controlled after 2 to 4 months. However, when diastolic BP is ≥120 mm Hg and/or systolic BP is ≥200 mm Hg, or if TOD is present, it is preferable to accelerate the process by making changes in the regimen every 2 or 3 weeks or to start with two drugs at once in combination or separate tablets. When diastolic BP is ≥130 mm Hg and/or systolic BP is ≥220 mm Hg, it may be advisable to initiate treatment with three drugs, and if TOD is present, referral to a specialist and/or hospitalization may be indicated.

Once hypertension has been controlled, follow-up visits are indicated 3 to 4 times a year for most patients.

Step-Down Therapy

After BP has been controlled effectively (eg, <135/85 mm Hg) for more than 1 year (and at least 4 consecutive office visits), it is reasonable to reduce doses or numbers of drugs. The clinician should proceed in a slow, deliberate fashion, monitoring the BP frequently, preferably at home as well as during office visits. Step-down therapy is more likely to succeed in patients who adhere to lifestyle modifications than in those who do not. Therapy can be discontinued entirely only in patients who can be trusted to have their BP measured at frequent intervals and return for follow-up visits, even if they are not receiving specific therapy. All too frequently, hypertension will recur within 1 to 2 years after therapy is discontinued, and serious complications may occur if it is not detected and treated promptly.

Adherence to Regimens

The large number of drugs now available to treat hypertension makes it possible to control BP with minimal adverse effects for most patients. Nevertheless, failure to adhere to prescribed regimens is still a major obstacle to achieving better control rates.

Although patient education is essential, even more important is a kind, sympathetic, and understanding attitude by the physician and his or her staff. The patient must be given the necessary time to discuss side effects and ask questions. Clinicians must be willing to alter regimens when necessary to minimize side effects. Every office visit should be an opportunity to educate the patient about his or her disease and the importance of treatment. These visits should offer a relaxed interchange between patient and health care provider that is so essential to promoting adherence. Other health professionals can play a significant role in office management of hypertensive patients. Finally, home monitoring of BP is helpful in fostering adherence and minimizing the frequency of office visits in many patients.

J Curve

Retrospective analyses of nonrandomized studies and randomized trials not originally designed to test the hypothesis have prompted concern that "excessive" reduction of diastolic BP, usually to levels <85 mm Hg, paradoxically increases coronary mortality. This phenomenon is described as the J- or U-shaped curve, because mortality rises as diastolic BP is reduced to <85 mm Hg. No J curve has been described for stroke mortality or for renal failure; in fact, it seems that maximal protection against stroke and renal failure may require reducing diastolic BP to <80 mm Hg.

The J curve has also been described for hypertensive patients on no treatment or on placebo, so it does not seem to be related to drug therapy. Moreover, J curves have been described for serum cholesterol, serum triglycerides, serum creatinine, and body weight. A rational explanation is that sick people approaching death tend to have low lipids and body weight, as well as low BP.

In contrast to diastolic BP, there is no J curve for systolic BP and any adverse outcome. Because cardiac work and myocardial oxygen consumption are proportionally reduced as systolic BP is reduced, it is reasonable to assume that one need not be concerned about the J curve if systolic BP is well controlled. Practically, if systolic BP is well controlled (eg, <130 mm Hg), there is not much to be gained by reducing diastolic BP to <80 to 85 mm Hg.

Additional Risk Factors

Hypertension is frequently found in association with other potentially treatable CV risk factors, including dyslipidemia, cigarette smoking, diabetes mellitus, obesity, and a sedentary lifestyle. If the goal of antihypertensive therapy is to reduce the risk of CV morbidity and mortality, the physician must identify and treat all other risk factors for the full benefits of antihypertensive treatment to be realized.

It is gratifying to realize that in the 25 years since the inception of the National High Blood Pressure Education Program in 1972, the mortality rate for coronary disease in the United States has decreased by 53% and the mortality rate for stroke has decreased by almost 60%. But there is still a large opportunity for improvement. According to the National Health and Nutrition Examination Survey of 1991–1994 (NHANES III Phase II), only 27.4% of the 50 million people in the United States with hypertension (≥140/90 mm Hg) have their BPs controlled to <140/90 mm Hg; this goal is probably not low enough.

SUGGESTED READING

1. Fletcher AE, Bulpitt CJ. How far should blood pressure be lowered? *N Engl J Med.* 1992;326:251–254.
2. Gueyffier F, Boutitie F, Boissel JP, et al. Effect of antihypertensive drug treatment on cardiovascular outcomes in women and men: a meta-analysis of individual patient data from randomized, controlled trials. The INDANA Investigators. *Ann Intern Med.* 1997;126:761–767.
3. Joint National Committee. The sixth report of the Joint National Committee on the Prevention, Detection, Evaluation and Treatment of High Blood Pressure (JNC-VI). *Arch Intern Med.* 1997;157:2413–2446.
4. Kaplan NM, Gifford RW Jr. Choice of initial therapy for hypertension. *JAMA.* 1996;275:1577–1580.
5. MacMahon S, Neal B, Rodgers A. Blood pressure lowering for the primary and secondary prevention of coronary and cerebrovascular disease. *Schweiz Med Wochenschr.* 1995;125:2479–2486.
6. Materson BJ, Reda DJ, Cushman WC. Department of Veterans Affairs single-drug therapy of hypertension study: revised figures and new data. Department of Veterans Affairs Cooperative Study Group on Antihypertensive Agents. *Am J Hypertens.* 1995;8:189–192.
7. Neaton JD, Grimm RH Jr, Prineas RJ, et al. Treatment of Mild Hypertension Study: final results. *JAMA.* 1993;270:713–724.
8. Psaty BM, Smith NL, Siscovick DS, et al. Health outcomes associated with antihypertensive therapies used as first-line agents: a systematic review and meta-analysis. *JAMA.* 1997;277:739–745.
9. SHEP Cooperative Research Group: Prevention of stroke by antihypertensive drug treatment in older persons with isolated systolic hypertension: final report of the Systolic Hypertension in the Elderly Program (SHEP). *JAMA.* 1991;265:3255–3264.
10. Staessen J, Fagard R, Thijs L. Morbidity and mortality in the placebo-controlled European Trial on Isolated Systolic Hypertension in the Elderly. *Lancet.* 1997;350:757–764.

Chapter 117

Treatment Goals in the Hypertensive Patient

Kenneth Jamerson, MD

KEY POINTS

- The target for achieving acceptable blood pressure control in a general population of hypertensive subjects is <149/90 mm Hg. Optimal BP control in the general population may be 138/83 at least according to one large clinical trial. Older persons with hypertension should be treated to a level of 140/90 mm Hg; however, an interim target of 160/90 mm Hg may be useful.

- Patients with diabetes should have control of their blood pressure to 130/85 mm Hg.

- Patients with hypertension and renal insufficiency should be treated to a goal of 130/85 mm Hg; those with >1 g/d of proteinuria should be treated to 120/75 mm Hg.

- Blacks with hypertension should have as their goal the normalization of blood pressure (130/85 mm Hg).

See also Chapters 116, 118, 121

Target for Optimal Control in a General Population of Hypertensive Subjects

The ultimate goal of controlling blood pressure is to reduce cardiovascular morbidity and mortality. The optimal blood pressure target to aim for in a general hypertensive population is not known. A consensus target of 140/90 mm Hg is based partly on epidemiological data, which demonstrated substantially higher risk above that level. It would appear, however, from the epidemiological data that the lower the blood pressure is, the better. There is, unfortunately, a paucity of data derived from clinical trials demonstrating that lowering blood pressure with antihypertensive medication to levels <140/90 mm Hg imparts improved or optimal cardiovascular protection. The majority of clinical data come from the subanalysis of clinical trials rather than prospective studies with adequate power and firm results from which therapeutic decisions can be made.

In a secondary analysis of the Treatment of Mild Hypertension Study (TOMHS), the investigators found a 20% improvement in cardiovascular end points in subjects who achieved a systolic blood pressure (SBP) of <126 mm Hg compared with those with an SBP of >132 mm Hg. There was not adequate statistical power in the secondary analyses, however, to provide firm treatment recommendations for a general hypertensive population. The secondary analyses of several clinical trials converge to suggest that aggressive blood pressure control (levels <140/90 mm Hg) may be beneficial, particularly for some subpopulations of hypertensive subjects.

Blood Pressure Targets in Subjects With Renal Insufficiency

In a secondary analysis of a study to determine whether captopril was beneficial for preserving renal function in subjects with type I diabetes, Lewis et al found an association between low blood pressure (120/75 mm Hg) and the prevention of decline in renal function. The data are not as clear for aggressive blood pressure control in subjects with hypertensive nephropathy.

The Medical Diet and Renal Disease (MDRD) Study provides evidence that hypertensive end-stage renal disease may benefit from aggressive blood pressure control. In subjects who attained the aggressive blood pressure control target, a mean arterial blood pressure (MAP) of 92 mm Hg (≤130/75 mm Hg), the rate in decline in renal function was reduced by 50% compared with the usual group, MAP of 102 to 107 (140/90 mm Hg). There was not enough statistical power in this trial to make clinical recommendations on the benefits of aggressive blood pressure control for the progression of renal dysfunction in hypertensive subjects. The significant improvement in renal function in this analysis provides a foundation for the consensus recommendation that control of blood pressure to 130/85 mm Hg (the target espoused by the Sixth Joint National Committee on the Prevention, Detection, and Treatment of Hypertension) may be renoprotective in hypertensive subjects with impaired renal function. A blood pressure level of 120/75 mm Hg is recommended for subjects with renal impairment and proteinuria of >1 g/d.

Optimal Blood Pressure Targets in Blacks

Renal failure secondary to essential hypertension occurs more frequently in blacks. The US Renal Data Registry has provided sound estimates demonstrating that within the age group 33 to 45 years, there is an 18-fold increase in hypertensive renal disease in blacks compared with their white counterparts. There is evidence from the Multiple Risk Factor Intervention Trial that renal function in blacks may not improve and may in fact progress even when the same level of blood pressure control is achieved as in white subjects.

The most effective drug regimen and appropriate blood pressure target to aim for in halting the progression to end-stage renal disease in blacks will be determined from the results of the African American Study of Kidney Disease and Hypertension (AASK). The study drugs are amlodipine, metoprolol, and ramipril. Preliminary data from this study confirm that aggressive blood pressure control is not deleterious to renal function. The final analyses from AASK on the benefits of lowering blood pressure for protecting renal function will not be available until 2002.

Current treatment strategies of targeting 140/90 mm Hg for control have been inadequate in stemming the near-epidemic rise in hypertensive end-stage renal disease in blacks. Blacks have significantly higher rates of congestive heart failure, stroke, and all-cause cardiovascular mortality. Preliminary clinical evidence shows that aggressive treatment of blood pressure may result in better target-organ protection. It seems judicious to target normalization of blood pressure to 130/85 mm Hg in this population, considering their high risk for hypertensive complications.

Hypertension Control in Older Subjects

Subjects in the Systolic Hypertension in the Elderly Program (SHEP) were randomized to treatment of isolated systolic hypertension with low-dose diuretics, followed by β-blockers or reserpine versus placebo. The goal of therapy was to reduce SBP to 160 mm Hg. There was a clear cardiovascular benefit in the active-treatment group. Furthermore, in subjects in whom SBP was reduced further, there appeared to be cardiovascular benefits to SBP levels as low as 120 mm Hg. Thus, in a cohort of elderly hypertensive subjects, the main results and secondary analyses of SHEP would suggest that the lower the SBP, the better.

Are There Any Deleterious Effects to Lowering Blood Pressure Too Far?

In theory, it is possible that aggressive lowering of blood pressure could exacerbate ischemic events rather than providing protection. The "J-curve" hypothesis is espoused most often in subjects with coronary artery disease who have very low diastolic blood pressures. The lack of perfusion through stenotic vessels during diastole is thought to incite ischemic events. In several retrospective analyses of clinical trials, there has been some evidence that coronary heart disease events increase when the diastolic blood pressure falls below 85 mm Hg.

The Hypertension Optimal Treatment (HOT) trial in more than 18000 subjects demonstrated that lowering BP to 138/83 is safe and that morbidity and mortality were further reduced by aspirin 75 mg/d. Major cardiovascular events were reduced by 30%, but this reduction did not achieve statistical significance. Lowering BP to a diastolic level of 70 mm Hg is safe but no additional cardiovascular benefit could be demonstrated. In subjects with diabetes, there was a statistically significant 52% reduction in major cardiovascular events and nonfatal stroke; cardiovascular mortality was reduced by more than 60%. Subjects in the HOT study with a history of ischemic heart disease showed no J-curve in regard to lowering BP and demonstrated a 43% reduction in stroke. Major cardiovascular events were 20% less when the diastolic BP target was <80 mm Hg compared with the <90 mm Hg group. The rate of cardiovascular events observed during the HOT study was much lower than that observed in previous prospective trials. The aggressive lowering of BP may be in part responsible for the lower mortality, yet the impact of improved treatment of other cormorbidities over the years. The effects of improved treatment cormorbidities, ie. cholesterol, may also contribute to improved mortality.

SUGGESTED READING

1. Collins R, MacMahon S. Blood pressure, antihypertensive drug treatment, and the risks of stroke and of coronary heart disease. *Br Med Bull.* 1994;50:272–298.
2. Farnett L, Mulrow CD, Linn WD, Lucey CR, Tuley MR. The J-curve phenomenon and the treatment of hypertension: is there a point beyond which pressure reduction is dangerous? *JAMA.* 1991;265:489–495.
3. Fogo A, Smith MC, Cleveland W, Deburge J, Agodoa L, for the ASSK Pilot Investigators. Renal biopsy findings in the African-American Study of Kidney Disease (AASK). *J Am Soc Nephrol.* 1994;5:560. Abstract.
4. Jamerson KA. Prevalence of complications and response to different treatments of hypertension in African Americans and white Americans in the US. *Clin Exp Hypertens.* 1993;15:979–995.
5. Klag MJ, Whelton PK, Randall BL, Neaton JD, Brancati FL, Stamler J. End-stage renal disease in African-American and white men: 16-year MRFIT findings. *JAMA.* 1997;277:1293–1298.
6. Lazarus JM, Bourgoignie JJ, Buckalew VM, Greene T, Levey AS, Milas NC, Paranandi L, Peterson JC, Porush JG, Rauch S, Soucie JM, Stollar C, for the Modification of Diet in Renal Disease Study Group. Achievement and safety of a low blood pressure goal in chronic renal disease. *Hypertension.* 1997;29:641–650.
7. Lewis EJ, Hunsicker LG, Bain RP, Rohde RD, for the Collaborative Study Group. The effect of angiotensin-converting-enzyme inhibition on diabetic nephropathy. *N Engl J Med.* 1993;329:1456–1462.
8. Liebson PR, Grandits GA, Dianzumba S, Prineas RJ, Grimm RH, Neaton JD, Stamler J, for the Treatment of Hypertension Study Research Group. Comparison of five antihypertensive monotherapies and placebo for change in left ventricular mass in patients receiving nutritional-hygienic therapy in the Treatment of Mild Hypertension Study (TOMHS). *Circulation.* 1995;91:698–670.
9. Systolic Hypertension in the Elderly Program Cooperative Research Group. Implications of the Systolic Hypertension in the Elderly Program. *Hypertension.* 1993;21:335–343.
10. US Renal Data System. *USRDS 1997 Annual Report.* Bethesda, Md: US Department of Health and Human Services, National Institute of Diabetes and Digestive and Kidney Disease; 1997.

Chapter 118

Lifestyle Modifications

Theodore A. Kotchen, MD; Jane Morley Kotchen, MD, MPH

KEY POINTS

- Cardiovascular disease risk factors typically cluster within individuals, and lifestyle modification should always address the overall risk of cardiovascular disease.

- On a population basis, relatively small reductions in blood pressure may significantly affect the incidence of cardiovascular disease, especially stroke.

- Strategies to decrease cardiovascular disease risk should include the following: the prevention and treatment of obesity; appropriate amounts of aerobic physical activity; an avoidance of diets high in NaCl, total fat, and/or cholesterol; meeting recommended dietary intakes for potassium, calcium, and magnesium; limiting alcohol consumption; and avoiding cigarette smoking.

See also Chapters 89, 99, 116, 117, 121

Blood pressure–associated risks are incremental over a wide range of blood pressure levels, and even among normotensive individuals, blood pressure levels are predictive of cardiovascular disease morbidity and mortality. It has been estimated that, if the diastolic blood pressure of a population were reduced by 2 mm Hg, the risk of stroke and transient ischemic attacks would be reduced by 15% and that of coronary heart disease by 6%.

Between 1971 and 1991, national health examination surveys in the United States documented a downward trend in both blood pressure levels and the prevalence of hypertension. Emphasis on adopting healthier lifestyles may have contributed to this favorable trend. Recognition of those lifestyles that most favorably impact blood pressure level has implications not only for the prevention and treatment of hypertension but also for developing population-based strategies to decrease cardiovascular disease risk by shifting the overall distribution of blood pressure values downward. Among hypertensive individuals, even when lifestyle modifications alone have not produced adequate reductions of blood pressure to avoid drug therapy, these maneuvers, if correctly applied, may reduce the number and/or dosage of antihypertensive medications required for blood pressure control.

Cardiovascular disease risk factors tend to cluster within individuals, and the presence of one or more such risk factors increases the likelihood of cardiovascular disease being expressed. Adolescents and adults with higher levels of blood pressure often have higher serum concentrations of total cholesterol, triglycerides, glucose, apolipoprotein B, and lower HDL cholesterol values. Hypertensive individuals have an increased prevalence of dyslipidemia and glucose intolerance. Data from the National Health and Nutrition Examination Survey II (NHANES II) show that 40% of adults <55 years of age with blood pressures >140/90 mm Hg have serum cholesterol concentrations >240 mg/dL, compared with a prevalence ≈50% of this found in normotensive age-matched control subjects. Likewise, of those individuals with blood cholesterol levels >240 mg/dL, ≈46% have blood pressure values >140/90 mm Hg. This clustering of risk factors within individuals is in part heritable, and resistance to insulin-stimulated glucose uptake may be the common link between hypertension and this pattern of dyslipidemia. On a practical level, the recognition that cardiovascular disease risk factors cluster within individuals has important implications for the prevention and treatment of hypertension and related cardiovascular diseases.

Body Weight

The association between obesity and hypertension has been demonstrated repeatedly. It has been estimated that as many as 60% of all hypertensives are >20% overweight. Longitudinal studies have shown a direct linear correlation between body weight and blood pressure even when salt intake is held constant. In both men and women, centrally located body fat is a more critical determinant of blood pressure elevation than is peripherally located body fat. This centripetal fat distribution is often associated with insulin resistance. In many patients, particularly during midlife, it is dangerous to ignore a 5- to 10-lb weight gain, because it may mean the patient has assumed a more sedentary lifestyle without a commensurate reduction in caloric intake. Subsequent weight gains are highly likely, and with this extra poundage, blood pressure readings assume an upward trajectory. Of note is the fact that in short-term trials in both hypertensive and normotensive individuals, even modest weight loss (a reduction of 5%) can lead to a reduction in blood pressure and an increase in insulin sensitivity. In situations in which a greater weight loss occurs (a reduction in mean body weight of 9.2 kg), 6.3 and 3.1 mm Hg changes in systolic and diastolic blood pressure, respectively, have been observed. Although a number of putative mechanisms have been proposed to explain the decrease in blood pressure with weight loss, the role of insulin resistance remains unclear in this process.

Physical Activity

Physical activity or planned exercise is an important part of any plan to prevent hypertension or reduce blood pressure. Regular aerobic physical activity can facilitate weight loss, decrease blood pressure, and reduce the overall risk of cardiovascular disease and all-cause mortality. It is likely that reducing cardiovascular disease mortality can best be accomplished by motivating the sedentary segment of the US population to perform some level of physical activity on at least a weekly basis. Further reductions in mortality may be achieved by encouraging people who are physically active occasionally to become active on a more regular basis. Sedentary individuals with normal blood pressure have a 20% to 30% increased risk of developing hypertension compared with their more active peers. For most people, blood pressure can be lowered with 30 minutes of moderately intense physical activity, such as brisk walking, 6 to 7 days a week. In instances when less time is available, then less frequent, more intense workouts are needed, such as running for 20 to 30 minutes 3 to 4 days a week. In either instance, if an exercise program is sufficiently well maintained, the long-term impact on blood pressure can be substantial.

Sodium Chloride

Both observational and interventional studies in a number of populations clearly document an association between NaCl intake and blood pressure. The effect of NaCl on blood pressure increases with age, with the level of blood pressure, and in normotensive individuals if a family history of hypertension exists. There may also be a modest association between a higher NaCl intake and raised blood pressure in children and adolescents. The Intersalt study described the relationship between blood pressure and 24-hour urine sodium excretion in >10 000 individuals at 52 centers around the world. Two principal findings of this study were that (1) a difference of 100 mEq/d in sodium intake was associated with a 3 to 6 mm Hg difference in systolic blood pressure and (2) lowering the sodium intake by 100 mEq/d attenuated the rise of systolic blood pressure by 10 mm Hg in individuals between the ages of 25 and 55 years.

Between 30% and 50% of hypertensives and a smaller percentage of normotensives are estimated to be sodium-sensitive (on the basis of results of acute sodium depletion/loading protocols) according to arbitrary criteria for defining sodium sensitivity. Low dietary intakes of potassium or calcium potentiates the effect of sodium on blood pressure, and the urine sodium/potassium ratio is a stronger correlate of blood pressure than either sodium or potassium excretion alone. Increasing clinical evidence now points to a genetic susceptibility to the effect of dietary NaCl on blood pressure.

In short-term intervention trials, the reduction of blood pressure derived from a moderate reduction in NaCl intake is relatively small. As reviewed in two recent meta-analyses, the lowering of blood pressure by reduction of NaCl intake is more evident in hypertensive than in normotensive individuals. Of note, many of the trials included in these analyses were of short duration, and the full impact of NaCl reduction on blood pressure may not have been realized, because this effect may increase over time. Nevertheless, it has been estimated that even these modest reductions of blood pressure in the population would reduce risks of stroke and coronary heart disease by 15% and 6%, respectively. In addition, moderate reduction of NaCl intake and weight loss, alone and in combination, have been shown to reduce blood pressure and attenuate the development of hypertension in adults with high-normal blood pressures.

Any population-based guidelines for an upper limit of NaCl are arbitrary and should represent a reduction that is both safe and palatable. For the general population, the American Heart Association recommends that the average daily consumption of NaCl in adults not exceed 6.0 g. There is no evidence that lowering NaCl consumption to this level poses any health risk, and this recommendation is consistent with guidelines of a number of other agencies both in the United States and abroad. Lower NaCl intakes may be recommended for hypertensive individuals, but the true risk-benefit ratio of this type of dietary manipulation is ill defined.

Potassium, Calcium, and Magnesium

Observational studies suggest inverse associations of blood pressure with dietary potassium, calcium, and magnesium consumption. For calcium, this inverse association is most convincing at low levels of calcium consumption (300 to 600 mg/d), and there is an increased prevalence of hypertension in societies consuming low-calcium or low-potassium diets. Results of two meta-analyses of available controlled clinical trials have shown that oral potassium supplements (60 to 120 mEq/d) lower both systolic and diastolic blood pressure. The magnitude of the blood pressure–lowering effect is greater in hypertensive than in nonhypertensive individuals and is more pronounced when subjects are on a high-NaCl diet. Except in patients who take a diuretic and need a potassium supplement, fruits and vegetables are the best source of this mineral. Meta-analyses suggest that calcium supplementation (1000 to 2000 mg/d) results in a small but statistically significant reduction of systolic but not of diastolic blood pressure. Despite evidence suggesting a benefit of calcium supplementation in high-risk pregnancy, results of a recent, randomized trial indicate that calcium supplementation does not prevent preeclampsia or pregnancy-associated hypertension in healthy, nulliparous women. Accordingly, calcium supplementation is not recommended as a means of controlling blood pressure or preventing its rise. Calcium intake in women, however, should be optimized to prevent osteoporosis. At best, the overall antihypertensive response to magnesium supplementation among hypertensives is small, and several trials have failed to show a significant effect of magnesium on blood pressure. Currently, no recommendation for magnesium supplementation is possible.

Overall Diet

Persons consuming vegetarian diets tend to have lower blood pressures than do nonvegetarians. The DASH (Dietary Approaches to Stop Hypertension) Trial is a randomized, multicenter study that evaluated the effects of three dietary patterns over a period of 8 weeks on blood pressure in 459 adults with high-normal blood pressure or mild hypertension. The dietary interventions were (1) normal diet, with potassium, calcium, and magnesium levels close to the 25th percentile of US consumption; (2) a diet rich in fruits and vegetables; and (3) a "combination" diet rich in fruits, vegetables, and low-fat dairy products. NaCl content was equivalent in all three diets (7.5 g/d). Systolic and diastolic blood pressures were significantly reduced by the fruit and vegetable diet (-2.8 and -1.1 mm Hg, respectively) and, compared with the control diet, were reduced to an even greater extent by the combination diet (-5.5 mm Hg and -3.0 mm Hg, respectively). Fruits and vegetables provide an enriched source of potassium, magnesium, and fiber, and dairy products are an important source of calcium. Although this study was not designed to identify the most effective dietary intervention, this trial clearly documents the importance of overall diet to blood pressure control.

Alcohol

Observational studies suggest a J-shaped relationship between alcohol consumption and blood pressure. Light drinkers have lower blood pressures than those who completely abstain from alcohol, whereas individuals who consume three or more drinks per day show a small but significant elevation of blood pressure compared with nondrinkers. In short-term studies of hypertensives, reduction of alcohol consumption has been associated with a reduction of 4 to 8 mm Hg in systolic blood pressure and a lesser reduction of diastolic pressure. Blood pressures of normotensives may also decrease in response to reduced alcohol consumption. JNC VI suggests that alcohol intake should be restricted to ≤1 oz of ethanol/d in men and 0.5 oz in women to optimize hypertension prevention efforts.

Stress

Emotional stress can raise blood pressure acutely. Chronic exposure to environmental and to occupational stress may also be associated with higher levels of blood pressure. It has been suggested that psychosocial stress contributes to the increased prevalence of hypertension among inner-city blacks. However, controlled trials of relaxation therapies have failed to document a consistent effect on blood pressure. At present, there is no compelling rationale for the use of relaxation therapies for the prevention or treatment of hypertension.

Conclusions

Lifestyle interventions for the prevention and treatment of hypertension should address overall cardiovascular risk. These include physical activity and diet. The beneficial effects of diet on blood pressure can be maximized by prevention and treatment of obesity; avoiding a high NaCl intake; ensuring adequate intakes of fruits, vegetables, and low-fat dairy products that are rich in potassium, calcium, and magnesium; and/or restricting alcohol consumption. Treatment of hypertension will often include more rigorous dietary interventions than those recommended for the general population. Additional strategies for prevention of cardiovascular disease include limitation of dietary fat to <30% of total daily caloric intake and dietary cholesterol to <300 mg/d. Finally, cigarette smoking is a powerful risk factor for cardiovascular disease and should be avoided whenever possible. The cardiovascular benefits of discontinuing tobacco use develop slowly, within a year. Those who continue to smoke may not receive the full degree of protection against cardiovascular disease from antihypertensive therapy.

SUGGESTED READING

1. Allender PS, Cutler JA, Follmann D, Cappuccio FP, Pryer J, Elliott P. Dietary calcium and blood pressure: a meta-analysis of randomized clinical trials. *Ann Intern Med.* 1996;124:825–831.
2. Appel LJ, Moore TJ, Obarzanek E, Vollmer WM, Svetkey LP, Sacks FM, Bray GA, Vogt TM, Cutler JA, Windhauser MM, Lin P-H, Karanja N, for the DASH Collaborative Research Group. A clinical trial of the effects of dietary patterns on blood pressure. *N Engl J Med.* 1997;336:1117–1124.
3. Bucher HC, Cook RJ, Guyatt GH, Lang JD, Cook DJ, Hatala R, Hunt DL. Effects of dietary calcium supplementation on blood pressure: a meta-analysis of randomized controlled trials. *JAMA.* 1996;275:1016–1022.
4. Burt VL, Whelton P, Roccella EJ, Brown C, Cutler JA, Higgins M, Horan MJ, Labarthe D. Prevalence of hypertension in the US adult population: results from the Third National Health and Nutrition Examination Survey, 1988–1991. *Hypertension.* 1995;25:305–313.
5. Cook NR, Cohen J, Hebert P, Taylor JO, Hennekens CH. Implications of small reductions in diastolic blood pressure for primary prevention. *Arch Intern Med.* 1995;155:701–709.
6. Cutler JA, Follmann D, Allender PS. Randomized trials of sodium reduction: an overview. *Am J Clin Nutr.* 1997;65(suppl):643S–651S.
7. Elliott P, Stamler J, Nichols R, Dyer AR, Stamler R, Kesteloot H, Marmot M, for the Intersalt Cooperative Research Group. Intersalt revisited: further analyses of 24-hour sodium excretion and blood pressure within and across populations. *BMJ.* 1996;312:1249–1253.
8. Midgley JP, Matthew AG, Greenwood CM, Logan AG. Effect of reduced dietary sodium on blood pressure: a meta-analysis of randomized controlled trials. *JAMA.* 1996;275:1590–1597.
9. The Trials of Hypertension Prevention Collaborative Research Group. Effects of weight loss and sodium reduction intervention on blood pressure and hypertension incidence in overweight people with high-normal blood pressure: the Trials of Hypertension Prevention, phase II. *Arch Intern Med.* 1997;157:657–667.
10. Whelton PK, He J, Cutler JA, Brancati FL, Appel LJ, Follmann D, Klag MJ. Effects of oral potassium on blood pressure: meta-analysis of randomized controlled clinical trials. *JAMA.* 1997;277:1624–1632.

Dose-Response Relationship and Dose Adjustments

Domenic A. Sica, MD; Todd W.B. Gehr, MD

KEY POINTS

- Dose-response relationships are dependent on the relationship between the pathophysiological basis for a hypertension variant and the mechanism of action for a medication.

- Several factors, most importantly physiological counterregulatory mechanisms, affect the dose-response relationships.

- An assessment of the dose-response relationship for an antihypertensive drug should include an evaluation of both its peak and trough effects.

- Combinations of different medications produce varying response relationships. Optimal responses occur when one member of a two-drug combination blocks counterregulatory responses triggered by the other.

See also Chapters 120, 121, 122, 123

Background

Several antihypertensive medications have been introduced into clinical practice at excessively high doses, including thiazide diuretics, β-blockers such as propranolol, α-methyldopa, hydralazine, and the ACE inhibitor (ACEI) captopril. This problem can be traced directly to the lack of a formal dose-response relationship for an antihypertensive medication. During developmental studies, drug doses were increased at regular intervals until the desired antihypertensive effect was achieved or until unacceptable side effects intervened. The downfall of such studies was either that the starting doses of the medication were too high, thus precluding identification of the dose necessary for a threshold effect, or that the intervals separating dose adjustments were too short. Subsequently, this approach of using either overly generous starting doses or excessive dose titrations of antihypertensive agents has become ingrained in clinical practice.

A result of the administration of these large doses is an impressive array of adverse effects, including dose-related adverse biochemical effects of thiazide diuretics; proteinuria, dysgeusia, and leukopenia with captopril; sedation and depression for α-methyldopa; and a lupus-like syndrome associated with hydralazine.

Dose-Response Relationships

A fundamental concept in therapeutics is the log-linear dose-response curve, which is critical to an accurate understanding of drug effect, whether it involves single-drug or multidrug therapy of hypertension. Otherwise stated, in the range of receptor occupancy from 0% to 100%, the effect of a drug is correlated with the logarithm of its concentration and, by extension, the logarithm of the dose. Thus, a 10-fold increase in dose is needed to double the effect (point A to B in the **Figure 119.1**). Doubling the dose would then be expected to increase the effect by the logarithm of 2 ($\approx$30%) (point A to C).

A corollary to this basic pharmacological principle is that a drug exhibits a log dose response for its toxic effects. This curve for adverse effect typically falls to the right of the curve constructed for therapeutic effect. Thus, at any given dose, a therapeutic effect greater than a toxic effect will be achieved (point B to B[1]). Decreasing the medication dose will decrease both the therapeutic and toxic effects and may allow an adequate therapeutic response with little or no toxic effect (point A to A[1]). It is only with more recently developed drug classes that effort has been expended to identify the lower portion of the dose-response relationship. With thiazides and other older drug classes, the low-end response dose was determined only by trial and error long after the agent was approved for use.

Dose-response relationships can be visualized in a number of ways. In the case of the angiotensin-receptor antagonists (AT$_1$-RAs), the character of the curve ranges from shallow to flat when the dose is increased beyond the initial-effect dose. Thiazide diuretics typically display a moderate response at low doses, which rapidly flattens thereafter. Short-acting dihydropyridines, such as the immediate-release form of nifedipine, have an uncharacteristically steep response. In virtually all cases, addition of a diuretic to a preexisting drug regimen will result in an additive response typically reflected by (1) a leftward shift of the curve (less drug required to effect the same reduction in blood pressure), (2) a greater peak response, or (3) a steepening of the response slope.

Factors Affecting the Pharmacodynamic Dose-Effect Curve

The time at which response is assessed is of considerable relevance in that it defines the magnitude and duration of the effect. In this regard, peak, trough, or peak-to-trough ratios for blood pressure response have been proposed as efficacy measures. Trough blood pressure readings are particularly useful in defining whether blood pressure control has been effectively maintained throughout a dos-

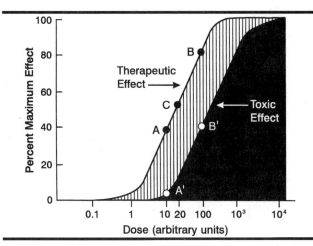

Figure 119.1. Theoretical therapeutic and toxic logarithmic-linear dose-response curves.

ing interval. Trough blood pressure readings are best ascertained with the use of home blood pressure monitoring.

Population Variation

A number of "host" factors are known to influence the response to a particular antihypertensive medication. For example, black hypertensives are generally less responsive to low doses of ACEIs, yet if doses are increased, their response differs little from that observed in white hypertensives.

Length of Therapy

An additional consideration for response to an antihypertensive medication relates to differences between acute and chronic dosing. In the case of the former, variables such as the formulation of a compound, circadian blood pressure rhythms, and inherent sensitivity to a medication dictate the extent to which blood pressure drops. In regard to the latter, it is now well recognized for several drug classes, such as ACEIs or AT_1-RAs, that their full blood pressure–lowering effects are not achieved until several weeks, perhaps even months, after therapy is begun. Thus, a dose-response relationship for an individual compound will vary as a function of time.

Counterregulation

Another major consideration in the pharmacodynamic dose-response relationship for an antihypertensive medication is the extent to which counterregulatory mechanisms are activated by its having lowered blood pressure. In this regard, the initial reduction in blood pressure as a primary medication effect can be abolished or significantly attenuated by volume expansion secondary to renal sodium retention, tachycardia triggered by baroreceptor stimulation, and peripheral vasoconstriction resulting from activation of the renin-angiotensin and/or sympathetic nervous systems. These responses are most likely to occur when arterial dilator drugs are used (hydralazine, minoxide, some calcium antagonists). Clinically, it is sometimes difficult to gauge the extent to which counterregulatory systems are activated. Most typically, a loss of previously established blood pressure control should point to this possibility. Baseline pulse

rates should generally be obtained at the time when therapy is begun. A clinically relevant increase in pulse rate ($\approx 10\%$) should prompt consideration of either lowering the dose of the provoking agent or adding a pulse rate–lowering compound. Sodium retention, as a means by which blood pressure control is lost, is easy to recognize if peripheral edema develops. Weight gain is only a rough and sometimes misleading clue to the degree of sodium retention.

Absorption

Daily dosing of most antihypertensive medications will generally lead to fairly predictable blood levels, once sufficient time has elapsed to reach a steady state. Problems relative to drug effect can arise if a medication is being given at the low end of its dose-response curve and day-to-day variance in absorption and/or a significant food effect exists. Furosemide is one such compound with the potential for marked variability in its day-to-day diuretic effect, a phenomenon related to its rather considerable absorptive variability.

Elimination

An additional dose-effect consideration arises from a review of how a compound is systemically eliminated. As a corollary to this, a specific drug dose may not always cause a predictable blood level. For example, most ACEIs, clonidine, and atenolol are eliminated primarily by renal mechanisms. Thus, these compounds will systematically accumulate in the setting of a diminished glomerular filtration rate if dosing has not been adjusted for the level of renal function. Failure to recognize this pharmacological nuance may result in an exaggerated and/or prolonged antihypertensive effect as well as a significant increase in the incidence of concentration-related side effects (eg, sedation with clonidine).

Route of Administration

A number of antihypertensive compounds must gain access to deep tissue compartments to achieve their desired effect. An example of one such drug is the central α-agonist, clonidine. When clonidine is administered orally, a peak-and-valley drug concentration is seen, whereas transdermal clonidine administration produces no such variation and typically results in persistent midrange blood levels throughout its dosing interval. When peak drug concentrations are avoided by a delivery system, far fewer side effects develop.

Salt and Water Balance

A final consideration in defining a dose-response relationship resides in the well-recognized influence of volume contraction on drug effect and thereby the extent to which blood pressure drops. When diuretic therapy is considered for adjunct therapy, two responses can be expected. First, the response to the diuretic and the other form of therapy will be either additive or possibly synergistic; second, the amount of the nondiuretic antihypertensive agent being administered can generally be reduced, consistent with the known amplifying effect of diuretic therapy.

Relationship Between Dose and Side-Effect Profile

Early in the treatment of hypertension, it was not uncommon to use high doses of a single drug. The price paid for this approach was frequent, severe, even fatal, side effects that were largely dose-related. For example, it is clear that for hydralazine, the dose-response curve for severe adverse effects (eg, the lupus-like syndrome) is certainly as pertinent as the dose-response curve for blood pressure efficacy. The ACEI captopril was also used in excessively high doses when first available, an approach accompanied by an assortment of peculiar connective-tissue abnormalities. In past years, it was quite common to administer hydrochlorothiazide in doses ranging from 100 to 200 mg. It took several years to appreciate that the peak effect of this medication occurred at a dose of only 25 mg. Although the dose-response relationship for blood pressure had already plateaued at these higher doses, the dose–side effect relationship for hypokalemia remained. Accordingly, the incidence rate of hypokalemia and hypomagnesemia was typically >50% with high-dose thiazide therapy, whereas at lower doses, these electrolyte abnormalities occurred with considerably lower frequency.

A lessening of such side effects occurred as the "stepped-care" approach to hypertension treatment became more widely accepted. In the process, relatively low doses of rational drug combinations were used to achieve a desired, additive antihypertensive effect. This was the foundation for a triple drug regimen in common use in the 1980s that was composed of hydralazine, propranolol, and hydrochlorothiazide.

Fixed-Dose Combination Products

Fixed-dose combination products for the treatment of essential hypertension have been available since the early 1960s, when the drug SER-AP-ES was first introduced. This fixed-dose combination of hydralazine, reserpine, and hydrochlorothiazide was in common use, in part because at that time there were a limited number of options for the treatment of hypertension. As the antihypertensive market evolved and different classes of drugs, such as ACEIs and calcium channel blockers, became available, enthusiasm waned for the use of fixed-dose combination products.

Some of the skepticism of the past several years surrounding the use of fixed-dose combination products has been replaced by cautious optimism as rational combinations of agents have become available in effective dose amounts. This resurgence in use coincides with the arrival of drug class combinations such as ACEIs and diuretics (diuretics lower blood pressure but activate the renin-angiotensin axis, whereas ACEIs decrease the activity of this axis), AT_1-RAs and diuretics, and calcium channel blockers and ACEIs (certain calcium channel blockers can increase central sympathetic outflow, and ACEIs decrease it). Thus, fixed-dose combination therapy can be viewed as being inherently rational. In addition, this form of therapy increases a patient's adherence to the treatment regimen.

SUGGESTED READING

1. Johnston GD. Dose-response relationships with antihypertensive drugs. *Pharmacol Ther.* 1992;35:53–92.
2. Meredith PA, Elliot HL. Concentration-effect relationships and implications for trough-to-peak ratio. *Am J Hypertens.* 1996;9:66S–70S.
3. Meredith PA, Reid JL. The use of pharmacodynamic and pharmacokinetic profiles in drug development for planning individual therapy. In: Laragh JH, Brenner BM, eds. *Hypertension: Pathophysiology, Diagnosis, and Management.* 2nd ed. New York, NY: Raven Press Ltd; 1995;2771–2783.
4. Sica DA. Fixed-dose combination antihypertensive drugs: do they have a role in rational therapy? *Drugs.* 1994;48:16–24.

Chapter 120

Variability in Individual Responses to Antihypertensive Drugs

Joseph L. Izzo, Jr, MD

KEY POINTS

- The heterogeneity of human hypertension, both essential and secondary, affects responses to monotherapy with antihypertensive drugs.

- Exaggerated homeostatic responses to blood pressure reduction, including renal sodium retention and baroreflex-mediated neurohumoral activation, tend to blunt the effectiveness of monotherapy.

- No single class of antihypertensive agents can control all cases of hypertension.

- Combination therapies are often more effective than monotherapy.

See also Chapters 45, 119, 121, 122, 123

If the desired initial antihypertensive response is achieved with a given drug, the clinician can simply monitor the continued efficacy and safety of that agent. If there is no initial response of blood pressure or if the initial response wanes or disappears, however, the clinician must play a detective role in assessing the reasons for apparent drug failure. In almost all cases of apparent drug failure, there are important clues that the astute clinician can use to improve therapeutic outcomes. Four major types of reasons account for apparent failure of standard antihypertensive therapy (**see Table 120.1**): (1) adherence problems (also sometimes called poor medication compliance), (2) physiological and population heterogeneity or "patient-drug mismatch" problems, (3) exaggerated homeostatic responses or "pseudotolerance," or (4) pharmacodynamic drug-related problems.

Adherence Problems

The major reason for apparent failure of blood pressure to respond to therapy is the fact that the majority of people self-discontinue therapy. Explanations for this behavior include psychological, economic, educational, and other causes. (see chapter 121)

Heterogeneity and Patient-Drug Mismatches

Three principles are central to understanding why monotherapy with a given antihypertensive drug may fail to lower blood pressure: (1) physiological redundancy (overlap) of blood pressure control mechanisms, (2) physiological and population heterogeneity (spectrum) within individual control mechanisms, and (3) specificity of antihypertensive drug classes for individual control mechanisms. These three principles can be recombined to explain the apparent variability of responses to each class of antihypertensive drugs within and between individuals.

Within-Individual (Physiological) Heterogeneity

The components of the blood pressure homeostatic system were conceptualized by Irvine Page as an overlapping, redundant, interac-

tive system he called the "mosaic." The human population is genetically diverse and is also physiologically highly adaptable. Thus, heterogeneity occurs both within individuals and between individuals. A good example of physiological variability or "within-individual variation" is the relationship of various antihypertensive drugs to hydration status. Homeostatic responses to dehydration or salt depletion include stimulation of the renin-angiotensin system and an enhanced blood pressure response to drugs that affect the renin-angiotensin system (central agents, β-blockers, ACE inhibitors, angiotensin receptor blockers). This interdependency of volume status and renin activity is the reason why the combination of diuretic and anti–renin-angiotensin drugs is so effective. Conversely, during expansion of the extracellular space, there are absent or diminished responses to anti–renin-angiotensin drugs.

Between-Individual (Population) Heterogeneity

Population heterogeneity ("between-individual heterogeneity") is also present in human hypertension because of genetic factors, aging effects, and disease. Perhaps the clearest examples of heterogeneity of hypertension mechanisms (components of the mosaic) lie within the syndromes of secondary hypertension (adrenal cortical, adrenomedullary, renovascular, and renal hypertension). The mechanisms of elevated blood pressure in these secondary forms of hypertension are relatively unique and act to predetermine a pattern of specific drug responses. For example, early in renovascular hypertension, the renin-angiotensin system plays an important part in the pathogenesis of blood pressure elevation. As would be expected, drugs that block the renin-angiotensin system are highly efficacious in these patients. By contrast, the catecholamine-induced hypertension present in pheochromocytoma responds preferentially to α-adrenergic receptor blockers. In steroid-induced hypertension, the complex mechanism of pressure and volume dysregulation is revealed by the relative efficacy of diuretic agents and sympatholytic agents.

Table 120.1. Reasons for Apparent Failure of Antihypertensive Drugs

Therapeutic adherence problems
Heterogeneity and patient-drug mismatches
  Within-individual heterogeneity (physiological responses)
  Between-individual heterogeneity (population differences)
Homeostatic overcompensation (pseudotolerance)
  Systemic pseudotolerance
  Renal pseudotolerance
Pharmacodynamic problems
  Pharmacokinetic variation (underdosing, drug metabolism differences)
  Drug-drug interactions

Within the category of essential hypertension, substantial heterogeneity also exists. In hemodynamic terms, the range of cardiac index seen in routine clinical practice spans values from ≈ 2 to 7 $L \cdot min^{-1} \cdot m^{-2}$. Those hypertensives with hyperdynamic (also known as hyperkinetic) circulatory states, who also have correspondingly low systemic vascular resistance values, respond favorably to β-adrenergic blocking agents, which act principally to lower cardiac output, and also to ACE inhibitors. Wide variation in activity of the renin-angiotensin system is also seen, with roughly 100-fold variation in plasma renin activity seen across the population. Although the correlation is imperfect, those individuals with the highest pretreatment plasma renin activity respond more favorably to monotherapy with ACE inhibition than those with low plasma renin activity.

Drug Specificity and Patient-Drug Mismatches

Also central to the operational understanding of antihypertensive drug effects is the notion that specific classes of drugs operate on well-defined targets within the blood pressure mosaic. The corollary to this assumption is that no single class of antihypertensive agents can normalize blood pressure in all persons with hypertension. These two related observations have far-reaching practical and pathophysiological implications. As will be discussed in the final section, the enlightened clinician can use these heterogeneous patterns to match the person being treated with the optimal agent for that individual. In the purest sense, the use of drugs that do not fit the "fingerprint" of that individual's blood pressure mosaic will lead to a patient-drug mismatch that can severely limit optimal therapeutic efficacy.

Homeostatic Overcompensation (Pseudotolerance)

Two principal types of pseudotolerance mechanisms exist: systemic homeostatic overcompensation, which generally involves baroreflex-mediated activation of the sympathetic nervous and renin-angiotensin systems, and renal pseudotolerance mechanisms, which are separate but closely related to systemic homeostatic overcompensations. These defense mechanisms for blood pressure and blood volume function equally well in hypertensive and normotensive individuals.

Systemic Pseudotolerance

An overly vigorous response of the two principal vasoconstrictive systems (sympathoadrenal and renin-angiotensin systems) to blood pressure decreases causes the phenomenon of systemic pseudotolerance. Pseudotolerance is most clearly seen when arterial dilator agents, such as thiazide diuretics, hydralazine, minoxidil, or calcium antagonists, are given as monotherapy. In most patients, these agents cause a mild degree of activation of aortocarotid and cardiopulmonary baroreceptors, which activates the sympathetic nervous system and thereby increases renal sympathetic nerve activity and renin release. In some individuals, however, this homeostatic response is so vigorous that the blood pressure returns nearly to pretreatment values. Such responses to vasodilators can actually increase myocardial oxygen consumption by as much as 20% to 25%. In this situation, lower blood pressure occurs at the expense of increased cardiac work, which may explain why arterial vasodilators (minoxidil, hydralazine, certain calcium antagonists) tend to increase the incidence of coronary events.

Clinical hallmarks of systemic pseudotolerance include tachycardia, edema, and a progressive loss of antihypertensive efficacy. As would be predicted, concomitant administration of β-blockers reduces the tendency for pseudotolerance to develop and tends to restore the antihypertensive efficacy of the original vasodilator. Similarly, combination with ACE inhibitors improves the incidence of edema caused by calcium antagonists.

Renal Pseudotolerance

Another phenomenon that is common with most antihypertensive drugs is increased salt and water retention at the lowered blood pressure, also called renal pseudotolerance. In chronic hypertension, afferent arteriolar disease (nephrosclerosis) necessitates a higher perfusion pressure for the hypertensive kidney to excrete a salt load normally. In this setting, any agent that lowers renal perfusion pressure will tend to favor excess salt and water retention, which in turn maintains an inappropriate level of cardiac output and favors a return of blood pressure to pretreatment values. In the strict sense, renal pseudotolerance mechanisms function independently of systemic mechanisms and are more directly related to phenomena of intrarenal blood and urine flow and pressure. Renal pseudotolerance is another major reason why thiazide diuretics are so useful as combination agents in the treatment of hypertension.

Pseudotolerance to loop diuretics (furosemide, bumetanide, torsemide) occurs in patients with normal renal function. Normally, exaggerated reflex antinatriuresis follows immediately after the initial loop diuretic effect. The subsequent reexpansion of plasma volume then limits both diuretic and antihypertensive efficacy. In patients with normal or near normal renal function, negative sodium balance can be achieved only when a low-salt diet is used in conjunction with loop diuretics. As a rule, there is no place for loop diuretics as initial therapy in patients with essential hypertension who have normal renal function. Loop diuretics are important agents in heart failure and in some patients with renal failure or with adverse reactions to thiazides.

Drug-Related Problems
Pharmacokinetic Variation and Underdosing

Apparent failure of drug therapy can also be due to failure of the clinician to recognize certain aspects of practical pharmacokinetics (drug dosages, dosing frequency, and, to a much lesser extent, potential variations in drug metabolism.) Underdosing, either because dosages are too small or because frequencies of administration are too long, is the most common pharmacokinetic reason for apparent drug failure. Underdosing is most problematic with ACE inhibitors and, to a lesser degree, β-blockers, apparently partly because of clinicians' poor understanding of pharmacodynamic dose-response and dose-duration relationships for these agents. The peak blood pressure–lowering effect of ACE inhibitors has a very steep dose-response relationship, so that maximal peak effects occur even with low doses (captopril 6.25 mg or equivalent doses of other ACE inhibitors). In contrast, the duration of these maximal effects of ACE inhibitors exhibits a relatively shallow dose-response curve, so that much higher doses of ACE inhibitors (captopril at least 50 mg twice daily, enalapril at least 20 mg daily, or their equivalents) are necessary to achieve a sustained 24-hour duration of action. Because most patients take their medications in the morning, the effects of low doses of ACE inhibitors usually have worn off by afternoon or evening. The problem is often undetected because measurement of blood pressures often occurs only in the morning.

Dosing frequency must be considered for other agents as well. For example, the antihypertensive effects of atenolol in doses of ≤50 mg/d (or the equivalents of metoprolol or propranolol unless formulated as extended-release preparations) do not generally span the full 24 hours. Short-acting calcium channel blockers, especially nifedipine, lower blood pressure for a few hours at most and are not indicated for the treatment of hypertension.

Pharmacogenetics

Genetic variation in drug metabolism (pharmacogenetics) does not cause a major clinical problem, largely because of the wide therapeutic ranges of modern antihypertensive drugs and the ability of the clinician to titrate dosages. There are phenotypic metabolic differences with a few drugs, but these have declining use patterns. Hydralazine, which is inactivated by acetylation, must be given in much higher doses to rapid acetylators than to slow acetylators, who can be identified for this heritable polymorphism. Potential deficiencies in oxidative metabolism of certain β-adrenergic blockers, such as propranolol and timolol, can be characterized by a polymorphism in debrisoquine metabolism. Although lower doses of these agents may be required in the slow oxidizers, there is often more practical advantage to reduced metabolism because 24-hour duration of action is improved.

An Integrated Therapeutic Approach

Knowledge of the basic heterogeneity of hypertension allows the astute clinician to individualize therapy and to use lower doses of fewer antihypertensive drugs. Side effects are therefore less likely, and it is probable that patient adherence will therefore be greater, although that premise has not been formally tested.

It is not difficult for a dedicated clinician to use this approach, which is closely related to the concept of the "controlled clinical trial with N = 1" as described by Guyatt and Sackett. According to this paradigm, each subject to be treated with antihypertensive therapy can be viewed as an individual clinical trial, providing that certain key

criteria are met. First, there must be adequate record-keeping, preferably in the form of a flow chart or spreadsheet that includes blood pressure and drug therapy organized by date of service. Second, the clinician should proceed with one step at a time, usually changing a single agent per visit. Third, an adequate follow-up period must be used, with at least 1 month allowed between visits (if the blood pressure is stage 1 or stage 2) to ensure that compensatory homeostatic responses will have stabilized.

This approach assumes that the ongoing or chronic response to a given class of agents functionally defines the contribution of that component of the mosaic to the elevated blood pressure in the patient being treated. Conversely, the failure of a given drug class to exhibit a sustained blood pressure effect identifies the relative lack of importance of that specific component within the mosaic of that particular patient. Assuming that there is an adequate baseline for comparison, the clinician uses each antihypertensive drug as a specific physiological probe to investigate the relative impact of a particular component of blood pressure regulation that should be blocked by that agent. For example, if a given patient exhibits a favorable response to a β-blocker, it can be assumed that the patient had a relatively high baseline cardiac output, that there was good adherence, that the dose was adequate, and that there was no significant pseudotolerance. In contrast, if a patient fails to respond to a β-blocker, assuming that there were no problems of drug adherence and that appropriate doses were used, there is a strong likelihood that the patient had a low baseline cardiac output (and probably plasma renin activity) and that the achievement of optimal blood pressure control in the future will require the use of a different class of antihypertensive drugs, perhaps a vasodilator or thiazide diuretic.

SUGGESTED READING

1. Case DB, Wallace JM, Klem HJ, Weber MA, Sealey JE, Laragh JH. Possible role of renin in hypertension as suggested by renin-sodium profiling and inhibition of converting enzyme. *N Engl J Med.* 1977;296:641–646.
2. Dustan HP, Tarazi RC, Bravo EL. Dependence of arterial pressure on intravascular volume in treated hypertensive patients. *N Engl J Med.* 1972;286:861–866.
3. Izzo JL Jr, Licht MR, Smith RJ, Larrabee PS, Radke KJ, Kallay MC. Chronic effects of direct vasodilation (pinacidil), alpha-adrenergic blockade (prazosin) and angiotensin-converting enzyme inhibition (captopril) in systemic hypertension. *Am J Cardiol.* 1987;60:303–308.
4. Frohlich ED, Dustan HP, Page IH. Hyperdynamic beta-adrenergic circulatory state. *Arch Intern Med.* 1966;117:614–619.
5. Guyatt G, Sackett D. The clinician's actions when N = 1. In: Melmon KL, et al, eds. *Clinical Pharmacology.* 3rd ed. New York, NY: McGraw Hill; 1992:942–950.
6. Laragh JH, Baer L, Brunner HR, Buhler FR, Sealey JE, Vaughan ED Jr. Renin, angiotensin, and aldosterone system in pathogenesis and management of hypertensive vascular disease. *Am J Med.* 1972;52:633–652.
7. Lennard MS, Tucker GT, Silas JH, Woods HF. Debrisoquine polymorphism and the metabolism and action of metoprolol, timolol, propranolol and atenolol. *Xenobiotica.* 1986;16:435–447.
8. Messerli FH. Hemodynamic and cardiac adaptation in essential hypertension: consequences for therapy. *J Clin Hypertens.* 1985;1:3–14.
9. Wilcox CS, Mitch WE, Kelly RA, Skorecki K, Meyer TW, Friedman PA, Souney PF. Response of the kidney to furosemide, I: effects of salt intake and renal compensation. *J Lab Clin Med.* 1983;102:450–458.
10. Yagil Y, Kobrin I, Stessman J, Ghanem J, Leibel B, Ben-Ishay D. Effectiveness of combined nifedipine and propranolol treatment in hypertension. *Hypertension.* 1983;5:II-113-II-117.

Chapter 121

Adherence to Antihypertensive Therapy

Martha N. Hill, RN, PhD

KEY POINTS

- Adherence, or compliance, is not an end in itself but rather a means to improved care and outcomes.

- The extent to which patients are able to adhere to treatment recommendations is a major issue in blood pressure control and depends on many factors.

- Effective strategies, with patients, providers, and healthcare organizations/systems taking action, can prevent, monitor, and address adherence problems.

See also Chapters 119, 120, 122, 123, 152

Therapeutic nonadherence, with patients not carrying out recommended therapy, is an important, costly, and pervasive problem that contributes to the low overall (27%) hypertension control rate in the United States. If patients are unable or unwilling to adhere to, or comply with, lifestyle modification or a medication regimen, long-term blood pressure control is impaired, and health may be adversely affected by complications such as stroke, heart failure, and end-stage renal disease.

"The extent to which the patient's behavior (in terms of taking medication, following a diet, or executing other lifestyle changes) coincides with the clinical prescription" is the commonly accepted definition of adherence (Sackett, 1979). Today, the terms adherence and compliance are commonly used interchangeably. Some prefer the term adherence because compliance connotes a paternalistic rather than collaborative relationship between physician and patient. More precise definitions of adherence vary according to the specificity of the recommended therapeutic behavior and the ability to measure the recommended behavior. For example, taking medication correctly ≥80% of the time is the most common definition of medication compliance found in the hypertension literature.

Medication nonadherence may begin with not having a prescription either filled or refilled on schedule. Taking the incorrect dose, taking a dose at the wrong time, forgetting to take a dose, or stopping a medication too early are additional forms of medication noncompliance. Different patterns of underdosing, particularly as 2- to 3-day drug-free holidays or omissions, are the most common form of medication nonadherence. The effects of missed doses on blood pressure depend on pharmacological parameters of the medication used. However, missed appointments, continuation of unhealthy habits such as tobacco smoking, a sedentary lifestyle, and a diet high in calories, fat, and sodium also are prevalent and important forms of nonadherence.

Detection

Measurement of nonadherence is problematic. Information can be collected by physical examination, interview, self-administered questionnaires, or pharmacy records. Objective changes in blood pressure, heart rate, and body weight may indicate adherence with recommendations. Alternative explanations, such as worsening comorbidity, may

be responsible for the observed changes. Asking patients to self-report is fraught with issues of recall bias and socially desirable responses. Counting returned, unused medication also may be unreliable, because medications may be shared or put into other containers.

Factors Associated With Adherence

The reasons for nonadherence and its variable patterns across blood pressure control behaviors are many and not fully understood. Problems with adherence are seen in patients of all ages, diseases, and severities of illness. Generally, adherence lessens over time, particularly in chronic conditions. Level of education, socioeconomic status, and sex are not predictive of nonadherence, whereas smoking, excessive alcohol intake, and other unhealthy behaviors are linked with nonadherence.

Seeing a doctor regularly, having other health conditions, and being on a simple medication regimen are associated with higher rates of adherence. The frequency of office visits for blood pressure monitoring is strongly associated with improved use of medication and blood pressure control. Social support from family members and friends, employment, and health insurance also have been shown to be determinants of improved high blood pressure control.

A knowledge of hypertension, its consequences if left untreated, and the benefits of therapy is important. However, although knowledge of the requirements of the treatment regimen is necessary, it is insufficient to ensure adherence. Patients' actual and perceived barriers to adherence influence adherence behavior. Healthcare providers need to consider patients' beliefs, attitudes, perceptions, and prior experiences as well as their goals, values, and motivation. It is important to assess the reasons why patients do not follow advice. Factors in the social environment often create other priorities in daily life. Additional frequently cited reasons for not filling prescriptions or not taking medication as prescribed include concerns about side effects, not believing medication is truly beneficial, a belief that the condition is improved, and cost.

Effective Strategies

Successful interventions that enhance compliance and lead to improved patient outcomes are primarily behavioral in nature. Patient knowledge is necessary but should be deemed inadequate if appropriate action does not follow. The relationship between the patient and the prescriber is of paramount importance.

The classic hypertension care and control clinical trials, such as MRFIT, HDFP, SHEP, and TOMHS, demonstrated that extensive and continuous interventions as provided by multidisciplinary teams could improve adherence. These and other studies designed to meet patient, provider, and organizational needs and minimize barriers to blood pressure control have been effective in a variety of clinical and community settings. Programs in which multidisciplinary teams address patients' beliefs and concerns and provide follow-up, feedback, and free medication if needed are the most successful. In these and other studies, blood pressure control within weeks of initiation of treatment was significantly associated with control at later periods of time. Adherence to antihypertensive therapy can be significantly improved by programs that focus on enhancing prioritized behaviors necessary for blood pressure control. Effective interventions use a variety of cognitive, educational, and behavioral strategies. A recent review of research on compliance with cardiovascular disease prevention strategies summarized a dozen successful approaches: signed agreements, behavioral skill training, self-monitoring, telephone/mail contact, spouse support, self-efficacy enhancement, contingency contracting, exercise prescription, external cognitive aids, persuasive communication, nurse-managed clinics, and work- or school-based programs.

From a behavioral perspective, adherence includes entering into and remaining in care, making and maintaining lifestyle changes, and taking medication. Achieving and maintaining goal blood pressure levels over time requires continuous educational and behavioral strategies so that patients have the knowledge, skills, motivation, and resources to carry out treatment recommendations with minimal relapses. Success adherence requires that patients know what steps to take and which skills to develop to address barriers and enhance memory in relation to problem identification and problem solving. Strategies to help patients develop these skills need to be adapted so that they are culturally salient and feasible for staff implementation.

A combination of strategies is most likely to maximize long-term adherence by preventing, recognizing, and responding to adherence problems. The effective strategies in **Table 121.1** appeared in the Report of the Fifth Joint National Committee on Detection, Evaluation, and Treatment of High Blood Pressure. These evidence-based strategies are clustered under the following approaches: educate the

---

Table 121.1. Preventing, Monitoring, and Addressing Problems of Adherence

Educate about conditions and treatment
  Assess patient's understanding and acceptance of the diagnosis and expectations of being in care.
  Discuss patient's concerns and clarify misunderstandings
  Inform patient of blood pressure level.
  Agree with patient on a goad blood pressure.
  Inform patient about recommended treatment and provide specific written information.
  Elicit concerns and questions and provide opportunities for patient to state specific behaviors to carry out treatment recommendations.
  Emphasize need to continue treatment, that patient cannot tell if blood pressure is elevated, and that control does not mean cure.
Individualize the regimen
  Include patient in decision making.
  Simplify the regimen.
  Incorporate treatment into patient's daily lifestyle.
  Set, with the patient, realistic short-term objectives for specific components of the treatment plan.
  Encourage discussion of side effects and concerns.
  Encourage self-monitoring.
  Minimize cost of therapy.
  Indicate that you will ask about adherence at next visit.
  When weight loss is established as a treatment goal, discourage quick weight loss regimens, fasting, or unscientific methods, because these are associated with weight cycling, which may increase cardiovascular morbidity and mortality.
Provide reinforcement
  Provide feedback regarding blood pressure level.
  Ask about behaviors to achieve blood pressure control.
  Give positive feedback for behavioral and blood pressure improvement.
  Hold exit interviews to clarify regimen.
  Make appointment for next visit before patient leaves office.
  Use appointment remainders and contact patients to confirm appointments.
  Schedule more frequent visits to counsel nonadherent patients.
  Contact and follow up patients who missed appointments.
  Consider clinician-patient contract.
Promote social support
  Educate family members to be part of the blood pressure control process and provide daily reinforcement.
  Suggest small-group activities to enhance mutual support and motivation.
Collaborate with other professionals
  Draw upon complementary skills and knowledge of nurses, pharmacists, dietitians, optometrists, dentists, and physician assistants.
  Refer patients for more intensive counseling.

The Fifth Joint National Committee on Detection, Evaluation, and Treatment of High Blood Pressure (JNC V). National High Blood Pressure Education Program. National Institutes of Health, National Heart, Lung, and Blood Institute. NIH publication 95–1088, March 1995. Reprinted with permission.

patient and the family about high blood pressure and its treatment, individualize the regimen, provide feedback to the patient, promote social support, and collaborate with other professionals.

Simplifying the regimen with once or twice daily dosing significantly improves adherence, although it does not resolve all problems with medication adherence. Self-monitoring of blood pressure levels at home or at the worksite increases patient involvement and provides feedback on the relationship between adherence and blood pressure levels. The pairing of adherence behavior with daily habits, for example, pill taking paired with brushing teeth or shaving, aids in minimizing missed medication. Reminders by telephone and/or mail or electronic aids enhance memory and stimulate appropriate behavior. Compliance packaging such as blister packaging helps patients remember when to take their medication and to notice if they have forgotten.

A multidisciplinary team approach to hypertension care and control permits flexibility in matching patients' needs with the competencies of staff with different but complementary skills and interests. Nonphysician health professionals, particularly nurses, pharmacists, and health educators, have demonstrated effective, safe, and well-

---

Table 121.2. Actions to Increase Compliance With Prevention and Treatment Recommendations

	SPECIFIC STRATEGIES
Actions by patients	
Patients must engage in essential prevention and treatment behaviors.	
Decide to control risk factors.	Understand rationale, importance of commitment.
Negotiate goals with provider.	Develop communication skills
Develop skills for adopting and maintaining recommended behaviors.	Use reminder systems.
Monitor progress towards goals.	Use self-monitoring skills.
Resolve problems that block achievement of goals	Develop problem-solving skills, use social support networks.
Patients must communicate with providers about prevention and treatment services.	Define own needs on basis of experience.
	Validate rationale for continuing to follow recommendations.
Actions by providers	
Providers must foster effective communication with patients	
Provide clear, direct messages about importance of a behavior or therapy	Provide oral and written instruction, including rationale for treatments.
	Develop skills in communication/counseling
Include patients in decisions about prevention and treatment goals and related strategies.	Use tailoring and contracting strategies.
	Negotiate goals and a plan.
	Anticipate barriers to compliance and discuss solutions.
Incorporate behavioral strategies into counseling.	Use active listening.
	Develop multicomponent strategies (ie, cognitive and behavioral).
Providers must document and respond to patient's progress toward goals.	
Create an evidence-based practice	Determine methods of evaluation outcomes.
Assess patient's compliance at each visit.	Use self-report or electronic data.
Develop reminder system to ensure identification and follow-up of patient status.	Use telephone follow-up.
Actions by healthcare organizations: healthcare organizations must:	
Develop an environment that supports prevention and treatment interventions.	Develop training in behavioral science, office setup for all personnel.
	Use preappointment reminders.
	Use telephone follow-up.
	Schedule evening/weekend office hours.
	Provide group/individual counseling for patients and families.
Provide tracking and reporting systems.	Develop computer-based systems (electronic medical records).
Provide education and training for providers.	Require continuing education courses in communication, behavioral counseling.
	Develop incentives tied to desired patient and provider outcomes.
Provide adequate reimbursement for allocation of time for all healthcare professionals.	
Adopt systems to rapidly and efficiently incorporate innovations into medical practice.	Incorporate nursing case management.
	Implement pharmacy patient profile and recall review systems.
	Use of electronic transmission storage of patient's self-monitored data.
	Obtain patient data on lifestyle behavior before visit.
	Provide continuous quality improvement training.

Miller NH, Hill MN, Kottke t, Ockene IS, The multilevel compliance challenge: recommendations for a call to action. *Circulation*. 1997;95:1085–1090. Reprinted with permission.

received contributions to improvement in compliance and blood pressure control. Nurse-supervised outreach workers, nurse case-managers, and nurse practitioners, in collaboration with physicians and other health professionals, in a variety of settings have effectively improved the outcomes of patients with hypertension. Involving family, friends, community resources, and other health professionals can help change lifestyle habits and maintain these changes over time.

Multilevel Approach

A multilevel approach is needed, with patients, providers, and healthcare organizations/systems taking action to increase compliance. The delivery of care needs to be organized to address potential and real problems with adherence at all levels simultaneously. **Table 121.2** presents the actions and strategies encouraged by the American Heart Association for patients, providers, and healthcare organizations to increase compliance with prevention and treatment recommendations. It is important to work with individual patients to ensure that they understand what is necessary to achieve treatment goals and that they participate in treatment decisions. Joint problem solving to prevent or minimize barriers to care and treatment is valuable. Provider responsiveness to patient concerns as well as reinforcement and support are also necessary. Provision of reminders, outreach, and follow-up services is beneficial. Use of one pharmacy to fill prescriptions improves surveillance and counseling. Identification of drug-drug interactions, particularly if there are multiple prescribers, and timeliness of prescription refills can be monitored. Integrated systems approaches with continuous quality improvement enhance the training and practice of providers and patient outcomes.

SUGGESTED READING

1. Burke LE, Dunbar-Jacob JE, Hill MN. Compliance with cardiovascular disease prevention strategies: a review of the research. *Ann Behav Med.* 1998. Volume 19, Number 3, pages 239–263.

2. National High Blood Pressure Education Program. The fifth report of the Joint National Committee on Prevention, Detection, Evaluation, and Treatment of High Blood Pressure. *Arch Intern Med.* 1993;153:154–183.

3. Hill MN, Miller NH. Compliance enhancement: a call for multidisciplinary team approaches. *Circulation.* 1996;93:4–6. Editorial.

4. Miller NH, Hill M, Kottke T, Ockene IS. The multilevel compliance challenge: recommendations for a call to action: a statement for healthcare professionals. *Circulation.* 1997;95:1085–1090.

5. Monane M, Bohn RL, Gurwitz JH, Glynn RJ, Levin R, Avorn J. The effects of initial drug choice and comorbidity on antihypertensive therapy compliance: results from a population-based study in the elderly. *Am J Hypertens.* 1997;10:697–704.

6. Roter, DL, Hall JA, Merisca R, Nordstrom B, Creten D, and Svarstad B. Effectiveness of interventions to improve patient compliance: a meta-analysis. Medical Care. 1998;36:1138–1161.

7. Royal Pharmaceutical Society of Great Britain. *From Compliance to Concordance: Achieving Shared Goals in Medicine Taking.* Great Britain; 1997.

8. Sackett DL, Haynes RB, eds. *Compliance With Therapeutic Regimens.* Baltimore, Md: The Johns Hopkins University Press; 1976.

9. The Sixth Report of the Joint National Committee on Prevention, Detection, Evaluation, and Treatment of High Blood Pressure (JNC VI). National High Blood Pressure Education Program. Bethesda, Md: National Institutes of Health, National Heart, Lung, and Blood Institute; 1997: NIH publication 98-4080.

10. Task Force for Compliance. *Noncompliance With Medications: An Economic Tragedy With Important Implications for Health Care Reform.* Baltimore, Md: The Task Force for Compliance; National Pharmaceutical Council of Reston, Virginia. 1993.

11. Working Group on Health Education and High Blood Pressure Control, National High Blood Pressure Education Program. *The Physician's Guide: Improving Adherence Among Hypertensive Patients.* Bethesda, Md: US Department of Health and Human Services, National Heart, Lung, and Blood Institute; 1987.

Chapter 122

When to Refer Patients For Hypertension Consultation

Gary L. Schwartz, MD

KEY POINTS

- Consider consultation if secondary hypertension is suspected, after hypertensive emergencies, and for treatment-resistant or complicated hypertension.

- Hypertension is considered resistant if blood pressure is not controlled to <140/90 mm Hg despite compliance with near-maximal doses of three drugs, one of which is a diuretic.

- Specialty advice may be helpful in the management of patients with hypertension and comorbidities or drug intolerance.

See also Chapters 119, 120, 121, 123

Hypertension is a common health problem that is most appropriately managed by primary-care professionals. However, in the course of patient evaluation and management, specific situations arise in which consultation with a hypertension specialist is likely to be beneficial.

Suspected Secondary Hypertension

Often, secondary hypertension is suspected at the time of initial evaluation on the basis of information from the history, physical examination, or screening laboratory studies (**Table 122.1**) that is inconsistent with essential hypertension. If evaluation for secondary hypertension is being considered, consultation with a specialist before further testing is appropriate. After confirming that further evaluation is reasonable, the specialist can facilitate the selection of a cost-efficient evaluation. For many secondary forms of hypertension, a variety of screening tests are available. The most appropriate test for a given patient is determined by a number of factors. In addition, tests need to be performed under specific conditions for proper interpretation. Making the best choice and performing the test under correct conditions will decrease the risk of both false-positive and false-negative results. False-positive results often lead to unnecessary further testing, and false-negative findings often result in failure to make the correct diagnosis.

A variety of therapeutic options are available for most forms of secondary hypertension. They include both invasive and conservative treatments. Once a diagnosis of secondary hypertension is made, the specialist can suggest the most appropriate management.

Resistant Hypertension

Hypertension is considered resistant if blood pressure is not controlled to <140/90 mm Hg despite compliance with near-maximal doses of three drugs, one of which is a diuretic. For older persons, resistant hypertension is defined by the inability of an adequate triple-drug regimen to lower systolic blood pressure to <160 mm Hg. Often, previously controlled hypertension progresses subacutely to a state of resistance.

Common causes for apparent drug-resistant hypertension include noncompliance with the diet or drug regimen, pseudotolerance (especially to monotherapy with vasodilators), use of interfering substances such as NSAIDs, office (white-coat) hypertension, and on rare occasions, pseudohypertension in older persons. Specialized laboratory studies and ancillary professional services available to the hypertension specialist may facilitate the identification of apparent drug-resistant hypertension.

Less than 1% of the general hypertension population is estimated to have secondary hypertension; a much higher percentage of patients with resistant hypertension will have an underlying secondary pathogenesis that either was previously unsuspected or is superimposed on a background of essential hypertension. Specialty advice may be helpful in assessing for secondary hypertension in patients for whom apparent causes of resistant hypertension have been excluded. If reversible or identifiable causes of resistant hypertension have been eliminated, the specialist may be helpful in designing an effective treatment plan that takes into consideration issues of cost, side effects, drug-drug interactions, and comorbidities.

Hypertensive Emergencies

Hypertensive emergencies are clinical situations associated with severe hypertension in which it is determined that immediate blood pressure reduction is necessary to prevent or limit target-organ damage. Most hypertensive emergencies are initially managed with parenteral therapy. These are high-risk situations because either overly aggressive or inadequate blood pressure reduction can cause organ damage. The need for specialty help in acute management depends on the knowledge and experience of the primary-care provider. After resolution of the emergency, an expanded evaluation is often indicated to determine the cause for the crisis, which typically includes a consideration of secondary hypertension.

Complicated Essential Hypertension

Complicated essential hypertension is defined as high blood pressure accompanied by significant target-organ disease (renal insuffi-

Table 122.1. Factors Inconsistent With Essential Hypertension

Age at onset <30 or >50 years
At time of diagnosis
  Blood pressure stage III
  Significant target organ damage: retinal hemorrhages or exudate, renal insufficiency, cardiomegaly on chest radiograph, left ventricular hypertrophy by ECG
Features suggesting specific secondary hypertension
  Hypokalemia
    Primary aldosteronism, Cushing's disease, Liddle's syndrome, renal vascular disease
  Labile blood pressure, headache, diaphoresis, tachycardia, pallor, neurofibromas, orofacial neuromas, hypercalcemia
    Pheochromocytoma
  Abdominal bruits
    Renal vascular disease
  Truncal obesity, pigmented stria, hypokalemia, glucose intolerance
    Cushing's disease
  Delayed or absent femoral pulses, claudication, headaches
    Coarctation of the aorta
  Abdominal or flank masses, family history of renal disease
    Polycystic renal disease

ciency, coronary heart disease, systolic or diastolic cardiac dysfunction, cerebrovascular disease) and cardiovascular risk factors (dyslipidemia, tobacco use, diabetes). Hypertension is often stage II or higher and requires multiple drugs for control. Patients with complicated hypertension are individually at high risk for morbidity and mortality, and the cost of their care accounts for a disproportionate amount of the total healthcare expense attributable to hypertension. Such patients may benefit from specialty advice to address proper blood pressure control, risk factor modification, and management of target-organ disease.

Among patients with complicated hypertension is a group who demonstrate a progressive decline in renal function. A search for potentially reversible factors is important to prevent progression to end-stage renal disease. An important, potentially reversible cause for a progressive decline in renal function is renal ischemia from bilateral atherosclerotic renovascular occlusive disease, which accounts for an unknown but potentially significant fraction of end-stage renal disease in older persons. Evaluation for and interventional management of renovascular disease is associated with risk of cardiovascular morbidity and mortality and further loss of renal function and is best managed by a specialty medical and surgical team experienced in the management of this complex clinical problem.

Other Situations

Control rates may improve, unnecessary iatrogenic morbidity may be avoided, and appropriate drug selection in specific clinical settings may be facilitated if specialty advice is more readily available to primary-care providers. Specialty advice regarding drug selection for patients on multiple medications may lessen the morbidity and cost due to adverse drug-drug interactions. Studies indicate that drugs established through clinical trials to have special efficacy in specific clinical settings are underused. Finally, the drug-intolerant patient may benefit from specialty advice to determine factors that contribute to intolerance and to construct an effective treatment program.

SUGGESTED READING

1. Appel RG, Bleyer AJ, Reavis S, Hansen KJ. Renovascular disease in older patients beginning renal replacement therapy. *Kidney Int.* 1995;48:171–176.
2. Gifford RW Jr, Kirkendall W, O'Connor DT, Weidman W. Office evaluation of hypertension: a statement for health care professionals by a writing group of the Council for High Blood Pressure Research, American Heart Association. *Circulation.* 1989;79:721–731.
3. Gordon RD, Klemm SA, Tunny TJ, Stowasser M. Primary aldosteronism: hypertension with a genetic basis. *Lancet.* 1992;340:159–161.
4. Joint National Committee on Prevention, Detection, Evaluation, and Treatment of High Blood Pressure. The Sixth Report of the Joint National Committee on Prevention, Detection, Evaluation, and Treatment of High Blood Pressure. *Arch Intern Med.* 1997;157:2413–2446.
5. Kincaid-Smith P. Malignant hypertension. *J Hypertens.* 1991;9:893–899.
6. Neusy AJ, Valeri A, Lowenstein J. Refractory hypertension: definition, prevalence, pathophysiology, and management. *Semin Nephrol.* 1990;10:546:546–551.
7. Scoble JE, Maher ER, Hamilton G, Dick R, Sweny P, Moorhead JF. Atherosclerotic renovascular disease causing renal impairment: a case for treatment. *Clin Nephrol.* 1989;31:119–122.
8. Yakovlevitch M, Black HR. Resistant hypertension in a tertiary clinic. *Arch Intern Med.* 1991;151:1786–1792.

Chapter 123

Management of Patients With Refractory Hypertension

Henry R. Black, MD

KEY POINTS

- The diagnosis of refractory or resistant hypertension should be reserved for those treated hypertensive patients whose blood pressure is not at goal even though they have received a regimen containing adequate doses of two or more appropriately chosen medications that have been given adequate time to be effective.

- The clinician evaluating a patient with refractory hypertension must be aware of the characteristic clinical presentation of those with secondary hypertension and should direct that evaluation toward finding the cause or causes most likely to be present.

- The most common exogenous substance that may interfere with an effective antihypertensive regimen is sodium.

- The most frequent reason for refractory hypertension in the primary care clinician's practice is nonadherence to the therapeutic regimen. Nonadherence should be suspected in all patients not at goal.

See also Chapters 119, 120, 121, 122, 158

The diagnosis of refractory or resistant hypertension should be reserved for those treated hypertensive patients whose blood pressure (BP) is not at goal even though they have received a regimen containing adequate doses of two or more appropriately chosen medications. The Sixth Joint National Committee on the Prevention, Detection, Evaluation, and Treatment of High Blood Pressure (JNC VI) has set a goal of <140 mm Hg for systolic BP and <90 mm Hg for diastolic BP in the office. The targets are even lower for those with diabetes mellitus (<130/85 mm Hg) or for those with renal insufficiency and ≥1 g proteinuria/d (<125/75 mm Hg). Other authors have characterized patients as refractory only when their BP is not controlled on three or even four drugs. With all of the highly effective and well-tolerated antihypertensive agents available, the diagnosis should be made and the search for specific reasons for the causes of refractory hypertension initiated once two appropriate agents have failed to get BP to goal. Untreated hypertensives and those who have not received an adequate regimen should never be considered to be refractory to treatment.

Only a small number of hypertensive patients, perhaps no more than 5% to 10% of patients cared for by a primary care physician, are truly resistant to treatment. In a tertiary care setting, however, the number has been as high as 25% to 30% in some series. With the lower goal for treatment recommended by JNC VI, the number of refractory hypertensives will undoubtedly be higher, but the principles of diagnosis and management remain unchanged.

Establishing the Diagnosis

The initial step in properly managing hypertensive patients, whether refractory or not, is to be certain that their BP has been properly measured. The sphygmomanometer used must be functioning and calibrated adequately; the observer must be trained and

his or her technique certified as accurate; and the cuff size used must be appropriate for the size of the patient's arm. The BP reading should be taken in a nonstressful environment after some time for rest and acclimation (usually ≥5 minutes of sitting in a quiet, if not darkened, room). Because both caffeine and nicotine acutely raise BP, the reading should not be done if the patient has had caffeine-containing products or has smoked within 30 minutes of the measurement.

In a few patients, indirect methods of measuring BP will not be accurate, and intra-arterial studies will be necessary to exclude "pseudohypertension." These measurements should be made only in patients with advanced atherosclerosis who have had no response to what should have been effective antihypertensive therapy and are having symptoms that suggest underperfusion of vital organs (dizziness, confusion, angina, intermittent claudication). The use of "Osler's maneuver" to help exclude those hypertensives with pseudohypertension whose lack of response to treatment is an artifact of the technique of indirect sphygmomanometry has proved to be disappointing and neither sensitive, specific, nor reproducible. If pseudohypertension is suspected and the establishment of the diagnosis absolutely necessary, intra-arterial readings may need to be done to be certain.

Those hypertensives who have normal readings outside of the office but are hypertensive when seen in the healthcare setting may have "white coat hypertension." They should not be characterized as being refractory unless this situation is reproduced once treatment has been initiated. Such patients have "office resistance." The term "white coat hypertension" should be reserved for untreated hypertensives.

Finding the Cause of Refractory Hypertension

Refractory hypertension should be classified according to the most likely etiology (**Table 123.1**). The clinician must appreciate

Table 123.1. **Causes of Refractory Hypertension**

1. Inaccurate measurement of BP
2. Identifiable secondary cause of hypertension
3. Ingestion of exogenous substances
4. Inadequate or inappropriate regimen
5. Complicating biological factors
6. Nonadherence

that several of these factors often contribute to the failure to control BP in the same patient.

Identifiable Secondary Causes

Although all hypertension has a cause, a specific cause can be identified in ≈5% of patients. Often such patients will appear to be refractory hypertensives because conventional therapy is often ineffective or unexpectedly troublesome. In a recent series, ≈5% of patients referred as refractory hypertensives had a secondary cause for their hypertension that was not suspected by the referring physician. Renovascular disease and mineralocorticoid excess hypertension were the two most common secondary causes not diagnosed by the referring clinician. Because patients with pheochromocytoma are often very symptomatic, this form of secondary hypertension, if refractory, was usually already considered before referral.

The clinician evaluating a patient with refractory hypertension must be aware of the characteristic clinical presentation of those with secondary hypertension and should direct that evaluation toward finding the cause or causes most likely to be present. An elderly individual with a long history of heavy cigarette smoking, clinically evident diffuse atherosclerosis, and renal insufficiency of uncertain cause, especially with a normal urinary sediment, has a reasonably high likelihood of having renovascular hypertension as the explanation for the refractory hypertension. Studies to evaluate this possibility and specific therapy, if available, are warranted. In a refractory hypertensive with unprovoked hypokalemia (serum K^+ <3.2 mEq/L without diuretic therapy) or "refractory hypokalemia" (serum K^+ <3.5 mEq/L while on potassium-sparing diuretics and/or ACE inhibitors or angiotensin receptor blockers [ARBs]), metabolic and imaging studies looking for hyperaldosteronism are appropriate.

Finding secondary causes for hypertension may not require extensive testing. For example, an elevated serum creatinine on the routine initial laboratory evaluation is evidence of renal parenchymal disease due to either primary renal disease, if the sediment is active and substantial proteinuria is present, or to essential hypertension. In either case, specific therapy to control the volume component of that patient's hypertension will be necessary if he or she is to reach goal BP.

The routine history and physical examination can also strongly suggest a secondary cause or the reason why a particular patient is not responding to treatment. Hypertensives with a history of loud snoring, daytime drowsiness, and somnolence, especially if they are obese, may well have sleep apnea. A formal sleep study may be needed to confirm this diagnosis. Treatment directed at improving the sleep apnea might help make the BP easier to control. The value of a careful and complete history to establish the use of exogenous substances that raise BP cannot be underestimated.

Exogenous Substances

The ingestion of exogenous substances or drugs, some legal and known to the clinician and patient and some illegal and not known to the clinician, can often interfere with a therapeutic regimen and make hypertension appear to be refractory to treatment (**Table 123.2**). Some of these drugs may still be required to treat a concomitant condition, even though the patient requires substantially more antihypertensive therapy to reach goal. Some of these compounds will directly raise BP, such as the sympathomimetic amines used in decongestants. Others will interfere with the action of certain antihypertensive agents, such as certain psychotropic drugs (eg, chlorpromazine) that interfere with the action of centrally acting sympatholytics. Some exogenous substances may do both. Nonsteroidal anti-inflammatory agents (NSAIDs) will interfere with the action of vasodilating prostaglandins in the kidney and may reduce the effectiveness of some ACE inhibitors. But NSAIDs also cause salt and water retention and may raise BP in volume-sensitive individuals regardless of what antihypertensive agent is prescribed. Hypertensive patients should be permitted to use NSAIDs or nasal decongestants so long as the use is strictly limited to periods when symptomatic relief is essential and the patients are not misclassified as being refractory to treatment. Drugs such as corticosteroids, erythropoietin, or cyclosporine may raise BP and interfere with what would have been an otherwise effective antihypertensive regimen. Frequently, these agents are necessary if no equally effective substitute can be found. The antihypertensive regimen must be adjusted accordingly.

Excess sodium intake is a particular problem for salt-sensitive hypertensives: the elderly, diabetics, blacks, and those with renal insufficiency. If this is considered to be the cause of a patient's resistance to therapy, a 24-hour urine analysis to assess sodium excretion will be very helpful to confirm the excess intake. Patients who ingest >100 mmol of sodium in 24 hours will often benefit from careful attention to a sodium-restricted diet or more aggressive diuretic therapy. Patients on all forms of antihypertensive therapy, even those on calcium antagonists (CAs), ACE inhibitors, or ARBs, will respond better to therapy if they are not ingesting excess sodium. Some hypertensives, when faced with the need to reduce sodium or take ad-

Table 123.2. **Exogenous Substances That Raise Blood Pressure**

1. Anabolic steroids
2. Caffeine
3. Cocaine
4. Ethanol
5. Nicotine
6. Sodium chloride
7. Sympathomimetic amines
8. Chlorpromazine
9. Corticosteroids
10. Cyclosporine
11. Erythropoietin
12. Monoamine oxidase inhibitors
13. Oral contraceptives
14. Tricyclic antidepressants
15. Anorectics

ditional antihypertensive medication, may opt to try to limit their intake of high-sodium food and their use of the salt shaker.

Excess alcohol intake and the use of illicit substances such as cocaine or amphetamines may elevate BP transiently and make the patient appear to be resistant to treatment. Phenylpropanolamine, which is used in some diet preparations, is still widely available and may be ingested by some hypertensive patients. If the use of certain anorectics, particularly sibutramine, that may raise BP in a small number of patients becomes more widespread, some hypertensive patients may appear to be resistant to treatment when using this drug.

Complicating Biological Factors

Certain biological factors may make BP difficult to control and refractory to treatment. In obese hypertensives and those with hyperinsulinemia and glucose intolerance, BP often fails to be reduced to goal with two drugs. Obesity-related hypertension is often volume-dependent, so adequate diuretic therapy is a necessity. Although the maintenance of weight as close to ideal body weight as possible is of value for all hypertensives, in those with refractory hypertension, modest weight loss (10 to 15 pounds) may make BP much easier to manage and obviate the need for a complex, expensive, and less-well-tolerated antihypertensive regimen. As with those hypertensives who eat too much sodium, the clear therapeutic benefit of reducing weight may provide the necessary motivation for a patient who has otherwise been reluctant to diet.

Some hypertensive patients will have certain comorbid conditions, such as asthma or gout, that will limit the therapeutic choices and make it impossible to use certain classes of what would otherwise be effective agents. In almost all instances, appropriate and effective alternatives are available.

It has recently become clear that anxiety and panic disorders can interfere with getting BP under control. Patients with these problems may blame their antihypertensive drugs for causing a wide variety of side effects, and so the clinician feels unable to use some effective agents to manage BP. The appreciation that psychological factors can interfere with therapy allows for a wider range of choices to reduce BP to goal.

Inappropriate or Inadequate Treatment

In our experience, the most common reason for apparent refractoriness to treatment in those referred to a tertiary center for evaluation of resistant hypertension was the use of an inappropriate or inadequate regimen. JNC VI has suggested that any of seven classes of antihypertensive agents (diuretics, β-adrenergic receptor blockers, ACE inhibitors, CAs, ARBs, α-adrenergic receptor blockers, or combined α- and β-adrenergic receptor blockers) are all appropriate as initial therapy in selected hypertensive patients. In others, low-dose, fixed-dose combinations are also recommended.

Too much has been made of what is appropriate as the initial choice for treatment and too little of what to do next. JNC VI has recommended titrating the starting dose in all patients who have tolerated the initial dose of the first choice and are still not at goal. The clinician should know not only what is the proper initial dose of a drug but also what he or she considers to be the maximum dose of that agent that is appropriate for that particular patient. He or she should not abandon the drug until that dose is reached. Substitution of a drug

from another class should be reserved for patients who have had no response once full dose has been reached or for those who have had intolerable side effects to the first agent selected. Should BP still not be at goal, then addition of an appropriate agent from another class with a different mechanism of action is recommended. This drug, too, should be titrated to full dose before the patient is considered refractory. Many hypertensives referred as resistant to therapy simply need their drugs titrated to higher or full dose to achieve goal.

In addition to inadequate therapy, the need to properly manage volume is underappreciated. Diuretic therapy is often underused or inappropriate. All antihypertensive agents are more effective if volume expansion is avoided either with sodium restriction, which is difficult to achieve, or with diuretics. It has been known for many years that thiazides are more effective antihypertensive agents than loop-active agents in hypertensives with normal renal function. Once the glomerular filtration rate falls to <30 to 50 mL/min, thiazides are often ineffective at eliciting natriuresis and reducing plasma volume. In hypertensives with this degree of renal insufficiency, loop-active agents become the diuretics of choice. In our recent series, the addition or adjustment of diuretic therapy was the single most important therapeutic change used to control BP.

Occasionally, unconventional combinations of therapeutic agents may significantly improve BP control and achieve goal. For example, the combination of dihydropyridine and nondihydropyridine CAs can be used. Although these drugs are both considered to be in the same therapeutic class, they have different effects in the heart and kidney, and their antihypertensive effect is often additive. Similarly, ACE inhibitors and ARBs also have additive antihypertensive effects.

Nonadherence to the Prescribed Regimen

In contrast to the tertiary care clinic, the most frequent reason for refractory hypertension in the primary care clinician's practice is nonadherence to the therapeutic regimen. This problem may be the primary reason in as many as 50% of refractory hypertension seen in that setting. The reason for the difference in the frequency of the causes of refractory hypertension may be that primary care clinicians are aware of the problem of nonadherence and do not refer to the specialist patients who are already known or suspected to not be taking their medication properly. Alternatively, it may indicate that hypertensives comply better with a regimen and come under control when faced with the prospect of seeing another physician.

Nonadherence should be suspected in all hypertensive patients who are not at goal. The likelihood of nonadherence increases in those who do not keep appointments and those who have no biochemical (lower potassium for those on thiazides) or physiological (slower heart rates for those on β-adrenergic receptor blockers) markers suggesting the use of prescribed agents. Unfortunately, these findings are not dependable and can only suggest, not prove, nonadherence. Patients' knowledge about hypertension or their level of education does not guarantee that they will take their antihypertensive medications properly. The clinician should strive to make the regimen simple and use as few daily doses of once-a-day medication as possible. It is also clear that an empathic and nonjudgmental approach will be particularly helpful in nonadherent patients. With the advent of newer agents, side effects are minimal and often similar to placebo, and so this reason for nonadherence need no longer be a vexing problem. The clinician must also be sensitive to economic issues and not prescribe drugs the patient cannot afford to purchase.

Finally, hypertensives who are truly refractory are likely to benefit from a referral to a hypertension specialist, who will presumably be better able to recognize and diagnose secondary hypertension and use available antihypertensive agents. It may be necessary to accept reducing BP to less than goal, because any BP reduction will benefit the patient.

Conclusions

Although some hypertensive patients will truly be unable to be treated to goal without excessive side effects, the overwhelming majority can be brought to goal or close to goal by following a few simple steps.

1. Be sure the measurement of BP is accurate and the patient is truly refractory.
2. Exclude identifiable secondary causes.
3. Be sure that the patient is not using exogenous substances that raise BP and prevent the regimen from being effective.
4. Evaluate sodium intake, and if it is high, get the patient to reduce it.
5. Get obese refractory hypertensives to lose weight.
6. Be sure that the regimen is appropriate, especially in the choice of diuretics, and that drugs are being used in adequate doses. Consider unconventional combinations.
7. Consider nonadherence and take steps to improve the patient's ability to comply with the therapeutic regimen.

8. Consider referral to a hypertension specialist.
9. Accept less than adequate control if goal BP is not obtainable.

SUGGESTED READING

1. Bravo EL, Tarazi RC, Dustan HP, Fouad FM, Textor SC, Gifford RW, Vidt DG. The changing clinical spectrum of primary aldosteronism. *Am J Med.* 1983;74: 641–651.
2. Davies SJ, Ghahramani P, Jackson PR, Hippisley-Cox J, Yeo WW, Ramsay LE. Panic disorder, anxiety and depression in resistant hypertension: a case-control study. *J Hypertens.* 1997;15:1077–1082.
3. Isaksson H, Cederholm T, Jansson E, Nygren A, Ostergren J. Therapy-resistant hypertension associated with central obesity, insulin resistance, and large muscle fibre area. *Blood Press.* 1993;2:46–52.
4. Kaplan NM. Anxiety-induced hyperventilation: a common cause of symptoms in patients with hypertension. *Arch Intern Med.* 1997;157:945–948.
5. Mezzetti A, Pierdomenico SD, Costantini F, Romano F, Bucci A, Di Gioacchino M, Cuccurullo F. White-coat resistant hypertension. *Am J Hypertens.* 1997;10: 1302–1307.
6. Modan M, Almog S, Fuchs Z, Chetrit A, Lusky A, Halkin H. Obesity, glucose intolerance, hyperinsulinemia, and response to antihypertensive drugs. *Hypertension.* 1991;17:565–573.
7. Ram CV, Garrett BN, Kaplan NM. Moderate sodium restriction and various diuretics in the treatment of hypertension: effects of potassium wastage and blood pressure control. *Arch Intern Med.* 1981;141:1015–1019.
8. Setaro JF, Black HR. Refractory hypertension. *N Engl J Med.* 1992;327:543–547.
9. Tarazi RC, Dustan HP, Frohlich ED, Gifford RW Jr, Hoffman GC. Plasma volume and chronic hypertension: relationship to arterial pressure levels in different hypertension diseases. *Arch Intern Med.* 1970;125:835–842.
10. Yakovlevitch M, Black HR. Resistant hypertension in a tertiary care clinic. *Arch Intern Med.* 1991;151:1786–1792.

Chapter 124

Diuretics

Jules B. Puschett, MD

KEY POINTS

- Diuretics continue to have, and should have, a prominent and important role in the therapy of hypertension.

- Lower dosages of the thiazides (eg, 12.5 mg to 25 mg of hydrochlorothiazide, or its equivalent, once daily) are effective and cause fewer side effects than larger doses but require a longer period of time (3 to 4 weeks) to reduce blood pressure.

- The concept advanced in the early to mid 1980s that the metabolic side effects of diuretics compromise expected beneficial effects of lowering blood pressure on coronary heart disease mortality has been refuted.

- The thiazides are not useful in renal insufficiency (glomerular filtration rate <30 mL/min).

See also Chapters 23, 123, 149

Thiazide diuretics, the first well-tolerated, orally effective antihypertensives, have enjoyed wide usage and popularity. More recently, it has been suggested that the treatment of hypertension with this class of drugs is largely responsible for the fact that markedly reduced deaths rates from stroke have been reported over the past 25 years. However the reduction in mortality from coronary artery disease has not fallen to the extent expected from epidemiological estimates. The possibility was raised that metabolic side effects—hypokalemia, hypomagnesemia, and a tendency toward elevated serum lipids—compromised the expected beneficial effects of lowering blood pressure. Several investigators suggested that thiazide use, especially as first-line agents, should be abandoned. It now seems clear, however, that diuretics continue to occupy a prominent and important role in the therapy of hypertension.

Mechanisms of Thiazide Diuretic Effects on Blood Pressure

Effects of thiazides on blood pressure may be categorized as having acute, subacute, and chronic phases **(Figure 124.1).** These three periods correspond roughly to 1 to 2 weeks, several weeks, and several months, respectively, after initial administration. The data suggest that early on, the major hypotensive effect of diuretics is to reduce extracellular fluid volume (Figure 124.1). Over time, these actions on volume become less important, although blood pressure remains lowered. The later or more chronic actions of diuretics result largely from a reduction in peripheral vascular resistance. In the "subacute" period, a transition phase occurs in which both of these factors play major roles. These pathophysiological facts have importance in at least two practical aspects of the therapy of hypertension with diuretics. First, to take full advantage of the early action of diuretics to reduce extracellular fluid volume, restriction of dietary sodium must be combined with the use of these agents. Second, in certain patient groups, particularly blacks, the elderly, and the obese, salt sensitivity appears to play a central role in the pathophysiology of hypertension. Accordingly, in these patients, diuretics are especially effective antihypertensive agents.

Diuretics are often helpful in combination with other antihypertensive agents, either when the latter are not completely effective as monotherapy or in the patient with edema. Concerns had been raised that diuretics might not protect hypertensive patients from the eventual development of heart failure. However, data obtained by the SHEP Cooperative Research Group **(Figure 124.2)** show that these fears appear to be unwarranted. As suggested previously and confirmed more recently, in older patients with isolated systolic hypertension or previous myocardial infarction, diuretic-based therapy for hypertension reduces the incidence of heart failure **(Figure 124.3).**

Therapeutic Recommendations

Dosage guidelines for diuretic therapy of hypertension are provided in **Table 124.1.** The thiazides or metolazone are preferred to the other more potent (but short-acting) loop-active agents (furosemide, ethacrynic acid, and bumetanide) because their duration of action is longer and because loop diuretics have less vasorelaxant effect on arterioles. Torsemide, which has a prolonged duration of action (up to 24 hours), is an exception. Thiazides do not cause rebound sodium retention, which is characteristic of short-acting loop-active agents, especially when the latter are given once daily.

It is now apparent that lower dosages of thiazides than those originally used are appropriate. In the elderly, a beginning dose of 12.5 mg and a maximum dose of 25 mg hydrochlorothiazide (or its equivalent) are recommended. In other groups of patients, it is rarely necessary or desirable to exceed 50 mg/d.

Sodium in the diet should be limited to "no added salt," because in the ambulatory patient, compliance with more severe restriction is difficult or impossible. Accordingly, the patient is asked to avoid obviously salty foods, to eliminate using the salt shaker at meals, and to not add salt during cooking.

If hypokalemia develops, it may be treated in one of three ways: (1) addition of potassium chloride, (2) addition of a potassium-sparing agent, or (3) use of a combination agent containing both a thiazide and a potassium-sparing drug (Table 124.1). Some use the combination drugs at the onset of therapy.

The thiazides are not useful in patients with renal insufficiency. In those who have glomerular filtration rates <30 to 40 mL/min, approx-

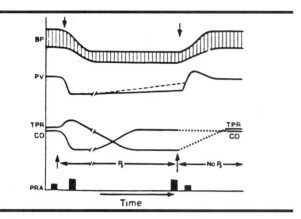

Figure 124.1. Diagrammatic representation of effects of diuretic administration on blood pressure (BP), plasma volume (PV), total peripheral resistance (TPR), and cardiac output (CO). PRA indicates plasma renin activity. Therapy was begun at arrow on left and discontinued at arrow on right. Adapted with permission from Tarazi RC, Dustan HP, Frohlich ED. Long-term thiazide therapy in essential hypertension. *Circulation.* 1970;41:709.

imately equivalent to a serum creatinine of 2.5 to 3.0 mg/dL, loop-active agents should be used. When used, furosemide, bumetanide, or ethacrynic acid should be given more than once daily in recognition of their much shorter duration of action (4 to 6 hours) than the thiazides (18 to 24 hours). Torsemide is effective when given once daily.

Side Effects and Complications
Volume Depletion

Volume depletion is unlikely with the thiazides and is ordinarily seen only with large doses of loop-active agents. When it occurs, there is an increase in blood urea nitrogen (BUN) without a proportional elevation in serum creatinine ("prerenal azotemia"). Reduction in dosage or discontinuation of the diuretic along with liberalization of sodium intake usually corrects this abnormality.

Hypokalemia

Hypokalemia results from the kaliuretic tendencies of natriuretic agents. Because hypokalemia may predispose patients to cardiac ar-

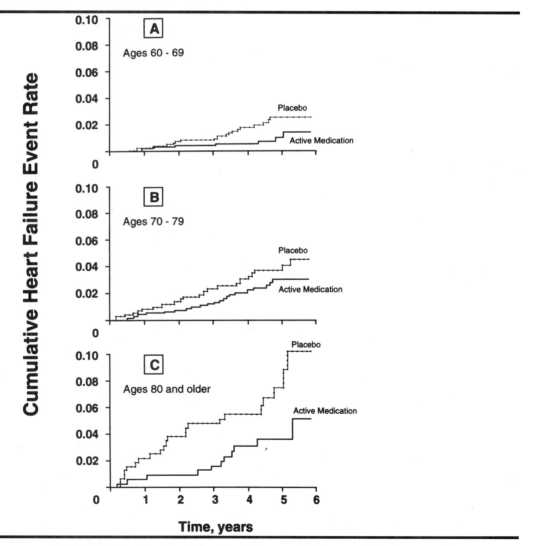

Figure 124.2. Total rates of occurrence of both fatal and nonfatal hospitalized heart failure in active therapy and placebo groups of patients in Systolic Hypertension in the Elderly Program categorized by age group. Therapy was with diuretic-based stepped-care treatment. Probability values for the three age groups comparing treated and untreated patients are A, *P*=.04; B, *P*=.14; and C, *P*=.04. Reproduced with permission from Kostis JB, et al. *JAMA.* 1997;278:212–216.

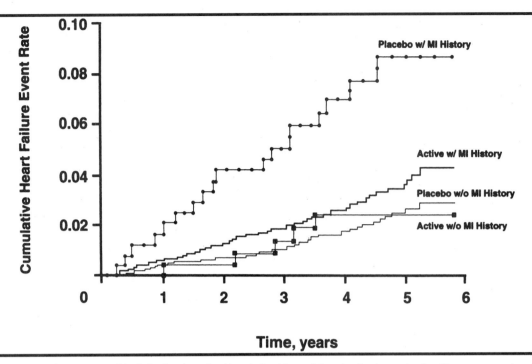

Figure 124.3. Total rates of occurrence of both fatal and nonfatal hospitalized heart failure in placebo and active-therapy groups in patients with and without previous myocardial infarction (MI). Therapy was with diuretic-based stepped-care treatment programs. In this study, use of atenolol (or reserpine) did not provide significant additional protection against development of heart failure compared with use of chlorthalidone alone. Reproduced with permission from Kostis JB, et al. *JAMA.* 1997;278:212–216.

rhythmias, especially in those taking digitalis or those with left ventricular hypertrophy, it should be corrected. As noted above, this can be done by administration of potassium chloride. Alternatively, a potassium-sparing agent may be added, or a combination drug (thiazide plus a potassium-sparing agent) may be administered.

Lipid Elevation

Increases in serum cholesterol are usually not seen with small doses of thiazides (≤25 mg hydrochlorothiazide or equivalent). The average increase, when it occurs, is small (6% to 7%), and the levels usually decline over time even if the thiazide is continued. This situation may be ameliorated by use of a low-fat diet, by addition of a lipid-lowering agent, or by discontinuation of the diuretic.

Glucose Intolerance

The sulfonamide-derivative diuretics (which includes the thiazides) rarely elevate the blood glucose level when given in small doses. However, they may worsen blood sugar control in some diabetics. They may, of course, be required for the therapy of edema in such patients. In some studies, thiazide diuretics have been shown to cause or worsen peripheral resistance to insulin.

Metabolic Alkalosis

Both the thiazides and the loop-active agents result in the excretion of both fluid and sodium, largely in association with chloride. In addition, both classes of drug present additional sodium ions to distal tubular sites for exchange with hydrogen and potassium ions. Accordingly, contraction metabolic alkalosis occurs, usually linked to

potassium loss. It is important not to replace the potassium deficit with a bicarbonate or gluconate salt because the chloride deficit will increase, will perpetuate or worsen the alkalosis, and will make it more difficult to replete potassium.

Hyponatremia

Hyponatremia, a complication of diuretic administration, is either idiosyncratic or dose-related. In the latter case, the patient becomes hemodiluted because the drug interferes with normal urinary diluting capacity (the mechanism by which solute-free water is excreted) while the patient continues to ingest excess solute-free water. Antidiuretic hormone is eventually stimulated by the volume contraction and the patient develops positive water balance and worsening hyponatremia. The exact mechanism by which acute idiosyncratic hyponatremia occurs with small amounts of drug is not completely understood. This has usually occurred in female patients given one of the thiazides or metolazone, often after only one or just a few doses. In both cases, the diuretic should be withdrawn.

Other Complications

Hyperuricemia occurs because of the effects of volume contraction and because uric acid and the diuretic compete for tubular secretion. In susceptible individuals, acute gouty arthritis may be precipitated, although it is rare. Hyperkalemia may be seen in patients given potassium-sparing agents. This is usually a problem only in patients with decreased rates of glomerular filtration, in whom potassium disposal is already a problem. Volume contraction exacerbates this problem because of its effects on glomerular filtration rate. Hy-

Table 124.1. Dosage Guidelines

DRUG	TOTAL DAILY DOSAGE/FREQUENCY	COMMENTS
Thiazides and similar drugs		
Hydrochlorothiazide	12.5–50 mg, QD	In the elderly, begin with 12.5 mg; a top dose of 25 mg is recommended. Exceeding 50 mg in any demographic group increases the likelihood of the development of hypokalemia. Treat hypokalemia with the chloride salt of potassium or add a potassium-sparing drug.
Chlorthalidone	12.5–50 mg, QD	Same as for hydrochlorothiazide. Chlorthalidone effect may last longer than that of hydrochlorothiazide (in some cases, up to 48 hours).
Metolazone	0.5–5.0 mg, QD	Unlike the thiazides, metolazone is effective in patients with significant reductions in glomerular filtration rate (<40 mL/min), although a higher dosage (10–20 mg) may be required than that which is effective in patients with normal renal function.
Loop-active diuretics		
Furosemide	40–240 mg, BID	With the exception of torsemide, the loop-active agents must be given more than once daily in order to avoid rebound sodium retention, because of the their shorter duration of action. In patients with renal insufficiency, it is usually necessary to give >40 mg/d of furosemide (or an equivalent dose of the other loop of Henle agents). The single effective dose should be determined, then repeated as necessary. In very edematous hypertensive patients, the intravenous route may be necessary. The same is true for pulmonary edema. Approximate drug dosage equivalencies are as follows:

furosemide 40 mg; bumetanide 1 mg; ethacrynic acid 50 mg; torsemide 20 mg.

DRUG	TOTAL DAILY DOSAGE/FREQUENCY	COMMENTS
Bumetanide	0.5–5.0 mg, BID	Comments (above) related to loop-active agents apply. Some patients who are not responsive to furosemide do respond to this agent and vice versa.
Ethacrynic acid	25.0–100 mg	See comments about. Ethacrynic acid has a chemical structure unlike furosemide and bumetanide, which are sulfonamide derivatives.
Torsemide	2.5–10 mg, QD	See comments above. Torsemide is equivalently bioavailable when given orally and intravenously. In the pulmonary edema patient, doses of up to 100 mg of torsemide have been used, and in patients with chronic renal failure who have both hypertension and edema, dosages up to 200 mg/d have been used successfully.
Potassium-sparing diuretics		
Spironolactone	25–100 mg, QD or BID	Used almost exclusively in combination with other agents (usually the thiazides to prevent or treat hypokalemia from the latter drug[s]). Fixed combinations with the thiazides are available and have been used frequently for therapy of hypertension. Should be used with great caution or not at all in patients with renal insufficiency. May contribute to the development of metabolic acidosis in the latter patient group.
Amiloride	5–10 mg, BID	Same as above. Amiloride is a sodium channel blocker, whereas spironolactone is a competitive inhibitor of aldosterone.
Trimterene	50–150 mg, QD or BID	Same as amiloride.

pomagnesemia can also occur with thiazides. Magnesium loss may increase the tendency toward the development of arrhythmias in patients with heart disease, and it may be impossible to replete potassium unless magnesium depletion is treated as well. Potassium-sparing diuretics also conserve magnesium.

SUGGESTED READING

1. Duke M. Thiazide-induced hypokalemia: association with acute myocardial infarction and ventricular fibrillation. *JAMA.* 1978;239:43–45.
2. Freis ED. Critique of the clinical importance of diuretic-induced hypokalemia and elevated cholesterol level. *Arch Intern Med.* 1989;149:2640–2648.
3. Kostis JB, et al. Prevention of heart failure by antihypertensive drug treatment in older persons with isolated systolic hypertension. *JAMA.* 1997;278:212–216.
4. Madias JE, Madias NE, Gavras HP. Nonarrhythmogenicity of diuretic-induced hypokalemia: its evidence in patients with uncomplicated hypertension. *Arch Intern Med.* 1984;144:2171–2176.
5. McVeigh G, Galloway D, Johnston D. The case for low dose diuretics in hypertension: comparison of low and conventional doses of cyclopenthiazide. *BMJ.* 1988;297:95–98.
6. Medical Research Council Working Party on Mild to Moderate Hypertension. Ventricular extrasystoles during thiazide treatment: substudy of MRC mild hypertension trial. *BMJ.* 1983;287:1249–1253.
7. Moser M, Setaro JF. Antihypertensive drug therapy and regression of left ventricular hypertrophy: a review with a focus on diuretics. *Eur Heart J.* 1991;12:1034–1039.
8. O'Donovan RA, Muhammedi M, Puschett JB. Diuretics in the therapy of hypertension: current status. *Am J Med Sci.* 1992;304:312–318.
9. Papademetriou V, Price M, Notargiacomo A, Gottdiener J, Fletcher RD, Freis ED. Effect of diuretic therapy on ventricular arrhythmias in hypertensive patients with or without left ventricular hypertrophy. *Am Heart J.* 1985;144:2171–2176.
10. Siegel D, Hulley SB, Black DM, et al. Diuretics, serum and intracellular electrolyte levels, and ventricular arrhythmias in hypertensive men. *JAMA.* 1992;267:1083–1089.

Chapter 125

β-Adrenergic Blockers

William H. Frishman, MD

KEY POINTS

- β-Adrenergic blockers differ in terms of presence or absence of intrinsic sympathomimetic activity, membrane stabilizing activity, β_1-selectivity, α-adrenergic blocking activity, relative potencies, and duration of action.

- β-Blockers are appropriate for initial as well as subsequent therapy of all degrees of arterial hypertension.

- Some β-adrenergic blockers reduce the risk of mortality and nonfatal reinfarction in survivors of acute myocardial infarction.

- β-Blockers with vasodilating properties may improve clinical outcomes in patients with left ventricular dysfunction and stable symptoms who are receiving conventional heart failure treatment.

See also Chapters 1, 44, 45, 126, 127

The Sixth Report of the Joint National Committee on Prevention, Detection, Evaluation, and Treatment of High Blood Pressure (JNC VI) from the National High Blood Pressure Education Program of the National Heart, Lung, and Blood Institute has reiterated the recommendation of JNC III, IV, and V that β-adrenergic blockers are appropriate alternatives as first-line treatment for hypertension. These recommendations are based on the reduction of morbidity and mortality when these drugs have been used in large clinical trials. Although there is no consensus as to the mechanisms by which β-blocking drugs lower blood pressure, it is probable that some or all of the modes of action listed in **Table 125.1** are involved.

Thirteen orally active β-adrenergic blockers are approved in the United States for treatment of hypertension **(Table 125.2)**. In addition, intravenous labetalol is approved for the management of hypertensive emergencies. Oral bisoprolol in combination with a very-low-dose diuretic has received approval as a first-line antihypertensive treatment, the first such β-blocker combination so approved for the treatment of hypertension.

The various agents differ in terms of the presence or absence of intrinsic sympathomimetic activity (ISA), membrane-stabilizing activity (MSA), β_1-selectivity, α-adrenergic blocking activity, relative potencies, and duration of action. Nevertheless, all β-blockers studied to date appear to have favorable blood pressure–lowering effects when used in appropriate dosages.

Pharmacodynamic Properties
Membrane-Stabilizing Activity

At concentrations well above therapeutic levels, certain β-blockers have a quinidine-like or local anesthetic membrane-stabilizing effect on the cardiac action potential. There is no evidence that MSA is responsible for any direct negative inotropic effect of the β-blockers, because drugs with and without this property (usually in high doses) can depress left ventricular function. However, MSA can manifest itself clinically with massive β-blocker intoxication.

β_1-Selectivity

When used in low doses, β_1-selective blocking agents such as acebutolol, betaxolol, bisoprolol, esmolol, atenolol, and metoprolol inhibit cardiac β_1-receptors but have less influence on bronchial and vascular β-adrenergic receptors (β_2). In higher doses, however, β_1-selective blocking agents also block β_2-receptors. Accordingly, β_1-selective agents may be safer than nonselective ones in patients with obstructive pulmonary disease, because β_2-receptors remain available to mediate adrenergic bronchodilatation. However, even selective β_1-blockers may aggravate bronchospasm in certain patients, and so these drugs should generally not be used in patients with bronchospastic disease.

A second theoretical advantage is that unlike nonselective β-blockers, β_1-selective blockers in low doses may not block the β_2-receptors that mediate dilatation of arterioles. It is possible that leaving the β_2-receptors unblocked and responsive to epinephrine may be functionally important in some patients with asthma, hypoglycemia, hypertension, or peripheral vascular disease treated with β-adrenergic blocking drugs.

ISA or Partial Agonist Activity

Certain β-adrenergic receptor blockers possess partial agonist activity at β_1-adrenergic receptor sites, β_2-adrenergic receptor sites, or both. In a β-blocker, this property is identified as a slight cardiac stimulation, which can be blocked by propranolol. The β-blockers with this property slightly activate the β-receptor, in addition to preventing the access of natural or synthetic catecholamines to the receptor. In the treatment of patients with arrhythmias, angina pectoris of effort, or hypertension, drugs with mild-to-moderate partial agonist activity appear to be as efficacious as β-blockers lacking this property. It is still debated whether the presence of partial agonist activity in a β-blocker constitutes an overall advantage or disadvantage in cardiac therapy. Drugs with partial agonist activity cause less slowing of the heart rate at rest than do propranolol and metoprolol, although the increments in heart rate with exercise are similarly blunted. β-Blocking agents with nonselective partial agonist activity reduce peripheral vascular resistance and may also cause less depression of atrioventricular conduction than drugs lacking this property.

α-Adrenergic Blocking Activity

Carvedilol and labetalol are β-blockers with antagonistic properties at both α- and β-adrenergic receptors, with direct vasodilator activity. Like other β-blockers, they are useful in the treatment of hypertension and angina pectoris. However, unlike most β-blocking drugs, the additional α-adrenergic blocking actions of carvedilol and labetalol lead to a reduction in peripheral vascular resistance that acts to maintain higher levels of cardiac output.

Pharmacokinetic Properties

Although the β-adrenergic blocking drugs as a group have similar therapeutic effects, their pharmacokinetics are markedly different **(Tables 125.3 and 125.4).** Their varied aromatic ring structures lead to differences in completeness of gastrointestinal absorption, amount of first-pass hepatic metabolism, lipid solubility,

protein binding, extent of distribution in the body, penetration into the brain, concentration in the heart, rate of hepatic biotransformation, pharmacological activity of metabolites, and renal clearance of a drug and its metabolites. These properties may then influence the clinical usefulness of β-adrenergic blockers in some patients.

The β-blockers can be divided by their pharmacokinetic properties into two broad categories: those eliminated by hepatic metabolism, which tend to have relatively short plasma half-lives, and those eliminated unchanged by the kidney, which tend to have longer half-lives. Propranolol and metoprolol are both lipid-soluble, are almost completely absorbed by the small intestine, and are largely metabolized by the liver. They tend to have highly variable bioavailability and relatively short plasma half-lives. A lack of correlation between the duration of clinical pharmacological effect and plasma half-life may allow these drugs to be administered once or twice daily.

In contrast, agents such as atenolol and nadolol are more water-soluble, are incompletely absorbed through the gut, and are eliminated unchanged by the kidney. They tend to have less variable bioavailability in patients with normal renal function, in addition to longer half-lives, allowing one dose a day. The longer half-lives may be useful in patients who find compliance with frequent β-blocker dosing a problem.

Extended-release formulations of metoprolol and propranolol are available that allow once-daily dosing of these drugs. Studies have shown that both long-acting propranolol and metoprolol provide much smoother curves of daily plasma levels than do comparable divided doses of conventional propranolol and metoprolol. Sublingual and nasal spray formulations that can provide immediate β-blockade are being tested in clinical trials.

Ultra–short-acting β-blockers are now available and may be useful when a short duration of action is desired (eg, in patients with questionable congestive heart failure). One of these compounds, esmolol, a β₁-selective drug, has been shown to be useful in the treatment of perioperative hypertension and supraventricular tachycardias. The short half-life (≈ 15 minutes) relates to the rapid metabolism of the drug by

---

Table 125.1 Proposed Mechanisms to Explain the Antihypertensive Actions of β-Blockers

1. Reduction in cardiac output
2. Central nervous system effect
3. Inhibition of renin
4. Reduction in venous return and plasma volume
5. Reduction in peripheral vascular resistance
6. Improvement in vascular compliance
7. Resetting of baroreceptor levels
8. Effects on prejunctional β-receptors: reduction in norepinephrine release
9. Attenuation of pressor response to catecholamines with exercise and stress

Adapted with permission from Frishman WH. *Clinical Pharmacology of the β-Adrenoceptor Blocking Drugs.* 2nd ed. Norwalk, Conn: Appleton-Century-Crofts; 1984.

Table 125.2 Pharmacodynamic Properties of β-Adrenergic Blocking Drugs Used in Hypertension

DRUG	β₁-BLOCKADE POTENCY RATIO (PROPRANOLOL = 1.0)	RELATIVE β₁-SELECTIVITY	INTRINSIC SYMPATHOMIMETIC ACTIVITY	MEMBRANE-STABILIZING ACTIVITY
Acebutolol	0.3	+	+	+
Atenolol	1.0	++	0	0
Betaxolol	1.0	++	0	+
Bisoprolol*	10.0	++	0	0
Carteolol	10.0	0	+	0
Carvedilol†	10.0	0	0	++
Labetalol‡	0.3	0	+?	0
Metoprolol	1.0	++	0	0
Nadolol	1.0	0	0	0
Penbutolol	1.0	0	+	0
Pindolol	6.0	0	++	+
Propranolol	1.0	0	0	+

Adapted with permission from Frishman WH. *Clinical Pharmacology of the β-Adrenoceptor Blocking Drugs.* 2nd ed. Norwalk, Conn: Appleton-Century-Crofts; 1984.
*Bisoprolol is also approved as a first-line antihypertensive therapy in combination with a very-low-dose diuretic.
†Carvedilol has additional α₁-adrenergic blocking activity without peripheral β₂-agonism.
‡Labetalol has additional α₁-adrenergic blocking activity and direct vasodilatory activity (β₂-agonism); it is available for use in intravenous form for hypertensive emergencies.

Table 125.3. Pharmacokinetic Properties of β-Adrenoceptor Blocking Drugs Used in Hypertension

DRUG	EXTENT OF ABSORPTION, % OF DOSE	EXTENT OF BIOAVAILABILITY, % OF DOSE	DOSE-DEPENDENT BIOAVAILABILITY (MAJOR FIRST-PASS HEPATIC METABOLISM)	INTERPATIENT VARIATIONS IN PLASMA LEVELS	β-BLOCKING PLASMA CONCENTRATIONS	PROTEIN BINDING, %	LIPID SOLUBILITY*
Acebutolol	≈70	≈40	No	7-fold	0.3–2.0 μg/mL	25	Moderate
Atenolol	≈50	≈40	No	4-fold	0.2–5.0 μg/mL	<5	Weak
Betaxolol	>90	≈80	No	2-fold	5–20 ng/mL	50	Moderate
Bisoprolol	>80	90	No		0.01–0.1 μg/mL	≈30	Moderate
Carteolol	≈90	≈90	No	2-fold	40–160 ng/mL	20–30	Weak
Carvedilol	>90	≈30	Yes	5- to 10-fold	10–100 ng/mL	98	Moderate
Labetalol	>90	≈33	Yes	10-fold	0.7–3.0 μg/mL	≈50	Weak
Metoprolol	>90	≈50	No	7-fold	50–100 ng/mL	12	Moderate
Long-acting metoprolol	>90	≈80	No	2-fold	70–400 ng/mL	12	Moderate
Nadolol	30	≈30	No	7-fold	50–100 ng/mL	30	Weak
Penbutolol	>90	≈90	No	4-fold		98	High
Pindolol	>90	≈90	No	4-fold	5–15 ng/mL	57	Moderate
Propranolol	>90	≈30	Yes	20-fold	50–100 ng/mL	93	High
Long-acting propranolol	>90	≈20	Yes	10 to 20-fold	20–100 ng/mL	93	High
Timolol	>90	≈75	No	7-fold	5–10 ng/mL	≈10	Weak

Adapted with permission from Frishman WH. *Clinical Pharmacology of the β-Adrenoceptor Blocking Drugs.* 2nd ed. Norwalk, Conn: Appleton-Century-Crofts; 1984.
*Determined by the distribution ratio between octanol and water.

Table 125.4. Elimination Characteristics of β-Adrenoceptor Blocking Drugs Used in Hypertension

DRUG	ELIMINATION HALF-LIFE, H	TOTAL BODY CLEARANCE, ML/MIN	URINARY RECOVERY OF UNCHANGED DRUG, % OF DOSE	TOTAL URINARY RECOVERY, % OF DOSE	PREDOMINANT ROUTE OF ELIMINATION	ACTIVE METABOLITES	DRUG ACCUMULATION IN RENAL DISEASE
Acebutolol	3–4*	480	≈40	>90	RE (≈40% unchanged & HM)	Yes	Yes
Atenolol	6–9	130	≈40	>95	RE	No	Yes
Betaxolol	15	350	15	>90	HM	No	Yes
Bisoprolol	9–12	260	50	>98	RE+HM	No	Yes
Carteolol	5–6	497	40–68	90	RE	Yes	Yes
Carvedilol	7–10	600†	<2	16	HM	Yes	No
Celiprolol	5	500	≈90	≈30	RE (≈50% unchanged & HM)	Yes	No
Labetalol	3–4	2700	<1	>90	HM	No	No
Metoprolol	3–4	1100	≈3	>95	HM	No	No
Long-acting metoprolol							
Penbutolol	27	350	50–70	>90	RE	No	No
Pindolol	3–4	400	≈40	>90	RE (≈40% unchanged & HM)	No	No
Propranolol	3–4	1000	<1	>90	HM	Yes	No
Long-acting propranolol	10	1000	<1	>90	HM	Yes	No
Timolol	4–5	660	20	65	RE (≈20% unchanged & HM)	No	No

Adapted with permission from Frishman WH. *Clinical Pharmacology of the β-Adrenoceptor Blocking Drugs.* 2nd. ed. Norwalk, Conn: Appleton-Century-Crofts; 1984.
RE indicates excretion; HM, hepatic metabolism.
*Acebutolol has an active metabolite with elimination half-life of 8 to 13 hours.
†Plasma clearance.

blood and hepatic esterases. Metabolism does not seem to be altered by disease states.

Effects on Blood Pressure
Clinical Use

β-Adrenergic blockers, alone and in combination with other antihypertensives, reduce blood pressure in patients with combined systolic and diastolic hypertension and in most patients with isolated systolic hypertension in the elderly. Uncommonly, there is a paradoxical elevation of systolic pressure during β-blockade in persons with severe aortic sclerosis, presumably due to the increased stroke volume caused by the rate-slowing effect of the agent.

β-Blockers are considered to be first-line treatment and are also indicated for patients having concomitant angina pectoris, hypertrophic cardiomyopathy, hyperdynamic circulations, essential tremor, and headaches. Some β-adrenergic blockers are also found to reduce the risk of mortality in survivors of acute myocardial infarction. The drugs can be used with caution in pregnancy and appear to be especially useful in treating perioperative hypertension.

Most antihypertensive drugs, including β-blockers, reduce left ventricular mass and wall thickness. It is not known, however, whether reversal of hypertension-induced cardiac hypertrophy improves the independent risk of cardiovascular morbidity and mortality associated with left ventricular hypertrophy.

There is evidence that some β-adrenergic blockers (those not having partial agonist activity) may not be as effective as other antihypertensive treatments in black patients. When combined with a diuretic, however, β-blockers appear to be as effective as other combination treatment regimens in black patients.

The combined α,β-blocker labetalol is the only β-blocker indicated for parenteral management of hypertensive emergencies and for treatment of intraoperative and postoperative hypertension. It can also be used in oral form to treat patients with hypertensive emergencies.

Adverse Effects and Contraindications

Most β-adrenergic blockers, at least in the usual antihypertensive dose range, should not be used in patients with asthma, chronic obstructive pulmonary disease, decompensated congestive heart failure with systolic dysfunction, heart block (greater than first degree), and sick sinus syndrome. The α,β-blocker carvedilol has been shown to reduce morbidity and mortality in patients with hypertension and stable New York Heart Association class II and III heart failure who are receiving diuretics, ACE inhibitors, and digoxin. Efficacy and safety experiences with metoprolol and other β-blockers in this population are limited, and clinical studies are currently in progress.

The drugs should be used with caution in insulin-dependent diabetes, because they may worsen glucose intolerance, mask the symptoms of hypoglycemia or prolong recovery from hypoglycemia, or increase the magnitude of the hypertensive response to hypoglycemia. There is probably a shorter recovery period from hypoglycemia with β_1-selective adrenergic blockers. β-Blockers should

not be discontinued abruptly in patients with known ischemic heart disease.

β-Blockers may increase levels of plasma triglycerides and reduce those of HDL cholesterol. Despite this effect, β-blockers without ISA are the only agents conclusively shown to decrease the rate of sudden death, overall mortality, and recurrent myocardial infarction in survivors of acute myocardial infarction. β-Blockers with ISA or α-blocking activity have little or no adverse effect on plasma lipids, but these agents have not been shown to have a protective effect after a myocardial infarction except in a limited study of high-risk patients.

There are special considerations when β-blockers are combined with other drugs. Combinations of diltiazem or verapamil with β-blockers may have additional depressant effects on the sinoatrial and atrioventricular nodes and may also promote negative inotropy. Addition of H_2-blocking agents to the combination of verapamil and β-blocker can also lead to myocardial depression. Combinations of β-blockers and reserpine may cause marked bradycardia and syncope. Combination with phenylpropanolamine, pseudoephedrine, ephedrine, and epinephrine can cause elevations in blood pressure due to unopposed α-receptor–induced vasoconstriction.

SUGGESTED READING

1. Devereux RB. Do antihypertensive drugs differ in their ability to regress left ventricular hypertrophy? *Circulation.* 1997;95:1983–1985.

2. Frishman WH, Bryzinski BS, Coulson LR, DeQuattro VL, Vlachakis ND, Mroczek WJ, Dukart G, Goldberg JD, Alemayehu D, Koury K. A multifactorial trial design to assess combination therapy in hypertension: treatment with bisoprolol and hydrochlorothiazide [published correction appears in *Arch Intern Med.* 1995; 155:709]. *Arch Intern Med.* 1994;154:1461–1468.

3. Frishman WH, Sonnenblick EH. β-Adrenergic blocking drugs and calcium channel blockers. In: Alexander RW, Schlant RC, Fuster V. *Hurst's The Heart.* 9th ed. New York, NY: McGraw-Hill Publishing Co; 1998:1583–1618.

4. Frishman WH. Alpha and beta-adrenergic blocking drugs. In: Frishman WH, Sonnenblick EH, eds. *Cardiovascular Pharmaco-therapeutics.* New York, NY: McGraw-Hill Publishing Co; 1997:59–94.

5. Frishman WH. *Clinical Pharmacology of the β-Adrenoceptor Blocking Drugs.* 2nd ed. Norwalk, Conn: Appleton-Century-Crofts; 1984.

6. Frishman WH. Postinfarction survival: role of β-adrenergic blockade. In: Fuster V, Ross R, Topol EJ, eds. *Atherosclerosis and Coronary Artery Disease.* Philadelphia, Pa: Lippincott Raven; 1996:1205–1214.

7. Mangano DT, Layug EL, Wallace A, Tateo I, for the Multicenter Study of Perioperative Ischemia Research Group. Effect of atenolol on mortality and cardiovascular morbidity after noncardiac surgery. *N Engl J Med.* 1996;335:1713–1720.

8. Materson BJ, Reda DJ, Cushman WC, Massie BM, Freis ED, Kochar MS, Hamburger RJ, Fye C, Lakshman R, Gottdiener J, Ramirez EA, Henderson WG, for the Department of Veterans Affairs Cooperative Study Group on Antihypertensive Agents. Single-drug therapy for hypertension in men: a comparison of six antihypertensive agents with placebo [published correction appears in *N Engl J Med.* 1994;330:1689]. *N Engl J Med.* 1993;328:914–921.

9. Psaty BM, Smith NL, Siscovick DS, Koepsell TD, Weiss NS, Heckbert SR, Lemaitre RN, Wagner EH, Furberg CD. Health outcomes associated with antihypertensive therapies used as first-line agents: a systematic review and meta-analysis. *JAMA.* 1997;277:739–745.

10. Systolic Hypertension in the Elderly Program Cooperative Research Group. Implications of the systolic hypertension in the elderly program. *Hypertension.* 1993; 21:335–343.

11. Gottlieb SS, McCarter RJ, Vogel RA, Effect of beta-blockade on mortality among high-risk and low-risk patients after myocardial infarction. N Engl J. Med 1998; 339:489–497.

Chapter 126

α-Adrenergic Blockers

R.H. Grimm, Jr, MD, PhD

KEY POINTS

- α_1-Antagonists inhibit the vasoconstrictor effects of norepinephrine, resulting in relaxation of blood vessels, particularly small arteries and arterioles, thus reducing peripheral vascular resistance and blood pressure (BP).

- α_1-Antagonists are effective agents for lowering BP. The degree of BP lowering is comparable to that with other major classes of BP drugs, with the exception that they are generally more potent when taken in the upright position than in the supine position. Used as monotherapy, α_1-antagonists lower systolic and diastolic pressures by 8% to 10%.

- Dizziness is the most common complaint, and it is usually mild and transient.

- α_1-Antagonists are the only class of antihypertensive drugs that have consistently been shown to favorably affect plasma lipids.

See also Chapters 1, 125, 127

α_1-Antagonists (α-blockers) are commonly used antihypertensive agents that safely and effectively lower blood pressure (BP). The first drug in this class introduced in the United States in 1976 was prazosin. Longer-acting agents such as doxazosin and terazosin are now more commonly used.

When α_1-antagonists were initially approved, the mechanism of action for lowering BP was considered to be phosphodiesterase inhibition. At the same time that the α-receptor antagonist activity was discovered, subtypes of α-receptors were identified. Nonselective α-blockers, such as phenoxybenzamine, were used in the 1960s but were largely abandoned because of serious side effects, in particular, syncope, orthostatic hypotension, limited efficacy in lowering BP, and the development of tolerance. When prazosin was initially marketed in the United Kingdom, the starting dose was higher than what was ultimately recommended, resulting in some patients developing syncope, dizziness, and orthostatic hypotension. The discovery that prazosin selectively blocked the α_2-activity afforded differentiation from the nonselective α-blockers while at the same time providing the rationale for clinical use.

Mechanism of Action

α_1-Antagonists inhibit the vasoconstrictor effects of norepinephrine, resulting in relaxation of blood vessels, particularly small arteries and arterioles, thus reducing peripheral vascular resistance and BP. α_1-Blockers do not appreciably influence cardiac output or renin release, in part because of a relatively balanced effect on arteries and veins. Although supine heart rate does not increase, postural change unmasks a tendency toward tachycardia. The effectiveness of α_1-antagonists is proportional to the degree of sympathetic activation, and most BP lowering occurs at the low- to mid-dose range (ie, 4 to 8 mg/d with doxazosin or 5 to 10 mg/d with terazosin).

Available Agents

Both nonselective and selective α_1-blockers are available for clinical use. Phenoxybenzamine is a noncompetitive, nonselective α-blocker that now is used primarily as a treatment for elevated BP due to pheochromocytoma. Phentolamine is a competitive, nonselective α-blocker that occasionally is used parenterally for severe hypertension. Prazosin was the first selective α-blocker, and it has the highest affinity for the α_1-receptor sites and also has a more rapid onset of action, which probably accounts for a relatively higher rate of syncope and orthostatic hypotension compared with doxazosin and terazosin. Prazosin has a relatively short duration of action and should be given twice daily. Doxazosin has the longest half-life (22 hours), making it a true once-a-day agent; it also has a smoother onset of action after surgery. Terazosin is similar to prazosin and has a longer half-life (12 hours), which allows symptoms to be controlled with once-daily dosing. The dose range for terazosin is 1 to 20 mg, and for doxazosin, 1 to 16 mg.

BP-Lowering Efficacy

α_1-Antagonists are effective agents for lowering BP. The degree of BP lowering is comparable to that of other major classes of BP drugs, with the exception that they are generally more potent when given with the patient in the upright position than supine. Used as monotherapy, α_1-antagonists lower systolic and diastolic pressures by 8% to 10%. α_1-Antagonists are also commonly used as add-on treatment in hypertensives with hard-to-control symptoms. Their BP-lowering efficacy has been demonstrated to be sustained over many years of treatment.

Side Effects

The incidence of side effects in long-term, well-controlled studies using doxazosin or terazosin has been low. The most visible effect has been first-dose hypotension and/or syncopy. In studies using the longer-acting agents, these effects have been rare ($<1\%$ to 2%), and in the Treatment of Mild Hypertension Study (TOMHS), in patients treated ≥ 4 years with doxazosin, the incidence of reported syncopy was no different from that with placebo.

In general, α_1-antagonists are tolerated similarly to other major

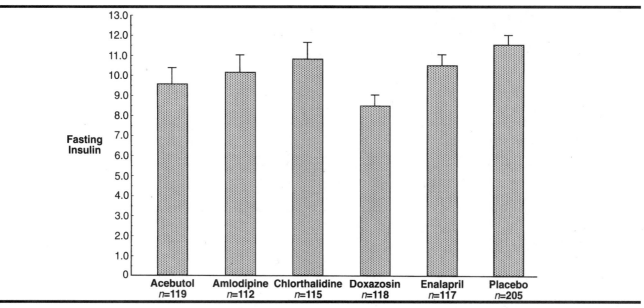

Figure 126.1. Fasting plasma insulin measured at fourth annual visit in the Treatment of Mild Hypertension Study (TOMHS).

classes of antihypertensive drugs. Dizziness is the most common complaint, and it is usually mild and transient (does not interfere with daily activities). Other complaints are lethargy, fatigue, and palpitations. In patients with a history of stress incontinence, urinary incontinence may be a problem. Rarely, α-blockers may exacerbate angina in patients with coronary disease. Priapism has also been reported rarely. In general, α₁-antagonists are tolerated similarly to other major classes of antihypertensive drugs.

Metabolic Effects: Lipids

α₁-Antagonists are the only class of antihypertensive drugs that have consistently been shown to favorably affect plasma lipids. Total cholesterol and LDL cholesterol are lowered by ≈5%, triglycerides are lowered by ≈10%, and some studies have reported an increase in HDL cholesterol. Virtually all α₁-antagonist lipid studies have demonstrated a favorable change in the total cholesterol/HDL cholesterol ratio, although no study to date has looked at the effect of α-blockers on cardiovascular disease mortality and morbidity. The Antihypertensive and Lipid Lowering Study to Prevent Heart Attack (ALLHAT) is studying >42 000 stage I and II higher-risk hypertensives treated blindly with either an α-blocker, a diuretic, a calcium antagonist, or an ACE inhibitor.

Other Effects

α₁-Antagonists have been shown to enhance insulin sensitivity. In the TOMHS study, doxazosin treatment over 4 years combined with lifestyle modification was associated with significantly lower fasting insulin compared with placebo or other antihypertensive agents **(Figure 126.1)**. Although the TOMHS 4-year data are cross-sectional, the randomized groups allow a reasonable between-group comparison.

α₁-Blockers do not adversely affect renal function, and, like many other types of antihypertensive agents, they allow regression of echocardiographic left ventricular mass in patients with left ventric-

ular hypertrophy. α₁-Antagonists do not cause impotence. In TOMHS, the incidence of erectile dysfunction on doxazosin was similar to that on placebo and had a higher rate of remission (compared with placebo) in men reporting erectile dysfunction at baseline. α-Blockers have become a common therapy for symptoms of benign prostatic hypertrophy. Both terazosin and doxazosin improve symptom scores and urinary flow parameters compared with placebo. These agents should also be considered for treating hypertensive men with benign prostatic hypertrophy.

SUGGESTED READING

1. Graham RM. Selective α₁-adrenergic antagonists: therapeutically relevant antihypertensive agents. *Am J Cardiol.* 1984;53:16A–20A.
2. Grimm RH Jr, Grandits GA, Prineas RJ, McDonald RH, Lewis CE, Flack JM, Yunis C, Svendsen K, Liebson PR, Elmer PJ. Long-term effects on sexual function of five antihypertensive drugs and nutritional hygienic treatment in hypertensive men and women: Treatment of Mild Hypertension Study (TOMHS). *Hypertension.* 1997;29:8–14.
3. Grimm RH Jr, Grandits GA, Cutlet JA, Stewart AL, McDonald RH, Svendsen K, Prineas RJ, Liebson PR, et al. Relationships of quality-of-life measures to long-term lifestyle and drug treatment in the Treatment of Mild Hypertension Study (TOMHS). *Arch Intern Med.* 1997;157:638–648.
4. Izzo JL Jr, Licht MR, Smith RJ, Larrabee PS, Radke KJ, Kallay MC. Chronic effects of direct vasodilation (pinacidil), alpha-adrenergic blockade (prazosin) and angiotensin-converting enzyme inhibition (captopril) in systemic hypertension. *Am J Cardiol.* 1987;60:303–308.
5. Koch-Weser J, Graham RM, Pettinger WA. Drug therapy: prazosin. *N Engl J Med.* 1979;300:232–236.
6. Materson BJ, Reda DJ, Cushman WC, Massie BM, Freis ED, Kochar MS, Hamburger RJ, Fye C, Lakshman R, Gottdiener J, et al. Single-drug therapy for hypertension in men: a comparison of six antihypertensive agents with placebo. *N Engl J Med.* 1993;328:914–921.
7. Neaton JD, Grimm RH Jr, Prineas RJ, Stamler J, Grandits GA, Elmer PJ, Cutler JA, Flack JM, Schoenberger JA, McDonald R, et al. The Treatment of Mild Hypertension Study: final results. *JAMA.* 1993;270:713–724.
8. The Treatment of Mild Hypertension Research Group. The Treatment of Mild Hypertension Study: a randomized, placebo-controlled trial of a nutritional-hygienic regimen along with various drug monotherapies. *Arch Intern Med.* 1991;151:1413–1423.

Chapter 127

α,β-Adrenergic Blockers

Mahboob Rahman, MD, MS; Jackson T. Wright, Jr, MD, PhD

KEY POINTS

- α,β-Blockers lower blood pressure by reducing heart rate and contractility (like the pure β-blockers), but via α-blockade they reduce systemic vascular resistance, resulting in little overall alteration in cardiac output or peripheral perfusion.

- Labetalol, available orally and parenterally, is effective in treating hypertensive urgencies and emergencies and clinical conditions associated with catecholamine excess.

- Carvedilol, in addition to its antihypertensive efficacy, is indicated for the treatment of congestive heart failure.

See also Chapters 1, 43, 125, 126

The distinguishing characteristic of this group of complex adrenergic blocking agents is their ability to competitively inhibit both α- and β-adrenergic receptors. Labetalol is a nonselective β-adrenergic blocker that also possesses selective α_1-blocking activity (at least with short-term administration) and weak partial β_2-agonist activity. Carvedilol is also a nonselective β-adrenergic inhibitor and selective α_1-blocker with no agonist activity.

Labetalol is available orally for the treatment of all stages of chronic hypertension. It is also available as a parenteral agent and is used to lower blood pressure in hypertensive urgencies and emergencies, especially those associated with catecholamine excess. Carvedilol is available in oral formulation only. It is indicated for the treatment of hypertension but is also indicated for use in patients with congestive heart failure.

Pharmacokinetics and Metabolism

After oral administration, both labetalol and carvedilol undergo extensive first-pass metabolism in the liver and intestinal mucosa, with bioavailability varying greatly among subjects, although averaging ≈33%. Increased bioavailability may be seen in the elderly, in patients with hepatic dysfunction, and in patients taking cimetidine concomitantly. Dosage modification may be necessary in these patients. Postprandial administration delays absorption but may increase bioavailability. Renal failure does not appear to significantly alter the pharmacokinetics of either agent.

Mechanism of Action

The acute hemodynamic properties of these agents are the result of their combined α_1- and nonselective β-adrenergic blocking activity. Labetalol is administered as a racemic mixture of four stereoisomers. The β-blocking and weak β_2-agonist activity reside on one isomer (RR) and the α-blocking properties on another (SR). Drug displacement studies indicate that labetalol affinity is ≈10 times higher for the β- than for the α-adrenergic receptor. Heart rate and blood pressure responses after isoproterenol and phenylephrine infusions demonstrate an in vivo β-to-α-adrenergic blocking ratio of 3:1 for oral administration and 7:1 for parenteral labetalol administration. This results in a dose-dependent reduction in blood pres-

sure, heart rate, and systemic vascular resistance. Acute intravenous administration of labetalol in normotensive and hypertensive subjects produces a rapid and substantial fall in blood pressure, primarily via a reduction in total peripheral resistance. However, the α-blocking properties of labetalol as measured by phenylephrine infusion decrease after 1 to 6 months of therapy.

The α-blockade produced by carvedilol is ≈50% as potent as that by labetalol. However, it may be longer lasting (stable for at least 3 weeks). Carvedilol does not demonstrate agonist activity. Hemodynamically, unlike pure β-blockers, which reduce heart rate and contractility, these compounds reduce total peripheral resistance, maintain cardiac output, and preserve peripheral blood flow, renal plasma flow, and glomerular filtration rate. In some studies, plasma renin activity acutely decreases after administration of these agents, whereas other studies have shown no effect on the renin-angiotensin system. Neither agent substantially increases plasma or urine catecholamine concentrations. However, labetalol has been reported to interfere with fluorometric methods of catecholamine determination and spectrophotometric assays of metanephrines, causing falsely high values for those substances. Therefore, these results should be interpreted with caution in patients on labetalol who are being evaluated for a pheochromocytoma unless radioenzymatic or chromatographic assays are used.

Clinical Applications of α,β-Blockers
Long-Term Treatment of Hypertension

Labetalol is safe and effective for the management of patients with mild, moderate, and severe hypertension. The oral dose for labetalol ranges between 200 and 1200 mg/d in two divided doses. The recommended dose for carvedilol is 6.25 to 25 mg twice daily, with peak antihypertensive action occurring 1 to 2 hours after a dose. The dosage of both agents may be titrated after 7 to 14 days.

The blood pressure–lowering effect of the α,β-blockers has been confirmed in multiple studies compared with either placebo or numerous other antihypertensive agents. There was early interest in evaluating labetalol in hypertensives of African descent, who generally respond less well to monotherapy with pure β-blockers. Some studies reported that black patients had better response to labetalol than to pure β-blockers, but this was not a consistent finding in all studies. In addition, the majority of these trials assessed standing blood pressure, which favored the α-blocking properties of these agents. Less difference between labetalol and pure β-blockers was seen when supine and seated blood pressure responses were compared. Because these trials were of relatively short duration, the potential reduction in α-blocking activity with chronic therapy was not evaluated as to its effect on blood pressure reduction. The α,β-blockers are very effective in lowering blood pressure in elderly hypertensives, including those with isolated systolic hypertension. Because bioavailability increases in older patients, lower drug doses may be required to control blood pressure. These agents, alone or in combination with diuretics, are also effective antihypertensive agents in patients with chronic renal insufficiency. Except for the trials documenting the benefit of carvedilol in patients with heart failure, there are no long-term clinical trial data to evaluate whether these agents have benefit aside from that expected of other β-blockers. In addition, post–myocardial infarction protection has not been demonstrated with the α,β-blockers, although the hemodynamic profile of the combined α,β-blockers is attractive for use in patients with myocardial ischemia, with or without hypertension.

Use in Hypertensive Urgencies and Emergencies

Labetalol can be used to treat hypertensive emergencies such as acute aortic dissection and postoperative hypertension. It may be administered as 20- to 80-mg IV boluses every 10 minutes or as a continuous infusion at 0.5 to 2 mg/min. All patients receiving parenteral therapy must be closely monitored. In addition, precautions should be taken with intravenous administration to avoid excessive orthostatic hypotension.

Use in the Treatment of Hypertension During Pregnancy

Several clinical trials with labetalol have demonstrated efficacy and safety in pregnant women with hypertension. However, the Food and Drug Administration has continued to classify labetalol in the "C" category with regard to pregnancy risk, indicating the continued need for risk/benefit assessment in considering the use of this drug during pregnancy.

Use in Conditions Associated With Catecholamine Excess

The α,β-blockers are useful in clinical conditions associated with catecholamine excess, uncontrolled hypertension, and/or a predisposition to cardiac arrhythmias. During the perioperative management of pheochromocytoma, the use of intravenous labetalol before surgical removal of these tumors may give adequate coverage for catecholamine release during the procedure. Severe hypertension after abrupt withdrawal of clonidine ("clonidine rebound") can be prevented or treated with labetalol. Intravenous labetalol is also effective in the management of cocaine crises.

Side Effects

In addition to the expected potential adverse reactions associated with β-blocker therapy (such as bronchospasm, atrioventricular conduction block, heart failure, etc), hepatotoxicity is a serious, although uncommon, side effect of therapy with labetalol and carvedilol. Other potential side effects with one or both agents include fatigue, dizziness, headache, gastrointestinal symptoms, scalp tingling, and postural hypotension (including first-dose syncope). Ejaculatory failure has been reported in a small number of patients. Many of these symptoms are transient and may not require discontinuation of the drugs. Appropriate laboratory testing should be done at the first symptom or sign of liver dysfunction, and both agents of this class should be used with caution in patients with liver disease.

SUGGESTED READING

1. Gay GR, Loper KA. The use of labetalol in the management of cocaine crisis. *Ann Emerg Med.* 1988;17:282–283.
2. Lund-Johansen P. Short and long term (six-year) hemodynamic effects of labetalol in essential hypertension. *Am J Med.* 1983;75;24–31.
3. Packer M, Bristow MR, Cohn JN, Colucci WS, Fowler MB, Gilbert EM, Shusterman NH. The effect of carvedilol on morbidity and mortality in patients with chronic heart failure. U.S. Carvedilol Heart Failure Study Group. *N Engl J Med.* 1996;334:1349–1355.
4. van Zweiten PA. An overview of the pharmacodynamic properties and therapeutic potential of combined alpha- and beta-adrenoceptor antagonists. *Drugs.* 1993;45:509–17.
5. Wallin JD, O'Neill WM Jr. Labetalol: current research and therapeutic status. *Arch Intern Med.* 1983;143:485–490.
6. Wright JT Jr, Douglas JG. Drug therapy in the black hypertensive. In: Fray J, Douglas JG, eds. *Pathophysiology of Hypertension in Blacks.* New York, NY: Oxford Press; 1993:271–291.

Chapter 128

Central and Peripheral Sympatholytics

Barry J. Materson, MD, MBA

KEY POINTS

- Central α_2-sympathetic agonists reduce blood pressure by decreasing central sympathetic outflow, peripheral vascular resistance, and heart rate.

- Major drawbacks to central sympatholytics include somnolence, dry mouth, rebound hypertension upon withdrawal, and sensitivity reactions (transdermal-delivery system for clonidine).

- Peripheral sympatholytics deplete nerve terminal norepinephrine, thereby decreasing reflex peripheral arterial and venous constriction during upright posture and predisposing to orthostatic hypotension.

- Sexual dysfunction and numerous drug-drug interactions further limit clinical use of peripheral sympatholytics.

See also Chapters 2, 33, 42, 43

Central Sympatholytics

The central sympatholytics (**Table 128.1**) have at least one common mechanism of action: central α_2-sympathetic agonism. Their principal side effects, sedation and dry mouth, are directly related to actions on cells with many interconnections within the brain stem. They are particularly useful for patients who have hypertension with associated anxiety, especially that which is manifested by sympathetic overactivity. Although they may be used as single-drug therapy, they are generally used in combination with a thiazide diuretic to block the salt and water retention that frequently accompanies their use. Clonidine, a representative of this class, was shown in the VA Cooperative Study to be somewhat more effective in whites than in blacks and is recognized as being more effective in older than younger blacks.

Mechanism of Action

All of these drugs stimulate α_2-receptors on the adrenergic neurons located within the rostral ventrolateral medulla, which controls sympathetic outflow. This action mimics the effect of local catecholamines, which act to decrease sympathetic nervous system outflow, thereby decreasing peripheral vascular resistance, heart rate, and systolic and diastolic blood pressure in a balanced fashion. Methyldopa, the first drug in this class, requires conversion to an active agonist, α-methylnorepinephrine, for its effect. The other drugs in this class do not require conversion for activity.

Side and Adverse Effects

Somnolence and dry mouth (40%) are the most common adverse drug reactions and are the major reason these medications are discontinued. Other central nervous system depressants and ethanol enhance sedative effects within this drug class. Dry mouth may be quite annoying to the patient, and decreased formation of saliva may increase the risk of dental caries or periodontal disease.

Drug Differentiation

Methyldopa is still widely used to treat pregnancy-induced hypertension. Treatment of hypertensive emergencies with intravenous methyldopa has been supplanted by more effective drugs. In this drug class, hypersensitivity reactions, including hepatitis and Coombs-positive hemolytic anemia, have been seen with methyldopa. Methyldopa and its metabolic products can interfere with some assays for catecholamines and can interfere with other therapeutic agents, such as levodopa, bromocriptine, and monoamine oxidase inhibitors.

Oral clonidine has a rapid onset of action (30 to 60 minutes) and is useful for managing hypertensive urgencies but is relatively short-acting. A transdermal patch delivery system (TTS patch) provides a constant dose of drug for 7 days, but it takes 1 to 2 days to attain peak effect, and the effect lingers from 8 to 24 hours after the patch is removed. Best absorption from the patch occurs when it is placed on the chest or upper arm. If clonidine is suddenly discontinued during treatment with high doses (usually $\geq$1.0 mg, though sometimes lower), rebound hypertension may occur secondary to an excessive sympathetic discharge. Rebound hypertension may be accentuated if β-blocker therapy is ongoing at the time of clonidine discontinuation. Skin hypersensitivity to the transdermal clonidine patch occurs in $\approx$15% to 20% of patients who use the TTS preparation.

Guanabenz is mechanistically similar to clonidine but is somewhat longer-acting and is slightly less prone to symptomatic hypertension with its sudden withdrawal. It is less likely to be associated with orthostatic hypotension.

Guanfacine differs from the other members of this class in that its prolonged (24 hours) duration of action typically allows dosing to be once daily. Its preferable dosing time is evening, to blunt the early morning surge in catecholamines and to allow for any sedative effect. As with other agents in this class, guanfacine works best when coadministered with a small dose of diuretic, which optimizes blood pressure lowering with minimum central nervous system adverse effects. Adverse effects increase significantly with doses >1 mg/d.

Peripheral Sympatholytics

These drugs have a common mechanism of action at postganglionic sympathetic nerve endings (**Table 128.2**). Reserpine has ad-

Table 128.1. **Central Sympatholytics: α_2-Agonists**

Methyldopa (Aldomet)	125-, 250-, 500-mg tablets, oral suspension, and parenteral (both 50 mg/mL); usual oral dose 500–2000 mg/d divided into 2 to 4 doses
Clonidine (Catapres)	0.1-, 0.2-, 0.3-mg tablets; usual dose, 0.2 to 0.6 mg in 2 doses. TTS 1, 2, and 3 (containing 2.5, 5.0, and 7.5 mg, respectively); patch to be applied once weekly
Guanabenz (Wytensin)	4- and 6-mg tablets; usual dose, 8 to 32 mg/d in 2 doses
Guanfacine (Tenex)	1-, 2-, and 3-mg tablets; usual dose, 1 to 3 mg at bedtime

Table 128.2. **Peripheral Sympatholytics: Rauwolfia Alkaloids**

Rauwolfia Alkaloids	
Reserpine (Serpasil)	0.1-, 0.25-mg tablets; usual dose, 0.1 to 0.25 mg/d
Deserpidine (Harmonyl)*	0.25-mg tablets; usual dose, 0.25 to 0.5 mg/d
Rauwolfia serpentina (Raudixin)*	50-mg tablets; usual dose, 50 to 200 mg/d
Post-ganglionic Adrenergic Blocking Agents	
Guanethidine (Ismelin)	10- and 25-mg tablets; usual dose, 10 to 50 mg/d
Guanadrel (Hylorel)	10- and 25-mg tablets; usual dose, 10 to 75 mg in 2 to 4 doses

*Rarely used in clinical practice.

ditional central nervous system mechanisms of action, so that their adverse effects are not entirely comparable. Reserpine remains a widely used agent on a worldwide basis. Nevertheless, all three drugs have important and potentially dangerous interactions with other drugs that affect postganglionic catecholamine metabolism, and their use has decreased since the advent of more powerful and safer antihypertensive drugs.

Mechanism of Action

Drugs of this class work by entering sympathetic neurons via catecholamine-hydrogen pump mechanism and depleting norepinephrine from storage granules in the postganglionic sympathetic nerves, thereby decreasing neurogenic vascular and cardiac tone. Because of reflex upregulation of peripheral adrenergic receptors, these agents cause exaggerated pressor responses to endogenous catecholamines. The ability to respond to upright postural change by reflex peripheral vasoconstriction is also impaired; thus, orthostatic hypotension may occur. In addition, reserpine depletes other tissue stores of catecholamines, including the heart, and it also reduces serotonin levels.

Side and Adverse Effects

Reserpine has been associated with significant depression. It can increase both gastric acidity and risk of acid-peptic disease and intestinal motility, which may exacerbate ulcerative colitis or precipitate biliary colic. Tricyclic antidepressants interfere with the norepinephrine pump mechanism and may decrease the hypotensive effect of guanethidine or guanadrel, which also require the same pump for their biological effects. If these drugs are added to monoamine oxidase inhibitors, a hypertensive crisis may be precipitated. This is important because monoamine oxidase inhibitors are being used increasingly in the management of Parkinson's disease. They may also trigger a hypertensive crisis if an occult pheochromocytoma is present. Frequent stools or diarrhea can be a problem, although less so with guanadrel. Retrograde ejaculation is another disturbing adverse reaction seen with these drugs.

Drug Differentiation

Reserpine is extremely long-acting and can be an effective and inexpensive antihypertensive agent when used in low doses (0.05 mg) with a diuretic. Most of its adverse effects occur with much higher dosage regimens. Guanethidine is difficult to titrate because of its wide therapeutic range and very long duration of action. This compound is sufficiently potent that some cases of resistant hypertension can be resolved by the addition of as little as 10 mg of guanethidine. Guanadrel is shorter-acting and easier to titrate than guanethidine and is observed to cause less diarrhea and orthostatic hypotension. Guanadrel is excreted renally and requires dosage adjustment in renally impaired patients. These drugs also typically cause salt and water retention, which attenuates their antihypertensive effect; thus, diuretic add-on therapy is almost always necessary in their long-term use. Guanfacine is the only α_2-agonist that can be given once daily.

SUGGESTED READING

1. Joint National Committee on Prevention, Detection, Evaluation, and Treatment of High Blood Pressure. The sixth report of the Joint National Committee on Prevention, Detection, Evaluation, and Treatment of High Blood Pressure. *Arch Intern Med.* 1997;157:2413–2446.
2. Materson BJ, Reda DJ, Cushman WC, et al. Single-drug therapy for hypertension in men: a comparison of six antihypertensive drugs with placebo. *N Engl J Med.* 1993;328:914–921.
3. Materson BJ, Kessler WB, Alderman MH, et al. A multi-center, randomized, double-blind dose-response evaluation of step-2 guanfacine versus placebo in patients with mild-to-moderate hypertension. *Am J Cardiol.* 1986;57:32E–37E.
4. Participating Veterans Administration Medical Centers. Low doses v standard dose of reserpine: a randomized, double-blind, multiclinic trial in patients taking chlorthalidone. *JAMA.* 1982;248:2471–2477.
5. Veterans Administration Cooperative Study Group on Antihypertensive Agents. Multi-clinic controlled trial of bethanidine and guanethidine in severe hypertension. *Circulation.* 1977;55:519–525.

Chapter 129

Angiotensin-Converting Enzyme Inhibitors

Domenic A. Sica, MD; Elizabeth Ripley, MD

KEY POINTS

- Angiotensin-converting enzyme inhibitors (ACEIs) decrease production of angiotensin II and sympathetic nervous system activity and increase bradykinin.

- Pharmacological properties proposed as distinguishing features for ACEIs include their tissue-binding potential and whether they are eliminated renally or renally and hepatically. .

- ACEIs are of clearly proven benefit in slowing the progression of chronic renal failure and have been demonstrated to have a powerful influence on the morbidity and mortality with progressive heart failure.

- ACEIs cause cough (which may occur in as many as 20% to 30% of treated patients), hyperkalemia, and a generally reversible form of renal insufficiency attributable to diminished glomerular filtration pressure in an angiotensin II–dependent kidney such as occurs with renal artery stenosis.

See also Chapters 3, 4, 5, 6, 41, 51, 130

In the treatment of hypertension, the renin-angiotensin-aldosterone (RAA) axis is an attractive target for pharmacological intervention. Therapies directed at this axis have either directly decreased angiotensin II concentrations, as is the case for angiotensin-converting enzyme inhibitors (ACEIs); or indirectly suppressed angiotensin II, as occurs with central agents or β-blocker therapy; or directly block angiotensin II receptor activation, as occurs with the angiotensin-receptor blockers (ARBs). The pivotal role for angiotensin II in hypertension derives not only from its being a potent vasoconstrictor substance but also from its ability to stimulate vascular smooth muscle cell hypertrophy. Angiotensin II is also an important contributor to the progressive deterioration in cardiac and renal function often observed in hypertensive patients. Thus, it seemed logical to seek additional indications for ACEIs in the areas of heart failure, post–myocardial infarction states, and diabetic nephropathy due to type 1 diabetes (**Table 129.1**).

Mechanism of Action

ACE is pluripotent in that it catalyzes both the conversion of angiotensin I to angiotensin II and the degradation of bradykinin (BK) as well as a range of other vasoactive peptides. Although ACEIs effectively curb the generation of angiotensin II from angiotensin I, they do not interrupt the production of angiotensin II by non–ACE-dependent pathways. Such pathways rely on chymase and other proteases to independently produce angiotensin II in myocardial and vascular tissue; the ensuing gradual rise in angiotensin II levels despite continuation of ACEIs is called "angiotensin escape." The presence of angiotensin II ordinarily dampens upstream activity in the RAA axis. When ACEIs are given, by virtue of their temporarily diminishing angiotensin II, this dampening influence disappears, with the result being a rise in both plasma renin activity (PRA) and angiotensin I concentrations. This excess of angiotensin I provides a substrate for alternative pathways.

Because ACEIs reduce angiotensin II levels only transiently (days to weeks), other mechanisms for their blood pressure–lowering effect need be considered, particularly if the pattern of blood pressure response to ACEIs is examined. When first administered, ACEIs very transiently reduce blood pressure, in parallel with the observed reduction in ACE activity. During chronic treatment, ACEIs provide a sustained drop in blood pressure, despite the aforementioned angiotensin II escape. The precise explanation for this persistent blood pressure drop is not yet available.

ACE participates in the processing of peptides other than angiotensin II, which, no doubt, has functional implications. For example, BK is broken down by kininases. One of these enzymes, kininase II, is identical to ACE. Thus, in theory, ACEI administration should increase tissue BK levels. In turn, BK is known to stimulate the production of endothelium-derived relaxing factor and to induce the release of prostacyclin. When circulating BK concentrations have been measured in ACEI-treated patients, the values obtained have been inconsistently elevated. It is possible, though, that tissue BK concentrations rise with ACEI therapy and locally influence vascular tone. This phenomenon may partially explain the chronically reduced blood pressure in ACEI-treated patients.

The precise contribution of prostaglandins (PGs) to the antihypertensive effect of ACEIs is still not fully understood. The evidence supporting a role for increased vasodilatory PGs in the blood pressure–lowering effect of ACEIs is circumstantial at best. Although circulating levels of PGE_2 and PGI_2 metabolites are inconsequentially changed by ACEIs, it has been observed that nonsteroidal anti-inflammatory drugs (NSAIDs) blunt the blood pressure-lowering effect of ACEIs. A portion of the ACEI effect is considered to be due to reduced activity in the sympathetic nervous system. ACEI administration does not produce a consistent change in circulating catecholamines but does attenuate sympathetically mediated vasoconstriction without altering circulatory reflexes. This

Table 129.1. FDA-Approved Indications for ACEIs

DRUG	HYPERTENSION	CHF	DIABETIC NEPHROPATHY	LEFT VENTRICULAR DYSFUNCTION
Captopril	X	X	X	X (post-MI)
Benazepril	X			
Enalapril	X	X		X (asymptomatic)
Fosinopril	X	X		
Lisinopril	X	X		
Moexipril	X			
Quinapril	X	X		
Ramipril	X	X		
Trandolapril	X	X (post-MI)		X (post-MI)

MI indicates myocardial infarction.

latter property explains why ACEIs are rarely associated with postural hypotension.

Pharmacology

ACEIs first became available in the early 1980s and soon became a mainstay of therapy for cardiovascular disease, with nine such compounds currently marketed in the United States. The first orally active ACEI was the drug captopril, a sulfhydryl-containing compound with a rapid onset and relatively short duration of action. Subsequently, a longer-acting compound, enalapril, became available. Enalapril, like all other ACEIs with the exception of lisinopril and captopril, must be metabolically converted to an active diacid form, a process that occurs in the liver.

ACEIs are structurally heterogeneous. For example, the active chemical side group or ligand for captopril is a sulfhydryl group, for fosinopril a phosphinyl group, and for the remaining ACEIs a carboxyl group. The presence of a particular side group on an ACEI has been associated with a wide range of pharmacological responses. For example, the sulfhydryl group is purported to act as a recyclable free-radical scavenger. For this reason, captopril may be more protective in atherogenesis, myocardial infarction, and diabetes, although this is not clinically substantiated. In addition, captopril directly stimulates PG synthesis, whereas other ACEIs accomplish this indirectly by increasing BK activity. The presence of a phosphinyl group on fosinopril has been suggested to be the reason for its low incidence of cough and its ability to improve diastolic dysfunction. In the latter instance, the phosphinyl group may enhance myocardial penetration of fosinopril.

Although ACEIs can be distinguished by differences in absorption, protein binding, half-life, and metabolic disposition, they behave quite similarly in how they lower blood pressure. Rarely, beyond the issue of frequency of dosing, do these pharmacological subtleties govern selection of an agent (**Table 129.2**).

A widely debated feature of the ACEIs involves the concept of tissue penetration and binding. Quinapril and ramipril are highly lipophilic and thereby bind to tissue sites for prolonged periods of time. It has been proposed that lipophilicity could favorably distinguish these compounds relative to blood pressure control or end-organ protection. Where comparisons between lipophilic and hydrophilic ACEIs have occurred, the results do not convincingly support the claim of superiority for lipophilic ACEIs.

Because there is very little that truly separates one ACEI from another, the cost of an ACEI has become a dominant theme. "Class effect" is a phrase often invoked to legitimatize use of a less-costly ACEI when a higher-priced agent has been the one specifically studied in a disease state, such as congestive heart failure (CHF) or diabetic nephropathy. The concept of class effect may be most germane in the treatment of diabetic nephropathy, in which the quantity of ACEI given is determined by the blood pressure response. In diabetic nephropathy, if dose equivalency for different ACEIs is established, then "an ACEI is an ACEI."

In CHF, dosage recommendations for ACEIs, such as enalapril and captopril, propose dose titration to amounts considerably in excess of what is ordinarily required for blood pressure control. This suggests that the success of an ACEI in CHF may derive from properties other than ACE inhibition. Myocardial binding, degree of change in plasma aldosterone, and changes in other neuropeptides degraded by ACE may contribute to their overall success. Because not all ACEIs have been thoroughly studied in CHF, particularly relative to these secondary response parameters, it is less likely that a specific class effect exists for ACEIs in the treatment of CHF.

Hemodynamic Effects

ACEIs cause a variety of interlinked hemodynamic effects (**Table 129.3**). When glomerular filtration rate (GFR) is reliant on efferent arteriolar tone (as in CHF, dehydration, and/or renal artery stenosis [RAS]) and an ACEI is administered, GFR may suddenly drop.

Blood Pressure–Lowering Effects

ACEI efficacy is comparable to that of most other drug classes, with response rates from 40% to 70% in stage I or II hypertension. There are few predictors of response to ACEIs. When hypertension is accompanied by high PRA values, as in RAS, the response to an ACEI can be brisk. Unfortunately, in most other cases there is a poorly defined relationship between the PRA value and the vasodepressor response to an ACEI.

Certain patient subsets demonstrate lower response rates to ACEI monotherapy, including low-renin, salt-sensitive individuals such as the diabetic, black, or elderly hypertensive. The low-renin state in elderly hypertensives is an exception in that it develops not as the result of volume expansion, although they are salt-sensitive, but because of age-related decreases in PRA. The elderly generally respond

Table 129.2. Pharmacokinetic Parameters of ACEIs

DRUG	ONSET/DURATION, H	PEAK HYPOTENSIVE EFFECT, H	PROTEIN BINDING, %	EFFECT OF FOOD ON ABSORPTION	SERUM HALF-LIFE, H	ELIMINATION
Benazepril	1/24	2–4	>95	None	10–11	Renal/some biliary
Captopril	0.25/dose-related	1–1.5	25–30	Reduced	<2	Renal, as disulfides
Enalapril	1/24	4–6	50	None	11	Renal
Fosinopril	1/24	2–6	95	None	11	Renal = hepatic
Lisinopril	1/24	6	10	None	13	Renal
Moexipril	1/24	4–6	50	Reduced	2–9	Renal/some biliary
Quinapril	1/24	2	97	Reduced	2	Renal>hepatic
Ramipril	1–2/24	3–6	73	Reduced	13–17	Renal
Trandolapril	2–4/24	6–8	80–94	None	16–24	Renal>hepatic

Table 129.3. Hemodynamic Effects of ACEIs

HEMODYNAMIC PARAMETER	EFFECT	CLINICAL SIGNIFICANCE
Cardiovascular		
Total peripheral resistance	Decreased	
Mean arterial pressure	Decreased	
Cardiac output	Increased or no change	These parameters contribute to a general decrease
Stroke volume	Increased	in systemic blood pressure
Preload and afterload	Decreased	
Pulmonary artery pressure	Decreased	
Right atrial pressure	Decreased	
Diastolic dysfunction	Improved	
Renal		
Renal blood flow	Usually increased	Contributes to the renoprotective effect of these agents
Glomerular filtration rate	Variable, usually unchanged, but may ↓ in renal failure	
Efferent arteriolar resistance	Decreased	
Filtration fraction	Decreased	
Peripheral Nervous System		
Biosynthesis of norepinephrine	Decreased	Enhances blood pressure–lowering effect and resets
Reuptake of epinephrine	Inhibited	baroceptor function
Circulating catecholamines	Decreased	

well to ACEIs, although interpretation of such a response is complicated by senescence-related renal failure having slowed the elimination of these drugs, resulting in higher plasma concentrations of an ACEI. The black hypertensive is also incorrectly perceived as poorly responsive to ACEIs. If sufficient dose titration occurs, blood pressure can often be lowered very effectively.

There are differences among ACEIs labeled as "once daily" in their ability to reduce blood pressure for a full 24 hours, as defined by a trough-to-peak ratio >50%. On the basis of a number of trials comparing trough-to-peak ratios with 24-hour ambulatory blood pressure monitoring, it appears that fosinopril, lisinopril, and trandolapril can truly be administered once daily. Other ACEIs, with the exception of captopril, can be given once daily to start with but may require twice-daily administration for optimal 24-hour blood pressure control. Considerable dosing flexibility exists with the available ACEIs. Enalaprilat is the only ACEI available in intravenous form **(Table 129.4).**

The question is often raised as to what to do if an ACEI does not normalize blood pressure. One approach is simply to increase the dose; however, the dose-response curve for ACEIs, like that for most antihypertensive agents, is fairly flat. Those who respond to ACEIs typically do so at doses well below those necessary for 24-hour suppression of ACE. Full vasodepressor response to an ACEI is not exhibited until several weeks after the beginning of therapy. Thus, only if there is complete failure to respond to an ACEI should it be replaced by a drug that interferes with a system other than the RAA axis. If a partial response has occurred, then therapy with an ACEI can be continued in anticipation of an additional drop in blood pressure over several weeks.

ACEIs in Hypertension Associated With Other Disorders

ACEIs, the agents of choice in the diabetic patient, exhibit a neutral effect on insulin resistance and hyperlipidemia. They also reduce urinary protein excretion in diabetics with renal involvement. In addition, compelling evidence exists that ACEIs improve survival in CHF patients and regression of left ventricular hypertrophy. Although ACEIs are not specific coronary vasodilators, they do decrease myocardial

Table 129.4. Dosage Strengths and Guidelines for Oral ACEIs

DRUG	STRENGTHS, MG	HYPERTENSION, MG/D / FREQUENCY	HEART FAILURE MG/D / FREQUENCY
Benazepril	5, 10, 20, 40	20–40 / QD → BID	Not FDA-approved
Captopril	12.5, 25, 20, 100	50–450 / BID → TID	18.75–150 / TID
Enalapril	2.5, 5, 10, 20	10–40 / QD → BID	5–20 / QD → BID
Fosinopril	10, 20	20–40 / QD → BID	20–40 / QD
Lisinopril	2.5, 5, 10, 20, 40	20–40 / QD	5–20 / QD
Moexipril	7.5, 15	7.5–30 / QD → BID	Not FDA-approved
Quinapril	5, 10, 20, 40	20–80 / QD → BID	20–40 / QD → BID
Ramipril	1.25, 2.5, 5, 10	2.5–20 / QD → BID	10 / BID
Trandolapril	1, 2, 4	1–4 / QD	1–4 / QD

oxygen consumption and thereby ischemia (Table 129.3); thus, they can be safely used in patients with coronary artery disease. ACEIs are also useful in patients with either isolated systolic hypertension or systolic-predominant forms of hypertension, because they improve arteriolar compliance. Finally, ACEIs are effective in the hypertensive patient with cerebrovascular disease because they maintain cerebral autoregulatory ability in the face of reduced blood pressure, which is of particular importance in the elderly hypertensive.

ACEIs in Combination With Other Agents

The antihypertensive effect of ACEIs are most predictably enhanced by the coadministration of a diuretic. This response pattern has spurred development of a number of fixed-dose combination products containing an ACEI and a diuretic. The rationale for this additivity derives from the observation that sodium depletion triggers renin release and thereby imparts an angiotensin II dependency to the hypertension. Very-low-dose diuretic therapy can evoke this additive response, suggesting that even subtle alterations in sodium balance are sufficient to bolster the effect of ACEIs.

The rationale behind combining an ACEI and a β-blocker is that the β-blocker will presumably blunt the hyperreninemia induced by an ACEI. Although this hypothesis seemed attractive, in practice only a marginal additional response occurs when these drug classes are combined. Alternatively, combining a peripheral α-antagonist or calcium antagonist with an ACEI generally results in a robust additional response.

Side Effects of ACEIs

Soon after their release, a syndrome of "functional renal insufficiency" was noted as a class effect with ACEIs. This process was initially recognized in patients with either a solitary kidney and RAS or bilateral RAS. Since these original reports, this phenomenon has been repeatedly observed in a number of other settings, including dehydration, CHF, and microvascular renal disease. The theme common to all of these conditions is that afferent arteriolar flow has diminished and GFR is being preserved by angiotensin II–mediated efferent arteriolar constriction. When the efferent arteriole constricts, upstream hydrostatic pressures within the glomerular capillary bed return to the "normal," abnormally low afferent arteriolar flow. The abrupt removal of angiotensin II (as occurs with ACEIs) causes this sustaining pressure increase in glomerular capillaries to dissipate and GFR to rapidly diminish. This "functional renal insufficiency" is

best treated by discontinuation of the ACEI, careful volume repletion if intravascular volume contraction is present, and consideration of the possibility that RAS is present. An additional renal side effect with ACEIs is hyperkalemia. Relevant degrees of hyperkalemia with ACEIs generally arise in predisposed patients, such as diabetics or CHF patients with renal failure, who are receiving potassium-sparing diuretics or potassium supplements. Otherwise, ACEIs will effectively decrease the degree of hypokalemia produced by diuretics.

A dry, nonproductive cough, seen in as many as 20% of patients, is an additional complication with ACEIs. This side effect is a class phenomenon and has ostensibly been attributed to increased BK levels or other vasoactive peptides such as substance P, which may play a second-messenger role in triggering the cough reflex. Although numerous therapies have been tried, few have proved successful in eliminating ACEI-induced cough. Typically, the cough will disappear 1 to 2 weeks after discontinuation of the ACEI. Nonspecific side effects are generally rare with ACEIs, with the exception of taste disturbances, leukopenia, and skin rashes. These are more frequent in captopril-treated patients and have been attributed to its sulfhydryl group.

Angioneurotic edema is a potentially life-threatening complication of ACEIs that occurs in <1% of treated patients. Angioneurotic edema can occur quite unpredictably and typically is not a first-dose phenomenon. It should be easily recognized because it characteristically involves the mouth, tongue, and upper airway. ACEIs can also cause birth defects. ACEIs are not teratogenic; rather, when administered during the second and third trimester of pregnancy, they can cause developmental defects, renal failure, or fetal death, in that the maturing fetus is heavily reliant on angiotensin II for proper development.

Class- and Agent-Specific ACEI Drug Interactions

Several class-specific drug interactions occur with ACEIs. Potassium supplements or potassium-sparing diuretics, when given with ACEIs, increase the probability of the patient's developing hyperkalemia. NSAIDS, such as indomethacin, reduce the antihypertensive effects of ACEIs, particularly in low-renin forms of hypertension. The administration of ACEIs with lithium is associated with a greater likelihood of lithium toxicity. Concomitant administration of captopril with allopurinol has been associated with a higher risk of hypersensitivity reactions in the form of the Stevens-Johnson syndrome. Quinapril reduces the absorption of tetracycline by ≈35%, which may be due to the high magnesium content of quinapril tablets.

SUGGESTED READING

1. Giatras I, Lau J, Levey SS. Effect of angiotensin-converting enzyme inhibitors on the progression of nondiabetic renal disease: a meta-analysis of randomized trials. *Ann Intern Med.* 1997;127:337–345.

2. Lewis EJ, Hunsicker LG, Bain RP, Rohde RD. The effect of angiotensin-converting enzyme inhibition on diabetic nephropathy. The Collaborative Study Group. *N Engl J Med.* 1993;329:1456–1462.

3. Sica DA. Kinetics of angiotensin-converting enzyme inhibitors in renal failure. *J Cardiovasc Pharmacol.* 1992;20(suppl 10):S13–S20.

4. The SOLVD investigators. Effect of enalapril on survival in patients with reduced left ventricular ejection fractions and congestive heart failure. *N Engl J Med.* 1991;325:293–302.

Chapter 130

Angiotensin II Receptor Blockers

Michael A. Weber, MD

KEY POINTS

- The efficacy of the angiotensin II receptor blockers (ARBs) is similar to that of the other major antihypertensive drug classes, but these agents have fewer side effects.

- The ARBs selectively block the AT_1 receptors.

- ARBs leave AT_2 receptors exposed to increased circulating concentrations of angiotensin II, but the effects of chronic AT_2 receptor stimulation are not known.

- The ARBs do not stimulate bradykinin and thus differ from ACE inhibitors.

See also Chapters 3, 4, 5, 6, 7, 8, 41, 51, 129

Blocking the renin-angiotensin system is a rational approach to treating hypertension. Angiotensin II contributes in two major ways to the clinical picture of hypertension: it raises blood pressure through its direct and indirect vasoconstrictor actions, and it has trophic (ie, growth-promoting) actions on the heart and blood vessels that might contribute directly to vascular structural change and to cardiovascular and renal events. The renin-angiotensin system can be interrupted by β-blockers or central sympatholytic drugs, which decrease renal renin secretion, or by ACE inhibitors, which limit conversion of angiotensin I to angiotensin II. The angiotensin receptor blockers, however, provide the most direct means for antagonizing this system.

Pharmacology

The angiotensin receptor blockers (ARBs) bind selectively to the AT_1 receptor, thereby blocking the vasoconstrictor and other actions typically exhibited by angiotensin II. The binding of these nonpeptidic, orally administered agents to the AT_1 receptors can be either competitive or nonsurmountable. Some ARBs are prodrugs that require conversion to an active metabolite. As yet, there is no evidence of clinical differences between drugs that work in their parent form and those that are prodrugs.

All the available ARBs are effective when given once daily, although there may be pharmacokinetic differences among them that could produce differences in blood pressure effects during the 24-hour treatment period. The effects of these agents on renal function, natriuresis, and metabolic factors have not been fully defined, and it is not possible to determine whether some agents might have advantages over others.

Angiotensin Receptors and Blockers

At least four angiotensin II receptors have been described: AT_1, AT_2, AT_3, and AT_4. Only the first two of these have been well defined. The AT_1 receptor mediates most of the known physiological actions of angiotensin II. The AT_2 receptor is found primarily during fetal development and appears to mediate programmed cell death or apop-

tosis. The AT_2 receptor can be expressed in normal adults in response to trauma or other injuries. It is possible that such stimuli as aging and high blood pressure could affect the vasculature sufficiently to evoke the expression of these receptors. When stimulated by angiotensin II, AT_2 receptors mediate vasodilation and inhibitory effects on cell growth. Recently, stimulation of these receptors has been shown to increase nitric oxide production.

Because administration of the ARBs increases circulating angiotensin II levels, it is possible that they work through a dual mechanism: first, direct blockade of the AT_1 receptor, and second, stimulation of the AT_2 receptor. Tissue culture studies have confirmed that AT_1 blockade reduces cell growth and that AT_2 blockade (with experimental agents) increases cell growth; simultaneous blockade of the AT_1 receptor and stimulation of the AT_2 receptor (the putative situation when an ARB is used) results in an enhanced antiproliferative effect. These interesting possibilities, which have yet to be documented in the clinical setting, are summarized in **Table 130.1.**

Use in Hypertension

The efficacy of the ARBs is similar to that found with other widely used antihypertensive drugs. Of more interest, though, is the question of whether the ARBs exhibit significant dose-response relationships. The lowest effective dose of losartan, the first of this class to be available, is 50 mg. Some studies, however, have indicated that the efficacy achieved with 100 mg is not greater and that doubling the dose of losartan in patients who do not respond adequately to 50 mg does not provide further benefit. Conversely, such agents as valsartan, irbesartan, telmisartan, eprosartan, and candesartan appear to have greater efficacy at higher doses, although even with these agents, the dose-response curves tend to be rather shallow. This poses an interesting but still unanswered question: when patients fail to respond fully to an initial dose, should a higher dose be given or should a second drug be added?

The ARBs work equally well in older and younger patients and in men and women. Preliminary data suggest that black patients might also respond to these agents, although a review of such data indicates

Table 130.1. Angiotensin II Receptors and Effects of Blockade

Vascular AT$_1$ Receptors
  Constantly expressed
  Mediates vasoconstriction
  Mediate angiotensin II arterial wall growth effects
Vascular AT$_2$ Receptors
  Expressed only after injury (sustained hypertension might provoke expression)
  Mediate vasodilation
  Mediate antiproliferative actions
  Activate other factors eg, nitric oxide
Potential Double Action of Selective AT$_1$ Blockers
  Directly block vasoconstrictor and growth actions of angiotensin II at AT$_1$ receptors
  Increase circulating angiotensin II levels
  Unblocked AT$_2$ receptors (if expressed), simulated by increased angiotensin II activity, mediate vasodilation and growth inhibition
  Net effects: AT$_1$ blockade plus AT$_2$ stimulation

that with agents such as valsartan and tasosartan, there is a shift in the dose-response curves such that higher doses are required to produce antihypertensive efficacies similar to those observed in whites. It is not clear whether different population response patterns reflect pharmacokinetic differences between the two population groups or lower levels of renin activity in black patients. Additional studies are important, particularly because black patients are especially vulnerable to the renal and other consequences of hypertension that might be addressed by this new drug class.

There have been relatively few studies of ARBs in combination with other antihypertensive agents. Like the ACE inhibitors, diuretics appear to be a logical addition to the ARBs. Experiences with combinations with such other drug classes as calcium channel blockers have not yet been published.

Side Effects

The absence of symptomatic and metabolic adverse events with ARBs is one of their strong attributes. The incidence of side effects is not different from that in placebo-treated patients.

Cough is less common than with ACE inhibitors, and its incidence is probably similar to that with other drug classes. It should be noted, however, that there have been rare case reports of angioedema with the ARBs. Like the ACE inhibitors, they should be avoided during pregnancy and in patients with bilateral renovascular disease.

Clinical End Points

It is too early for definitive data. Studies of heart effects have been inconsistent: left ventricular hypertrophy has been shown to be regressed, worsened, or unchanged by ARBs in different trials (all, unfortunately, characterized by small patient numbers and methodological flaws). Studies in congestive heart failure have shown that ARBs have effects on hemodynamics and symptoms similar to those with ACE inhibitors. There have been no studies of the effects of ARBs on arteries in humans, but these drugs have reversed arterial wall hypertrophy in such animal models as the spontaneously hypertensive rat. ARBs (most commonly losartan) have significantly reduced proteinuria in nephrotic patients and also in hypertensive patients with or without diabetes mellitus. Some early studies indicate that candesartan and losartan might improve insulin sensitivity in hypertension.

Comparison With ACE Inhibitors

In addition to their comparable efficacies, there are potentially important differences between ARBs and ACE inhibitors. The ACE inhibitors do not fully interrupt the renin-angiotensin system; during chronic treatment, such enzymes as chymase might substitute for ACE and convert angiotensin I to angiotensin II. Conversely, the ACE inhibitors reduce bradykinin breakdown, thus increasing bradykinin availability and thereby increasing vasodilatory prostaglandins and nitric oxide. These substances may contribute to both the hemodynamic and cardioprotective effects of the ACE inhibitors.

Because of their differences, combinations of ACE inhibitors and ARBs have been studied both in congestive heart failure (no endpoint data yet available) and in hypertension. Because of flaws in study design, it is not known whether the effects of the two classes may indeed be additive. In one small study (ELITE), losartan was associated with a lower mortality rate than the ACE inhibitor captopril in patients with congestive heart failure. In a second small study, losartan produced greater survival benefits than placebo.

Clinical Trials

Several outcome studies in hypertension are being sponsored by manufacturers. For example, losartan is being compared with atenolol, and valsartan with amlodipine, in older high-risk hypertensive patients with respect to fatal and nonfatal cardiovascular events and strokes. Irbesartan and losartan are being studied for their renoprotective and cardiovascular effects in patients with diabetic nephropathy and type II diabetes.

SUGGESTED READING

1. Almazov VA, Shlyakhto EV, Conrady AO, Brodskaya IS, Zaharov DV. Effects of losartan on left ventricular mass and heart rate variability in hypertensive patients. *Cardiovasc Drugs Ther.* 1997;11(suppl 2):406.
2. Azizi M, Guyene TT, Chatellier G, Wargon M, Menard J. Additive effects of losartan and enalapril on blood pressure and plasma active renin. *Hypertension.* 1997;29:634–640.
3. Benz J, Oshrain C, Henry D, Avery C, Chiang YT, Gatlin M. Valsartan, a new angiotensin II receptor antagonist: a double-blind study comparing the incidence of cough with lisinopril and hydrochlorothiazide. *J Clin Pharmacol.* 1997;37:101–107.
4. Bermann MA, Walsh MF, Sowers JR. Angiotensin-II biochemistry and physiology: update on angiotensin-II receptor blockers. *Cardiovasc Rev.* 1997;15:75–100.
5. Chan JC, Critchley JA, Tomlinson B, Chan TY, Cockram CS. Antihypertensive and anti-albuminuric effects of losartan, potassium and felodipine in Chinese elderly hypertensive patients with or without non–insulin-dependent diabetes mellitus. *Am J Nephrol.* 1997;17:72–80.
6. DeGasparo M, Bottari S, Leven NR. Characteristics of angiotensin II receptors and their role in cell and organ physiology. In: Laragh JH, Brenner BM, eds. *Hypertension: Pathophysiology, Diagnosis, and Management.* 2nd ed. New York, NY: Raven Press; 1995:1695–1720.
7. Messerli FH, Weber MA, Brunner HR. Angiotensin II receptor inhibition: a new therapeutic principle. *Arch Intern Med.* 1996;156:1957–1965.
8. Paolisso G, Tagliamonte MR, Gambardella A, Manzella D, Gualdiero P, Varricchio G, Verza M, Varricchio M. Losartan mediated improvement in insulin action is mainly due to an increase in non-oxidative glucose metabolism and blood flow in insulin-resistant hypertensive patients. *J Hum Hypertens.* 1997;11:307–312.
9. Pitt B, Segal R, Martinez FA, Meurers G, Cowley AJ, Thomas I, Deedwania PC, Ney DE, Snavely DB, Chang PI. Randomised trial of losartan versus captopril in patients over 65 with heart failure (Evaluation of Losartan in the Elderly Study, ELITE). *Lancet.* 1997;349:747–752.
10. Weber MA. Angiotensin II receptor antagonists in the treatment of hypertension. *Cardiol Rev.* 1997;5:72–80.

Chapter 131

Dihydropyridine Calcium Antagonists

Matthew R. Weir, MD

KEY POINTS

- Dihydropyridine calcium antagonists (CAs) are primarily arteriolar dilators.

- All CAs have been shown to be similarly effective and safe antihypertensive drugs in their approved dosing range, with monotherapy response rates from 55% to 84% in all age ranges.

- The antihypertensive properties of CAs remain robust despite increased dietary salt intake, which makes them useful in patients who find it difficult to reduce dietary salt consumption.

See also Chapters 25, 32, 132, 133

Dihydropyridine calcium antagonists (CAs) exert their clinical effects by blocking the L class of voltage-gated calcium channels in a variety of tissues. Because calcium plays a critical role in cellular communication, regulation, and function, any manipulation of transmembrane calcium flux can affect a variety of cellular regulatory processes and functions. Normally, cells maintain a low resting intracellular concentration of ionized calcium in the face of large and inwardly directed concentrations of extracellular calcium. As calcium enters the cell in the presence of calcium-binding proteins, it stimulates a number of second messenger systems within the cell, which then couples calcium entry to cellular response.

Calcium channels have both activator and antagonist binding sites, which may be regulated and altered experimentally and in disease states. Calcium entry blockers are both quantitatively and qualitatively distinct, in that they have differential sensitivity and selectivity for binding the pharmacological receptors along the calcium channel in various tissues. This differential selectivity of action has important implications for the use of these drugs in clinical medicine.

Pharmacokinetics

Calcium entry blockers have been divided into four different classes on the basis of their structural properties (dihydropyridine, phenylalkylamine, benzothiazepine, tetralene). This chapter will focus exclusively on the dihydropyridine group. Dihydropyridine calcium entry blockers are reasonably well absorbed, but they tend to undergo extensive first-pass metabolism and biotransformation in the liver (**Table 131.1**). In general, the metabolites are inactive, with the possible exception of nifedipine. Amlodipine does not have an extensive hepatic first-pass metabolism like other CAs, and this results in a much more prolonged drug effect. Many of these drugs have been reformulated into sustained-release preparations to facilitate once-daily administration.

Several studies have demonstrated a consistent concentration-effect relationship for many of the calcium entry blockers, including nifedipine, amlodipine, felodipine, and nisoldipine. This helps predict the effectiveness of long-term therapy from the first-dose response. In addition, the concentration-effect relationship illustrates the importance of pharmacokinetic differences between drugs and the influence of aging and disease on absolute drug effect.

Mechanisms of Action

Dihydropyridine CAs have attracted interest as antihypertensive agents because they uniformly reduce vascular resistance. There is no significant effect on cardiac output except in patients with impaired systolic ventricular function. The ability of calcium entry blockers to diminish cytosolic calcium concentrations within vascular smooth muscle cells probably explains their vasodilatory properties. CAs interfere with both angiotensin II and α_2-adrenergic receptor–mediated vasoconstriction and may affect α_1-adrenergic receptor–mediated vasoconstriction. Experimental maximal vasodilator responses are inversely related to the patient's plasma renin activity and angiotensin II concentration. In general, the vasodilation associated with CAs is usually not associated with reflex-mediated sympathoneural activation, although at higher doses, such activation is more likely.

CAs are more effective in constricted than in nonconstricted vascular beds, and greater vasodepressor responses occur in patients with higher levels of blood pressure. Calcium entry blockers facilitate natriuresis, probably by improving renal blood flow, diminishing renal tubular sodium reabsorption, and interfering with aldosterone secretion.

Cardiac Effects

The primary hemodynamic effect of calcium entry blockers is vasodilation (**Table 131.2**). Numerous studies have demonstrated that total peripheral resistance and regional vascular resistance are reduced both acutely and chronically with therapy. Cardiac function is unaffected by calcium entry blockers, with the exception of patients who have ejection fractions of <30%. Dihydropyridine calcium entry blockers are less likely than nondihydropyridines to induce a fall in cardiac output in patients with systolic dysfunction of the heart. Amlodipine and felodipine have been demonstrated to be safe when used in patients with systolic cardiac dysfunction. CAs may be useful for the treatment of diastolic dysfunction, in which an improvement in ventricular compliance frequently results in improved cardiac output. Such an improvement, however, is more likely to occur with rate-lowering CAs, such as verapamil.

Dihydropyridine CAs have variable effects on heart rate. Acutely, these drugs tend to induce a reflex tachycardia, but long-term

379

Table 131.1. Pharmacokinetics of the Dihydropyridine Calcium Entry Blockers

	ORAL ABSORPTION, %	BIOAVAILABILITY, %	PROTEIN BINDING, %	PLASMA HALF-LIFE, H	HEPATIC METABOLISM	ACTIVE METABOLITE
Amlodipine	>90	60–65	>95	45	Yes	No
Felodipine	>90	10–25	>95	2.8	Yes	No
Isradipine	>90	20	>95	8.3	Yes	No
Nicardipine	>90	35	>95	4.8	Yes	No
Nifedipine	>90	30–60	>90	3.4±10.4 (capsule)	Yes	?Yes
Nisoldipine	>90	5	99	7–12	Yes	No

Table 131.2. Cardiac and Hemodynamic Effects of the Dihydropyridine Calcium Entry Blockers in Patients with Normal Ejection Fractions

EFFECT	AMLODIPINE	FELODIPINE	ISRADIPINE	NICARDIPINE	NIFEDIPINE	NISOLDIPINE
Arteriolar dilation	++++	++++	++++	++++	++++	++++
Coronary vasodialtion	++++	++++	++++	++++	++++	++++
Cardiac afterload	↓↓	↓↓	↓↓	↓↓	↓↓	↓↓
Cardiac contractility*	0	0	0	0	0/↓†	0
Heart rate	→ or ↑ (acute) then →	→ or ↑ (acute) then →	↑ (acute) then →	↑ (acute) then →	↑	→ or ↑ (acute) then →
Atrioventricular conduction	0	0	0	0	0	0
Sinoatrial automaticity	0	?	↓ (slight)	0	0	0

*Net effect (direct cardiac effect plus influence of activation of sympathetic nervous system, etc.)
†Depends on type of patient and extent of sympathetic stimulation; nifedipine may decrease contractility in susceptible patients.

studies show similar heart rates before and during therapy. Higher doses of these drugs can be expected to be associated with an increase in pulse rate. Calcium entry blockers do not reduce exercise capacity.

Clinical Use

CAs have been shown to be similarly effective and safe antihypertensive drugs in their approved dosing range, with monotherapy response rates from 55% to 84%. The drugs appear to be well tolerated but do tend to have dose-dependent side effects, such as headache, tachycardia, and edema. The peripheral edema seen with these compounds relates not to salt and water retention but rather to a greater arteriolar than venous dilation and increased transcapillary pressure gradients. This phenomenon is dose-independent and is linked to excessive upright posture. The drugs are rarely associated with abnormalities in electrolyte, carbohydrate, or lipid metabolism and can be used in a wide variety of patients. There is similar efficacy in younger or older patients, despite earlier reports suggesting that CAs were more efficacious in older patients. The drugs also work well in both black and white hypertensive patients. CAs are useful in hypertensive patients with a wide variety of concomitant conditions, including ischemic heart disease, peripheral vascular insufficiency, asthma, chronic pulmonary disease, chronic renal disease, hypertrophic cardiomyopathy, left ventricular hypertrophy, or variant angina. Recently, concern has been raised about the relative safety of dihydropyridine calcium antagonists compared with ACE inhibitors in hypertensives with type II diabetes. Further studies are needed before this issue can be resolved.

The antihypertensive effect of calcium entry blockers is additive with other antihypertensive drugs, including diuretics. More studies are necessary to determine whether CAs of the dihydropyridine and nondihydropyridine classes can be used together for increased antihypertensive efficacy. If CAs are to be combined with β-blockers, it is preferable to use a dihydropyridine to avoid atrioventricular block or systolic dysfunction.

CAs do not cause rebound hypertension, but rapid withdrawal may induce coronary artery spasm or angina pectoris, especially in patients with ischemic heart disease. CAs are effective independent of sodium intake, making them especially useful in patients who have difficulty adhering to dietary sodium restriction.

Safety

Controversy has recently arisen in the medical and lay press concerning the safety of calcium entry blockers with respect to coronary heart disease, cancer, and bleeding. A subcommittee of the Liaison Committee of the World Health Organization and the International Society of Hypertension has recently reviewed available data and concluded that the current evidence does not prove the existence of either additional beneficial or harmful effects of CAs on coronary heart disease events, including fatal or nonfatal myocardial infarctions and other deaths from coronary heart disease. Available evidence from observational studies does not provide good evidence of an adverse effect of CAs on cancer risk or bleeding risk. If anything, more recent data demonstrate that these drugs may be used safely even in patients with systolic heart failure

Table 131.3. Selected Pharmacokinetic Interactions of Dihydropyridine Calcium Entry Blockers

INTERACTING DRUG	CALCIUM ENTRY BLOCKER	RESULT
Cardiovascular drugs		
α-Blockers	Dihydropyridines	Excessive hypotension
Propranolol	Dihydropyridines	Increased propranolol levels
Noncardiovascular drugs		
Cimetidine	Dihydropyridines	Increased area under the curve and plasma levels of calcium entry blocker
Cyclosporine	Nicardipine Amlodipine	Increased levels of cyclosporine

Table 131.4. Dosage and Administration of Currently Available Dihydropyridine Calcium Entry Blockers

	DAILY DOSE RANGE, MG	FREQUENCY OF ADMINISTRATION, PER DAY
Amlodipine (Norvasc)	2.5–10	Once
Felodipine (Plendil)	5–20	Once
Isradipine (Dynacirc)	5–20	Twice
Isradipine CR (Dynacirc CR)	5–20	Once
Nicardipine SR (Cardene SR)	60–120	Twice
Nifedipine XL (Procardia XL)	30–120	Once
Nifedipine CC (Adalat CC)	30–120	Once
Nisoldipine CC (Sular)	10–60	Once

(amlodipine, felodipine). Prevention of stroke-related morbidity and mortality in elderly patients with systolic hypertension was demonstrated in the Syst-Eur trial. Careful ongoing review of new clinical trial data examining for positive/negative outcomes with dihydropyridine remains a prudent consideration for these agents.

Drug Interaction

Calcium entry blockers may interact with a variety of drugs, and appropriate caution needs to be used (**Table 131.3**).

Dosage and Administration

The preferred formulations of these drugs for hypertension are designed in a way that allows once- or twice-daily administration (**Table 131.4**).

SUGGESTED READING

1. Ad Hoc Subcommittee of the Liaison Committee of the World Health Organization and the International Society of Hypertension. Effects of calcium antagonists on the risks of coronary heart disease, cancer and bleeding. *J Hypertens.* 1997; 15:105–115.
2. Epstein M. Calcium antagonists in the management of hypertension. In: Epstein M, ed. *Calcium Antagonists in Clinical Medicine.* Philadelphia, Pa: Hanley & Belfus Inc; 1992:213–230.
3. Lydtin H, Trenkwalder P. *Calcium Antagonists: A Critical Review.* New York, NY: Springer-Verlag; 1990:1–241.
4. Morris AD, Meredith PA, Reid JL. Pharmacokinetics of calcium antagonists: implications for therapy. In: Epstein M, ed. *Calcium Antagonists in Clinical Medicine.* Philadelphia, Pa: Hanley & Belfus Inc; 1992:49–67.
5. Piepho RW, Culbertson VL, Rhodes RS. Drug interactions with the calcium-entry blockers. *Circulation.* 1987;75(suppl V):V-181–V-194.
6. Triggle DJ. Calcium antagonists. In: Antonaccio MJ, ed. *Cardiovascular Pharmacology.* 3rd ed. New York, NY: Raven Press; 1990:107–160.

Chapter 132

Non-dihydropyridine Calcium Antagonists

T. Barry Levine, MD; Domenic Sica, MD

KEY POINTS

- Nondihydropyridine calcium antagonists (verapamil and diltiazem) are agents whose primary hemodynamic effect (like that of the dihydropyridines) is vasodilation.

- In contrast to dihydropyridines, verapamil and diltiazem have significant effects on the cardiac conduction system and tend to slow the heart rate.

- Side effects and drug-drug interactions are not uncommon with these compounds.

See also Chapters 24, 32, 131, 133

The calcium antagonists (CAs) have traditionally consisted of a structurally and pharmacologically diverse group of compounds that fit into three classes: phenylalkylamines, benzothiazepines, and 1,4-dihydropyridines; the prototypes of these classes are verapamil, diltiazem, and nifedipine, respectively. The common pharmacological mechanism of action of these drugs is to decrease cellular calcium entry via the L-type channel. The CAs vary considerably in their effects on regional circulatory beds, sinus and atrioventricular nodal functions, and myocardial contractility; thus, the CAs have quite different clinical applications, contraindications, drug-drug interactions, and side-effect profiles.

Cellular Mechanisms of Action

Verapamil and diltiazem exert their primary effects at the cellular level by blocking the transmembrane movement of calcium ions through voltage-gated L-type calcium channels. The ensuing decrease in cytosolic calcium concentration is a probable explanation for their vasodilatory effects. The complex relationship between the blockade of T-type channels and the resultant clinical effects has not yet been fully elucidated. CAs also blunt the effects of angiotensin II– and α_1- and α_2-adrenergic receptor–mediated vasoconstriction, although the clinical significance of these properties remains unknown. These CAs (but not all CAs) may exhibit negative inotropic effects, particularly if systolic function is already impaired.

CAs also dilate different arterioles and modify renal tubular sodium absorption, causing a modest natriuresis in some patients. This phenomenon occurs even as blood pressure is reduced, augments the vasodilatory effects of these compounds in reducing blood pressure, and may occasionally be associated with nocturia.

Pharmacokinetics and Pharmacodynamics

The pharmacokinetic properties of these compounds are somewhat similar **(Table 132.1)** The bioavailability of verapamil and diltiazem increases with chronic dosing, most likely secondary to saturable metabolism. This process (among other factors) allows immediate-release verapamil or diltiazem to be effective when administered twice daily. Verapamil and diltiazem are both currently

available in a number of different sustained-release formulations **(Table 132.2)** that allow once-daily dosing. Some of these delivery systems result in precisely timed drug delivery that coincides with circadian rhythm–related blood pressure peaks.

The pharmacokinetics of the CAs are affected by age and intercurrent disease. In patients with renal insufficiency, the pharmacokinetics of these drugs are minimally changed. In hepatic disease states, each of these compounds may have diminished systemic clearance, necessitating dosage adjustments. Aging slows the metabolism of these drugs, presumably secondary to the accompanying decrease in hepatic blood flow. As a consequence of this, lower doses of CAs may prove to be more than adequate for obtaining blood pressure control in the elderly.

Systemic Hemodynamic Effects

CAs reduce total peripheral resistance, and thereby arterial pressure, in both the short and the long term. CAs dilate constricted more than nonconstricted vascular beds, and vasodepressor responses to CAs are greatest in patients with the highest pretreatment blood pressures. CAs increase coronary blood flow to a variable extent and can be effective antianginal agents. CAs preferentially induce arteriolar vasodilation while leaving mechanisms of venoconstriction intact. This property is a prominent factor in the development of lower-extremity peripheral edema in susceptible subjects. Nondihydropyridines can act as negative inotropes, but this property is most apparent when there is preexisting cardiac dysfunction (ejection fraction <30%).

Cardiac Effects

Although verapamil has the greatest negative inotropic effect, its ability to act as a coronary vasodilator, to decrease afterload, and to effectively treat diastolic dysfunction can effectively counterbalance any deleterious consequences of negative inotropism.

Diltiazem tends to reduce sinoatrial nodal conduction, whereas diltiazem is more active in blocking the atrioventricular node. Both diltiazem and verapamil are widely used in the treatment of supraventricular arrhythmias. In the dose range used for the treatment of hypertension, these drugs usually have no effect on pulse rate. In some patients, pulse rate may be decreased by as much as 10%, but this is usually less than the pulse rate reduction observed with β-blocker therapy (a reduction of 20% to 30%). In contrast, dihydropyridine CAs can induce a dose-dependent duration of treatment-related reflex tachycardia. Exercise performance, when it is studied, is well preserved with these drugs, but they do not block peak systolic BP response to exercise stress.

Clinical Use

When used in their approved dosing range, verapamil and diltiazem have demonstrated monotherapy response rates between 50% and 80%, with each compound displaying a moderately steep dose-response curve. The higher the blood pressure at the inception of therapy with these compounds, the greater the observed reduction in blood pressure. Abrupt discontinuation of these compounds does not result in rebound hypertension.

Although there are few head-to-head comparisons, it seems that there is little if any difference in blood pressure–lowering potency among the various agents, provided that adequate doses are given. CAs seem to have a more powerful effect in patient types characterized by a low plasma renin activity, as in the case of many black hypertensives. An early belief that CAs had a distinct age effect has not been verified in all studies. CAs exhibit their vasodepressor response independent of salt intake, with some investigators suggesting that CAs have an even more potent antihypertensive effect when salt intake is high. Patients who respond well to diuretic therapy are likely to respond to CAs. The antihypertensive effect of CAs is additive with a number of other agents, including diuretics, peripheral α-blockers, and ACE inhibitors. The concomitant use of β-blockers with drugs in this class is to be discouraged, particularly in the presence of an already reduced heart rate. If β-blocker therapy is considered necessary for a patient, then a dihydropyridine CA is a more prudent choice of concomitant agent. Finally, the antihypertensive effects of CAs are not offset by the concomitant administration of nonsteroidal anti-inflammatory agents, as is the case for a number of other antihypertensive drug classes, such as diuretics, β-blockers, or ACE inhibitors.

The use of CAs is not accompanied by any deterioration in electrolyte status or lipid/glucose control. These compounds have also been shown not to reduce glomerular filtration rate and/or renal blood flow in the hypertensive patient; in fact, they may increase these parameters in certain such patients. Unlike dihydropyridine CAs, the nondihydropyridine CAs have been reported to reduce proteinuria in patients with diabetic renal disease.

CAs can be safely used in patients with a wide variety of comorbid conditions, including ischemic heart disease, peripheral vascular disease, chronic obstructive pulmonary disease, left ventricular hypertrophy or hypertrophic cardiomyopathy, and variant angina. The concerns raised about the safety of dihydropyridine CAs in diabetics have not been an issue for nondihydropyridine CAs. These compounds are also useful in the primary treatment of variant angina and/or diastolic dysfunction, although their abrupt discontinuation may sometimes result in a crescendo angina pattern.

Verapamil and diltiazem are both used in the treatment of acute and/or chronic supraventricular arrhythmias. Alternatively, verapamil is contraindicated in patients with preexcitation syndrome and a rapid ventricular response, because it may accentuate conduction through the accessory tract. Verapamil has also been demonstrated to reduce reinfarction rate and postmyocardial infarction morbidity and mortality when administered 1 to 2 weeks after a myocardial infarction. In this regard, verapamil is probably the drug of choice in

Table 132.1. Pharmacokinetic Properties of Diltiazem and Verapamil in Humans

	VERAPAMIL	DILTIAZEM
Absorption, %	>90	90
Bioavailablity, %	10–20	24–74
Protein binding, %	85–95	77–86
Therapeutic plasma concentration, ng/mL	80–300	≈ 100–200
Elimination half-life, h		
Acute	2–6	
Chronic	8–12	2.0–6.0
Volume of distribution, L/kg	4.0	3.0–8.0
Active metabolite	Norverapamil	Desethyldiltiazem

Table 132.2. Nondihydropyridine Calcium Channel Blockers: Dosing Recommendations

GENERIC (TRADE) NAME	DOSE, MG	FREQUENCY, DOSES PER DAY	PHYSIOLOGICAL EFFECTS	COMMENTS AND PROBABLE SIDE EFFECTS
Diltiazem SR (Cardizem SR)	120–360	2	Block inward movement of calcium ions across cell membranes and cause smooth-muscle relaxation. Peripheral resistance ↓; blood pressure ↓; heart rate ↔↓	Block slow channels in heart and may reduce sinus rate; increase degree of arteriovenous block; constipation
Diltiazem CD (Cardizem CD, Dilacor XR, Tiazac)	120–360	1		
Verapamil LA (Calan SR, Isoptin SR Verelan Covera-HS*)	90–360	1		

*Specifically indicated for bedtime dosing.

Table 132.3. Drug-Drug Interactions With Nondihydropyridine Calcium Channel Blockers

CALCIUM ANTAGONIST	INTERACTING DRUG	RESULT
Verapamil	Digoxin	↑ Digoxin levels by 50%–90% ↑ Digoxin levels by 40%
Verapamil	β-Blockers	↑ AV nodal blockade, hypotension, bradycardia, asytole
Verapamil, diltiazem	Cyclosporine	↑ Cyclosporine levels by 30%–40%
Verapamil, diltiazem	Cimetidine	↑ Verapamil and diltiazem levels by decreased metabolism
Verapamil	Rifampin/phenytoin	↓ Verapamil levels by enzyme induction

the post–myocardial infarction patient, in whom β-blocker therapy either is not tolerated or is contraindicated.

Adverse Reactions

Side effects differ considerably among the different CAs and frequently relate to the amount of drug being administered. Commonly observed events include flushing, headache, and peripheral edema, with the latter finding being somewhat more common with dihydropyridine CAs. In patients with CA-related peripheral edema, the addition of an ACE inhibitor (secondary to its venodilatory effect) will frequently cause the peripheral edema either to remit or to diminish significantly. Constipation is a very common side effect with verapamil therapy, and diltiazem sometimes causes headaches.

A recent debate has developed concerning the role of CA treatment in increasing cardiovascular morbidity and mortality and/or increasing the risk of cancer. The issues surrounding this debate include the type of CA used (dihydropyridine versus nondihydropyridine) and whether the compound is short-acting or not. Ongoing clinical trials may distinguish dihydropyridine from nondihydropyridine CAs in respect to their increasing cardiovascular morbidity and mortality. A careful review of available information concerning the risk of cancer with CAs suggests that their use is unrelated to the overall risk of cancer or to the development of a specific type of cancer. Several drug-drug interactions occur with nondihydropyridine CAs (**Table 132.3**).

Dosage and Administration

Current formulations for drugs in this class permit once-daily, or at most twice-daily, dosing (Table 132.2). Currently available sustained-release formulations are more effective in blood pressure control than were the immediate-release formulations. The optimal timing of administration of these CAs is poorly delineated. One sustained-release form of verapamil (Covera-HS) is specifically designed for nocturnal dosing because its drug-release rate peaks in the early morning hours at the time of the natural circadian peak in blood pressure.

SUGGESTED READING

1. Hansen JF. Treatment with verapamil after an acute myocardial infarction: review of the Danish studies on verapamil in myocardial infarction (DAVIT I and II). *Drugs.* 1991;42(suppl 2):43–53.
2. Materson BJ, Reda DJ, Cushman WC, Massie BM, Freis ED, Kochar MS, Hamburger RJ, Fye C, Lakshman R, Gottdiener, et al. Single drug therapy for hypertension in men: a comparison of six antihypertensive agents with placebo. The Department of Veterans Affairs Cooperative Study Group on Antihypertensive Agents. *N Engl J Med.* 1993;328:914–921.
3. Pool PE. Diltiazem. In: *Cardiovascular Drug Therapy.* 2nd ed. Philadelphia, Pa: WB Saunders; 1996:931–971.
4. Rosenberg L, Rao RS, Palmer JR, Strom BL, Stolley PD, Zauber AG, Warshauer ME, Shapiro S. Calcium channel blockers and the risk of cancer. *JAMA.* 1998;279: 1000–1004.
5. Saunders E, Weir MR, Kong BW, Hollifield J, Gray J, Vertes V, Sowers JR, Zemel MB, Curry C, Schoenberger J, et al. A comparison of the efficacy and safety of a β-blocker, a calcium channel blocker, and a converting enzyme inhibitor in hypertensive blacks. *Arch Intern Med.* 1990;150:1707–1713.

Chapter 133

Direct Vasodilators

C. Venkata S. Ram, MD

KEY POINTS

- Drugs that directly relax resistance vessels are particularly useful in the management of severe or refractory hypertension.

- Reflex increases in sympathetic nervous activity, renin-angiotensin activation, and salt retention occur during monotherapy (pseudotolerance mechanisms).

- Combining vasodilators with antiadrenergic drugs and diuretics limits side effects and counteracts pseudotolerance mechanisms.

- Although minoxidil is extremely effective, its adverse effects have limited its utility in clinical practice, and its use is recommended only in hypertensive patients who are refractory to all other drugs.

See also Chapters 32, 130, 131

Chronic hypertension is characterized by increased peripheral vascular resistance, and therefore, drugs that directly relax resistance vessels would seem to be desirable in the pharmacological management of high blood pressure. However, the efficacy of direct vasodilators, such as hydralazine and minoxidil, as monotherapy is blunted by physiological reflex responses that limit their effects (pseudotolerance). Direct arterial dilation triggers baroreceptor-mediated sympathetic activation, resulting in tachycardia and increased cardiac output and myocardial oxygen demand, making it risky to use these agents alone in patients with known or possible coronary artery disease. Second, direct vasodilators cause unpleasant side effects such as flushing, headache, and palpitations. Third, direct vasodilators cause significant fluid retention, which may decrease their long-term therapeutic effectiveness. These disadvantages, however, can be overcome by combining direct vasodilators with antiadrenergic agents and diuretics **(see Figure 133.1)**. When used in this fashion, vasodilators can be remarkably useful in the long-term management of refractory or severe hypertension.

Hydralazine

Hydralazine, a classic direct vasodilator, was introduced in the early 1950s for clinical use in hypertension. Although hydralazine reduces blood pressure, the problems mentioned above limited its use as monotherapy until β-adrenergic receptors were developed. These drugs, together with diuretics, typically block the pseudoresistance that characterizes long-term hydralazine use. Therapy with hydralazine should generally be combined with an antiadrenergic drug and a diuretic.

Pharmacokinetics

After oral administration, 90% of hydralazine is absorbed from the gastrointestinal tract. Very little of the unchanged drug appears in the urine. A number of hydralazine metabolites have been identified, and the relative amounts of each may depend on the acetylation status of the individual.

Acetylation of hydralazine is genetically determined by the concentration of *N*-acetyltransferase. "Slow" acetylators have a higher plasma concentration after a given dose than "fast" acetylators. The incidence of drug-induced toxicity is greater in patients who are slow acetylators, which includes approximately one half of the US population. The plasma half-life of hydralazine is only 4 hours, but its clinical action lasts from 8 to 12 hours after oral dosing. An oral dose of 75 to 100 mg is equipotent to 10 to 25 mg given parenterally.

Mechanism of Action

The predominant mode of action of hydralazine is to induce direct relaxation of vascular smooth muscle in the resistance vessels. This leads to a fall in peripheral vascular resistance. The hypotensive effect of hydralazine is accompanied by a reflex activation of the autonomic reflexes, with resultant increases in the heart rate and cardiac output. Hydralazine also stimulates the renin-angiotensin system, leading to aldosterone release, sodium retention, and expansion of plasma volume.

Clinical Use

Because the efficacy of hydralazine therapy is best sustained in combination with a β-blocking drug and a diuretic, its use is restricted to patients who require multiple-drug therapy. The drug can be given twice daily, despite its short half-life. The total daily dose should be limited to 200 to 300 mg because higher doses clearly pose a risk of inducing a lupus-like syndrome (see below). In fast acetylators, higher doses may be used because the risk of this reaction is less. Usually, hydralazine is added as the third agent to patients unresponsive to diuretics and β-blockers. Some authors recommend using hydralazine and β-blockers first and adding a diuretic if necessary. When a β-blocker is contraindicated, other antiadrenergic drugs, usually central α-agonists, are appropriate alternative choices to facilitate pulse rate reduction.

Side Effects and Toxicity

Hydralazine causes numerous bothersome and sometimes serious side effects. In addition to the side effects described above, some

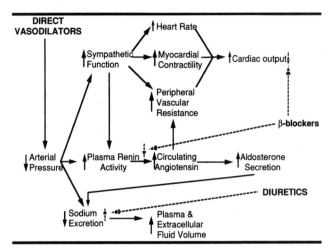

Figure 133.1. Hemodynamic consequences of direct vasodilators and the influence of concomitant therapy with a diuretic and a β-blocker. (Effects of concomitant therapy shown by dashed arrows.)

patients develop nausea and vomiting and occasionally peripheral neuropathy. Fluid retention can cause not only edema but also pseudotolerance to the vasodepressor effect of hydralazine, an effect that can be overcome by diuretic therapy and/or dietary restriction of salt intake.

Hydralazine-induced lupus usually presents with arthralgia and may be accompanied by malaise, weight loss, skin rash, splenomegaly, and pleural and pericardial effusion. Rare patients with hydralazine-induced lupus have associated glomerulonephritis. The syndrome occurs mainly in slow acetylators and is more common in women. Hydralazine-induced lupus appears between 6 and 24 months after the therapy is begun. The risk is proportional to the dosage; chronic therapy of >200 mg/d clearly enhances the risk. The syndrome is reversible after discontinuation of therapy, and full recovery occurs within weeks. In contrast to systemic lupus erythematosus, hydralazine-induced lupus is associated with antibodies directed against single-stranded DNA rather than against the native double-stranded DNA. Antibodies to histones are also frequently present.

Dosage and Administration

Therapy with hydralazine can be initiated with 10 to 25 mg BID, which can be increased at weekly intervals to 200 to 400 mg/d.

Intramuscular or intravenous administration of hydralazine is used for hypertensive crises. The dose requirements to achieve the therapeutic goal are unpredictable. The usual dose is 20 to 40 mg, which may be repeated as necessary. Although an effect on the blood pressure may be seen in a few minutes, the maximum decrease occurs between 15 and 75 minutes. Parenteral hydralazine therapy is successfully and safely applied to the management of severe hypertension in pregnancy.

Minoxidil

Minoxidil is a more potent vasodilator than hydralazine but is similar in its overall hemodynamic actions. Although minoxidil is extremely effective, its adverse effects have limited its utility in clinical practice, and its use is recommended only in hypertensive patients who are refractory to all other drugs.

Pharmacokinetics

Minoxidil is completely and rapidly absorbed from the gastrointestinal tract. In patients with advanced renal failure, the absorption of the drug is delayed. It is metabolized predominantly in the liver. The elimination half-life of minoxidil varies from 3 to 4 hours, although the duration of action may be as long as 12 to 72 hours.

Mechanism of Action

Like hydralazine, minoxidil dilates the resistance vessels directly and lowers peripheral vascular resistance. There is some evidence that minoxidil may act by opening potassium channels at the vascular smooth muscle cellular level. The dominant action of minoxidil is on the arterial side of the circulatory system. Venodilation does not occur; thus, postural hypotension is rare.

As a result of marked reduction in peripheral vascular resistance, minoxidil causes considerable activation of the sympathetic nervous and renin-angiotensin systems, with resultant reflex tachycardia and secondary hyperaldosteronism, consequences that may blunt its antihypertensive potential.

Hemodynamic Effects

Monotherapy with minoxidil is accompanied by a fall in peripheral vascular resistance and an increase in heart rate, stroke volume, and cardiac output.

Clinical Use

Minoxidil is frequently necessary in patients with renal insufficiency, who are often refractory to all other drugs. Minoxidil therapy is effective regardless of the severity or etiology of hypertension and the status of renal function. An unsatisfactory response to minoxidil is extremely rare in our clinical experience. Before the availability of minoxidil, bilateral nephrectomy was the only therapeutic option in patients with uncontrolled hypertension and renal damage.

Minoxidil should always be administered with a β-blocking drug and a potent diuretic, usually of the loop-active variety. β-Blocker and diuretic doses should be adjusted as needed to prevent tachycardia and edema formation, respectively, even if high doses are necessary. Rarely, a loop-active diuretic and a thiazide or metolazone need to be used to treat otherwise refractory edema. In the event of contraindications to a β-blocker, a centrally acting α-agonist can be used.

Some studies have shown that prolonged minoxidil therapy stabilizes or improves renal function in hypertensive patients with renal failure, and sustained blood pressure control with minoxidil occasionally has resulted in the discontinuation of dialysis in patients with an "acute" or chronic component of hypertensive nephrosclerosis. The improvement in renal function is primarily due to aggressive and effective blood pressure control, rather than a specific renoprotective effect of minoxidil.

Side Effects

In addition to fluid retention and symptoms due to the reflex activation of sympathetic tone, other specific adverse reactions occur. ST-segment depression and T-wave flattening or inversion of the ECG are sometimes seen in patients receiving minoxidil. Whether this observation represents cardiac ischemia or is a manifestation of left ventricular hypertrophy is unclear.

Pericardial effusion, including tamponade, has also been reported in patients receiving minoxidil therapy. The true incidence of this side effect is not known, because many patients receiving minoxidil are already predisposed to develop fluid retention as a result of cardiac or renal dysfunction. Elevated pulmonary artery pressures have been documented in patients receiving chronic minoxidil therapy, an effect less likely to occur in patients receiving β-blockers concurrently.

Hypertrichosis occurs in nearly all patients treated with minoxidil. This is particularly evident on the face, which is a serious limitation to the use of this drug in women. The specific mechanism for minoxidil-induced hair growth is not known, but it is probably related to increased blood flow in affected areas. Hypertrichosis disappears within a few weeks after discontinuation of the drug. Hypertrichosis can be treated with depilatory agents.

Dosage and Administration

The usual starting dose of minoxidil is 5 mg/d, and the maintenance dosage for most patients is 10 to 40 mg/d given once or in two divided doses. A few patients, particularly those with advanced renal failure, require doses >40 to 50 mg/d to achieve the necessary therapeutic effect.

SUGGESTED READING

1. Campese VM. Minoxidil: a review of its pharmacological properties and therapeutic use. *Drugs.* 1981;22:257–278.
2. Handler RP, Federman JS. Hydralazine-induced lupus. *NY State J Med.* 1982;82:1288.
3. Katila M, Frick MH. Combined dihydralazine and propranolol in the treatment of hypertension. *Int Z Klin Pharmakol.* 1970;4:111–114.
4. Koch-Weser J. Medical intelligence drug therapy. *N Engl J Med.* 1976;295:320–323.
5. Lundeen TE, Dolan DR, Ram CV. Pericardial effusion associated with minoxidil therapy. *Postgrad Med.* 1981;70:98–100.
6. Mitchell HC, Pettinger WA. Renal function in long-term minoxidil treated patients. *J Cardiovasc Pharmacol.* 1980;2(suppl 2):S163–S172.
7. Ram CV. Clinical considerations in combined drug therapy of hypertension. *Prac Cardiol.* 1984;10:83–105.
8. Ram CV. Management of essential and secondary hypertension. In: Martinez-Maldonado M, ed. *Handbook of Renal Therapeutics.* New York, NY: Plenum Medical Book Co; 1983:263–299.
9. Ram CV. Clinical applications of beta-adrenergic blocking drugs: a growing spectrum. *Heart Lung.* 1979;8:116–123.
10. Zacest R, Gilmore E, Koch-Weser J. Treatment of essential hypertension with combined vasodilation and beta-adrenergic blockage. *N Engl J Med.* 1972;286:617–622.

Other Agents

Potassium Channel Openers, Serotonin-Related Agents, Dopamine Agonists, Renin Inhibitors, Imidazolines, Neutral Endopeptidase Inhibitors, and Endothelin-Receptor Antagonists

William J. Elliott, MD, PhD

KEY POINTS

- Potassium channel openers and serotonin antagonists are already marketed in several countries, but low efficacy as monotherapy and frequent side effects limit their appeal.

- Dopamine agonists appear to have specific advantages when intravenous antihypertensive medications are warranted.

- Renin inhibitors, newer imidazolines, neutral endopeptidase inhibitors (which retard hydrolysis of atrial natriuretic peptide and also inhibit ACE), and endothelin-receptor antagonists are being investigated for potential use in human hypertension.

See also Chapters 18, 20, 24

Potassium Channel Openers

Several compounds that directly "open" ATP-sensitive potassium channels, including cromakalim, pinacidil, minoxidil, and nicorandil, are potent vasodilators in humans. The large number of different subtypes of potassium channels in vivo is both a challenge and an opportunity, so that more selective agents than those available would be desirable to minimize adverse effects. Several organ systems are affected by potassium channel openers, including the cardiovascular, respiratory, reproductive, genitourinary, gastrointestinal, peripheral muscular, and central nervous systems, as well as the skin and eye. Currently available agents have limited utility as antihypertensive monotherapies because of the range of side effects in multiple organ systems in humans.

Serotonin-Related Agents

Several molecules that affect either peripheral or central serotonin metabolism have been studied in humans, including ketanserin (which is thought to lower blood pressure by α_1-adrenergic blockade rather than 5-hydroxytryptamine agonism), flesinoxan, urapidil, and 5-methylurapidil. Beneficial effects on platelet function and fibrinolysis may account for improved outcomes in long-term trials (Prevention of Atherosclerotic Complications with Ketanserin [PACK] and Prognosis of Ischemic Risk in Atheromatous Patients under Mediatensyl [PRIHAM], with urapidil). Other similar compounds are still in clinical development.

Dopamine Agonists

Several decades of research have resulted in the synthesis of molecules with more selective pharmacological actions than dopamine, which activates dopaminergic, β-adrenergic, and α-adrenergic re-

ceptors in a dose-dependent fashion. Because the vasculature has a high density of vasodilatory dopaminergic receptors, dopamine and related agonists effectively lower blood pressure at relatively low doses. The first of these drugs to reach market is fenoldopam mesylate. Because it has limited oral bioavailability and a very short elimination half-life (5 to 9 minutes), fenoldopam is given as an intravenous infusion for hypertensive emergencies. Several studies of fenoldopam have shown that it is as effective as sodium nitroprusside but that it does not produce toxic metabolic products, such as cyanide and thiocyanate. Fenoldopam acutely improves many renal parameters, including urinary flow and sodium, potassium, and creatinine clearance in a dose-dependent fashion.

Fenoldopam is useful for intraoperative control of blood pressure and possibly for its salutary effect on renal blood flow. Fenoldopam would be expected to have interactions with other drugs that affect the dopaminergic system, including monoamine oxidase inhibitors, metoclopramide, bromocriptine, most antipsychotics, and tricyclic antidepressants. Fenoldopam increases intraocular pressure slightly, but this is unlikely to prohibit its use in most patients.

Fenoldopam is administered intravenously, beginning with a dose of $0.1 \ \mu g \cdot kg^{-1} \cdot min^{-1}$, by constant infusion. Doses are increased by 0.05 to $0.1 \ \mu g \cdot kg^{-1} \cdot min^{-1}$ every 10 to 20 minutes as necessary to reduce blood pressure to the desired level. Doses >1.5 $\mu g \cdot kg^{-1} \cdot min^{-1}$ are not recommended; the average dose in the largest series of 142 patients was $0.40 \ \mu g \cdot kg^{-1} \cdot min^{-1}$.

Renin Inhibitors

Blockade of the initial step of the renin-angiotensin-aldosterone cascade has been achieved with a new class of poorly bioavailable, intravenously administered drugs, which have been given the generic suffix "-kiren." Early work with these compounds in Europe has shown promise not only for reduction in blood pressure in salt-depleted or diuretic-treated patients but also for the treatment of heart failure or renal disease. The challenge now is to find an orally bioavailable compound.

Imidazolines

Compounds chemically related to clonidine have recently been shown to interact with a novel I_1-receptor in animal experiments. In early clinical studies, moxonidine and rilmenidine have been shown to effectively reduce blood pressure. This presumably occurs by a more specific central mechanism than with clonidine-like drugs. The major advantage of newer imidazolines is the potential avoidance of nonspecific central nervous system depression, including sedation and dry mouth.

Neutral Endopeptidase Inhibitors

Blockade of atrial natriuretic peptide metabolism offers the possibility of manipulating volume regulation in hypertension and heart failure and may also help in the management of atrial dysrhythmias. The most promising approach so far is not to use synthetic analogues of the natural peptide but rather to prolong the pharmacological effects of the endogenous hormones by blocking their degradation. Several such "neutral endopeptidase inhibitors" have now been synthesized and studied in animals, but their use in humans has only recently begun. The most attractive new compounds not only block atriopeptin degradation but also inhibit ACE (mixanpril or omipatrilat) or endothelin-converting enzyme (thiorphan).

Endothelin-Receptor Antagonists

Blood pressure is affected by several compounds designed to block endothelin-1 receptors of the ET_A and ET_B subclasses. At present, it is unclear whether both subtypes must be blocked for sustained efficacy. The first of these agents to show efficacy in large groups of patients is bosentan, which lowers seated blood pressure in a dose-dependent fashion without reflex sympathetic stimulation. Development of additional ET-1 blockers for hypertension and heart failure is expected.

SUGGESTED READING

1. Everitt DE, Boike SC, Piltz-Seymour JR, Van Coevorden R, Audet P, Zariffa N, Jorkasky D. Effect of intravenous fenoldopam on intraocular pressure in ocular hypertension. *J Clin Pharmacol.* 1997;37:312–320.
2. Godeau P, Allaert FA, Barrier J, Bletry O, Chamontin B, Devulder B, Godin M, Guillevin L, Guilmot JL, Luccioni R, Ninet J, Serise JM, Zannad FM. Course of ischemic risk in treated atheromatous hypertensive patients: the PRIHAM Study. (Prognosis of Ischemic Risk in Atheromatous Patients under Mediatensyl). [In French]. *Ann Med Interne (Paris).* 1996;147:403–407.
3. Goldberg ME, Cantillo J, Nemiroff MS, Subramoni J, Munoz R, Torjman M, Schieren H. Fenoldopam infusion for the treatment of postoperative hypertension. *J Clin Anesth.* 1993;5:386–391.
4. Kleinert HD. Hemodynamic effects of renin inhibitors. *Am J Nephrol.* 1996;15:252–260.
5. Krum H, Viskoper RJ, Lacourcière Y, Charlon V, for the Bosentan Hypertension Investigators. The effect of an endothelin-receptor antagonist, bosentan, on blood pressure in patients with essential hypertension. *N Engl J Med.* 1998;338:784–790.
6. Lawson K. Is there a therapeutic future for "potassium channel openers?" *Clin Sci (Colch).* 1996;91:651–663.
7. McCall RB, Clement ME. Role of serotonin$_{1A}$ and serotonin$_2$ receptors in the central regulation of the cardiovascular system. *Pharmacol Rev.* 1994;46:231–243.
8. Shusterman NH, Elliott WJ, White WB. Fenoldopam, but not nitroprusside, improves renal function in severely hypertensive patients with impaired renal function. *Am J Med.* 1993;95:161–168.
9. Turner AJ, Murphy LJ, Medeiros MS, Barnes K. Endopeptidase-24.11 (neprilysin) and relatives: twenty years on. *Adv Exp Med Biol.* 1996;389:141–148.
10. Ziegler D, Haxhiu MA, Kaan EC, Papp JG, Ernsberger P. Pharmacology of moxonidine, an I_1-imidazoline receptor agonist. *J Cardiovasc Pharmacol.* 1996;27(suppl 3):S26–S37.

Chapter 135

Management of Orthostatic Hypotension, Hypertension, and Tachycardia

David H.P. Streeten, MB, DPhil, FRCP

KEY POINTS

- Normally, rising from a recumbent position causes blood pooling in dependent veins with consequent decreases in stroke volume and systolic blood pressure (BP) and increases in systemic vascular resistance, diastolic BP, and heart rate.

- Hypovolemia in the absence of other disease usually causes orthostatic tachycardia that is apparent within seconds to minutes, often accompanied by a decrease in BP; saline infusion rapidly corrects the problem.

- Excessive venous pooling, autonomic failure, states of reduced cardiac function, diabetes, and adrenal insufficiency can cause immediate or delayed orthostatic hypotension, which often appears after 10 or more minutes of upright posture.

- Certain individuals with excessive venous pooling manifest a syndrome of exaggerated orthostatic *hypertension,* which is also corrected by volume repletion.

See also Chapters 115, 136

Normal Postural Adaptation

When a normal individual stands up or is tilted head-up after recumbency, there is a >2-fold increase in the pooling of blood in the dependent veins, which diminishes venous return and cardiac output and stimulates sympathetically mediated arteriolar and venous constriction. The results are a slight fall in systolic blood pressure (BP) and a slight rise in diastolic BP, with a mild increase in heart rate. The normal limits of these changes are shown in **Table 135.1.** When one or more of these limits are exceeded, there is objective evidence of an orthostatic disorder: systolic or diastolic hypotension, diastolic hypertension, or tachycardia.

Excessive reduction of cardiac output in the upright posture is the proximate mechanism of almost all forms of orthostatic hypotension, orthostatic hypertension, and orthostatic tachycardia. This may be caused by (1) reduced venous return resulting from intravascular hypovolemia (plasma or erythrocyte), excessive orthostatic pooling of blood in the lower body veins, resulting from impaired orthostatic venoconstriction or diffuse autonomic failure or (2) intrinsic mechanisms of impaired cardiac output. When the sympathetic innervation of the heart and peripheral vasculature is intact, the initial response to excessive postural decreases in venous return (venous pooling) is tachycardia and arteriolar constriction, which is stimulated mainly through cardiopulmonary (low-pressure) baroreceptor reflexes. In a few individuals, an exaggerated increase in diastolic BP (orthostatic hypertension) is caused by an exaggerated postural sympathetic activation. This syndrome is characterized by a small (if any) postural increase in systolic BP, marked increases in heart rate (frequently an increase exceeding 27 bpm or to above 108 bpm), and excess diastolic BP increases (a rise of more than 22 mm Hg or to above 97 mm Hg) in the erect posture.

When the hypovolemia or the orthostatic pooling is severe, cardiac output may fall so profoundly in the upright posture that intense

arteriolar constriction and tachycardia fail to prevent orthostatic hypotension and neurocardiogenic syncope. Either orthostatic hypotension or orthostatic diastolic hypertension may result from the hypovolemic effect of rapid diuresis and may be corrected by repletion of the extracellular fluid **(Figure 135.1)**. Diffuse autonomic failure usually causes a severe orthostatic fall in systolic and diastolic BP and can be differentiated from hypovolemic syndromes by the absence of heart rate changes in the erect posture.

Evaluation of Patients With Orthostatic Hypotension and Hypertension
Clinical Presentation

Symptoms result mainly from reduced cerebral blood flow. In orthostatic hypertension, these may be occasional or precipitated only during diuretic therapy. Patients with mild orthostatic hypotension complain of intermittent lightheadedness. More severe orthostatic hypotension may cause unsteadiness of gait, severe fatigue, "weakness," blurred vision, impaired cognition, chest pain in the upright posture, or syncope, all of which are rapidly relieved by lying down. Palpitations and excessive sweating suggest "hyperadrenergic" orthostatic hypotension. Impotence, loss of bladder or bowel control, or shoulder pain suggest diffuse autonomic failure, with or without multiple system atrophy (the Shy-Drager syndrome, parkinsonism, or olivopontocerebellar disease).

Clinical Testing

Physical examination discloses abnormal orthostatic changes in BP and heart rate from measurements made in recumbency to standing (or head-up tilt, or even sitting with legs dangling) for more than 3 minutes. However, to exclude delayed orthostatic hypotension, and in patients with tachycardia but no significant fall in BP after 3 to 5 minutes of orthostasis, it is necessary to continue these measurements for up to 10 to 90 minutes.

Table 135.1. Orthostatic Blood Pressure and Heart Rate Changes in Health and Disease

Normal orthostatic changes

Systolic BP, −19 to +11 mm Hg (mean, −6.5 mm Hg)

Diastolic BP, −9 to +22 mm Hg (mean, +5.6 mm Hg)

Heart rate, −6 to +27 bpm (mean, +12.3 bpm)

Abnormal orthostatic changes

Orthostatic systolic hypotension: decrease of at least 20 mm Hg in systolic BP

Orthostatic diastolic hypotension: decrease of at least 10 mm Hg in diastolic BP

Orthostatic diastolic hypertension: diastolic BP ≤90 mm Hg in recumbency and ≥98 mm Hg in the standing position

Orthostatic tachycardia: increase in heart rate by >27 bpm or to >108 bpm

BP indicates blood pressure. Values are based on observations in 92 healthy subjects.

Reprinted with permission from Streeten DHP. *Orthostatic Disorders of the Circulation.* New York, NY: Plenum Press Inc; 1987:118.

When BP is measured in the upright posture, the arm in which the BP is being measured should be passively elevated, that is, held or supported in abduction, at the approximate horizontal level of the atria. A transient fall in BP while standing for <1 minute may be normal. Sustained, progressive, or delayed (evident only after >10 minutes) falls or rises in BP or increases in heart rate are required to diagnose orthostatic hypotension, orthostatic hypertension, or orthostatic tachycardia (the latter now called orthostatic intolerance or postural orthostatic tachycardia syndrome, POTS). Criteria for the diagnosis of these disorders are shown in Table 135.1.

Proof that excessive orthostatic pooling of blood is causing orthostatic hypertension, hypotension, or tachycardia can be obtained by preventing excessive venous pooling with a medical antishock trouser (MAST) pressure suit inflated to 45 mm Hg. Hyperadrenergic orthostatic hypotension or hypertension heralded by the presence of orthostatic tachycardia can be confirmed by plasma norepinephrine measurements that are normal (90 to 300 pg/mL) after recumbency for 30 minutes and at least doubled after the patient

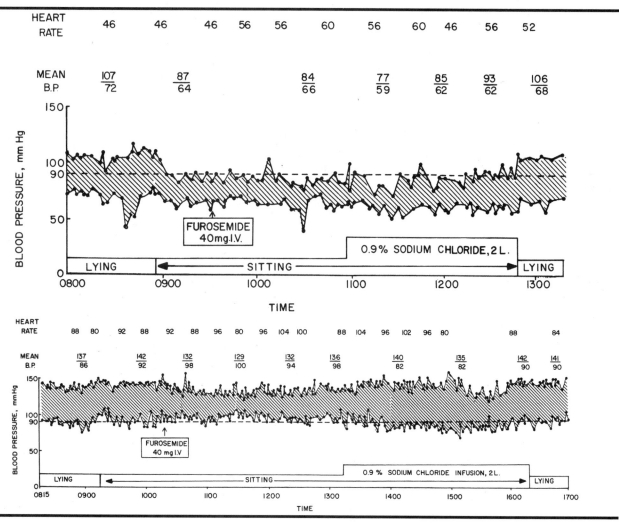

Figure 135.1. Studies showing the effects of volume reduction (after furosemide diuresis) and expansion (during 0.9% NaCl infusion). Top, Effects on sitting blood pressure measurements in a patient with orthostatic systolic hypotension in whom diuresis resulted in both diastolic and systolic hypotension, while saline infusion overcame the pathological orthostatic changes. Bottom, Effects in a patient with diastolic hypertension in the standing posture (not shown), in whom volume depletion raised the diastolic blood pressure to a mean value of 98 to 100 mm Hg in the sitting posture. Volume repletion with saline lowered diastolic blood pressure to 82 to 90 mm Hg. From Streeten DHP. *Orthostatic Disorders of the Circulation.* New York, NY: Plenus Press Inc; 1987:138 and 141. Reproduced with permission.

stands for 3 to 15 minutes. In contrast, impaired sympathetic innervation of the heart and the entire vasculature, which occurs in *diffuse autonomic failure,* causes orthostatic hypotension with negligible increases in heart rate or in plasma norepinephrine concentration.

Causes of excessive venous pooling and orthostatic hypotension include autonomic failure, which may be diffuse or localized exclusively to the innervation of the lower limb veins. Venomotor abnormalities can also be found in adrenal insufficiency, hypopituitarism, pheochromocytoma, diabetes mellitus, and such relatively rare disorders as amyloidosis, hyperbradykininism, and porphyria, all of which may be diagnosed by standard procedures. Excessive tachycardia as the exclusive abnormality in the upright posture may result predominantly from hypovolemia of plasma and/or red blood cell mass. Prolonged orthostasis in these patients is frequently followed by hypotension, presyncope, or syncope.

Drug Therapy for Chronic Orthostatic Hypotension and Hypertension

Medical therapy for *orthostatic hypotension* depends on the cause. Discontinuation of diuretics and liberalization of salt intake may be helpful in some patients. Chronic mineralocorticoid (fludrocortisone) administration is frequently useful in doses of 0.05 to 1.0 mg BID. This treatment may cause edema, headaches, and hypokalemia; higher doses have caused severe supine hypertension with left ventricular hypertrophy. Fludrocortisone treatment may fail to improve upright BP chronically, perhaps because of "mineralocorticoid escape," in which renal natriuretic mechanisms overcome the initial steroid-induced volume expansion, thereby lowering extracellular volume to pretreatment levels. β-Blockade has been useful in some patients with orthostatic intolerance and postural tachycardia,

but many patients fail to benefit. More recently, methylphenidate and midodrine (ProAmatine®) have been used in orthostatic syndromes, particularly orthostatic hypotension and tachycardia. In the most refractory patients, erythropoietin has been combined with fludrocortisone and ferrous sulfate to improve upright BP.

Chronic orthostatic hypertension may respond to cessation of diuretic therapy or acute volume repletion. In some individuals, an elastic leotard or abdominal binder may be useful. Low doses of fludrocortisone (0.05 to 0.1 mg/d) to expand blood volume or low doses of clonidine (0.05 to 0.1 mg/d) to blunt excess sympathetic responses may also be used. The natural history of this syndrome and the long-term efficacy of these therapies remain unclear at this time.

SUGGESTED READING

1. Bannister R, ed. *Autonomic Failure: A Textbook of Clinical Disorders of the Autonomic Nervous System.* 2nd ed. Oxford, UK: Oxford University Press; 1988.
2. Campbell IW, Ewing DJ, Clarke BF. Therapeutic experience with fludrocortisone in diabetic postural hypotension. *Br Med J.* 1976;1:872–874.
3. Hoeldtke RD, Streeten DH. Treatment of orthostatic hypotension with erythropoietin. *N Engl J Med.* 1993;329:611–615.
4. Jankovic J, Gilden JL, Hiner BC, Kaufmann H, Brown DC, Coghlan CH, Rubin M, Fouad-Tarazi FM. Neurogenic orthostatic hypotension: a double-blind, placebo-controlled study with midodrine. *Am J Med.* 1993;95:38–48.
5. Low PA, ed. *Clinical Autonomic Disorders: Evaluation and Management.* Boston, Mass: Little Brown; 1993.
6. Streeten DHP. Pathogenesis of hyperadrenergic orthostatic hypotension: evidence of disordered venous innervation exclusively in the lower limbs. *J Clin Invest.* 1990; 86:1582–1588.
7. Streeten DHP, Anderson GH Jr. Delayed orthostatic intolerance. *Arch Intern Med.* 1992;152:1066–1072.
8. Streeten DHP, Auchincloss JH Jr, Anderson GH Jr, Richardson RL, Thomas FD, Miller JW. Orthostatic hypertension: pathogenetic studies. *Hypertension.* 1985;7: 196–203.

Chapter 136

Management of Baroreflex Failure

David Robertson, MD

KEY POINTS

- Acute baroreflex failure presents as severe episodic hypertension, headache, tachycardia, and diaphoresis, closely resembling pheochromocytoma. Such pressor crises alternate with periods of hypotension.

- Baroreflex failure results from bilateral damage to glossopharyngeal and vagal nerves or their medullary interconnections. Common causes include trauma, neck irradiation, and bilateral paragangliomata.

- Baroreflex failure is usually accompanied by significant collateral damage to vagal parasympathetic efferent fibers. In the absence of such damage (selective baroreflex failure), hypotensive crises may be accompanied by malignant vagotonia with cardiac arrest of 10 seconds or more.

- Treatment with central (clonidine, methyldopa) or peripheral (guanadrel, guanethidine) sympatholytic agents can be useful.

See also Chapters 34, 115, 135

Baroreflex failure presents in several ways **(Figure 136.1)**. Acute baroreflex failure occurs after sudden loss of baroreflex afferent innervation and causes severe sustained hypertension (blood pressure 170 to 300/100 to 140 mm Hg) and tachycardia in both supine and upright postures, usually accompanied by subjective sensations of warmth or flushing, palpitations, severe headache, and diaphoresis. The initial clinical impression is usually pheochromocytoma, but this diagnosis can be excluded by computed tomography or MIBG scanning, venous sampling for norepinephrine, or arteriography. After a few days, the "sustained hypertension" gives rise to a more chronic "labile blood pressure" phase. The hallmark of this phase is hypertension and tachycardia alternating with periods of hypotension, with or without bradycardia **(Figure 136.2)**. During the pressor crises, which usually last less than an hour, patients experience hot flushing with pallor rather than redness. The crises can be brought on by even minor emotional or physical perturbations. It is as though the cardiovascular effects of emotional stimuli are fully expressed in the absence of buffering by intact baroreflex mechanisms. Patients sometimes exhibit emotional volatility, but it is not always clear whether the emotional volatility is the result of the pressor crisis or the cause of it. Late in the disorder, the hypotensive phase may gradually become more pronounced or the hypertensive crises more attenuated.

Diagnosis

The hallmark of baroreflex failure is a failure of pressor and depressor drugs to alter heart rate in a patient who can raise and lower heart rate in response to endogenous sympathetic activation and withdrawal. Physiological testing of patients with baroreflex failure reveals supranormal pressor responses to the handgrip test, the cold pressor test, and especially the mental arithmetic test. Pharmacological testing reveals a pressor response to phenylephrine without a compensatory fall in heart rate. The corresponding depressor response to intravenous nitroprusside also is pronounced, but heart

rate may not change. The response to atropine is typically that of no change in blood pressure and no increase in heart rate, usually due to concomitant damage to vagal parasympathetic efferent fibers to the heart. In occasional patients with selective baroreflex failure **(Figure 136.3)**, such damage to efferent parasympathetic fibers is absent or minimal. In these patients, profound bradycardia and cardiac arrest may occur during the hypotensive phase. Propranolol's ef-

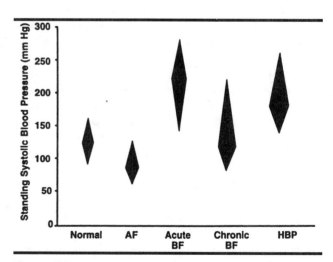

Figure 136.1. Representative standing systolic blood pressures recorded in inpatients and normal subjects. The widest point of each diamond depicts the most common standing systolic pressure seen in typical patients, while the height depicts the range of pressures seen throughout the day. Patients with autonomic failure (AF) have the lowest standing pressure. In the acute phase of baroreflex failure (acute BF), usually days to weeks immediately after acute bilateral damage to cranial nerves IX and X, extremely high pressures are similar to essential hypertension (HBP). After several months (chronic BF), the standing systolic pressure is usually near normal, but great variability is still seen. (Used with permission from, Academic Press Inc.)

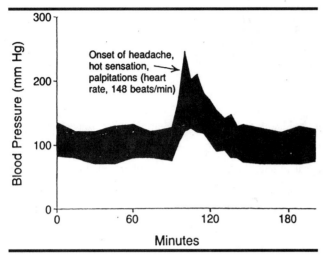

Figure 136.2. Blood pressure monitoring in a 43-year-old man approximately 2 weeks after surgical removal of a carotid-body tumor and 5 years after removal of a contralateral carotid-body tumor. While blood pressure was being monitored, the patient's right hand was immersed in ice water for 60 seconds. The blood pressure immediately rose and continued to rise for several minutes after discontinuation of the cold stimulus. Symptoms appeared during this time and then resolved as blood pressure and heart rate returned to normal during the following 30 minutes. On some occasions, the patient had spontaneous paroxysms of similar magnitude. (From Robertson D et al. The diagnosis and treatment of baroreflex failure. *N Engl J Med.* 1993;329:1449–1455. Used with permission. Copyright 1993 Massachusetts Medical Society. All rights reserved.)

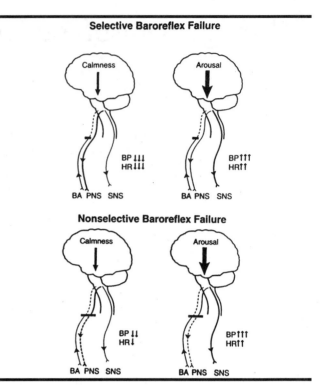

Figure 136.3. Selective baroreflex failure (top) contrasted with nonselective baroreflex failure (bottom). Efferent sympathetic (SNS) and parasympathetic (PNS) nerves are intact in selective baroreflex failure. In nonselective baroreflex failure, efferent parasympathetic nerves were damaged. Baroreflex afferents (BA) were damaged in selective and nonselective baroreflex failure. BP indicates blood pressure and HR, heart rate. (Used with permission from *Hypertension.*)

fect on heart rate is more variable and depends on the prevailing activity of the sympathetic nervous system. Perhaps the most helpful agent in diagnosing baroreflex failure is clonidine. A small dose of clonidine (for example, 0.1 to 0.2 mg PO) often lowers blood pressure precipitously in patients with baroreflex failure, especially during the pressor phase.

Causes for baroreflex failure include trauma, irradiation for cancer of the throat, familial paraganglioma syndrome (a genetic disorder in which affected subjects develop benign, non–catecholamine-producing tumors of the glomus vagale, glomus jugulare, or the carotid body, which physically damage nearby vagal and glossopharyngeal nerves), and bilateral cell loss in the nuclei of the solitary tract due to a degenerative neurological disease. In some patients, no cause can be documented. In patients with baroreflex failure after radiation therapy, the syndrome develops weeks to months after the initial radiation, perhaps in response to fibrotic injury. Patients whose nerve damage occurs slowly in this fashion do not usually experience the dramatic initial severe sustained hypertensive phase and may have more difficulties with hypotension than with pressor crises.

Between crises, plasma norepinephrine levels are often normal, although they may be low during periods of quiet rest or sedation. In contrast, plasma norepinephrine concentrations during attacks are dramatically elevated, often in the range (1000 to 3000 pg/mL) seen in pheochromocytoma. Over time, the pressor crises in baroreflex failure tend to become attenuated, whereas worsening occurs more commonly in pheochromocytoma, an important long-term differential sign. Urinary norepinephrine levels in baroreflex failure are usually at

the upper border or slightly above normal range, averaging 110 µg/24 hours in our series.

Therapy

The treatment of baroreflex failure is difficult. The initial sustained hypertension phase may require hospitalization in an intensive care unit and control with nitroprusside and sympatholytic agents. In the first 2 or 3 days, apneic spells occasionally occur when powerful pain medications are employed, so monitoring is necessary. Once the chronic labile phase is reached, clonidine, either orally or in the form of a clonidine patch, can be extremely effective, but high doses (0.6 to 2.5 mg daily in divided doses) are sometimes required. Such agents may make hypotension episodes worse in some patients. A practical point in the management of patients in the early phase of baroreflex failure is recognition of the relationship between emotional upset and pressor crises. Patients may over time learn to control the onset of the pressor crises (usually recognized by flushing or headache) and may be able to exert calming self-control. Thus, in some cases, patients may develop a spontaneous biofeedback treatment that may result in a reduction in both the number and severity of attacks. In the chronic phase, some patients may be switched from clonidine to benzodiazepine with continued adequate control.

The patient with selective baroreflex failure may have the additional problem of episodic malignant vagotonia. In such patients, placement of a cardiac pacemaker may be required to prevent cardiac arrest. Long-term management of hypertension by guanethidine or guanadrel with concomitant attenuation of hypotension by fludrocortisone may also be required.

SUGGESTED READING

1. Aksamit TR, Floras JS, Victor RG, Aylward PE. Paroxysmal hypertension due to sinoaortic baroreceptor denervation in humans. *Hypertension.* 1987;9:309–314.
2. Jordan J, Shannon JR, Black BK, Costa F, Ertl AC, Furlan R, Biaggioni I, Robertson D. Malignant vagotonia due to selective baroreflex failure. *Hypertension.* 1997;30: 1072–1077.
3. Kuchel O, Cusson JR, Larochelle P, Buu NT, Genest J. Posture- and emotion-induced severe hypertensive paroxysms with baroreceptor dysfunction. *J Hypertens.* 1987;5:277–283.
4. Robertson D Goldberg MR, Hollister AS, Wade D, Robertson RM. Baroreceptor dysfunction in man. *Am J Med.* 1984;76:A49–A58.
5. Robertson D, Hollister AS, Biaggioni I, Netterville JL, Mosqueda-Garcia R, Robertson RM. The diagnosis and treatment of baroreflex failure. *N Engl J Med.* 1993;329: 1449–1455.

Chapter 137

Management of Hypertensive Patients With Cerebrovascular Disease

Robert D. Brown Jr, MD

KEY POINTS

- Precipitous decline in blood pressure after ischemic stroke may lead to increased infarction size, and agents such as sublingual nifedipine should be avoided.

- In acute ischemic stroke, moderate blood pressure elevation can usually be managed conservatively.

- Blood pressure must be tightly controlled if intravenous t-PA is used for acute ischemic stroke.

- In intracerebral and subarachnoid hemorrhage, hypertension should be treated if it is of moderate to marked severity.

See also Chapters 60, 72, 76, 108, 151

Hypertension is an important risk factor for transient ischemic attack, cerebral infarction, and intracerebral hemorrhage and is also commonly noted in conjunction with asymptomatic cerebrovascular occlusive disease. Optimal blood pressure management differs on the basis of the nature of the cerebrovascular ischemic symptoms, the cause of the ischemic event, and presence of intracerebral hemorrhage or subarachnoid hemorrhage.

For patients with asymptomatic, noncritical carotid stenosis or in those who have recovered from a cerebral infarction or intracerebral hemorrhage, blood pressure should be managed aggressively, as in persons without cerebrovascular occlusive disease. Persons with asymptomatic high-grade carotid or vertebrobasilar system stenosis who have not had previous cerebral ischemic symptoms are candidates for moderate blood pressure management.

Cerebral Ischemia

Management of hypertension in the setting of acute ischemic stroke is controversial because there are no randomized trials that guide optimal management in this setting. Management is currently based on anecdote, animal studies, knowledge of intracranial vascular autoregulation, and clinical experience.

Hypertension after cerebral infarction is quite common. The causes of the elevated blood pressure include pain, undiagnosed or undertreated preexisting hypertension, anxiety or agitation, reaction to artificial ventilation, hypoxia, or increased intracranial pressure. In the setting of cerebral infarction, cerebral blood flow is dependent on the systemic blood pressure because of the lack of autoregulation in the area of the infarct. Thus acute decrease in blood pressure may cause further damage.

Although there are no large trials defining the best management after cerebral infarction, it is believed that mild-to-moderate elevations of blood pressure after cerebral infarction should be left untreated. There is no evidence that the risk of hemorrhagic transformation or other deleterious outcomes is increased with a conservative approach to moderate hypertension in the acute ischemic stroke setting. In persons with a prior history of hypertension, more aggressive management of acutely elevated blood pressure is more likely to increase infarct size, leading to poorer outcome.

For more marked elevations of blood pressure in the acute period, there are no strict criteria as to what level of blood pressure mandates aggressive management. In the NINDS intravenous t-PA stroke study, patients were excluded from receiving intravenous t-PA for acute ischemic stroke if the blood pressure was >185 mm Hg systolic or 110 mm Hg diastolic or if ongoing aggressive management was needed to meet these criteria. If intravenous t-PA is used, the goal blood pressure should be <185 mm Hg systolic and 110 mm Hg diastolic (**Table 137.1**). In general, diastolic blood pressure >140 mm Hg precludes candidacy for intravenous t-PA for acute ischemic stroke. In addition, persons in whom more than two doses of labetalol or other ongoing aggressive maneuvers are necessary to bring blood pressure to <185 mm Hg systolic or 110 mm Hg diastolic are not considered optimal candidates for intravenous t-PA.

If intravenous t-PA is not used, then antihypertensive drugs should be withheld unless the mean blood pressure [(sum of systolic pressure plus double the diastolic pressure) divided by 3] is >130 mm Hg or the systolic blood pressure is >220 mm Hg (Table 137.1). If less severe high blood pressure (systolic 185 to 220 or diastolic 121 to 130 or mean pressure >130 mm Hg) is associated with hemorrhagic transformation, myocardial infarction, renal failure secondary to accelerated hypertension, or dissection of the thoracic aorta, then parenteral drugs must be initiated.

The best agent to be used in the setting of acute ischemic stroke is also not defined. Aggressive management with agents such as intravenous sodium nitroprusside is typically not needed but should be initiated if diastolic blood pressure is >140 mm Hg (Table 137.1). Parenteral agents that are easily titrated with immediate-onset, minimal effect on cerebral blood vessels and low likelihood of causing precipitous decline in blood pressure should be initiated, eg, intravenous labetalol or low-dose enalapril. Sublingual use of calcium channel blockers should be avoided because of the risk of precipitous decline in blood pressure.

Table 137.1. Hypertension Management in Acute Cerebrovascular Disorders

BLOOD PRESSURE LEVEL, MM HG	MANAGEMENT
Cerebral infarction	
Diastolic >140	Sodium nitroprusside, 0.5 to 1.0 mcg·kg·min IV
Systolic >220 or diastolic 121 to 140, or Mean BP >130 with diastolic <140	Labetalol, 10 mg IV over 1 to 2 minutes, repeat or double every 10 to 20 minutes, up to 300 mg. Alternative: enalapril, 1 mg over 5 minutes, then 1 to 5 mg every 6 hours
Systolic 185 to 220 or diastolic 105 to 120	No acute treatment, unless hemorrhagic transformation, myocardial infarction, renal failure from accelerated hypertension, or aortic dissection
Systolic <185 or diastolic <105	No acute treatment
Intracerebral hemorrhage	
Diastolic >140	Sodium nitroprusside, 0.5 to 1.0 mcg·kg·min IV
Mean BP >130, or Systolic >180 and Diastolic <140	Labetalol, 10 mg IV over 1 to 2 minutes, repeat or double every 10 to 20 minutes, up to 300 mg. Alternative: enalapril, 1.0 mg over 5 minutes, then 1 to 5 mg every 6 hours
Mean BP <130 and Systolic <180	No acute treatment
Subarachnoid hemorrhage	
Diastolic >140	Sodium nitroprusside IV
Mean BP >130 and diastolic <140	Labetalol or enalapril IV as noted above
Mean BP <130	No acute treatment

BP indicates blood pressure.

Intracerebral Hemorrhage

Blood pressure elevation is common after intracerebral hemorrhage. It is uncertain whether aggressive blood pressure management in the setting of intracerebral hemorrhage will lessen the chance of increased hemorrhage size or recurrent hemorrhage or will lead to other deleterious outcomes, such as worsening diffuse cerebral ischemia or an increased zone of ischemia surrounding the hemorrhage. For persons with intracerebral hemorrhage, antihypertensive medications are typically not initiated acutely unless the mean arterial pressure is >130 mm Hg or the systolic blood pressure

is >180 mm Hg. The initial management goal should not be to rapidly achieve normotension; an appropriate initial goal would be to reduce mean arterial pressure to 110 to 130 mm Hg or systolic pressure to 140 to 160 mm Hg. Patients with a prior history of hypertension should be managed with particular care, and the goal levels may not be as strict. Increased intracranial pressure is also more common in intracerebral hemorrhage than in cerebral infarction, and a higher blood pressure is necessary to maintain a stable cerebral perfusion pressure. The antihypertensive agents recommended are similar to those used for cerebral infarction (Table 137.1).

Subarachnoid Hemorrhage

The management of hypertension after subarachnoid hemorrhage is controversial. Studies have not consistently defined a higher rate of rebleeding or death from rebleeding in persons with increased systolic blood pressure. Among those with persistently elevated blood pressure (mean arterial pressure >130 mm Hg), very careful reduction in blood pressure by use of agents such as labetalol is reasonable (Table 137.1). Should any evidence of clinical deterioration or vasospasm occur, emergent reconsideration of the antihypertensive medications and fluid resuscitation must be undertaken.

SUGGESTED READING

1. Adams HP, Brott TG, Crowell RM, Furlan AJ, Gomez CR, Grotta J, Helgason CM, Marler JR, Woolson RF, Zivin JA, Feinberg W, Mayberg M. Guidelines for the management of patients with acute ischemic stroke: a statement for healthcare professionals from a special writing group of the Stroke Council, American Heart Association. *Stroke.* 1994;25:1901–1914.
2. Broderick J, Brott T, Barsan W, Haley EC, Levy D, Marler J, Sheppard G, Blum C. Blood pressure during the first minutes of focal cerebral ischemia. *Ann Emerg Med.* 1993;22:1438–1443.
3. Broderick J, Brott T, Zucarelb M. Management of intracerebral hemorrhage. In: Batjer H, ed. *Cerebrovascular Disease.* Philadelphia, Pa: Lippincott-Raven; 1996: 1–17.
4. Brott T, Reed RL. Intensive care for acute stroke in the community hospital setting: the first 24 hours. *Stroke.* 1989;20:694–697.
5. Lisk DR, Grotta JC, Lamki LM, Tran HD, Taylor JW, Molony DA, Barron BJ. Should hypertension be treated after acute stroke? a randomized controlled trial using single photon emission computed tomography. *Arch Neurol.* 1993;50:855–862.
6. Mayberg MR, Batjer HH, Dacey R, Diringer M, Haley EC, Heros RC, Sternau LL, Torner J, Adams HP Jr, Feinberg W, Thies W. Guidelines for the management of aneurysmal subarachnoid hemorrhage: a statement for healthcare professionals from a special writing group of the Stroke Council, American Heart Association. *Circulation.* 1994;90:2592–2605.
7. The National Institute of Neurological Disorders and Stroke rt-PA Stroke Study Group. Tissue plasminogen activator for acute ischemic stroke. *N Engl J Med.* 1995; 333:1581–1587.
8. Powers WJ. Acute hypertension after stroke: the scientific basis for treatment decisions. *Neurology.* 1994;43:461–467.
9. Wiebers DO, Feigen VL, Brown RD Jr. *Handbook of Stroke.* Philadelphia, Pa: Lippincott-Raven; 1997.
10. Wijdicks EF, Vermeulen M, Murray GD, Hijdra A, van Gijn J. The effects of treating hypertension following aneurysmal subarachnoid hemorrhage. *Clin Neurol Neurosurg.* 1990;92:111–117.

Chapter 138

Management of Hypertensive Patients With Ischemic Heart Disease

Jay M. Sullivan, MD, Charles K. Francis, MD

KEY POINTS

- Evaluation must be linked with therapeutic goals and directed toward assessment of overall cardiovascular risk, degree of target-organ damage, and degree of coronary artery disease.

- The principal imperative in the management of the hypertensive patient with myocardial ischemia is the reduction of absolute cardiovascular risk, with particular attention to the combined management of hypertension and ischemic symptoms.

- Agents that reduce myocardial oxygen requirements or increase coronary blood flow are the agents of choice for treating hypertension and CAD; β-blockers, nitrates, and calcium antagonists are preferred therapy in patients with angina.

- Aspirin is recommended adjunctive therapy.

See also Chapters 65, 75, 109, 110, 111

Major coronary events often occur without warning and in patients in whom overt signs and symptoms of coronary artery disease have not been previously appreciated despite the fact that preclinical myocardial ischemia usually antedates most coronary events. In the patient at significant coronary risk, whether because of multiple coronary risk factors or due to symptoms, detection and quantification of myocardial ischemia are critical for the formulation of appropriate diagnostic and treatment strategies. In the patient with established evidence of myocardial ischemia, further risk stratification is required based on the extent and severity of myocardial ischemia and the degree of left ventricular functional impairment.

Evaluation: Risk Factors, Other Than Target-Organ Damage, and Extent of Coronary Disease

Management of patients with hypertension and confirmed or suspected coronary artery disease requires a global evaluation of the patient, including an assessment of three major areas: (1) the extent of target-organ damage (cardiac disease, cerebrovascular disease, peripheral vascular disease, renal disease, retinopathy) or presence of diabetes; (2) the overall cardiovascular risk factor status (age, sex, postmenopausal status, cholesterol status, glucose intolerance, cigarette smoking); and (3) the extent and severity of coronary artery disease. The principles for the first two of these requirements are nicely summarized in the Sixth Report of the Joint National Committee on the Prevention, Detection, Evaluation, and Treatment of High Blood Pressure (1997).

Information derived from a thorough history and physical examination provides the foundation for management of hypertension and for the quantification of myocardial ischemia in hypertensive patients. The probability of significant coronary artery disease may be estimated on the basis of age, sex, symptoms, ECG, stress testing,

and coronary risk factor assessment. Also useful are various resting and stress-monitoring forms of echocardiography and nuclear imaging. These techniques are discussed in detail in other parts of this Section.

Treatment

Treatment Goals and General Considerations

The goal of treatment for patients with hypertension and coronary artery disease (CAD) is more complex than simply lowering BP. Additional goals in patients with hypertension and CAD are control of ischemic symptoms and retarding disease progression. It is particularly important to enhance quality of life by reducing the frequency and severity of attacks of angina pectoris. Concomitant conditions that can serve as aggravating factors should be corrected, such as thyrotoxicosis and anemia, which increase cardiac workload and myocardial oxygen demand. Stress modification programs should be considered when appropriate. Regular aerobic exercise, according to an exercise prescription guided by the results of exercise testing, is useful for conditioning skeletal muscles and cardiovascular reflexes and enables an individual to exert a greater level of physical effort without a corresponding increase in cardiac workload and myocardial oxygen requirements.

The level of target BP in patients with ischemic heart disease continues to be debated. Meta-analyses had identified an apparent increase in CAD mortality in patients whose treated diastolic BPs were <85 mm Hg. This increased mortality at lower diastolic BP levels (the so-called J-curve) has been attributed to reduced myocardial perfusion when diastolic pressure is lowered to a point inadequate to maintain flow across stenotic coronary lesions. Recent data from the Hypertension Optimal Treatment trial, however, indicate that the optimal BP value for risk reduction in a cohort of 19 000 hypertensive patients was 138/83 mm Hg, with no evidence of a significant increase in mortality when treated diastolic BP fell below 85 mm Hg. Nevertheless, it makes sound clinical sense to lower BP gradually in patients with hypertension and angina pectoris, paying particular attention to new symptoms and other evidence that ischemic manifestations are improved and myocardial workload is diminished.

General Risk Factor Management

In the hypertensive patient with myocardial ischemia, reduction of coronary risk factors is the foundation of management. To achieve optimal benefit in patients with myocardial ischemia, the goal of BP lowering must be linked to nonpharmacological, as well as pharmacological, strategies for effective reduction of absolute cardiovascular risk. Reduction of the total ischemic burden (ie, symptomatic plus silent ischemia), repair of endothelial dysfunction, and regression and stabilization of atherosclerotic plaque are additional considerations. Individualized therapeutic strategies that address general cardiovascular health as well as control of BP and myocardial ischemia are of paramount importance. These approaches, which are discussed in detail in other sections of this book, include reduced intake of saturated fat and cholesterol, smoking cessation, weight reduction, moderation of alcohol intake, increased physical activity, reduced sodium intake, and maintenance of adequate dietary intake of potassium, calcium and magnesium, as recommended in JNC VI.

Other adjunctive therapies such as antioxidants, while showing some positive benefit on cardiovascular morbidity and mortality in some studies, are considerably less effective in reducing heart attack rates than aspirin, lipid lowering, and HRT.

Aspirin Therapy

Because unstable angina pectoris and acute myocardial infarction are usually associated with acute thrombus formation atop an atherosclerotic lesion, efforts to prevent adherence of platelets and propagation of thrombi are essential. Aspirin has been shown to improve survival of patients who have had an acute myocardial infarction, to lower the reinfarction rate by as much as 50%, and to reduce mortality in patients with unstable angina. Aspirin therapy also reduces the infarction and mortality rates in patients with stable angina and has been shown to lower the myocardial infarction rate among healthy middle-aged men who take 325 mg every other day. Two studies examining the effect of aspirin in healthy men have noticed an increase in the number of fatal hemorrhagic strokes. While statistically insignificant, this finding is still worrisome and calls for careful control of BP in hypertensive patients with coronary disease treated with aspirin. Optimal doses of aspirin have not been established at this time, with benefits in various studies confirmed in the dose range of 80 to 325 mg daily.

Antihypertensive Anti-Ischemic Therapy
General Considerations

The challenge in antihypertensive drug selection is choosing a pharmacological agent that will minimize the incidence of myocardial ischemia and reduce the risk of adverse coronary heart disease events, as well as control BP. Thus, metabolic and anti-atherosclerotic features of the drug influence the choice. It is important to keep the goal of lowering BP as the highest priority, because in virtually all major trials the level of BP was the primary independent predictor of coronary heart disease events and prognosis.

In choosing optimal therapy, it is imperative to avoid using drugs that may aggravate myocardial ischemia. Direct-acting vasodilators, while effective antihypertensive agents, cause profound vasodilatation with reflex stimulation of the baroreceptors, leading to an increase in heart rate, myocardial contractility, peripheral vascular resistance, and venous tone. This sequence results in increased myocardial work, thus increasing oxygen demand and worsening angina when this demand cannot be met by an increase in coronary blood flow. In addition, hydralazine appears to have a direct stimulatory effect on the heart, increasing contractility and oxygen demand. The dihydropyridine type of calcium antagonists, specifically nifedipine, also can cause profound vasodilatation, reflex cardiac stimulation, and aggravation of angina pectoris. Thus, they should be used with caution in patients with angina pectoris but are appropriate in the treatment of severe coronary spasm or Prinzmetal's angina.

Specific Drugs

β-Blockers. β-Blockers are the most effective agents available for the primary and secondary (postinfarction) protection of the heart. β-blockers are recommended by JNC VI as the agents of choice for treating hypertension and coronary artery disease concomitantly. β-Blockers reduce heart rate and contractility, thus lowering myocardial oxygen demands. They also lower BP, thus further reducing wall tension and further reducing myocardial oxygen demands. β-Blockers prevent a rise in systolic BP during exercise, which enables the hypertensive patient with coronary disease to enjoy a greater level of activity than would be possible otherwise, despite the fact that the blockers do not increase coronary blood flow. They reduce arterial sheer stress, suppress ventricular arrhythmias, reduce total mortality, help minimize infarct size, and decrease incidence of sudden death and nonfatal ischemic complications. These same cardioprotective features have not been established for those β-blockers with intrinsic sympathomimetic activity.

Long-acting β-blockers may be helpful in reducing early-morning angina and may be preferred in patients with supraventricular arrhythmias and hypertension. Although the antihypertensive efficacy of β-blockers may not be as great in blacks as in whites, the anti-ischemic effects are comparable in all racial groups. β-Blockers may have a limited acute adverse effect on lipid levels, increasing triglycerides and LDL cholesterol and decreasing HDL levels. Agents with intrinsic sympathomimetic activity have minimal impact on lipids and do not reduce heart rate and cardiac output. In patients with symptoms of myocardial ischemia, the benefits of β-blockers appear to exceed any negative metabolic consequences. β-Blockers were initially thought to be detrimental in patients with left ventricular dysfunction, but more recent data, particularly with newer agents with both β- and α-blocking properties, have suggested that these agents are beneficial in patients with ischemic as well as non-ischemic cardiomyopathy.

Nitrates. The efficacy of nitrates in myocardial ischemia is due to their metabolism by endothelial cells to nitric oxide, which causes vascular smooth muscle relaxation, venodilatation, reduced arteriolar and arterial tone, dilation of epicardial coronary arteries, and antiplatelet aggregation effects. Nitrates also variably lower BP, particularly in the upright position, principally because they cause significant venodilation. They may thus cause or exacerbate orthostatic hypotension. At higher doses, they can reduce afterload by causing arterial vasodilatation, especially in the cerebral and coronary circulations. Nitrates also increase coronary flow by dilating the large epicardial coronary vessels. This action increases luminal area in patients who do not have a concentric or "napkin ring" type of coronary artery stenosis, which can no longer dilate. Nitrate compounds also block coronary spasm and increase collateral blood flow in the coronary tree, thus improving regional perfusion distal to coronary stenoses.

Nitroglycerin and other organic nitrate therapy, either in sublingual, transdermal, or long-acting oral preparations, has been a mainstay of the treatment of myocardial ischemia for many years. The sublingual preparations have proven to be effective in the termination of acute anginal episodes and may be used prophylactically in patients with chronic angina pectoris. Longer-acting preparations are effective in reducing the frequency of anginal episodes, improving exercise tolerance, and lessening the total ischemic burden by decreasing silent ischemia. "Nitrate tolerance," the diminution of efficacy with chronic administration, may occur with longer-acting preparations with sustained plasma nitrate level; tolerance development may be avoided by incorporating a nitrate-free period into the dosing schedule.

Calcium antagonists. Calcium antagonists have gained wide usage in the treatment of hypertension and angina pectoris on the basis of predictable effects and a relatively favorable side-effect profile in uncomplicated hypertension. A diverse class of agents, they variably block L-type channels in vascular smooth muscle, reducing systemic BP and dilating *normal* coronary vessels. Calcium antagonists may reduce myocardial oxygen requirements in three ways. They reduce afterload, and thereby myocardial oxygen requirements, by lowering BP. They dilate veins slightly, reducing venous return to the heart and thus reducing preload or end-diastolic pressure and size. They also reduce myocardial contractility. The calcium antagonists also decrease coronary vascular resistance, and nondihydropyridine calcium blocking agents decrease heart rate and myocardial contractility, thus lowering oxygen requirements. They also have variable anti-platelet and possibly antiatherogenic properties. Numerous clinical trials have demonstrated reduction of angina pectoris and control of hypertension with calcium antagonist therapy. Calcium antagonists may be particularly useful in hypertensive patients with chest pain who cannot tolerate β-blockers. The heart rate–slowing effects of diltiazem or verapamil may also exert a cardioprotective effect in patients with normal ventricular function.

Calcium antagonists are not suitable for all patients with ischemic heart disease. In patients after infarction, dihydropyridines have been shown to have an unfavorable effect on reinfarction and mortality rates, and thus they should be avoided in the management of acute myocardial infarction. Studies of diltiazem in post–myocardial infarction (MI) patients with left ventricular dysfunction have not demonstrated a beneficial effect on mortality; however, reinfarction rates were improved in patients with normal ventricular function. The favorable impact on reinfarction rates of verapamil may be greater in hypertensive than normotensive patients. Verapamil improved survival after acute MI in one study but not others.

An association of excess MI incidence in dihydropyridine-treated hypertensive patients has led to concern about the cardioprotective efficacy of this group, including both long-acting and short-acting dihydropyridines. A meta-analysis of several trials involving the use of calcium antagonists for the treatment of hypertension has found that the chronic use of high doses of rapidly acting nifedipine is associated with increased risk of MI. The use of rapid-acting nifedipine in the urgent or emergent treatment of severe hypertension has been associated with abrupt hypotension and the precipitation of MI or severe myocardial ischemia and is strongly discouraged. Nifedipine in the setting of acute MI has been shown to increase mortality compared with results in placebo-treated patients.

ACE inhibitors. In patients with coronary disease, the initial demonstration of the mortality benefit of ACE inhibition was confined to patients with reduced left ventricular function after MI. More-recent clinical experience in asymptomatic post-MI patients with impaired ventricular function has confirmed reduced mortality, lower reinfarction rates, and decreased incidence of coronary events with ACE-inhibitor treatment. The addiction of ACE inhibitors to aspirin and β-blockers further improves the favorable impact of these agents on mortality and coronary events after infarction. In patients with preserved left ventricular function there is limited evidence of benefit of ACE inhibitor therapy prescribed early in the course of acute MI. Even though ACE inhibitors have been shown in experimental models to improve endothelial function, impede the progression of atherogenesis, and cause coronary arterial dilatation, studies in humans have shown no consistent antiarrhythmic, anti-anginal efficacy or long-term benefit in the chronic ischemic syndromes.

Drug combinations for hypertension and myocardial ischemia. Effective combinations of lower doses of two antihypertensive agents can often achieve effective BP control with fewer side effects than high doses of a single agent. The same statement can be made for angina, although there is less clinical trial evidence in support. Combinations of antihypertensive and anti-anginal agents with different mechanisms of action are often the best way to control concomitant angina and hypertension. For example, combining nitrates and β-blockers or β-blockers and calcium antagonists is often effective at achieving control of chest pain and BP while minimizing side effects. In patients with bradycardia, AV nodal disease, or left ventricular dysfunction, the combination β-blockers with nondihydropyridines is contraindicated because of the additive suppressive effects of these agents in the conducting system and on the contractility of cardiomyocytes.

Revascularization

In patients at low risk (ie, single-vessel disease, mild symptoms, or minimal inducible ischemia), medical therapy is an appropriate therapeutic strategy. In more complex or severe cases, the decision to consider coronary revascularization is based on assessment of the extent and severity of myocardial ischemia, refractoriness of symptoms, and the degree of impairment of left ventricular dysfunction. A thorough discussion of the relative merits and indications of coronary angioplasty, coronary stenting, and coronary artery bypass graft (CABG) surgery is beyond the scope of this chapter. CABG is the most widely accepted therapeutic option in the high-risk patient with three-vessel or left main coronary disease, ventricular dysfunction, and severe angina pectoris refractory to maximal medical therapy. There is also evidence that revascularization is useful in patients with preserved left ventricular function, inducible ischemia, and left main, three-vessel disease or two-vessel and left anterior descending disease. Revascularization is also appropriate in patients with multivessel disease and mild or moderate symptoms, abnormal ventricular function, or significant myocardial ischemia inducible with exercise or pharmacologic stress testing if medical therapy has failed.

The choice of revascularization technique, usually CABG or percutaneous transluminal coronary angioplasty (PTCA) depends on patient characteristics (operative and cardiovascular risk status, characteristics of the coronary lesions, coronary anatomy, the severity of left ventricular dysfunction, the necessity of complete revascularization, and patient preference) and on institutional experience and expertise. However, in patients with isolated proximal left anterior descending artery disease, greater improvement in 5-year survival has been observed with PTCA than with medical therapy. Angioplasty has become a preferred approach in patients with critical single-vessel disease, significant inducible ischemia, and moderate to severe symptoms, even though there is minimal evidence from randomized trials supporting PTCA rather than medical therapy for these patients.

SUGGESTED READING

1. Bonow RO, Bohannon N, Hazzard W. Risk stratification in coronary artery disease and special populations [published erratum appears in *Am J Med.* 1997;102:322]. *Am J Med.* 1996;101(suppl 4A):17S–24S.
2. Brush JE Jr, Cannon RO III, Shenke WH, Bonow RO, Leon MB, Maron BJ, Epstein SE. Angina due to coronary microvascular disease in hypertensive patients without left ventricular hypertrophy. *N Engl J Med.* 1988;319:1302–1307.
3. Fuster V. Lewis A Conner Memorial Lecture: Mechanisms leading to myocardial infarction: insights from studies of vascular biology [published erratum appears in *Circulation.* 1994;90:2126–2146.
4. Merz CN, Rozanski A, Forrester JS. The secondary prevention of coronary artery disease. *Am J Med.* 1997;102:572–581.
5. Pfeffer MA, Braunwald E, Moyé LA, Basta L, Brown EL Jr, Cuddy TE, Davis BR, Geltman EM, Goldman S, Flaten GC, et al. Effect of captopril on mortality and morbidity in patients with left ventricular dysfunction after myocardial infarction: results of the Survival and Ventricular Enlargement Trial (SAVE). *N Engl J Med.* 1992;327:669–677.
6. Psaty BM, Heckbert SR, Koepsell TD, Siscovick DS, Raghunathan TE, Weiss NS, Rosendaal FR, Lemaitre RN, Smith NL, Wahl PW, et al. The risk of myocardial infarction associated with antihypertensive drug therapies. *JAMA.* 1995;274: 620–625.
7. Solomon AJ, Gersh BJ. Management of chronic stable angina: medical therapy, percutaneous transluminal coronary angioplasty, and coronary artery bypass graft surgery: lessons from the randomized trials. *Ann Intern Med.* 1998;128: 216–223.
8. Yusuf S, Peto R, Lewis J, Collins R, Sleight P. Beta-blockade during and after myocardial infarction: an overview of the randomized trials. *Prog Cardiovasc Dis.* 1985;27:335–371.
9. Gradman AH. Hypertension and ischemia: evolving concepts. *J Am Coll Cardiol.* 1992;19:816–817.
10. Sullivan JM. Hypertension. In: Sobel BE, ed. *Medical Management of Heart Disease.* New York, NY: Marcel Dekker Inc; 1996:101–144.

Chapter 139

Management of Hypertensive Patients with Left Ventricular Hypertrophy and Diastolic Dysfunction

Edward D. Frohlich, MD

KEY POINTS

- Left ventricular hypertrophy (LVH) prevalence depends upon the technological means by which it is diagnosed; ECG changes are relatively specific but echocardiography is the most precise widely available method for detection.

- The best treatment for LVH is prevention via effective BP control; in those patients with established LVH, effective BP control and electrolyte balance remain the primary goals.

- Clinical trials are in progress to establish whether reversal of LVH and reduction of LV mass affect outcomes; effective BP control with any class of antihypertensive agents reduces LV mass.

See also Chapters 68, 77, 140

As the left ventricle progressively hypertrophies, its contractile (systolic) pumping reserve becomes diminished. Even before systolic dysfunction becomes clinically evident, the hypertrophic left ventricle becomes "stiffer" or less distensible, and diastolic filling becomes impaired. The left atrium adapts structurally to provide a "booster pump" that improves diastolic filling at the expense of increased left atrial size, demonstrable by ECG and by echocardiogram. Some hypertensive patients with diastolic dysfunction (primarily elderly patients, diabetics, and those with ischemic heart disease) develop cardiac failure without apparent systolic dysfunction. This condition results from increased collagen deposition, from ventricular ischemia that results from hypertensive coronary arteriolar disease, or from occlusive atherosclerotic disease of epicardial coronary arteries.

LVH resulting from pressure overload is not always evident clinically in hypertension, but when present it is usually an "appropriate" concentric hypertrophy. When hypertension is associated with a relative volume overload, the structural type of hypertrophy may be more eccentric in shape. This latter form of hypertrophy may be expected in obese patients or in chronic renal insufficiency or when a volume overload and pressure overload occur together.

Clinical Considerations

The primary factors responsible for the development of LVH are pressure or volume overload. A number of nonhemodynamic factors, including a variety of hormonal and humoral mechanisms and growth factors (eg, catecholamines, angiotensin II, endothelins) are also associated with vascular and cardiac myocytic growth. Other clinical considerations include state of hypertensive disease; demographic factors such as age, sex, and race; coexistence with other diseases (eg, obesity, diabetes mellitus, atherosclerotic coronary arterial disease); and coincident pharmacological therapies.

The precise explanation for the increased risk associated with LVH is not known with certainty and a number of mechanisms may contribute. LVH is associated with progressive impairment in coronary blood flow and flow reserve, increased coronary vascular resistance, endothelial dysfunction, and impaired arteriolar dilator capacity. Epicardial and microvascular arteriolar diseases are exacerbated by the atherogenic process in patients with hypertensive disease. In addition, there is a progressive contraction of intravascular (plasma) volume in proportion to the increasing arterial pressure (and vascular resistance), which exacerbates the abnormal rheology and viscosity alterations of the coronary microcirculation. Each of these changes may contribute to the development of congestive heart failure, coronary arterial insufficiency, angina pectoris, lethal cardiac dysrhythmias, and sudden death. Finally, compounding these factors is an increased deposition of collagen that increases stiffness of the ventricular chamber and the likelihood of developing cardiac failure.

Diagnosis

Comparison of Available Techniques

Detection of LVH may be accomplished by various techniques. The chest x-ray is not nearly as sensitive as the ECG and may be associated with changes that reflect not only LVH but ventricular chamber dilation as well. The ECG is more precise, but it also falls short of detecting early LVH. The best and most sensitive clinical means of the three for detecting early LVH as well as changes in left ventricular function is the echocardiogram. Recently, less-costly limited echocardiography has been suggested. Other, more-costly techniques that provide a more clear-cut definition of LVH are magnetic resonance and positron emission imaging techniques.

For routine evaluation of the patient with hypertension the ECG remains the most useful and cost-effective method. Echocardiogram should be reserved for patients with questionable LVH (particularly in children, adolescents, and young athletes), severe hypertension with exercise but not at rest, persistently high office arterial pressures with normal ECGs, severe retinopathy, renal functional impairment without apparent cardiac involvement, chest pain, or cardiac dysrhythmias. Finally, the existence of a fourth heart sound and the presence of at least two ECG criteria of left atrial abnormality are highly concordant with early development of LVH (which has been confirmed by the echocardiogram).

ECG Criteria

There are 30 or more indices of LVH by the ECG. Commonly used criteria are the Sokolow-Lyons criteria (sum of the negative deflection in V_1 and positive deflection in V_5 or V_6 >35 mV) and the Cornell criteria (product of the QRS duration and the sum of the positive deflection in aVL and negative deflection in V_3 >2400 mV·msec). Highly sensitive is the McPhee index (sum of the tallest precordial R wave and deepest S wave ≥ 4.5 mV) and the left ventricular strain pattern (ie, the QRS complex and T-wave vectors are 180 degrees apart), which also provides few false negative diagnoses. The latter "strain pattern" is associated with severely diminished vascularity of the hypertrophied ventricle, which has been correlated with coronary arteriography evidence of ischemic disease. As indicated, enhancing the diagnostic ability of the ECG, particularly in early LVH, are left atrial abnormalities. Among these criteria are: P wave ≥ 0.12 second in duration, bipeak interval of notched P waves ≥ 0.04 second, a P-wave duration to PR segment ratio of ≥ 1.6 (in lead II), and terminal atrial forces (V_1) ≥ 0.04 second. Presence of two or more of these criteria is highly concordant with the presence of cardiac dysrhythmias and echocardiographic evidence of left atrial enlargement and LVH.

Echocardiogram

The M-mode, two-dimensional echocardiogram (with or without Doppler flow measurements) provides a highly precise means of detecting LVH clinically. Intraventricular septal hypertrophy (≥ 1.0 cm) may be the first finding; and an increased width of the left ventricular free wall to ≥ 1.1 cm also indicates LVH. Increased left ventricular mass suggests LVH, but this index takes into consideration left ventricular diastolic volume, which is different in men and women (<100 and ≥ 131 g/m², respectively), and even varies with intravascular and ventricular volume (which change with weight reduction). Also important are changes in early and late ventricular filling ("E-A wave reversal").

Therapy
LVH

The best treatment for LVH is prevention. Vigorous use of antihypertensive therapy as soon as a persistently elevated BP is established provides the best assurance that LVH may be prevented. In this regard, all classes of antihypertensive agents will prevent or diminish LVH as long as BP is well controlled.

In those patients who already have LVH, the cornerstone therapy remains continuous and effective control of arterial pressure. As indicated, every class of antihypertensive agent will diminish LVH, including diuretics and direct-acting vasodilators. Other agents (eg, centrally acting adrenergic inhibitors, β-adrenergic receptor blocking agents, ACE inhibitors, angiotensin receptor antagonists, and cal-

cium antagonists) have been shown experimentally and clinically to reduce LV mass most rapidly—even within 3 to 8 weeks. Potential superiority of one class over another remains to be confirmed by prospective clinical trials demonstrating favorable effects on morbidity and mortality related to LVH, however.

Particular care should be exercised with use of diuretics to prevent hypokalemia and associated hypomagnesemia in patients with LVH, because the hypertrophied ventricle is predisposed to cardiac dysrhythmias and sudden death. Proper electrolyte balance is even more important if digitalis is used concomitantly.

Diastolic Dysfunction

Although diastolic dysfunction may occur in the absence of systolic dysfunction, when systolic dysfunction already exists there is also some degree of impaired diastolic function. Treatment of systolic functional impairment will also improve to some degree the diastolic dysfunction. In those cases, the major factor in improving systolic function is the excellent control of both systolic and diastolic arterial pressure, ideally to a goal of <140 and 90 mm Hg, respectively. Although there has been some concern expressed by reducing arterial pressures to levels of 80 to 85 mm Hg (for fear of impairing left ventricular blood flow in diastole, the so-called J-curve), recent studies have not borne out the existence of such a curve in prospective clinical studies. These studies have related to the isolated Systolic Hypertension in the Elderly Study (SHEP) and similar studies in Sweden and Great Britain (the STOP-Hypertension and MRC Trials), the SAVE and SOLVD studies, and more recently with the HOT Study.

Thus, treatment of systolic and diastolic dysfunction will result in reduction of left ventricular mass and in both ECG and echocardiographic evidence of LVH. This response also improves diastolic distensibility and relaxation, thereby enhancing diastolic function. With respect to reducing left ventricular mass, all forms of antihypertensive therapy (as already discussed) will reduce LV mass.

However, when diastolic dysfunction already exists in the absence of systolic dysfunction, it usually occurs in the elderly patient with collagen deposition in the ventricular wall or in patients with myocardial ischemia. Experimental studies have demonstrated the efficacy of the ACE inhibitors, angiotensin II receptor antagonists, and calcium antagonists in reducing the hydroxyproline and collagen content of the ventricle. This deposition occurs with aging as well as with hypertension in the hypertrophied and nonhypertrophied ventricles and is also associated with reduced left ventricular coronary blood flow reserve. Unfortunately, well-controlled clinical trials have not yet been conducted or reported to extrapolate the existing experimental findings.

It has been proposed that phenylalkylamines (verapamil) improve diastolic function to a greater degree than other antihypertensive agents because of their specific role in modifying myocyte calcium concentrations during cardiac relaxation. Well-controlled trials have yet to be performed to understand the potential clinical significance of this observation, however.

Impact of Therapy

Even though there is ample evidence to relate LVH and increased cardiovascular risk, there still is no adequate evidence available, at present, to indicate that LVH reversal actually reduces risk, although multicenter studies are in progress. Reduction of risk with

LVH reversal must be disassociated from the pharmacological actions in reducing arterial pressure, improving coronary blood flow and flow reserve, or even preventing arrhythmias.

SUGGESTED READING

1. Frohlich ED. Is reversal of left ventricular hypertrophy in hypertension beneficial? *Hypertension.* 1991;18(suppl 1): I-33-I-38.
2. Frohlich ED, Apstein C, Chobanian AV, Devereux RB, Dustan HP, Dzau V, Fouad-Tarazi F, Horan MJ, Marcus M, Massie LB, Pfeffer MA, Re RN, Roccella EJ, Savage D, Shub C. The heart in hypertension [published erratum appears in *N Engl J Med.* 1992;327:1768]. *N Engl J Med.* 1992;327:998–1008.
3. Roman MJ, Saba PS, Pini R, Spitzer M, Pickering TG, Rosen S, Alderman MH, Devereux RB. Parallel cardiac and vascular adaptation in hypertension. *Circulation.* 1992;86:1909–1918.
4. Dunn FG, Pringle SD. Sudden cardiac death, ventricular arrhythmias and hypertensive left ventricular hypertrophy. *J Hypertens.* 1993;11:1003–1010. Editorial.
5. Treasure CB, Klein JL, Vita JA, Manoukian SV, Renwick GH, Selwyn AP, Ganz P, Alexander RW: Hypertension and left ventricular hypertrophy are associated with impaired endothelium-mediated relaxation in human coronary resistance vessels. *Circulation.* 1993;87:86–93.
6. Siscovick DS, Raghunathan TE, Psaty BM, Koepsell TD, Wicklund KG, Lin X, Cobb L, Rautaharju PM, Copass MK, Wagner EH. Diuretic therapy for hypertension and the risk of primary cardiac arrest. *N Engl J Med.* 1994;330:1852–1857.
7. Levy D, Larson MG, Vasan RS, Kannel WB, Ho KK The progression from hypertension to congestive heart failure. *JAMA.* 1996;275:1557–1562.
8. Nunez E, Hosoya K, Susic D, Frohlich ED. Enalapril and losartan reduces cardiac mass and improves coronary hemodynamics in SHR. *Hypertension.* 1997;29:519–524.
9. Sheps SG, Frohlich ED. Limited echocardiography for hypertensive left ventricular hypertrophy. *Hypertension.* 1997;29:560–563.
10. Susic D, Nunez E, Hosoya H, Frohlich ED. Coronary hemodynamics in aging spontaneously hypertensive and normotensive Wistar-Kyoto rats. *J Hypertens.* 1998;16:231–237.

Chapter 140

Management of Hypertensive Patients With Dilated Cardiomyopathy (Systolic Dysfunction)

Jay N. Cohn, MD

KEY POINTS

- Congestive heart failure is a common complication of chronic hypertension because of a variety of hemodynamic and neurohormonal mechanisms affecting the vasculature and the myocardium. Reducing the elevated blood pressure is critical for effective therapy.

- Ventricular remodeling resulting in a dilated chamber with a low ejection fraction carries a poor prognosis and requires therapy to inhibit or reverse the remodeling process.

- Aggressive treatment of uncomplicated hypertension and other associated risk factors can prevent heart failure and its poor prognosis.

See also Chapters 69, 77, 139

Patients with long-standing hypertension are at markedly increased risk of developing heart failure, for the following reasons. (1) Increased impedance to left ventricular (LV) ejection may impair ventricular systolic shortening during ejection. (2) Coexistent coronary disease may impair myocardial perfusion and aggravate contractile dysfunction. (3) Concentric hypertrophy and fibrosis, perhaps aggravated by subendocardial ischemia, may impair LV filling (diastolic dysfunction). (4) Ventricular remodeling related to pressure elevation and/or activated hormonal systems may result in chamber enlargement, increased wall stress, and aggravation of ischemia. (5) Vascular remodeling induced by pressure elevation or neurohormonal activation may lead to reduced arterial compliance that places a further impedance burden on the dysfunctional myocardium.

The adverse effects on the left ventricle of long-standing hypertension also may persist even if the blood pressure normalizes as a consequence of myocardial damage, as after a myocardial infarction. Therefore, normalization of blood pressure is an important therapeutic strategy in hypertensive heart failure, but traditional antihypertensive drugs may also exert a favorable effect in normotensive individuals with LV dysfunction. In these individuals, vasodilator drugs that lower impedance can improve systolic emptying and raise cardiac output without necessarily lowering blood pressure.

Ventricular Dilation

Dilation of the left ventricle in a hypertensive individual indicates that the myocardial hypertrophy has become eccentric rather than concentric. This implies that in addition to thickening, the myocyte has lengthened, and this lengthening may be associated with some reduction of fractional shortening. Under these circumstances, the LV ejection fraction is reduced, and the patient is described as having systolic dysfunction **(Figure 140.1)**. Echocardiography or ventriculography (dye or radionuclide) is mandatory to detect this structural and functional alteration. The process of ventricular hy-

pertrophy and dilation is often referred to as ventricular remodeling. The therapeutic challenge is to prevent further remodeling of the chamber, because this progressive remodeling process is associated with a poor prognosis related to both pump failure and ventricular arrhythmias.

Both pressure overload and hormonal stimulation may contribute to the remodeling process, and both should ideally be addressed in the therapeutic plan. Systolic load, identified by the systolic blood pressure, should be aggressively lowered to low normal levels, if tolerated, in the presence of heart failure. In the therapeutic range, it is not uncommon to have systolic pressures in the range of 70 to 90 mm Hg. Such values are appropriate as long as the patient feels well. It should also be recognized that cuff pressures may underestimate the magnitude of late systolic pressure augmentation from reflected waves in the root of the aorta. LV diastolic pressure contributes to diastolic wall stress and also should be normalized by pharmacological means.

Hormonal contributors to LV remodeling may include angiotensin, norepinephrine, endothelin, and other mediators of myocyte and interstitial cell growth. Therapies that interfere with these systems may be more effective in inhibiting hypertrophy and remodeling than drugs that exert only a hemodynamic effect to reduce LV wall stress.

Treatment of the Patient With a Dilated Ventricle

Therapy should be aimed at relieving symptoms and slowing or reversing the ventricular remodeling process that has caused the dilated ventricle. Symptom relief involves diuretics to relieve congestion, vasodilator drugs to improve LV hemodynamics, and digoxin to exert a beneficial effect on symptoms through positive inotropic or antiadrenergic effects. The goal of slowing cardiac remodeling (dilation) and prolonging life requires aggressive intervention to interfere with the myocardial process.

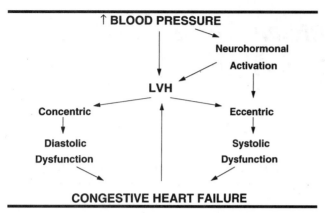

Figure 140.1. Schematic of mechanisms contributing to congestive heart failure in hypertensive individuals.

ACE inhibitors exert a number of favorable effects, including mild regression or slowing of ventricular remodeling and a vasodilator effect to improve hemodynamics. These drugs are first-line therapy for dilated cardiomyopathy and should be administered to all individuals with heart failure and LV dilation. Underdosing remains a major problem; the dose should be titrated up to that demonstrated in clinical trials to prolong life (enalapril 10 mg BID, captopril 50 mg TID, etc). In patients who cannot tolerate ACE inhibitors (intractable cough, progressive renal dysfunction, or allergy to the drug), the combination of isosorbide dinitrate and hydralazine administered 3 or 4 times daily can replace the ACE inhibitors.

Symptom relief can be achieved with diuretics, which should be dosed to normalize cardiac filling pressure, usually monitored by evaluating the jugular venous pressure and its response to abdominal pressure (hepatojugular reflux). Thiazide diuretics when fluid retention is mild or loop-active diuretics in more severe congestive states are appropriate. A second diuretic, such as metolazone, may be added to the loop-active diuretic to augment the effect in resistant congestive states. Potassium levels need to be protected by coadministration of ACE inhibitors, potassium supplementation, or potassium-sparing diuretics. Renal function needs to be monitored to help avoid excessive diuresis.

Other drugs are also useful. β-Blockers have recently been shown to cause regression of LV remodeling with long-term therapy in slowly escalating doses. Although this therapy has not yet been evaluated in a hypertensive heart failure population, it is likely that these drugs will exert a favorable effect on this subpopulation with heart failure. Angiotensin receptor blockers have not yet been evaluated adequately for treatment of heart failure. These and a number of newer drugs are currently under investigation as possible additives

to current conventional therapy for heart failure. Digoxin in low doses appears to be safe in dilated heart failure and exerts a modestly favorable effect on symptoms. In the absence of contraindications, it may be added to the regimen. In acute decompensation with severe pump failure, short-term intravenous infusion of dobutamine or milrinone may improve pump function and relieve tissue underperfusion. Long-term infusion of these drugs may increase the risk of arrhythmic death, and this therapy does not appear to slow or reverse the LV remodeling process.

Prevention of Heart Failure in Hypertension

One of the goals of treatment of hypertension is to prevent heart failure. Early and adequate control of elevated blood pressure prevents or slows the development of LV hypertrophy (LVH), which precedes the onset of heart failure. ACE inhibitors appear to exert a more marked benefit on regression of LVH when LVH already exists in a hypertensive patient. Other drugs, including diuretics, β-blockers, and calcium antagonists, also are effective in reversing LVH.

Treatment of coexistent risk factors also may forestall the development of heart failure. Lipid control with statin drugs in patients with an elevated LDL appears to reduce the risk of heart failure. Smoking cessation, weight reduction, and diabetes control also may contribute to prevention of cardiovascular events, including heart failure. The goal is to use blood pressure as well as other risk factors to identify the at-risk population who need aggressive treatment.

SUGGESTED READING

1. Cohn JN. Drug therapy: the management of chronic heart failure. *N Engl J Med.* 1996;335:490–498.
2. Cohn JN. Prevention of heart failure: a new agenda. *N Engl J Med.* 1992;327:725–727. Editorial.
3. Cohn JN. Structural basis for heart failure: ventricular remodeling and its pharmacological inhibition. *Circulation.* 1995;91:2504–2507. Editorial.
4. Cohn JN. Vasodilator therapy for heart failure: the influence of impedance on left ventricular performance. *Circulation.* 1973;48:5–8.
5. Cohn JN, Archibald DG, Ziesche S, Franciosa JA, Harston WE, Tristani FE, Dunkman WB, Jacobs W, Francis GS, Flohr KH, Goldman S, Cobb FR, Shah PM, Saunders R, Fletcher RD, Loeb HS, Hughes VC, Baker B. Effect of vasodilator therapy on mortality in chronic congestive heart failure: results of a Veterans Administration Cooperative Study (V-HeFT). *N Engl J Med.* 1986;314:1547–1552.
6. Digitalis Investigation Group. The effect of digoxin on mortality and morbidity in patients with heart failure. *N Engl J Med.* 1997;336:525–533.
7. Kannel WB, Castelli WP, McNamara PM. Role of blood pressure in the development of congestive heart failure: the Framingham Study. *N Engl J Med.* 1972;287:781–787.
8. Kjekshus J, Pedersen TR, Olsson AG, Faergeman O, Pyörälä K. The effects of simvastatin on the incidence of heart failure in patients with coronary heart disease. *J Card Fail.* 1997;3:249–254.
9. SOLVD Investigators. Effect of enalapril on survival in patients with reduced left ventricular ejection fractions and congestive heart failure. *N Engl J Med.* 1991;325:293–302.

Management of Hypertensive Patients With Chronic Renal Insufficiency

Marc A. Pohl, MD

KEY POINTS

- Progressive renal insufficiency worsens hypertension, and uncontrolled blood pressure hastens the decline in glomerular filtration rate.

- Good blood pressure control is essential to prevent or slow the progression of CRI toward end-stage renal disease (ESRD).

- Loop-active diuretics are generally required to control blood pressure in pre-ESRD patients, and adequate fluid removal is necessary in dialysis patients.

- Patients with hypertension, CRI, and proteinuria ($>$1 g/24 h) should receive an ACE inhibitor unless contraindicated.

See also Chapters 51, 74, 78, 112, 146,153

The association of hypertension and chronic renal insufficiency (CRI) has been appreciated since the observations of Richard Bright in the 1830s. When hypertension develops consequent to primary renal disease, elevated arterial pressure is the predominant factor promoting continued loss of renal function. There is a vicious circle when hypertension and CRI coexist, each aggravating the other and contributing to the adverse sequelae of hypertensive cardiovascular disease and progressive renal failure. Therapeutic interruption of this circle is critical to retarding progression of renal disease and reducing cardiovascular morbidity and mortality before and after initiation of renal replacement therapy.

Effective antihypertensive therapy retards the progression of CRI. The Sixth Report of the Joint National Committee on Prevention, Detection, Evaluation, and Treatment of High Blood Pressure (JNC VI) has recommended that "blood pressure should be controlled to 130/85 mm Hg—or lower (125/75 mm Hg) in patients with proteinuria in excess of 1 gr/24 hr—with whatever antihypertensive therapy is necessary." Although all classes of antihypertensive drugs are effective in lowering blood pressure (BP) in CRI, ACE inhibitors are most effective in reducing proteinuria.

Nonpharmacological Therapy

General measures recommended in the treatment of essential hypertension may require modification in the management of hypertension in CRI. Dietary sodium restriction (ie, reducing dietary sodium to $<$100 mEq/d) is the single most important nonpharmacological approach in these patients. Because the failing kidney is characterized by obligated renal losses of sodium, however, overly aggressive dietary salt restriction or diuretic use may contribute to volume contraction and increased azotemia. As renal failure worsens, regular exercise can improve functional status but is more difficult for these patients because of generalized fatigue, anemia, and central circulatory congestion. There is no consensus regarding treating hyperlipidemic patients with CRI (with or without the

nephrotic syndrome) to prevent coronary artery disease. However, the use of lipid-lowering drugs is reasonable for patients with markedly abnormal lipid levels and for younger (ie, $<$65 years old) individuals with CRI.

Pharmacological Therapy

Antihypertensive drugs should be introduced at low doses and titrated upward as necessary. Modification of drug dosage based on routes of drug elimination is usually not necessary for patients with CRI. With several exceptions, the effective antihypertensive drug dose and tolerance of these drugs are similar in patients with and without impaired renal function.

Diuretics

Given the central role of volume expansion in renal parenchymal hypertension, thiazide or loop-active diuretics should be used as first-line drug therapy. Thiazide diuretics are not effective with advanced CRI (serum creatinine level $\geq$2.5 mg/dL), and loop-active diuretics are frequently needed in this situation, often at relatively large doses. As glomerular filtration rate (GFR) decreases, the dose of loop-active diuretics usually must be increased. In patients with a GFR $<$20 mL/min, the upper plateau of the dose-response curve is attained with 160 mg furosemide (or its equivalent) given intravenously, which corresponds to an oral dose of 320 to 400 mg. If an oral daily dose of 400 mg of furosemide is ineffective, there is little to be gained by increasing the dose further, and deafness may occur at high doses of furosemide. The addition of a thiazide diuretic such as hydrochlorothiazide or metolazone may be a useful adjunct to control plasma volume and hyperkalemia in patients with CRI, but this tandem use of diuretics (diuretics acting at different sites in the nephron) carries the hazard of excessive volume contraction and increased azotemia. Potassium-sparing diuretics should be avoided in patients with CRI unless there is coexisting significant hypokalemia (ie, serum potassium $<$3.5 mEq/L).

As renal function declines and the patient approaches the need for hemodialysis, diuretics become ineffective, and combinations of other antihypertensive agents are required. As this situation supervenes, hemodialysis is required to control the expanded extracellular fluid volume usually present with severe CRI and corroborated by features of volume expansion upon physical examination.

Adrenergic Blocking Agents

β-Blockers are of particular value in patients with concomitant coronary disease. Prolonged use of propranolol has been reported to produce a 10% to 20% reduction in GFR and renal blood flow, whereas nadolol has been reported to increase GFR. Lipid-soluble β-Glockers are metabolized largely by the liver, and an alteration in dose is not required in renal failure, whereas hydrophilic β-Blockers, such as atenolol, have a prolonged elimination and are best avoided in patients with severe renal insufficiency. β-Blockers may increase triglycerides and lower HDL cholesterol levels, but the long-term clinical significance of these effects in patients with CRI is unclear. Labetalol, which combines β- and α-Blockade, is quite effective when combined with a diuretic. Plasma lipids are not adversely affected, no reduction in dosage in renal insufficiency is required, and significant alteration of renal hemodynamics is not observed with labetalol. Labetalol, however, may produce profound orthostatic hypotension, particularly when used in combination with diuretics.

The α-adrenergic blockers have no significant effect on renal hemodynamics and have been used successfully in patients with CRI. These agents may produce significant orthostatic hypotension (usually after the first dose but sometimes chronically), particularly in the elderly or in diabetic patients with impaired autonomic reflexes. Increased sensitivity to prazosin has been reported in patients with CRI; therefore, the initial dose should be reduced and upward titration carried out cautiously with this agent.

Sympatholytic Agents

Centrally acting α_2-adrenergic agonists (clonidine, guanfacine, guanabenz, methyldopa) are effective in lowering BP with CRI, are not associated with changes in renal hemodynamics, and suppress the hyperactive sympathetic nervous system found in chronic renal disease. Modest doses of these agents may produce lethargy in a significant proportion of patients, which may mimic uremic encephalopathy.

Direct Vasodilators

Hydralazine, and particularly minoxidil, may be required for severe hypertension or refractory hypertension in patients with CRI. Because both drugs are associated with reflex tachycardia and an increase in cardiac output, the concomitant use of a β-adrenergic blocker or clonidine is recommended. The amount of diuretic must usually be increased when minoxidil is added to the antihypertensive regimen to counteract salt and water retention. Both agents may increase renal blood flow but have no significant effect on GFR. Minoxidil requires no dosage modification in CRI, but its use may be limited because of tachycardia, salt and water retention, hirsutism, and an increased incidence of pericardial effusion in patients with CRI.

Calcium Antagonists

Calcium antagonists are widely used in the management of hypertension in CRI. With chronic use, the calcium antagonists have neither deleterious effects on renal function nor clinically significant effects on sodium metabolism. Calcium antagonists, particularly the benzothiazopines (diltiazem) and phenylalkylamines (verapamil), may provide a renoprotective effect above and beyond their ability to lower BP in CRI patients. The antihypertensive effect of calcium antagonists is additive with other antihypertensive drugs. They do not cause rebound hypertension, and because they are metabolized by the liver, dosage adjustments with CRI are not required.

Dihydropyridine calcium antagonists, in contrast to nondihydropyridine calcium antagonists, have failed to show a consistent pattern in either attenuating or worsening albuminuria or progressive glomerulosclerosis in either experimental or clinical studies. Because calcium antagonists, particularly dihydropyridine calcium antagonists, are so effective in lowering both systolic and diastolic BP, they are widely used early in the management of hypertension in patients with CRI and are relatively free of significant side effects. These drugs may be associated with a disproportionate incidence of untoward cardiovascular events in patients with renal failure. Because it has been proposed that activation of the sympathetic nervous system can be caused by dihydropyridine, concomitant use of central sympatholytic drugs seems to be justified, particularly in patients with serum creatinine levels >3 mg/dL, in whom BP control is critically important.

ACE Inhibitors

These agents are particularly indicated for patients with type I diabetic nephropathy and are strongly suggested when proteinuria (>1 g/d) is present in patients with type II diabetic nephropathy or other renal diseases. In addition to their antihypertensive effect, ACE inhibitors are renoprotective in proteinuric patients, presumably because of their ability to lower glomerular filtration pressure. The recently completed GISEN Study demonstrated that the ACE inhibitor ramipril markedly retarded the rate of GFR decline in patients with urinary protein excretion >3 g/d, an effect not accounted for by BP reduction. Renal protection with benazepril, in a study enrolling more than 500 nondiabetic patients with creatinine clearances ranging from 30 to 60 mL/min, was greatest in those with greater degrees of proteinuria. Meta-analysis of a number of clinical trials comparing ACE inhibitor with non–ACE inhibitor therapy with at least 1 year of follow-up suggests that ACE inhibition is associated with a significant risk reduction for end-stage renal disease (ESRD). These observations, however, are confounded by lower BPs associated with ACE therapy.

ACE inhibitors are well tolerated in patients with CRI, with only a minority of patients experiencing hypotension, reversible hemodynamically induced renal dysfunction, cough, or angioedema. ACE inhibitors are excreted primarily by the kidney (except for fosinopril) and require significant dose reduction in CRI.

Two additional precautions need to be taken when ACE inhibitors are used in patients with CRI. Because high-normal serum potassium levels are frequently seen in CRI and because ACE inhibitors predictably increase the serum potassium concentration (often above the upper limit of normal at GFR levels <30 mL/min/1.73 m², close monitoring of the serum potassium is mandatory. ACE inhibitor–induced hyperkalemia may be blunted by concomitant diuretic therapy, especially by a combination of loop-active diuretics and thiazides or by a reduction of the dose. Hyperkalemia is usually completely reversible with discontinuance of the ACE inhibitor. If bilateral renal artery stenosis or renal artery stenosis involving a solitary kidney is present, acute deterioration in renal function may occur, particularly in the setting of concomitant heart failure or volume contraction. Renal function is usually restored with discontinuation of the drug but not by substitution of another ACE inhibitor or angiotensin receptor blocker. Patients with CRI without renal artery stenosis occasionally show a reversible decrease in GFR when treated with an ACE inhibitor, usually in the setting of volume contraction or overzealous use of diuretics. In these patients, acute renal failure occurs because of impaired renal autoregulation secondary to severe intrarenal nephrosclerosis or compression of the intrarenal arterial tree by large renal cysts. After volume repletion, ACE inhibitors may be reinstituted with monitoring.

Angiotensin II Receptor Blockers

These agents appear to be as effective as ACE inhibitors in lowering both systolic and diastolic BP in patients with CRI. The angiotensin receptor blockers are well tolerated and do not produce cough or angioedema. Renal protective effects appear to be similar to ACE inhibitors in experimental models, including reduction in proteinuria and amelioration of glomerulosclerosis, independent of BP reduction.

Precautions regarding the use of angiotensin receptor blockers in hypertensive patients with CRI are the same as those for ACE inhibitors.

Hypertension in Dialysis Patients

Hypertension is present in 80% to 100% of patients who reach ESRD. Two broad patterns of BP response have been recognized in hemodialysis patients: about 85% of well-dialyzed patients achieve sustained normal BP when free of edema and become hypotensive with further volume removal (achievement of dry weight). The other 10% to 15% of hypertensive ESRD patients have sustained hypertension in the euvolemic state and may become hypertensive with further volume removal. In dialysis patients who become more hypertensive at "dry weight," plasma renin levels may be elevated, and the term "renin-dependent hypertension" has been used. Although bilateral nephrectomy makes BP easier to control, it is rarely necessary. Plasma norepinephrine concentrations are elevated in hypertensive hemodialysis patients and may correlate with BP levels. Erythropoietin therapy also raises BP, and a significant number of patients who had been normotensive on dialysis have required antihypertensive medications.

With the exception of diuretics, antihypertensive drugs used to treat CRI before ESRD may be used in hemodialysis patients. Dialysis and ultrafiltration are necessary to control volume, because most patients on chronic dialysis are severely oliguric or anuric. Dietary salt and potassium restriction are also important. Therapy with antihypertensive drugs is indicated primarily for the minority of patients in whom elevated BP persists despite seemingly adequate volume control. Goal BPs for individual dialysis patients may be based on their clinical status, age, cardiac condition, neuropathy, and propensity for dialysis-related hypotension. Within this context, one should attempt to maintain the BP level close to a mean ambulatory BP of 135/85 mm Hg. Ideally, antihypertensive medication should be taken in the evening as a once-a-day dose, with drugs that do not cause reflex cardiac neurohumoral stimulation. Control of interdialytic weight gain and adequate dialysis (total number of hours dialyzed per week) are equally important in BP control in these patients.

SUGGESTED READING

1. Blythe WB. Natural history of hypertension in renal parenchymal disease. *Am J Kidney Dis.* 1985;5:A50–A56.
2. Galla JH, Luke RG. Hypertension in renal parenchymal disease. In: Brenner BM, ed. *Brenner and Rector's The Kidney.* Philadelphia, Pa: WB Saunders Co; 1996: 2126–2147.
3. Giatras I, Lau J, Levey AS, for the Angiotensin-Converting-Enzyme Inhibition and Progressive Renal Disease Study Group. Effect of angiotensin-converting enzyme inhibitors on the progression of nondiabetic renal disease: a meta-analysis of randomized trials. *Ann Intern Med* 1997;127:337–345.
4. GISEN Group. Randomised placebo-controlled trial of effect of ramipril on decline in glomerular filtration rate and risk of terminal renal failure in proteinuric, nondiabetic nephropathy. The GISEN Group (Gruppo Italiano di Studi Epidemiologici in Nefrologia). *Lancet.* 1997;349:1857–1863.
5. Lazarus JM, Bourgoignie JJ, Buckalew VM, Greene T, Levey AS, Milas, NC, Paranandi L, Peterson JC, Porush JG, Rauch S, Soucie JM, Stollar C. Achievement and safety of a low blood pressure goal in chronic renal disease. The Modification of Diet in Renal Disease Study Group. *Hypertension.* 1997;29:641–650.
6. Maschio G, Alberti D, Janin G, Locatelli F, Mann JFE, Motolese M, Ponticelli C, Ritz E, Zucchelli P, and the Angiotensin-Converting-Enzyme Inhibition in Progressive Renal Insufficiency Study Group. Effect of the angiotensin-converting-enzyme inhibitor benazepril on the progression of chronic renal insufficiency. *N Engl J Med.* 1996;334:939–945.
7. National High Blood Pressure Education Program (NHBPEP) Working Group. 1995 update of the working group reports on chronic renal failure and renovascular hypertension. *Arch Intern Med.* 1996;156:1938–1947.
8. Peterson JC, Adler S, Burkart JM, Greene T, Hebert LA, Hunsicker LG, King AJ, Klahr S, Massry SG, Seifter JL. Blood pressure control, proteinuria, and the progression of renal disease: the Modification of Diet in Renal Disease Study. *Ann Intern Med.* 1995;123:754–762.
9. Tomita J, Kimura G, Inoue T, Inenaga T, Sanai T, Kawano Y, Nakamura S, Baba S, Matsuoka H, Omae T. Role of systolic blood pressure in determining prognosis of hemodialyzed patients. *Am J Kidney Dis.* 1995;25:405–412.
10. Vertes V, Cangiano JL, Berman LB, Gould A. Hypertension in end-stage renal disease. *N Engl J Med.* 1969;280:978–981.

Chapter 142

Management of Hypertensive Patients With Peripheral Arterial Disease

Jeffrey W. Olin, DO

KEY POINTS

- β-Adrenergic blocker therapy does not worsen intermittent claudication in most subjects with peripheral arterial disease.

- A structured walking program has been shown to significantly increase the pain-free walking distance and maximum walking distance in patients with intermittent claudication.

- In patients with an abdominal aortic aneurysm, β-blocker therapy is the preferred antihypertensive treatment.

- All patients with evidence of peripheral atherosclerosis should be screened for the presence of coronary artery disease.

See also Chapters 65, 79, 113

There is little published information regarding the treatment of hypertension in patients with peripheral arterial disease (PAD). In the sixth report of the Joint National Committee on Prevention, Detection, Evaluation, and Treatment of High Blood Pressure (JNC VI), there are no specific recommendations regarding treatment of high blood pressure in patients with PAD. Although treating hypertension clearly has a beneficial effect on the incidence of myocardial infarction, stroke, and congestive heart failure, no available data suggest that treating hypertension alters the course of PAD. The Treatment of Mild Hypertension Study (TOMHS) did show, however, that drug treatment in combination with nutritional-hygienic interventions was superior to nutritional-hygienic treatment alone (placebo) in preventing the development of intermittent claudication and PAD over an average follow-up period of 4.4 years.

Recognition of PAD

Patients with PAD usually present with the symptom complex of intermittent claudication: aching, pain, or tiredness in the buttocks, hip girdle, thighs, or calf muscles brought on by exercise and relieved by rest. There are three major clinical features in patients with intermittent claudication: (1) Claudication is reproducible with a consistent level of exercise from day to day. (2) The discomfort completely resolves within 2 to 5 minutes after exercise has been stopped unless the patient has walked to the point of severe leg pain. (3) The discomfort occurs again at approximately the same distance once walking has been resumed.

Treatment of Hypertension in PAD Patients

Direct-acting vasodilators, calcium channel antagonists, α_1-blockers, and ACE inhibitors are all effective arteriolar vasodilators, but these agents will not dilate atherosclerotic vessels and therefore will not improve the symptoms of intermittent claudication. Most studies show that these agents have no measurable effect on walking distance or calf blood flow. However, in a recent report, verapamil was shown to increase treadmill walking dis-

tance in patients with claudication, but only after individual dose titration.

β-Blockers in PAD

The commonly held belief that β-blocking agents worsen intermittent claudication and shorten the amount of exercise required to bring on discomfort in the extremity has now been challenged. In a carefully performed meta-analysis of 11 randomized, controlled trials, Radack and Deck concluded that β-adrenergic blocker therapy does not worsen intermittent claudication in subjects with PAD. Only 1 of 11 studies in this meta-analysis showed that pain-free and maximal treadmill walking distances were decreased by atenolol, labetalol, and pindolol but not captopril.

Nevertheless, some patients may experience the onset of claudication after starting β-blocker therapy. In these instances, the β-blocker should be discontinued and another agent tried. If the patient has advanced PAD with ischemic rest pain and is not surgically reconstructible, β-blocker therapy should be discontinued with the hope that this may improve the peripheral circulation enough to avoid amputation. A comprehensive review of the peripheral vascular effects of β-blocker therapy is nicely summarized by the work of Heintzen and Strauer.

Patients with vasospastic diseases (Raynaud's phenomenon or disease, chronic pernio) and hypertension should not receive β-blockers, because the extent of vasospasm may increase with the use of these drugs. Under these circumstances, calcium antagonists and α-blockers may lower the blood pressure and decrease the severity and frequency of the vasospasm.

ACE Inhibitors in PAD

Uncontrolled observations suggest that ACE inhibitors may improve walking distance in patients with intermittent claudication. Although ACE inhibitors can effectively lower blood pressure in many patients with PAD, the overall consensus of investigators is that they do not alter walking distance significantly. Renal function should be followed closely in patients with PAD who are on ACE inhibitors because the prevalence of atherosclerotic renal artery sclerosis is so high in this patient population. We have demonstrated that anatomically significant renal artery sclerosis may be present in 39% of patients with peripheral arterial occlusive disease and 38% of patients with abdominal aortic aneurysm. High-grade bilateral disease was present in ≈13% of patients.

Role of Exercise in PAD

A structured walking program has been shown to significantly increase the pain-free walking distance and maximum walking distance in patients with intermittent claudication. In 26 trials of exercise conditioning summarized by Hiatt and Regensteiner, claudication pain improved an average of 134% (range, 44% to 290%) and peak walking time increased an average of 96% (range, 25% to 183%). Recent studies using validated disease-specific questionnaires have shown that exercise in PAD improves the quality of life for the patient. In addition, a regular walking program can lower blood pressure, improve survival, lower triglycerides, raise HDL cholesterol, and improve glucose intolerance and insulin resistance **(Table 142.1)**.

The initial period of walking should be 35 minutes long, with subsequent increases of 5 minutes each session until a 50-minute session is possible. During the exercise sessions, the patient walks on the treadmill (or outside) until a mild or moderate level of pain is reached, followed by a rest period until the pain abates. After the pain is gone, the patient resumes walking until a moderate level of claudication pain is reached again, followed by another rest period. This process is repeated until the 50-minute exercise period has elapsed. In our experience, actual treadmill exercise constitutes ≈35 minutes and rest periods ≈15 minutes of the 50-minute exercise time. The beneficial effects of walking disappear quickly once the patient stops walking on a regular basis.

Smoking Cessation

Discontinuing cigarette smoking may be the single most important factor that determines whether PAD progresses. In addition, discontinuation of smoking may have a favorable effect on walking tolerance. It is important to encourage and help patients to discontinue smoking.

Abdominal Aortic Aneurysms

Both animal and human data suggest that β-blockers may slow the rate of expansion of abdominal aortic aneurysms more than any other class of antihypertensive drug. Therefore, in the patient with an abdominal aortic aneurysm, β-blocker therapy is the antihypertensive treatment of choice if there are no contraindications to its use. Resection of the abdominal aortic aneurysm should be considered

for all symptomatic patients and in the asymptomatic patient with an aneurysm ≥5.0 cm.

Special Considerations

Coronary Artery Disease

The mortality rate for patients with PAD is ≈30% at 5 years, 50% at 10 years, and 75% at 15 years. More than 90% of these deaths are due to myocardial infarction and stroke. The relative risk of dying of coronary heart disease in patients with PAD was 6.6 times that of a control population. The relative risk of dying from any cardiovascular disease was 5.9 times that of the control population. Several investigators have shown that the resting ankle/brachial index is an important predictor of cardiovascular mortality **(Figure 142.1)**. In this study, there was an ≈25% mortality rate at 4 years in women with an ankle/brachial index of <0.9. This increased mortality occurred even in the absence of symptomatic PAD.

We believe that all patients with evidence of peripheral atherosclerosis should be screened for the presence of coronary heart disease with one of the noninvasive screening modalities.

Lipid Abnormalities

Data from our institution have shown that ≈87% of patients with PAD have abnormalities in their lipid profile. Patients may exhibit increased serum triglycerides, increased total and LDL cholesterol, and/or decreased HDL cholesterol. A nonpharmacological approach (weight loss, exercise) to the treatment of hypertension and dyslipidemia would have the most beneficial effect on the patient with PAD (Table 142.1).

Guidelines from the National Cholesterol Education Program Adult Treatment Panel II should be followed. The goal LDL cholesterol for patients with PAD should be <100 mg/dL. The statins are a very effective class of cholesterol-lowering drugs that have been shown to decrease coronary event rates, allow for regression of atherosclerosis, and help to normalize endothelial function.

Glucose Intolerance and Diabetes Mellitus

In individuals with PAD who are also overweight, especially if the weight is distributed in the central portion of the body (android obesity), there may be some degree of glucose intolerance and/or insulin resistance. Again, exercise and weight reduction are important. Approximately 35% of patients with PAD have diabetes mellitus. Aggressive management of the diabetes is indicated.

Table 142.1. Beneficial Effects of Exercise in Peripheral Arterial Disease

Lowers blood pressure
Improves claudication symptoms
   Increases pain-free walking distance
   Increases maxiumum walking distance
Improves quality of life
Improves survival
Lowers triglycerides and raises HDL cholesterol
Improves glucose tolerance and insulin resistance

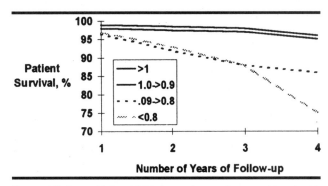

Figure 142.1. Ankle/brachial index and mortality. Reproduced with permission from Vogt MT, et al. Decreased ankle/arm blood pressure index and mortality in elderly women. *JAMA*. 1993;270:465–469. Copyright 1993, American Medical Association.

Our approach is to use an angiotensin-converting inhibitor as the drug class of choice in patients with PAD, diabetes, and hypertension. If hyperkalemia or worsening renal dysfunction limits the use of this class of drugs, a calcium channel antagonist is a reasonable alternative.

SUGGESTED READING

1. Criqui MH, Langer RD, Fronek A, Feigelson HS, Klauber MR, McCann TJ, Browner D. Mortality over a period of 10 years in patients with peripheral arterial disease. *N Engl J Med.* 1992;326:381–386.

2. Ernst E, Fialka V. A review of the clinical effectiveness of exercise therapy for intermittent claudication. *Arch Intern Med.* 1993;153:2357–2360.

3. Hiatt WR, Regensteiner JG, Hargarten ME, Wolfel EE, Brass EP. Benefit of exercise conditioning for patients with peripheral arterial disease. *Circulation.* 1990;81:602–609.

4. McInnes GT. Role of ACE inhibitors in hypertension complicated by vascular disease. *Br Heart J.* 1994;72(suppl):S33–S37.

5. Olin JW, Cressman MD, Young JR, Hoogwerf BJ, Weinstein CE. Lipid and lipoprotein abnormalities in lower-extremity arteriosclerosis obliterans. *Cleve Clin J Med.* 1992;59:491–497.

6. Olin JW, Melia M, Young JR, Graor RA, Risius B. Prevalence of atherosclerotic renal artery stenosis in patients with atherosclerosis elsewhere. *Am J Med.* 1990;88:46N–51N.

7. Radack K, Deck C. Beta-adrenergic blocker therapy does not worsen intermittent claudication in subjects with peripheral arterial disease: a meta-analysis of randomized controlled trials. *Arch Intern Med.* 1991;151:1769–1776.

8. Roberts DH, Tsao Y, McLoughlin GA, Breckenridge A. Placebo-controlled comparison of captopril, atenolol, labetalol, and pindolol in hypertension complicated by intermittent claudication. *Lancet.* 1987;2:650–653.

9. Vogt MT, Cauley JA, Newman AB, Kuller LH, Hulley SB. Decreased ankle/arm blood pressure index and mortality in elderly women. *JAMA.* 1993;270:465–469.

10. Working Group on Management of Patients with Hypertension and High Blood Pressure. National Education Programs Work Group Report on the management of patients with hypertension and high blood cholesterol. *Ann Intern Med.* 1991;114:224–237.

Chapter 143

Management of Minority Patients With Hypertension

Keith C. Ferdinand, MD

KEY POINTS

- The prevalence of hypertension in various minority populations is greatly affected by socioeconomic status and lifestyle habits.

- Minority populations benefit from culturally sensitive educational interventions for prevention of hypertension and assistance with blood pressure control.

- Blacks in the U.S. have hypertension rates among the highest in the world, with greater degrees of target-organ damage, including end-stage renal disease, stroke mortality, and heart disease mortality.

- It is important not to use race or ethnicity as a marker for poor response to any antihypertensive agent and also important to recognize evidence-based survival advantages.

See also Chapters 87, 88

The United States is an increasingly diverse nation of individuals from various racial and ethnic origins. In 1990, the US population was 0.8% American Indians, Aleuts, and Inuits; 2.9% Asians and Pacific Islanders; 9% persons of Hispanic origin; 12.1% blacks; and 80.3% US whites (US Census Bureau by self report). The United States has experienced a continued growth in the number of immigrants in the past decade, and a continued marked increase in minority populations is expected. Although race and ethnicity are useful categories for social scientists and demographers, they are usually without any documented biological or physiological markers. In virtually all racial groups, there is a demonstrated rise in blood pressure with age, and hypertension is largely attributable to potentially modifiable risk factors, such as increased body mass index. Hypertension prevention and treatment, therefore, should focus on shared environment and lifestyle habits.

Hispanics

Hispanics are heterogeneous with regard to racial origins. Overall, they have higher rates of unemployment and lower educational attainment and income levels than the general population. Blood pressure control rates in Mexican Americans are among the lowest in the United States. Low socioeconomic status is compounded by language barriers, which may affect preventive and primary health care. However, despite a greater prevalence of obesity and diabetes, the prevalence of hypertension in the Hispanic population is generally lower than in the general population. Management should therefore include careful risk assessment and appropriate therapy. Because of the high prevalence of diabetes, educational materials using a bilingual format and focusing on diabetes could be helpful for Hispanics.

Asians

Two thirds of Asian Americans and Pacific Islanders in 1990 were foreign born, with many recent immigrants and the highest percent-

age of any ethnic group with <5 years of education. Obesity is very high in native Hawaiians and American Samoans. For recent immigrants, emphasis on lifestyle modification and overcoming limited English language skills is important. Asian Indian immigrants have higher rates of type 2 diabetes and insulin resistance than other ethnic groups, with increased coronary heart disease in men. Management should therefore include careful evaluation of glucose tolerance and cardiac status. Asian Americans may respond to lower doses of antihypertensive drugs than are needed in other ethnic groups.

Native Americans

American Indians (Native Americans) and Alaskan natives experience adverse socioeconomic conditions, lower educational levels, higher unemployment, and lower income than other ethnic groups. Among some Native American populations, hypertension is associated with obesity, age, and diabetes. Early detection and prevention is very important to diminish the effects of untreated hypertension, including increased cardiovascular mortality. No studies currently demonstrate increased efficacy of a particular drug type.

Blacks

The prevalence of hypertension among American blacks is among the highest in the world. Blacks develop hypertension earlier in life and have higher rates of stage 3 hypertension than other ethnic groups. There is a greater increase in target-organ damage, including 320% increase in hypertension-related end-stage renal disease, 80% higher stroke mortality rates, and 50% higher heart disease rate.

Various biochemical and endocrine characteristics of black hypertensives have been suggested. However, a recent study in seven populations of West African descent, including African, Caribbean, and US populations, that used a highly standardized protocol demonstrated a consistent effect of environmental factors, most notably obesity and a high urinary sodium-to-potassium ratio, as strong predictors of hypertension prevalence.

In blacks as well as in whites diuretics are a first pharmacological step in the absence of conditions that prohibit their use. Many blacks require multidrug therapy. The addition of a diuretic should be considered in any drug regimen in which there is poor control. Calcium channel blockers effectively lower blood pressure in blacks, although these agents have no reports of decreased mortality and morbidity in this ethnic group. β-Blockers, angiotensin-converting enzyme inhibitors, and angiotensin receptor blockers are less effective as antihypertensive monotherapy in blacks. Diuretic therapy, however, increases the efficacy of these drugs in blacks to equal that seen in whites. Nevertheless, ACE inhibitors are attractive choices in blacks because of their higher rates of end-organ damage, especially renal disease with diabetic nephropathy, left ventricular systolic dysfunction, and heart failure. Both ACE inhibitors and β-blockers are specifically indicated, regardless of ethnicity, when heart failure or coronary artery disease is present. Blacks may have increased sensitivity to bradykinin and therefore have increased rates of cough and angioedema when treated with ACE inhibitors. α + β-Blockers remain effective antihypertensive drugs in blacks.

When blacks are treated aggressively, their blood pressure response is equal to that of whites, with a greater overall reduction in cardiovascular disease. In blacks with renal insufficiency and urinary protein excretion >1 g/d, a target blood pressure equivalent to 125/75 mm Hg can be achieved safely and may decrease the progression of renal failure. However, blacks are often not treated effectively until blood pressure has been elevated for a prolonged period and target-organ damage is already present. Lifestyle interventions should be administered in a culturally competent manner, with appropriate resources to overcome barriers to compliance.

Dietary customs, including cultural identification with high-salt, high-fat meals, greater acceptance of the obese female, and decreased levels of exercise, may be a causative factor in poor blood pressure control in blacks. Salt sensitivity, which increases with age and perhaps with body weight and is largely heritable, has been demonstrated in as much as 75% of hypertensive black patients. Sodium restriction augments the reduction in blood pressure in most of these patients. Interestingly, one study in blacks showed a significant decrease in systolic and diastolic blood pressure at 3 months with relaxation therapy. Social, cultural, and socioeconomic factors most likely explain the excess hypertension rates in blacks, rather than any postulated genetic determinants.

Although for some purposes it may be useful to classify members of the population on the basis of race or ethnicity, it is important not to use these categories as markers for poor response to an antihypertensive agent and also to recognize evidence-based survival advantages.

SUGGESTED READING

1. Chen MF, Chen CC, Chen WJ, Wu CC, Liau CS, Lee YT. Dose titration study of isradipine in Chinese patients with mild to moderate essential hypertension. *Cardiovasc Drugs Ther.* 1993;7:133–138.
2. Cooper R. A note on the biologic concepts of race and its application in epidemiologic research. *Am Heart J.* 1984;108:715–722.
3. Crespo CJ, Loria CM, Burt VL. Hypertension and other cardiovascular risk factors among Mexican Americans, Cuban Americans, and Puerto Ricans from the Hispanic Health and Nutritional Examination Survey. *Public Health Rep.* 1996;111 (suppl 2):7–10.
4. Enas EA, Garg A, Davidson MA, Nair VM, Huet BA, Yusef S. Coronary heart disease and its risk factors in first-generation immigrant Asian Indians to the United States of America. *Indian Heart J.* 1996;48:343–353.
5. Falkner B. Differences in blacks and whites with essential hypertension: biochemistry and endocrine. *Hypertension.* 1990;15:681–686.
6. Havas S, Sherwin R. Putting it all together: summary of the NHLBI workshop on the epidemiology of hypertension in Hispanic American, Native American, and Asian/Pacific Islander American populations. *Public Health Rep.* 1996;111(suppl 2):77–79.
7. Howard BV. Blood pressure in 13 American Indian communities: the Strong Heart Study. *Public Health Rep.* 1996;111(suppl 2):47–48.
8. Lazarus JM, Bourgoignie JJ, Buckalew VM, Greene T, Levey AS, Milas NC, Paranandi L, Peterson JC, Porush JG, Rauch S, Soucie JM, Stollar C. Achievement and safety of a low blood pressure goal in chronic renal disease: the Modification of Diet in Renal Disease Study Group. *Hypertension.* 1997;29:641–650.
9. Svetkey LP, McKeown SP, Wilson AF. Heritability of salt sensitivity in black Americans. *Hypertension.* 1996;28:854–858.
10. The National Heart, Lung, and Blood Institute. *Latino Community Cardiovascular Disease Prevention and Outreach Initiative: Background Report.* Washington, DC: National Institutes of Health; March 1996.

Chapter 144

Management of the Obese Hypertensive Patient

Efrain Reisin, MD

KEY POINTS

- Obesity—specifically central adiposity—is an important determinant of hypertension.

- An understanding of the metabolic, endocrinological, and hemodynamic mechanisms of obesity-induced hypertension is essential to determine the best approach to the treatment of hypertension in the obese population.

- Moderate weight reduction of ≈ 20 pounds in obese hypertensive patients is an effective and well-tolerated long-term treatment for reducing blood pressure and correcting some of the abnormalities that occur in these individuals.

- If a pharmacological approach to obesity-induced hypertension is necessary, ACE inhibitors, calcium antagonists, and α-adrenergic receptor blocking agents may offer an efficient and safe antihypertensive effect.

See also Chapters 46, 47, 93, 94

Past studies have found that obesity—specifically central adiposity—is a strong determinant of hypertension. Recent reports reveal important differences in the metabolic, endocrinological, and hemodynamic mechanisms of obesity-induced hypertension and also have described cardiac and renal changes effected by obesity-induced hypertension. An understanding of these mechanisms and the related morphological changes is essential to determine the best approach to the treatment of hypertension in obese patients.

Mechanisms of Obesity-Induced Hypertension
Fluid Volume Distribution and Systemic Hemodynamic Changes

Compared with lean hypertensives, patients with obesity-induced hypertension have a higher absolute total blood volume that is redistributed chiefly in the cardiopulmonary area. This leads to augmented venous return and higher cardiac output, yet total peripheral resistance in obese hypertensives remains "inappropriately" normal. However, when hypertension is associated with but not induced by obesity, total peripheral resistance was found to be elevated.

Insulin Resistance

The large accumulation of lipolytic hyperactive abdominal cells and the release of large amounts of free fatty acids into the portal vein in obese persons cause excessive hepatic synthesis of triglycerides, inhibition of insulin intake, hyperinsulinemia, and insulin resistance. Insulin increases absorption of sodium in the diluting segment of the distal nephron, with consequent water retention, and it also increases adrenergic activity. These mechanisms link hyperinsulinemia and insulin resistance to the development of hypertension. Although some authors have found a correlation only between the characteristics of hyperinsulinemia, insulin resistance, and elevated blood pressure in obese individuals, they do not believe that a cause-and-effect relationship has been clearly established, nor do they support the concept that hyperinsulinemia is a major cause of hypertension.

Sympathetic Nervous System Activity

Chronic overeating may induce adrenergic stimulation via increased insulin concentration, which increases the reactivity of tissues to catecholamines. However, most investigators have not proved that the catecholamine level or sympathetic activity is greater in obese individuals than they are in the nonobese.

Na$^+$,K$^+$-ATPase

Obese hypertensives may have increased concentrations of sodium in their cells, as demonstrated by changes in sodium levels in erythrocytes. This defect may be induced by Na$^+$,K$^+$-ATPase inhibitors that decrease calcium efflux and increase both intracellular calcium and sodium concentrations, changes that may enhance smooth muscle tone and vascular resistance.

Plasma Renin Activity and Serum Aldosterone Levels

Opinions differ concerning the changes in the renin-angiotensin-aldosterone system that occur in obese hypertensive patients. Some investigators believe that the level of plasma renin activity is not abnormally high but that hyperaldosteronism occurs instead and triggers sodium and water retention in obese hypertensive patients, with consequent hypervolemia and increased cardiac output.

Cardiac and Renal Changes

In obese individuals, chamber dilatation prompts the myocardium to adapt by adding contractile elements in series. When hypertension occurs in obese patients, the myocardium restores wall stress to a normal level by thickening, a process that adds contractile elements in parallel. Consequently, the presence of obesity-hypertension will induce both eccentric and concentric left ventricular hypertrophy, a pathological process that may increase the risk for congestive heart failure.

Compared with lean patients, obese individuals, whether or not they are hypertensive, have elevated renal blood flow, an increased glomerular filtration rate, and a higher filtered sodium load, all changes that induce glomerular hyperfiltration with hyperfunction and increased proteinuria. These hemodynamic renal characteristics increase glomerular volume and may also induce changes in the renal medulla that elevate intrarenal pressure and shift pressure natriuresis to higher blood pressure, a hemodynamic change that is necessary to maintain sodium balance.

Weight Reduction in the Management of Obesity-Induced Hypertension

Several studies of large numbers of patients have shown that weight reduction is an effective and well-tolerated long-term treatment for reducing blood pressure in obese patients with hypertension, regardless of race or sex. Weight loss is also a very important tool in the prevention of cardiovascular complications.

Mechanistic and Morphological Changes Induced by Weight Reduction

Moderate weight loss (20 pounds) in obese hypertensives decreases intravascular volume and reduces cardiac output and left ventricular work but does not change total peripheral resistance. Echocardiographic studies done after weight loss have shown a decrease in interventricular septum and posterior wall thickness and in left ventricular mass. Weight reduction reduces plasma insulin levels by increasing the number of insulin receptors and the affinity of those receptors for insulin. In addition, sympathetic activity is reduced, which, in turn, conserves calories by diminishing metabolism and heat production. The effects of weight reduction on plasma renin activity, plasma aldosterone levels, and Na^+,K^+-ATPase activity are still controversial, but several investigators have reported decreased plasma renin activity, plasma aldosterone levels, and intracellular sodium levels after weight loss. **Figure 144.1** outlines the physiological changes that are linked to weight reduction.

Compliance With the Weight-Loss Approach

Some studies suggest that dropout rates in weight-loss programs range from 50% to 70% within 1 to 2 years. Consequently, the American Dietetic Association is refocusing its recommendations from weight loss alone to weight management, which is defined as "the adoption of healthful and sustainable eating and exercise behaviors indicated for reduced disease risk and improved feelings of energy and well being." The association recommends that to enhance long-term maintenance of goals, all weight management programs should include the following: (1) a gradual change to a healthful eating style, with increased intake of whole grain, fruits, and vegetables; (2) a nonrestrictive approach to eating based on internal regulation of food (hunger and satiety); and (3) gradual increase to at least 30 minutes of physical activity each day.

Pharmacological Interventions

In patients with initial moderate or severe hypertension or in those unable to lose weight, a pharmacological approach to obesity-induced hypertension that meets the specific requirements of this complex pathological condition is recommended. **Table 144.1** outlines the potential benefits and side effects of selected pharmacological approaches to hypertension in the obese hypertensive patient.

Diuretics

Hydrochlorothiazide (HCTZ) and other diuretics lead to decreased intravascular and extracellular fluid volume and decreased cardiac output and total peripheral resistance, which may lower blood pressure. A recent large prospective cooperative study that compared the use of HCTZ with lisinopril in obese hypertensive subjects demonstrated that HCTZ significantly reduced systolic and diastolic blood pressure in obese hypertensive patients, but nearly half of these patients (46%) required the highest dose (50 mg/d) to maintain blood pressure control. HCTZ therapy was more effective in blacks than in whites. Treatment increased plasma glucose and significantly reduced serum potassium levels after 12 weeks of therapy, and when long-term therapy is necessary, the high doses required to control blood pressure may generate more side effects.

Adrenergic Blocking Agents

Adrenergic blocking agents reduce blood pressure by lowering cardiac and sympathetic activity. Consequently, they may be effective

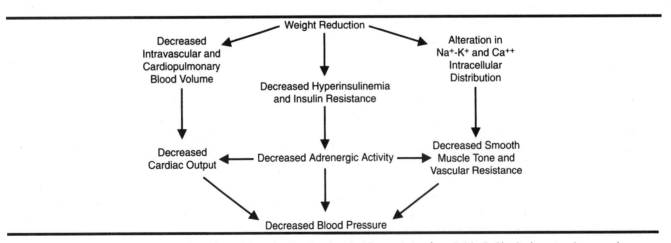

Figure 144.1.   Physiological changes induced by weight reduction. Reprinted with permission from Reisin E. Obesity hypertension: nonpharmacologic and pharmacologic therapeutic modalities. In: Laragh JH, Brenner BM, eds. *Hypertension: Pathophysiology, Diagnosis and Management.* New York, NY: Raven Press; 1995:2683–2691. Originally modified with permission from Reisin E, Frohlich ED. Hemodynamics in obesity. In: Zanchetti A, Tarazi RC, eds. *Handbook of Hypertension.* New York, NY: Elsevier; 1987:280–297.

Table 144.1. Potential Benefits and Side Effects of Antihypertensive Drugs in Obesity Hypertension

DRUG CLASS	POTENTIAL BENEFITS IN OBESE HYPERTENSIVES	POTENTIAL SIDE EFFECTS IN OBESE HYPERTENSIVES
Diuretics	Diuresis, natriuresis; decreased cardiac output and total peripheral resistance	Increased triglycerides, LDL, and VLDL; decreased insulin sensitivity
β-Blockers	Decreased cardiac output and sympathetic nervous system tone	Increased triglycerides; decreased HDL and insulin sensitivity
Centrally acting agents	Decreased total peripheral resistance and sympathetic nervous system tone	Decreased fatty acid mobilization; fatigue, sedation; interference with weight loss
α_1-Blockers	Decreased total cholesterol, VLDL, triglycerides, and insulin resistance; vasodilation	Orthostatic hypotension
Calcium antagonists	Natriuresis; decreased total peripheral resistance and left ventricular mass; improved insulin metabolism	Edema
ACE inhibitors	Decreased total peripheral resistance and left ventricular mass; increased insulin sensitivity	Cough, angioedema

Adapted with permission from Richards RJ, et al. Obesity-related hypertension. *J Hum Hypertens.* 1996;10:S59–S64.

in controlling hypertension in obese patients. Two different studies of metoprolol yielded conflicting results, with only one demonstrating efficacy in lowering blood pressure via doses of up to 100 mg/d. Another cardioselective agent, atenolol, also has a beneficial effect on blood pressure. However, the use of these agents is not without potential problems, because they may reduce glucose tolerance and induce worsening of insulin resistance.

Centrally Acting Agents

Centrally acting agents have been shown to inhibit the release of epinephrine as well as the cardiac response to postganglionic adrenergic nerve stimulation. A study that sought to compare the effect of clonidine, a centrally acting α-adrenergic stimulator, with that of a diuretic concluded that the diuretic was more effective than clonidine in obese hypertensive subjects.

α-Adrenergic Receptor Blockers

α-Adrenergic receptor blocking agents may reduce the early insulin response and increase insulin sensitivity. An early study in a small number of obese hypertensive subjects showed that prazosin, an α_1-adrenergic receptor blocking agent, significantly reduced blood pressure, increased insulin-mediated glucose disposal, and decreased the insulin response to an intravenous glucose load. A study that included a large number of obese hypertensives treated with doxazosin monotherapy showed a beneficial effect on blood pressure in those subjects.

Calcium Antagonists

The calcium antagonists are a heterogeneous group of drugs that reduce blood pressure by reducing peripheral vascular resistance, and some of them may also promote natriuresis. Calcium antagonists apparently do not affect insulin sensitivity. A large study with

nifedipine in obese hypertensive patients showed a 70% to 80% rate of efficacy in controlling blood pressure.

ACE Inhibitors

Among other effects, ACE inhibitors block the renin-angiotensin-aldosterone system. They reduce total peripheral vascular resistance and may improve insulin sensitivity, reverse increased left ventricular mass, and protect the kidneys from adverse effects. A large, prospective cooperative study previously mentioned showed that compared with HCTZ, lisinopril effectively lowered systolic and diastolic blood pressure in obese hypertensive subjects. Treatment with lisinopril may show greater efficacy as monotherapy at lower doses than HCTZ; lisinopril also was more effective in white than in black subjects and may generate a more rapid rate of response with fewer side effects.

SUGGESTED READING

1. Reisin E. Obesity hypertension: nonpharmacologic and pharmacologic therapeutic modalities. In: Laragh JH, Brenner BM, eds. *Hypertension: Pathophysiology, Diagnosis and Management.* New York, NY: Raven Press; 1995:2683–2691.
2. Hall JE. Louis K. Dahl Memorial Lecture: Renal and cardiovascular mechanisms of hypertension in obesity. *Hypertension.* 1994;23:381–394.
3. Reisin E, Abel R, Modan M, Silverberg DS, Eliahou HE, Modan B. Effect of weight loss without salt restriction on the reduction of blood pressure in overweight hypertensive patients. *N Engl J Med.* 1978;298:1–5.
4. Davis BR, Blaufox MD, Oberman A, Wassertheil-Smoller S, Zimbaldi N, Cutler JA, Kirchner K, Langford HG. Reduction in long-term antihypertensive medication requirements: effects of weight reduction by dietary intervention in overweight persons with mild hypertension. *Arch Intern Med.* 1993;153:1773–1782.
5. Cummings MS, Kenneth Goodrick G, Foreyt JP. Position of the American Dietetic Association: weight management. *J Am Diet Assoc.* 1997;97:71–74.
6. Reisin E, Weir MR, Falkner B, Hutchinson HG, Anzalone DA, Tuck ML, for the Treatment in Obese Patients With Hypertension (TROPHY) study group. Lisinopril versus hydrochlorothiazide in obese hypertensive patients: a multicenter placebo-controlled trial. *Hypertension.* 1997;30:140–145.

Chapter 145

Management of the Hypertensive Patient with Lipid and Lipoprotein Abnormalities

Michael D. Cressman, DO

KEY POINTS

- Coronary heart disease risk increases progressively as total and low-density lipoprotein cholesterol levels increase.

- Total and high-density lipoprotein cholesterol levels should be measured during the basic laboratory evaluation of all hypertensive patients.

- The presence of hypothyroidism or type II diabetes mellitus should be considered in hypertensive patients who have elevated serum cholesterol or triglyceride levels.

- Cholesterol lowering drug treatment, especially with HMG-CoA reductase inhibitors, has been shown to reduce the risk of stroke and myocardial infarction.

See also Chapters 64, 65, 75, 79, 118

Coronary heart disease (CHD) risk increases progressively as systolic blood pressure, diastolic blood pressure, or total cholesterol (TC) levels increase. The association of systolic blood pressure and TC levels with CHD death rates in the 316 000 middle-aged men free of preexisting CHD who were screened for the Multiple Risk Factor Intervention Trial (MRFIT) is summarized in **Table 145.1.** Thus, a single TC measurement provides information that improves the accuracy of CHD risk assessments in both normotensive and hypertensive patients.

Classification of TC and LDL Cholesterol Levels

Measurement of TC and HDL cholesterol (HDL-C) levels has been recommended by the second Adult Treatment Panel (ATP-II) of the National Cholesterol Education Program (NCEP) for all adults ≥20 years old. Initial classification of TC and HDL-C is summarized in **Table 145.2.** This information is used in an overall assessment of CHD risk, which uses risk factors other than LDL cholesterol (LDL-C) and HDL-C as well as a classification based on the presence or absence of clinical manifestations of atherosclerotic vascular disease. Definitions of the "positive" risk factors are provided in **Table 145.3.** An HDL-C ≥60 mg/dL is considered to be a "negative" risk factor (ie, it confers protection) in the ATP-II risk classification scheme.

Decisions for use of lipid-lowering therapy in an overall cardiovascular risk reduction program require determination of LDL-C levels. These values are calculated from determinations made on a fasting lipid profile, which includes measurements of TC, triglyceride (TG), and HDL-C levels. The formula that is generally used in this calculation is LDL-C = [(TC − HDL-C) − TG/5]. The approach to treatment decisions based on LDL-C levels and CHD status is summarized in **Table 145.4.**

Secondary Causes of Hypercholesterolemia

The most important causes of altered lipoprotein metabolism that occur in hypertensive patients that are correctable include (1) drugs, (2) hypothyroidism, and (3) diabetes mellitus. Drugs that should be considered as potential causes or contributing factors to elevated serum TC, LDL-C, or TG levels include the thiazide-type diuretics, β-adrenergic receptor blocking agents, oral contraceptives (particularly those with a high progestational agent content), and prednisone or other steroid hormones. Obtaining 2 on-treatment and 2 post-treatment lipid profiles (≈4 to 6 weeks after discontinuation of a potentially offending drug) provides a reasonable assessment of the role of antihypertensive or other drugs on blood lipid levels.

Although the effects of antihypertensive drugs (particularly the thiazide diuretics and β-adrenergic receptor blockers) on blood lipid levels have been extensively studied, it is not clear whether any of the lipoprotein changes that occur in patients receiving these agents influence CHD risk. Lasser and coworkers reported the effects of diuretics on TC, TG, HDL-C, and LDL-C levels in men receiving a low-saturated-fat

Table 145.1. Age-Adjusted CHD Death Rates (per 10> 000 Person-Years) by Systolic Blood Pressure and TC Levels in Nonsmoking MRFIT Screencees (12-Year Follow-up)

SYSTOLIC BLOOD PRESSURE, MM HG	TOTAL CHOLESTEROL LEVELS, MG/DL				
	<182	182–202	203–220	221–244	>245
<118	3.1	4.3	5.5	5.9	12.2
118–124	3.4	6.0	6.3	9.6	12.7
125–131	5.6	7.9	8.6	8.3	17.1
132–141	5.0	7.9	10.7	12.3	21.0
≥142	13.7	16.7	17.7	22.6	33.7

Adapted from Marin MJ, Hulley SB, Browner WS, et al. Serum Cholesterol, blood pressure, and mortality: implications from a cohort of 361,662 men. *Lancet.* 1986;2:933–936. Reprinted with permission.

and low-cholesterol diet in the special intervention group of the MRFIT trial. In this study, 1917 participants received diuretics for a period of 6 years. The mean reduction of TC levels in these study participants was 4.3 mg/dL less than that observed in 2537 participants receiving a similar diet but no diuretics. This difference in the cholesterol-lowering response to diet was largely explained by the increase in VLDL-C concentrations (rather than LDL-C levels) in participants receiving diuretics. Thus, changes in LDL-C levels were similar in participants who received or did not receive a diuretic during the currently recommended dietary approach to treatment of hypercholesterolemia.

The effect of β-blockers on blood lipids depends on the type of β-blocker used; β-blockers with intrinsic sympathomimetic activity and those with α-receptor blocking do not affect blood lipid levels. The effects of 1 year of treatment with propranolol on TC and TG levels were reported in more than 100 patients in a Veterans Administration multicenter study. Although no significant change in TC levels was observed, TG values increased by 42 mg/dL.

Nonpharmacological Therapy for Hypertensive Patients With Hypercholesterolemia (Table 145.4)

The principal nutritional goals for hypercholesterolemic hypertensive patients are shown in **Table 145.5**. Alcohol intake should be restricted to <2 oz/d of ethanol, and sodium intake should be <2 g/d. These measures, combined with reduction of total fat, saturated fat, and cholesterol intake, may be particularly beneficial and should be especially encouraged in hypertensive patients who have hypercholesterolemia. Although many patients find it difficult to make dietary and other lifestyle changes, the clinician should still provide appropriate counseling and/or referral to facilities in which information related to lifestyle changes can be obtained.

Pharmacological Treatment of Hypercholesterolemia in the Hypertensive Patient (Table 145.4)

No major alteration in the currently recommended approach to pharmacological management of hypercholesterolemia in adults is required in patients with coexisting hypertension. The patient's overall cardiovascular risk status is the most important factor to consider in selection of candidates for lipid-altering drug treatment. In addition, the LDL-C–lowering goal of treatment depends primarily on whether the patient has or does not have preexisting evidence of advanced atherosclerosis.

The concept that lowering LDL-C levels reduces CHD risk, slows progression of established coronary artery lesions, and decreases the risk of developing new coronary artery lesions has been firmly established. Clinical trials of LDL-C treatment using certain 3-hydroxy-3-methylglutaryl coenzyme A (HMG-CoA) reductase inhibitors (lovastatin, pravastatin, or simvastatin) have also shown reductions in the risk of stroke. Evidence of these benefits is particularly strong in the population of patients with established CHD. This justifies the recommendation to be particularly aggressive with cholesterol-lowering therapy in the CHD patient population.

HMG-CoA reductase inhibitors (lovastatin, pravastatin, simvastatin, fluvastatin, atorvastatin) have become the cornerstone of

Table 145.2. Classification of TC and HDL-C Levels in Adults

INITIAL CLASSIFICATION	TC	HDL-C
Desirable blood cholesterol	<200 mg/dL	
Borderline-high blood cholesterol	200–239 mg/dL	
High blood cholesterol	≥240 mg/dL	
Low HDL-C		<35 mg/dL

Adapted from the ATP-II guidelines. *JAMA.* 1993; 269:3015–3023.

Table 145.3. Risk Status Based on Presence of CHD Risk Factors Other Than LDL Cholesterol

POSITIVE RISK FACTORS

Age
  Male ≥45 years
  Female ≥55 years or premature menopause without estrogen replacement therapy
Family history of premature CHD (definite myocardial infarction or sudden death before 55 years of age in father or other male first-degree relative or before 65 years of age in mother or other female first-degree relative)
Current cigarette smoking
Hypertension (blood pressure ≥140/90 mm Hg or taking antihypertensive medication)
Low HDL cholesterol (<35 mg/dL [0.9 mmol/L])
Diabetes mellitus

Adapted from the ATP-II guidelines. *JAMA.* 1993;269:3015–3023.

Table 145.4. Treatment Decisions Based on LDL Levels and CHD Status

PATIENT CATEGORY	INITIATION LEVEL, MG/DL (MMOL/L)	LDL GOAL, MG/DL (MMOL/L)
Dietary therapy		
Without CHD and with <2 risk factors	≥160 (4.1)	<160 (4.1)
Without CHD and with ≥2 risk factors	≥130 (3.4)	<130 (3.4)
With CHD	≥100 (2.6)	≤100 (2.6)
Drug treatment		
Without CHD and with <2 risk factors	≥190 (4.9)	<160 (4.1)
Without CHD and with ≥2 risk factors	≥160 (4.1)	<130 (3.4)
With CHD	≥130 (3.4)	≤100 (2.6)

Adapted from the ATP-II guidelines. *JAMA.* 1993;269:3015–3023.

Table 145.5. Nutritional Guidelines for Management of Hypertensive Patients with Hypercholesterolemia

	NUTRITIONAL GOALS
Total calories	Body weight within 15% of desirable weight
Alcohol	<2 oz/d ethanol
Sodium	<2 g/d
Total fat	<30% of total calories
Saturated fat	<10% of total calories
Cholesterol	<300 mg/d

Table 145.6. Comparison of Lipid-Lowering Effects and Cost of HMG-CoA Reductase Inhibitors Across a Typically Used Dose Range

DRUG	DOSE, MG	LDL-C, %	TG, %	AWP COST/D, $
Lovastatin	20–40	−(24–34)	−(10–16)	2.24–4.04
Pravastatin	20–40	−(32–34)	−(11–24)	1.89–3.19
Simvastatin	5–40	−(24–40)	−(10–19)	1.78–3.67
Fluvastatin	20–40	−(25–31)	−(10–11)	1.21–1.36
Atorvastatin	10–40	−(39–50)	−(19–29)	1.82–3.40
Cerivastatin	0.3	−28	−13	1.32

Adapted from Kellick et al. *Formulary.* 1997; 32:352–363.

cholesterol-lowering drug therapy because of their favorable tolerability profile and unparalleled efficacy in lowering LDL-C levels. Comparisons of the lipid-lowering effects and cost of the currently marketed statins through their typically prescribed dose range are given in **Table 145.6.** The most feared complication of treatment with the HMG-CoA reductase inhibitors is rhabdomyolysis. Although this is uncommon when these agents are administered alone, coadministration of drugs such as cyclosporine, erythromycin, gemfibrozil, niacin, and the calcium channel blocker mibefradil have been shown to increase the risk of development of rhabdomyolysis.

The bile acid sequestrants nicotinic acid and the fibric acid derivative gemfibrozil now have a limited role in the therapeutic armamentarium for management of patients with dyslipidemia. It should be recognized that the HMG-CoA reductase inhibitors are primarily LDL-lowering agents although they do tend to reduce TG and raise HDL concentrations. In contrast, gemfibrozil reduces TGs and raises HDL but is only modestly effective in reducing LDL concentrations. The unfavorable side effect profiles of the bile acid sequestrants and niacin severely limit their use in the management of most patients.

SUGGESTED READING

1. Ginsberg HN. Update on the treatment of hypercholesterolemia, with a focus on HMG-CoA reductase inhibitors and combination regimens. *Clin Cardiol.* 1995;18: 307–315.
2. Gotto AM. Statin therapy and reduced Incidence of stroke: implications of cholesterol-lowering therapy for cerebrovascular disease. *Arch Intern Med.* 1997; 157: 1283–1284.
3. Gotto AM. Results of recent large cholesterol-lowering trials and implications for clinical management. *Am J Cardiol.* 1997; 79:1663–1666.
4. Kellick KA, Burns K, McAndrew E, Haberl E, Hook N, Ellis, AK. Focus on atorvastatin: an HMG-CoA reductase inhibitor for lowering both elevated LDL cholesterol and triglycerides in hypercholesterolemic patients. *Formulary.* 1997;32:352–363.
5. Neaton JD, Wentworth D, for the Multiple Risk Factor Intervention Trial Research Group. Serum cholesterol, blood pressure, cigarette smoking, and death from coronary heart disease: overall findings and differences by age for 316,099 white men. *Arch Intern Med.* 1992;152:56–64.
6. Lasser NL, Grandits G, Caggiula AW, Cutler JA, Grimm RH Jr, Kuller LH, Sherwin RW, Stamler J. Effects of antihypertensive therapy on plasma lipids and lipoproteins in the Multiple Risk Factor Intervention Trial. *Am J Med.* 1984;76:52–66.
7. Summary of the second report of the National Cholesterol Education Program (NCEP) Expert Panel on Detection, Evaluation, and Treatment of High Blood Cholesterol in Adults (Adult Treatment Panel II). *JAMA.* 1993;269:3015–3023.
8. Veterans Administration Cooperative Study Group on Antihypertensive Agents. Comparison of propranolol and hydrochlorothiazide for the initial treatment of hypertension. II: results of long-term therapy. *JAMA.* 1982;248:2004–2011.

Chapter 146

Management of Hypertensive Patients With Diabetic Nephropathy

George L. Bakris, MD

KEY POINTS

- Diabetes and hypertension are the two most common causes of renal failure in patients starting renal replacement therapy (dialysis) in the United States.

- Blood pressure in diabetic patients should be reduced to levels substantially below 130/85 mm Hg to maximally preserve renal function.

- Goals of therapy are to normalize blood pressure and reduce renal and cardiovascular morbidity and mortality.

- Reduction of blood pressure by use of combinations of ACE inhibitors, nondihydropyridine calcium antagonists, and diuretics provides the best overall protection against nephropathy progression.

See also Chapters 74, 78, 141

More than two thirds of patients starting renal replacement therapy (dialysis) in the United States have hypertension with or without diabetes. Hypertension accelerates the progression of diabetic renal disease and increases associated cardiovascular events (stroke, myocardial infarction). Thus, the most common cause of death in these patients results from cardiovascular causes. Reduction of blood pressure to levels <140/90 mm Hg slows nephropathy progression and reduces cardiovascular events. However, recent data support the concept that patients with diabetic nephropathy require blood pressure reduction to levels <130/85 mm Hg to maximally slow nephropathy progression; this may require multiple antihypertensive drugs as well as lifestyle modifications.

Antihypertensive drugs have varied effects on risk factors that predict adverse renal and cardiovascular outcomes **(Table 146.1).** Combinations of certain antihypertensive drug classes, however, minimize adverse effects on metabolic, cardiovascular, and renal markers of cardiovascular and renal disease outcome.

The vascular and intrarenal effects of antihypertensive medications should also be considered when they are selected to lower blood pressure **(Table 146.2).** Antihypertensive agents such as ACE inhibitors, angiotensin II receptor blockers (ARBs), and nondihydropyridine calcium antagonists (non-DHPCAs) such as verapamil or diltiazem attenuate both the morphological progression (mesangial matrix expansion) and accentuated glomerular membrane permeability associated with diabetic renal disease (Table 146.2). Moreover, only ACE inhibitors and ARBs reduce intraglomerular pressure, whereas CAs do not (Table 146.2). CAs produce outcome differences in renal morphology as summarized in **Table 146.3.**

In addition to race and ethnicity, a number of preexisting conditions can also influence selection of antihypertensive medications in diabetic patients **(Table 146.4).** Blacks do not have the same antihypertensive response to a given dose of an ACE inhibitor or ARB as whites. However, ACE inhibitors should not be denied to this patient group. Rather, these patients should be started on higher-than-usual

---

Table 146.1. Effects of Antihypertensive Therapy on Metabolic, Cardiovascular, and Renal Markers Associated with Increased Morbidity and/or Mortality in the Patient With Diabets and Hypertension

	CENTRAL AGONISTS	α-BLOCKERS	α, β-BLOCKER	VASODILATOR	β-BLOCKERS	ACEI	ARBS	CAS	DIURETICS
Metabolic									
Cholesterol (LDL)	→	→	→	→	→↑*	→	→	→	→↑
Insulin resistance	→	↓	→↑	→↑	→↑	↓	↓	→	→↑
Glucose control	→	→	→	→	→↓	→↑	→	↑*→	→↓
Cardiovascular									
Left ventricular hypertrophy	↓	↓	↓	→↑	↓	↓	↓	↓	→↓
Renal									
Microalbuminuria	→	→	→↓	→	→↓	↓	↓	↓†→	→↓

ACEI indicates ACE inhibitor; ARB, angiotenisn II receptor antagonist; →, no effect; ↑, increase; and ↓, decrease. Note, this table summarizes the general trends in the literature.
Only β-blockers with intrinsic sympathomimetic activity; only when used in high doses (eg, 480 mg/d diliazem, 480 mg/d verapamil, 90 mg/d nifedipine).
†Only nondihydrophyridine calcium antagonists (CA's, verapamil, diltiazem).

Table 146.2. Intrarenal and Vascular Alterations in the Diabetic Hypertensive Patient With Associated Effects of Antihypertensive Agents*

	ANTIHYPERTENSIVE EFFECT ON ALTERATIONS	
PATHOPHYSIOLOGICAL ALTERATIONS	REVERSE OR IMPROVE	POTENTIATE OR WORSEN
Increases in		
Vascular		
Vascular reactivity	ARBs, ACEI, CAs	None
Intrarenal		
Intraglomerular pressure	ARBs, ACEI, ?non-DHPCAs	None ?DHPCAs
Glomerular volume	?ARBs, ACEI, CAs	None
Mesangial matrix	?ARBs, ACEI, non-DHPCAs	DHPCAs (no effect)
		α-blocker (no effect)
Glomerular capillary permeability	ACEI, ARBs, non-DHPCAs	DHPCAs (no effect)
		?Minoxidil, ?hydralazine
Decreases in		
Intrarenal		
Natriuretic response to hormones	ACEI, CAs, diuretics	Hydralzaine/minoxidil, β-blockers
Autoregulation	None	DHPCAs (abolish)

ARB indicates angiotensin II receptor blockers; ACEI, ACE inhibitor; CAs, calcium channel blockers; Non-DHPCAs, nondihydrohyridine calcium antagonists (verapamil, diltiazem); and DHPCAs, dihydrophyridine calcium antagonists (amlodipine-like agents).
*These effects occur in addition to blood pressure reduction, some of which may also be independent of blood pressure reduction. These agents generally do not reduce intraglomerular pressure, and only the dihydropyridine-type CAs do not have effects on permeability, because they have no effect on albuminuria.

Table 146.3. Intrarenal Actions of Calcium Antagonists in Animal Models of Diabetes That Help Explain Renal Outcomes

	DIABETES (UNTREATED)	NON-DHPCAS (VERAPAMIL, DILTIAZEM)	DHPCAS (AMLODIPINE-LIKE AGENTS)
Autoregulatory ability	↓	→	(Abolished)
Glomerular membrane permeability	↑	↓	→
Mesangial matrix expansion	↑	↓	→
Transcapillary glomerular pressure	↑	↓*	→

DHPCAs indicates dihydropyridine calcium antagonists; ↓, decreased; ↑, increased; and →, no effect.
*Decreased relative to DHPCAs.

Table 146.4. Factors to Consider Before Selection of Antihypertensive Therapy in the Diabetic Patient

FACTOR	PREFERRED	AVOID
Hyperkalemia	Non-DHPCAs, diuretic, α-blocker	ACEI, β-blockers
Renal failure* (GFR ≤30)	Non-DHPCAs, loop-active diuretic, ACEI with diuretic	High dose ACEIs, ?ARBs
Nephrotic syndrome	Non-DHPCAs, ?loop-active diuretic, ?ARB	Minoxidil, hydralazine, ?α-blockers
Coronary artery disease	ACEI, Non-DHPCAs, β-blockers	Minoxidil, hydralazine
Autonomic neuropathy	Central α-agonists, ?β-blockers	α-Blockers, hydralazine, minoxidil
Microalbuminuria	ARBs, ACEI, non-DHPCAs	DHPCAs, minoxidil, hydralazine
Side-effect profile	ARB, ACEI, CAs	β-Blocker, diuretic, central α-agonists, minoxidil, hydralazine
Peripheral vascular disease	ARBs, ACEI, non-DHPCAs, α-blockers	β-Blockers

GFR indicates glomerular filtration rate; DHPCAs, dihydropyridine calcium antagonists; ACEI, ACE inhibitors; ARBs, angiotensin receptor blockers; and central α-agonists, clonide, methyldopa.
*This population usually need diuretic therapy in addition to other antihypertensive therapy for edema control. All CAs increase renal blood flow in early diabetes, which may not be of benefit. Only non-DHPCAs agents have been shown to consistently decrease albuminuria.

doses, eg, 20 mg of benazapril or enalapril. If blood pressure is subsequently not controlled, a non-DHPCA or low-dose diuretic should be added. If renal insufficiency or significant edema is present, diuretics are preferred as the second choice.

Several small (n<50), randomized, long-term (≥3 years) studies in patients with diabetic nephropathy demonstrate that if an ACE inhibitor is included in the "antihypertensive cocktail" and adequate blood pressure reduction is achieved, renal disease progression is slowed by 40% to 60% compared with a control group that received no ACE inhibition. Seven different large-scale, long-term, randomized, clinical studies in patients with diabetic nephropathy confirm this observation. Moreover, studies that compared CAs with ACE inhibitors report differences in renal outcome, depending on the CA used. More precisely, in patients with renal insufficiency (serum creatinine values between 1.4 and 3.1 mg/dL), blood pressure control regardless of agents used will slow renal disease progression. However, non-DHPCAs and ACE inhibitors provide relatively greater benefits on both slowing the rate of decline in renal function and reducing albuminuria compared with other agents.

Reduction in proteinuria strongly correlates with a slowed progression of diabetic nephropathy. Fixed-dose combinations of an ACE inhibitor with a non-DHPCA have additive antiproteinuric effects. Fixed doses of an ACE inhibitor/DHPCA in combination reduce proteinuria to the same degree as ACE inhibition alone. Renal outcome data with any combination agent, however, are lacking.

The key to slowing progression of diabetic nephropathy rests with appropriate blood pressure reduction by use of agents shown to be "renoprotective" such as ACE inhibitors. Not all agents, however, have been extensively studied in this regard. No long-term data on "renoprotection" are available with central α-agonists, α-blockers, or α,β-blockers. With the exception of the long-acting α-blockers, however, these drugs are generally poorly tolerated. Furthermore, no specific intrarenal effects have been observed with these agents in animal models of diabetes. Finally, DHPCAs should generally not be used in the absence of an ACE inhibitor in patients with diabetic nephropathy. This recommendation results from clinical trial data showing that DHPCAs do not reduce the rate of cardiovascular or renal morbid events in patients with diabetic nephropathy.

SUGGESTED READING

1. Bakris GL, Mehler P, Schrier R. Hypertension and diabetes. In: Schrier RW, Gottschalk CW, eds. *Diseases of the Kidney.* 6th ed. Boston, Mass: Little Brown & Co; 1996:1455–1464.

2. Bakris GL, Weir, MR, Sowers JR. Therapeutic challenges in the obese diabetic patient with hypertension. *Am J Med.* 1996;101:33S–46S.

3. Bakris GL. Combination therapy for hypertension and renal disease in diabetes. In: Mogensen CE, ed. *The Kidney and Hypertension in Diabetes Mellitus.* 4th ed. Boston, Mass: Kluwer Academic Publishers; in press.

4. Bakris GL. Pathogenesis of hypertension in diabetes. *Diabetes Rev.* 1995;3: 460–476.

5. National High Blood Pressure Education Program Working Group. 1995 update of the working group reports on chronic renal failure and renovascular hypertension. *Arch Intern Med.* 1996;156:1938–1947.

6. Sixth report of the Joint National Committee on prevention, detection, evaluation, and treatment of high blood pressure (JNC VI). *Arch Intern Med.* 1997;157:2413–2446.

7. Tarif N and Bakris GL Preservation of renal function: the spectrum of effects by calcium-channel blockers. *Nephrol Dial Transplant.* 1997;12:2244–2250.

Chapter 147

Management of Hypertensive Children and Adolescents

Bonita Falkner, MD

KEY POINTS

- Hypertension is not a rare problem in children and adolescents, although its prevalence is lower than in adults.

- Children with severe blood pressure elevation usually have secondary hypertension and therefore warrant careful clinical evaluation.

- Blood pressure levels at the upper limits (95th percentile) for age depict a high-risk condition for developing hypertension.

- The higher the blood pressure and the younger the child, the greater the possibility that the hypertension has a secondary cause.

See also Chapters 56, 65

Hypertension is not a rare clinical problem in children or adolescents, although its prevalence is lower than in adults. Compared with adults, children with severe blood pressure (BP) elevation more often have secondary hypertension and therefore warrant careful clinical evaluation. Essential hypertension in children and adolescents is generally expressed by mild BP elevation and is associated with other risk factors for cardiovascular disease. The management of a child or an adolescent with elevated BP involves a series of clinical decisions that include confirming the presence of high BP, determining the extent of a clinical evaluation for each child, and selecting the most beneficial intervention for optimal BP control. Epidemiological studies on BP and growth in childhood, as well as more frequent measurement of BP in the young, have refined the perspective on individual management.

Detection

Normally there is an increase in BP throughout childhood. Within this normal distribution of BP for age, such factors as weight, height, and maturation also correlate positively with BP. Published standards for BP are helpful in determining whether or not BP is elevated for a given age. BP levels at the upper limits (95th percentile) for age depict a high-risk condition for developing hypertension. BP levels that are consistently 5 to 9 mm Hg above the upper limit constitute mild hypertension in children. BP levels that are consistently ≥10 mm Hg above the upper limit of normal for age reflect significant hypertension in childhood.

BP should be measured during routine health examinations, beginning at 3 years of age. However, a child of any age, including infants, should have his or her BP measured when acutely ill or symptomatic. To avoid measurement error, it is important that the size of the BP cuff is appropriate for the size of the child. Standard guidelines for BP cuff size relative to the length and circumference of the child's arm are available. As a general rule, the widest cuff that will comfortably encircle the upper arm without covering the antecubital fossa should be used in BP measurements on children <10 years of age. In overweight children, as in obese adults, care should be taken to use a cuff that is large enough so that readings are not erroneously elevated.

The BP measurement in a child should be compared with the childhood BP reference data. These standards are based on age, sex, and height. To use the tables, the child's height is measured and the height percentile determined. The 95th percentile for systolic BP and diastolic BP at the child's sex, age, and height percentile are compared with the child's BP to determine whether the BP is normal. The reference BP tables for children now use the fifth Korotkoff sound (K5) to define the diastolic BP. **Table 147.1** provides an abbreviated guide to BP levels at the 95th percentile for boys and girls with height at the 50th and 75th percentile for age. Complete tables are published in the Working Group Report from the National High Blood Pressure Education Program (NHBPEP). For infants in whom accurate measurements by auscultation are uncertain, an electronic device using a Doppler technique can be used. These instruments have been shown to generate reliable and reproducible measurements of systolic BP.

When an elevated reading is obtained, repeat measurements at different times are necessary to determine the stability of the elevation. However, with a symptomatic or acutely ill child with significantly elevated BP, evaluation and intervention should begin immediately. In asymptomatic children with marginal or slight BP elevations, measurements of the BP should be repeated in 3 to 6 months; any child or adolescent whose BP is elevated ≥10 mm Hg above the upper limits of normal should have repeat measurements within a week, and if the BP remains elevated, further evaluation should begin immediately.

Evaluation

The purpose of a diagnostic evaluation of elevated BP in a child is to identify underlying causes of hypertension, establish the presence of target organ damage, and develop a plan for the most appropriate

Table 147.1. 95th Percentile of Blood Pressure by Selected Ages in Girls and Boys by the 50th and 75th Height Percentiles*

AGE, Y	SBP/DBP, GIRLS		SBP/DBP, BOYS	
	50TH PERCENTILE FOR HEIGHT	75TH PERCENTILE FOR HEIGHT	50TH PERCENTILE FOR HEIGHT	75TH PERCENTILE FOR HEIGHT
1	104/58	105/59	102/57	104/58
6	111/73	112/73	114/74	115/75
12	123/80	124/81	123/81	125/82
17	129/84	130/85	136/87	138/88

SBP indicates systolic blood pressure; DBP, diastolic blood pressure.
*Adapted with permission from the report by the NHBPEP Working Group on Hypertension Control in Children and Adolescents.

management. Some of the underlying causes of hypertension are reversible. More typical secondary causes of hypertension in the young are summarized in **Table 147.2.** The major portion (70% to 80%) of secondary hypertension in childhood is of renal origin. Cardiovascular and renovascular causes are second in frequency. Endocrine and neurological causes of hypertension in childhood are uncommon.

A careful medical history and physical examination are essential in detecting clues to secondary hypertension. The basic pediatric principles of growth and development should be incorporated into the medical history. The growth pattern should be considered to determine whether growth is delayed (failure to thrive), because this may occur with underlying chronic disease. Children with either hyperthyroidism or hypothyroidism may have failure to thrive. Failure to gain weight or weight loss may occur in cases of pheochromocytoma and other tumors. The adrenal disorders with Cushing's syndrome from excessive cortisone production cause excessive weight gain. Extremely short stature is present in Turner's syndrome. Variations in sexual development occur in several of the adrenocortical enzyme defects. Precocious puberty in boys and virilization in girls are seen in the 11α-hydroxylase defect. Delayed secondary sexual development and amenorrhea occur in girls affected with the 17α-hydroxylase deficiency. The medical history should include an assessment of cardiovascular risk factors, such as hypertension in the parents or a family history of early stroke, myocardial infarction, or cardiac-related death. A positive family history of hypertension in adult relatives is typical in essential hypertension. However, the history of hypertension in several generations with onset at a young age may be a clue for the autosomal dominant disorder dexamethasone-suppressible hyperaldosteronism. The history should also include questions of drug usage, including prescription, over-the-counter, and illicit substances. Amphetamines, ephedrine compounds in cold remedies, oral contraceptives, and anabolic steroids can elevate BP in children and adolescents.

Chronic hypertension in childhood is usually asymptomatic; the presence of significant clinical symptoms should raise suspicion of possible secondary causes. Headaches, dizziness, and epistaxis are nonspecific symptoms associated with more significant hypertension. Episodes of sweating, palpitations, or weakness, with periodic anxiety, are typical of a pheochromocytoma. Fevers, joint pain, or peripheral edema suggest collagen vascular disease, possibly with renal involvement. General weakness, fatigue, muscle cramps, and abdominal pain may be symptoms of metabolic abnormalities resulting from an endocrine disorder such as hyperaldosteronism. The advan-

Table 147.2. Secondary Causes of Hypertension in the Young

Cardiovascular
  Patient ductus arteriosus
  Coarctation of the aorta
Endocrine
  Hyperthyroidism
  Adrenal adenomas
  Congenital adrenal hyperplasia
  11α-Hydroxylase deficiency
  17 α-Hydroxylase deficiency
  Dexamethasone-suppressible hyperaldosteronism
  Apparent mineralocorticoid excess*
  Hyperaldosteronism*
  Pheochromocytoma
Renal
  Unilateral pyelonephritis (chronic)
  Hydronephrosis
  Glomerulonephritis (acute and chronic)
  Renal dysplasia
  Hereditary nephritis
  Renal cystic disease
  Renal vascular stenosis
Other
  Tumors
  Turner's syndrome
  Neurofibromatosis (renal vascular lesions)
  Burns
  Central nervous system lesions

*Rare

tage of a careful medical history is that the history elicits or eliminates findings that are useful guides in the rest of the diagnostic evaluation.

The diagnosis of cardiac defects that cause hypertension in childhood can be made by physical examination. Patent ductus arteriosus has a typical loud machinery-like murmur over the precordium in a child with physical signs of cardiac failure. This defect in children is almost always detected in newborns. Coarctation of the aorta may be undetected in infancy and early childhood. These children are generally asymptomatic, with normal growth and development. Elevated BP is frequently the only indication of abnormality. On physical examination, the pulses over the femoral arteries and the arteries in the lower extremities are absent or barely detectable by palpation, and the leg BP will be markedly lower than the BP in the upper arm. The diagnosis can be confirmed by echocardiography. The coarctation should be corrected, because this generally cures the hypertension.

When an endocrine disorder is suspected, laboratory studies will be necessary to confirm the diagnosis. Most children with hyperthyroidism will have an enlarged thyroid gland, and frequently a thyroid bruit can be auscultated over the gland. A serum thyroxine level will verify the diagnosis. Tumors or metabolic defects in adrenal gland function can result in glucocorticoid excess, mineralocorticoid excess, enzymatic defects with androgen excess, or catecholamine excess (Table 147.2). Procedures and laboratory studies used to delineate the defect in adrenal function and determine the diagnosis are provided in Table 147.3. When the presence of a pheochromocytoma is determined by the presence of elevated catecholamine levels in urine and serum, specialized radiographic studies are necessary to localize the tumor for surgical removal. Measurement of other adrenal hormones, including cortisol, deoxycorticosterone, and 11-deoxycortisol, is necessary to determine the type of enzymatic defect in the congenital adrenal hyperplasia syndrome.

Renal causes of chronic hypertension may have no clinical manifestations detectable on history and physical examination except for hypertension. Some children with occult urological lesions such as reflux nephropathy may have a history of urinary tract infections. Because renal disorders also account for the majority of the identifiable causes of hypertension in childhood (Table 147.2), additional renal diagnostic studies are appropriate, especially in asymptomatic children. Preliminary tests include a urinalysis, urine culture, serum creatinine, and renal ultrasound. These basic studies will determine whether the hypertension is due to a defect in renal parenchyma such as glomerulonephritis, chronic pyelonephritis, or renal dysplasia. If these basic studies are all normal and the child has significant hypertension, additional studies will be necessary to determine whether the hypertension is due to a renal vascular lesion or some other lesion **(Table 147.3)**.

An echocardiogram is particularly helpful in determining whether the elevated BP has induced changes in cardiac dimensions and function. The presence of increased left ventricular mass, posterior ventricular wall thickening, or intraventricular septal thickening signifies cardiac strain due to a high pressure load and is an indication for more direct intervention to lower BP.

Isolated systolic hypertension is unusual in children but can be seen in hyperthyroidism, coarctation of the aorta, or patent ductus arteriosus. In the absence of these underlying causes, mild isolated systolic hypertension should be considered a risk factor for essential hypertension.

Significant BP elevation in younger children usually warrants intensive evaluation. In adolescents with significant BP elevation, the extent of the evaluation is more limited and is determined by whether cardiovascular risk factors are present, eg, obesity, positive family history. As advances in genetic detection for specific types of hypertension become clinically applicable, families with multiple hypertensive relatives, including children, may benefit from genetic screening.

Treatment

The cause of the hypertension determines the direction for treatment. If the underlying cause of hypertension is not correctable or if

---

Table 147.3. **Specialized Diagnostic Studies**

Endocrine studies
  Measurement of adrenal cortical hormones (cortisol, 18-hydroxycortisone)
  Measurement of cortisol and aldosterone from adrenal veins
  Measurement of peripheral plasma renin activity and serum aldosterone
  Measurement of urine aldosterone and electrolytes before and after salt loading
  Measurement of urine catecholamines and metabolites
  Measurement of plasma catecholamines before and after clonidine suppression
Radiological studies
  Renal ultrasound
  Excretory urography
  Renal radionuclide studies of flow and function
  Renal angiography with renal vein renin measurement
  Computerized tomography of kidneys
  Computerized tomography of adrenal glands and abdomen

---

no cause is determined, treatment to control the BP is necessary to prevent hypertension-related end-organ damage. In cases of mild BP elevation, lifestyle interventions such as diet, weight control, and exercise are appropriate first steps in treatment. Pharmacological therapy should be instituted for more severe hypertension if there is insufficient response to lifestyle modifications. The choices of drugs for children are similar to those for adults. However, the dosages of antihypertensive medications should be determined on the basis of the child's body weight. Recommended dosages are provided in the Working Group Report from the NHBPEP.

Uncomplicated BP elevation alone is not an indication to restrict asymptomatic children from participating in sports or physical activities. Aerobic exercise may be beneficial for children or adolescents with primary hypertension. Smoking should be discouraged in children and adolescents, as well as use of anabolic steroid hormones for the purpose of bodybuilding. Follow-up BP monitoring is appropriate to enforce life-style behaviors that reduce cardiovascular risk and, when medications are prescribed, to adjust dosages.

SUGGESTED READING

1. Brownell KD, Kelman JH, Stunkard AJ. Treatment of obese children with and without their mothers: changes in weight and blood pressure. *Pediatrics*. 1983;71: 515–523.

2. Lifton RP, Dluhy RG, Powers M, Rich GM, Gutkin M, Fallo F, Gill JR Jr, Feld L, Ganguly A, Laidlaw JC, et al. Hereditary hypertension caused by chimeric gene duplications and ectopic expression of aldosterone synthase. *Nat Genet*. 1992;2:66–74.

3. Loggie JMH, ed. *Pediatric and Adolescent Hypertension*. Boston, Mass: Blackwell Scientific Publications; 1992.

4. National High Blood Pressure Education Program Working Group Report on Hypertension Control in Children and Adolescents. Update on the 1987 Task Force Report on High Blood Pressure in Children and Adolescents: a working group report from the National High Blood Pressure Education Program. *Pediatrics*. 1996;98:649–658.

5. Rich GM, Ulick S, Cook S, Wang JZ, Lifton RP, Dluhy RG. Glucocorticoid-remediable aldosteronism in a large kindred: clinical spectrum and diagnosis using a characteristic biochemical phenotype. *Ann Intern Med*. 1992;116:813–820.

6. Rocchini AP, Key J, Bondie D, Chico R, Moorehead C, Katch V, Martin M. The effect of weight loss on the sensitivity of blood pressure to sodium in obese adolescents. *N Engl J Med*. 1989;321:580–585.

Chapter 148

Management of Pregnant Hypertensive Patients

Phyllis August, MD

KEY POINTS

- Therapy for suspected or diagnosed preeclampsia consists of hospitalization with bed rest, control of blood pressure, seizure prophylaxis when signs of impending eclampsia are present, and timely delivery. The overall goal of therapy is to deliver a mature fetus without compromising maternal health.

- During pregnancy, blood pressure decreases in the first and second trimesters; thus, in women with chronic hypertension, antihypertensive medications may be reduced or in some cases withheld, provided that patients are closely monitored.

- Methyldopa is considered by some to be the drug of choice in pregnancy, but β-blockers can be effective.

- ACE inhibitors and angiotensin receptor blockers should not be used during pregnancy.

See also Chapter 59

Appropriate treatment of hypertension in pregnancy requires the accurate distinction of preeclampsia from chronic hypertensive disorders that antedated pregnancy. Preeclampsia is a potentially life-threatening condition, which may lead to explosive maternal complications as well as fetal death. Thus, proper treatment involves diagnosis, close monitoring of maternal and fetal condition, appropriately timed delivery, and prevention of maternal complications. Treatment of chronic hypertension during pregnancy involves close maternal surveillance for signs of superimposed preeclampsia and maintaining blood pressure (BP) at levels that are safe for the mother.

Prevention of Preeclampsia

In the past decade, thousands of pregnant women have been enrolled in clinical trials investigating the ability of low-dose aspirin to prevent preeclampsia. Despite the encouraging results of earlier, small trials, none of the large multicenter trials of aspirin demonstrated any benefit compared with placebo. Only one single-center trial reported a significantly lower incidence of preeclampsia in aspirin-treated women. Thus, the current consensus is that low-dose aspirin is not indicated for the prevention of preeclampsia, even in high-risk groups. Women with the antiphospholipid antibody syndrome, who are at increased risk for preeclampsia, may be an exception, and low-dose aspirin is considered part of the treatment of this disorder.

Another preventive strategy that has received considerable attention is calcium supplementation. The rationale for calcium supplementation stems from the observations that a low calcium intake is associated with an increased risk of preeclampsia and that alterations in calciotropic hormones are involved in the pathogenesis of preeclampsia. A recent NIH-sponsored trial of 2 g of calcium supplementation compared with placebo in >4589 normotensive nulliparas did not demonstrate any difference in the incidence of preeclampsia in the groups. Additional studies in high-risk women are pending.

Thus, at present there are no "magic bullets" that have documented efficacy with respect to prevention of preeclampsia. The recommended strategy is to identify women at increased risk (primigravidas; women with multiple gestations; women with preexisting hypertension, renal disease, or diabetes; positive family history) and follow such individuals closely so that if preeclampsia develops, it is diagnosed in the early stages when interventions (bed rest) are more likely to be beneficial.

Preeclampsia: Management

Therapy for suspected or diagnosed preeclampsia consists of hospitalization with bed rest, control of BP, seizure prophylaxis when signs of impending eclampsia are present, and timely delivery. Therapeutic intervention is palliative and does not appear to alter the underlying pathophysiology of preeclampsia. At best, it may slow the progression of the condition. When patients are close to term and fetal maturity is certain, delivery is appropriate, because preeclampsia is completely reversible and begins to abate with delivery. Difficulties arise when preeclampsia develops before the fetus is mature, when it may be difficult to decide on the proper timing of delivery. If the infant is very premature (<32 weeks gestation), BP is only moderately elevated, and there are no other signs of severe maternal disease, then valuable time may be gained by postponing delivery. When the gestational age is between 32 and 36 weeks, the maternal risks of postponing delivery must be carefully weighed against the fetal risks of prematurity. It must be recognized that it is unusual for preeclampsia to remit spontaneously, and in most cases the disease worsens. Thus, close maternal and fetal surveillance on a daily basis is mandatory. Regardless of gestational age, delivery should be strongly considered when there are signs of fetal distress, including intrauterine growth retardation or signs of maternal jeopardy, including uncontrolled severe hypertension; hemolysis, elevated liver function tests, and low platelet count (designated as the HELLP syndrome); evidence of deteriorating renal function; visual disturbances; headache; and epigastric pain.

Preeclampsia: Antihypertensive Therapy

The use of antihypertensive therapy in women with preeclampsia is controversial. This is because abnormalities in the circulation in the placenta leading to decreased placental perfusion are believed to be important in the pathogenesis of the disorder. The impact of acute lowering of BP on placental perfusion is difficult to assess, and because of the concern that antihypertensive agents will unfavorably affect uteroplacental blood flow, these medications should be used cautiously. It is clear that lowering maternal BP does not cure or reverse preeclampsia; thus, the consensus is that antihypertensive therapy should be prescribed only for maternal safety. There is considerable disagreement regarding what level of BP should be treated: the National Institutes of Health Working Group on Hypertension in Pregnancy recommends beginning therapy when diastolic BP is $\geq$100 to 105 mm Hg (Korotkoff phase V). Excessive BP reduction should be avoided, because this may compromise uteroplacental blood flow and possibly predispose to placental abruption. It is also important to emphasize that many women with preeclampsia were previously normotensive, with BPs in the range of 100 to 110/70 mm Hg. Thus, acute elevations of BP to the range that might be considered only mild in a chronic hypertensive individual (eg, 150/100 mm Hg) might actually result in symptoms and require treatment. As with any hypertensive illness, decisions regarding treatment should be individualized and all aspects of the patient's condition taken into consideration.

When delivery is imminent, parenteral agents are practical and effective. Both intravenous hydralazine (5 mg initial bolus, followed by subsequent doses in 20 minutes as needed) and intravenous labetalol (starting with 10- to 20-mg doses, which may be increased every 20 minutes depending on response) have been used successfully to treat preeclamptic hypertension. Although small studies of the use of short-acting nifedipine have been reported in women with preeclampsia, this agent should be used with caution, because it may lower BP precipitously, especially when magnesium sulfate is being administered concomitantly. Intravenous diazoxide in small doses (30-mg boluses) is restricted to rare resistant cases. The use of diuretics is not recommended in preeclampsia except in rare cases of pulmonary edema.

When delivery is not anticipated for several days, an oral agent is preferable. It must be emphasized that antihypertensive therapy is largely for maternal benefit. The benefit to the fetus is that control of BP may permit prolongation of pregnancy to a point at which the fetus is more mature. Methyldopa is considered by many to be the drug of choice, because there is extensive experience with this agent in pregnancy. If it is not tolerated, β-blockers, combined α- and β-blockers, long-acting calcium channel blockers, and hydralazine are reasonable additions or alternatives. Some experts discourage the use of thiazide diuretics during pregnancy because of the concern that any contraction of extracellular fluid volume may predispose toward vasoconstriction and adverse maternal and fetal outcomes.

Chronic Hypertension: Rationale for Treatment

The majority of women with chronic hypertension in pregnancy have mild to moderate elevations in BP; therefore, the risk of acute cardiovascular complications due to elevated BP during pregnancy is low. In fact, BP may normalize by the second trimester because of the physiological vasodilation of pregnancy. Therefore, in many women, antihypertensive medications may be reduced or in some cases withheld, provided that patients are closely monitored.

Women with chronic hypertension have an increased risk of developing superimposed preeclampsia, and there is evidence that most if not all of the increased perinatal morbidity and mortality associated with chronic hypertension are attributable to this complication. At the present time, there is no evidence that antihypertensive therapy reduces the incidence of superimposed preeclampsia; therefore, medication should not be prescribed for this indication. With regard to fetal well-being, there is still controversy regarding the benefits of lowering BP with medication. Given the potential hazards of antihypertensive treatment during pregnancy (the possibility that medication may reduce placental blood flow, possible adverse effects of drugs on the fetus), treatment of mild to moderate hypertension must be undertaken cautiously. Excessive BP reduction is to be avoided. If diastolic BP in the first trimester is between 90 and 100 mm Hg, then it is reasonable to await the expected physiological decrease in BP in the second trimester before using antihypertensives. If diastolic BP is <90 mm Hg in a patient already on medication early in pregnancy, then a reduction in medication can be contemplated. Most authorities would begin treatment when diastolic BPs are consistently $\geq$100 mm Hg.

Treatment of Chronic Hypertension: Nonpharmacological Therapy

During pregnancy, the nonpharmacological approach to hypertension basically consists of restriction of activity. Strategies such as weight reduction and exercise are not recommended during pregnancy. If a hypertensive woman is overweight and planning pregnancy, then weight reduction before pregnancy is advisable. Sodium restriction is recommended only to those women who have been successfully treated with this approach before pregnancy. Preliminary studies of calcium supplementation suggest that BP may be lowered by this method; however, this is considered experimental. Because close medical supervision is important during pregnancy, home BP monitoring is a useful adjunct to management of hypertensive pregnant women.

Chronic Hypertension: Antihypertensive Therapy

If the decision is made to lower BP with antihypertensive medication, then it is necessary to consider both antihypertensive efficacy and effects on the fetus. To date, the drug that has been most extensively evaluated in pregnancy is methyldopa; therefore, some consider this agent the "drug of choice" in pregnancy. If there is inadequate response to methyldopa or if it is poorly tolerated, then there are several acceptable alternatives.

Both β blockers, and combined α,β-blockers have been shown to be, for the most part, safe and effective during pregnancy. These agents have compared favorably with methyldopa in controlled trials, although some prefer methyldopa in the first trimester because one recent study suggested that use of β-blockers early in pregnancy may be associated with smaller babies.

Calcium antagonists have not been studied sufficiently in pregnancy to be recommended as first-line agents. However, growing clinical experience has led some to use them as second-line drugs, in addition to either methyldopa or β-blockers.

Although diuretics are not recommended in women with

preeclampsia, if a pregnant woman with chronic hypertension has been treated successfully with these agents before pregnancy, it is not necessary to discontinue them. Rather, it may be possible to reduce the dose while carefully monitoring the patient.

ACE inhibitors and angiotensin receptor blockers should be avoided in pregnancy. Although no teratogenic effects have been observed, use of these agents in the second and third trimesters has been associated with acute renal failure in neonates. The adverse effects of these agents on fetal renal function are believed to be due to hemodynamic effects.

Little information is available regarding the effects of maternal ingestion of antihypertensive agents on the breast-fed infant. It should be assumed that most agents will be detectable in breast milk, although it is not known what effects this has on the baby. If BP is only mildly elevated, it may be possible to withhold medication for a few months. If hypertension is more severe, then medication is advisable, and if multiple agents are necessary, then breast-feeding is not recommended.

SUGGESTED READING

1. National High Blood Pressure Education Program Working Group Report on High Blood Pressure in Pregnancy. *Am J Obstet Gynecol.* 1990;163:1691–1712.
2. Barron WM. Hypertension. In: Barron WM, Lindheimer MD, eds. *Medical Disorders in Pregnancy.* Chicago, Ill: Mosby-Year Book; 1991:1–42.
3. Fletcher AE, Bulpitt CJ. A review of clinical trials in pregnancy. In: Rubin PC, ed. *Handbook of Hypertension: Hypertension in Pregnancy.* New York, NY: Elsevier Science Publishing Co; 1988:186–201.
4. Lindheimer MD. Pre-eclampsia—eclampsia 1996: preventable? Have disputes on its treatment been resolved? *Curr Opin Nephrol Hypertens.* 1996;5:452–458.

Chapter 149

Management of Hypertension in Older Persons

Henry R. Black, MD

KEY POINTS

- Older patients benefit from antihypertensive therapy even more than younger individuals.

- The value of therapy extends to those >80 years of age and is evident whether the patient has diastolic or stage 2 to 3 isolated systolic hypertension ($\geq$160/<90 mm Hg).

- The elderly often metabolize drugs differently from younger individuals, and so the recommended starting dose and the maximum doses are lower and the duration of action is longer than for younger hypertensives.

- Many elderly people are on fixed incomes, making the cost of therapy a particularly crucial issue.

See also Chapters 86, 124

There can no longer be any doubt that treating hypertension reduces most, although perhaps not all, of the cardiovascular (CV) and renal complications attributable to having an elevated blood pressure (BP). The benefits of antihypertensive therapy were unequivocally shown in the 1960s, 1970s, and 1980s for middle-aged and younger elderly people (up to the age of 74 years), but considerable skepticism remained about whether treatment would help or harm older individuals. Only one trial from that era, the European Working Party in the Elderly, enrolled only older hypertensives. In that study, CV mortality and events were reduced by treatment, but many felt that the results were not convincing enough to recommend treatment for all older persons with high BP.

In the 1990s, four large prospective randomized clinical trials were completed: the Systolic Hypertension in the Elderly Program (SHEP), the Swedish Trial in Old Patients with Hypertension (STOP-1), the Medical Research Council Elderly Trial (MRC-E), and the European Trial on Isolated Systolic Hypertension in the Elderly (SYST-EUR). These trials unequivocally showed that older patients benefit from antihypertensive therapy even more than younger individuals do. These results are consistent with the concept that those individuals whose absolute risk is highest (in the case of hypertension and CV disease, the elderly) will benefit the most from effective therapy. The value of therapy extends to the those >80 years of age and is evident whether the patient has diastolic or stage 2 to 3 isolated systolic hypertension ($\geq$160/<90 mm Hg).

Lifestyle Modifications

The Sixth Joint National Committee on the Prevention, Detection, Evaluation, and Treatment of High Blood Pressure (JNC VI) suggested that lifestyle modification be part of the initial regimen for all hypertensives, including older patients. Of the many types of lifestyle modifications available, only four (weight loss, sodium restriction, isotonic exercise, and alcohol restriction) have been shown to reduce BP.

In the elderly, some of these techniques may be particularly helpful. Because many elderly hypertensive persons are obese, weight loss should be encouraged. Reduction to ideal body weight is rarely

necessary, and 10 pounds of weight loss may be adequate. Because the elderly tend to have sodium-sensitive hypertension, limiting daily sodium intake to 2.3 g/d (100 mEq) is often especially helpful. Isotonic exercise, such as 30 minutes of vigorous walking at least three to four times per week, is feasible for most elderly people and can have many other health benefits in addition to its antihypertensive effect. Limiting the use of alcohol to no more than one to two drinks per day in those elderly individuals who drink excessively can lower BP.

Although potassium supplementation has not been persuasively shown to be an effective antihypertensive therapy, many elderly people do not eat adequate amounts of potassium-rich foods and thus should be encouraged to do so, even if BP reduction does not specifically result from supplementation. Even though calcium supplements do not reduce BP, the elderly, who are at great risk of osteoporosis, should be sure to have an adequate intake regardless of the effect on BP. Though the Dietary Approaches to Stop Hypertension (DASH) study was not done in older individuals, it is likely that a diet high in calcium, magnesium, and fiber and also low in saturated fat and cholesterol will help prevent the progressive increase in BP that will be applicable to older people.

Considerations for the Choice of Antihypertensive Drug Therapy in the Elderly

The factors that dictate the choice of antihypertensive therapy in the elderly and the drugs we recommend are the same as in younger individuals.

First, in view of the greater prevalence of target-organ damage and other CV risk factors in older patients, the clinician must be especially careful not to aggravate these conditions. He or she should not miss the opportunity to select an agent that can also treat a comorbid condition, should such a choice be feasible.

Second, the elderly often metabolize drugs differently from younger individuals because of alterations in hepatic blood flow and renal function with aging. Thus, the recommended starting dose and the maximum dose of drugs used in older persons are characteristically lower and the duration of action longer than in other demographic groups.

Third, the elderly may be especially sensitive to certain types of adverse reactions, in particular CV and neurological reactions. The enhanced risk of these side effects limits the usefulness of some classes of agents in the elderly.

Fourth, the drugs that work for diastolic hypertension are also effective for isolated systolic hypertension. More information about the risks and benefits of therapy is still needed for elderly with stage 1 isolated systolic hypertension (systolic BP from 140 to 159 mm Hg and diastolic BP <90 mm Hg).

Last, many elderly are on fixed incomes, and so the cost of therapy is a particularly crucial issue. No drug will work if the patient cannot afford to buy it.

Efficacy of Therapy
Clinical End Points

The data from multiple clinical trials have proved that treating hypertension in the elderly reduces the incidence of clinical end points related to hypertension, such as coronary artery disease (CAD), cerebrovascular disease, and heart failure. Thiazide diuretics and/or chlorthalidone were almost always the initial drugs used in these studies and the agents for which we have the most evidence of the value of therapy. In SHEP, STOP-1, and MRC-E, low doses of diuretics (with potassium-sparing agents in STOP-1 and MRC-E) were used, and serum potassium was carefully monitored to avoid hypokalemia. This strategy may explain why these drugs were so successful at reducing not only cerebrovascular disease but also CAD. In SHEP, a β-adrenergic receptor blocker was added in the active therapy group if needed to reduce BP to target levels. In MRC-E and STOP-1, thiazides were compared with β-adrenergic receptor blockers. Although β-adrenergic receptor blockers reduce clinical events in younger patients, in the MRC-E trial, these agents were no more effective than placebo and surprisingly inferior to diuretics at preventing CAD. The most recently published trial of treatment of hypertension in older persons, SYST-EUR, initiated therapy with a moderately long-acting dihydropyridine calcium antagonist (DHP-CA), nitrendipine. The study showed a benefit for fatal and nonfatal stroke and all CV events almost identical to that for SHEP. Probably because it was stopped early, SYST-EUR did not show that a regimen beginning with a DHP-CA (and adding an ACE inhibitor [ACE-I] and thiazide if needed to reduce BP to target levels) was as beneficial as the SHEP regimen, a diuretic plus β-adrenergic receptor blocker if needed. Therefore, JNC VI recommended diuretics as preferred initial therapy for older persons with isolated systolic hypertension but considered a DHP-CA an alternative, unless there was a specific reason to choose another class of drugs, such as benign prostatic hypertrophy, in which peripheral α_1-adrenergic receptor blockers would improve both conditions.

Surrogate End Points

Surrogate end points are functional correlates of target-organ damage, such as left ventricular hypertrophy, atherosclerosis, or proteinuria, and biochemical abnormalities (dyslipidemias or glucose intolerance) that are altered by drugs in ways that could reduce or increase the frequency of clinical end points. Although it is likely that drugs that favorably affect surrogate end points would also benefit clinical end

points if tested, this is not necessarily the case. JNC VI also recommended that ACE-Is, calcium antagonists (CAs), peripheral α_1-adrenergic receptor blockers, combined and β-adrenergic receptor blockers, and the newly released angiotensin receptor blockers (ARBs) could also be used for initiating therapy for hypertension. All of these drugs are effective and well tolerated but have not been shown to reduce clinical end points, with the exception of DHP-CAs and ACE-Is.

For the elderly, it is especially important to consider both the beneficial and adverse effects of our choice of treatment on surrogate end points. Diuretics and β-adrenergic receptor blockers worsen glucose tolerance and may precipitate diabetes mellitus, very common problems with advancing age. Peripheral α_1-adrenergic receptor blockers and some ACE-Is may improve insulin sensitivity, making them potentially good choices for older patients. High-dose but probably not low-dose diuretics raise total cholesterol and triglycerides, and β-adrenergic receptor blockers lower HDL cholesterol and raise triglycerides. Peripheral α_1-adrenergic receptor blockers improve the lipid profile. CAs and ARBs have no effect on either glucose or insulin metabolism and are lipid-neutral.

Left ventricular hypertrophy is much more common in older hypertensive persons than it is in those <60 years of age. Data from both the recent Treatment of Mild Hypertension Study (TOMHS) and the Department of Veterans Affairs Trial of Monotherapy indicated that all classes of antihypertensive agents reduce left ventricular mass. In both trials, diuretics were most effective.

Other forms of target-organ damage are also very common in the elderly. Non-DHP-CAs and β-adrenergic receptor blockers may be useful for those with diastolic dysfunction, in whom diuretics and ACE-Is are valuable if systolic dysfunction is present. β-Adrenergic receptor blockers and perhaps ACE-Is may be specifically indicated after an acute myocardial infarction. ACE-Is, ARBs, and non-DHP-CAs appear to reduce proteinuria and may reduce the progression of renal insufficiency, very important issues in elderly hypertensive patients. ACE-Is may be particularly effective at preventing CV morbidity and mortality in type II diabetics. The combination of these agents with CAs may be better still.

Safety

Most classes of antihypertensive agents are surprisingly well tolerated in the elderly as long as doses are not too high. Drugs that may cause postural hypotension (peripheral α_1-adrenergic receptor blockers and sympatholytics) must be given with special care, because many elderly have baroreceptor dysfunction. Excessive volume depletion must be avoided, but the elderly tolerate diuretics very well if a low dose is used. Although cardiac output is often reduced, β-adrenergic receptor blockers can be given safely in many elderly patients. The elderly, especially women, are more likely to get a cough from ACE-Is and may be especially bothered by constipation from verapamil and the vasodilator side effects and edema commonly seen with DHP-CAs. Drugs that adversely affect cognition, such as central sympatholytics and reserpine, are best avoided unless other considerations take precedence.

Comorbidity

The high prevalence of CV diseases such as CAD, heart failure, and cerebrovascular disease, and other conditions such as chronic renal failure, diabetes mellitus, dementia, depression, osteoporosis, and osteoarthritis means that the clinician treating an elderly patient must be especially aware of the need to consider these and other conditions when choosing treatment.

Demography

All antihypertensive agents are effective in some patients from any demographic group, but certain agents are thought to be more effective in whites than in blacks, and others are more effective in blacks than in whites. Diuretics reduce BP better in elderly blacks than in whites, and β-adrenergic receptor blockers, ACE-Is, and ARBs work better in whites. CAs are equally effective in both groups. The Department of Veterans Affairs Monotherapy Study confirmed this construct and showed that for elderly whites (≥60 years of age), β-adrenergic receptor blockers and ACE-Is were the most effective, whereas CAs and diuretics were best for blacks, at least with respect to BP control.

Dosage Schedule

BP control must be maintained throughout a 24-hour period. Recent data suggest that the relatively steep increase in BP that accompanies awakening may precipitate coronary artery plaque rupture, meaning that BP during sleep cannot be ignored. It may be prudent to choose agents that do not lower BP excessively during sleep. Japanese investigators have shown an increase in "white matter lesions" in elderly who are "excessive dippers" (nighttime systolic BP decreases of >20% compared with daytime BP). More study is needed to see whether chronotherapeutically designed delivery symptoms provide special benefit compared with homeostatic regimes. Although the duration of action of some drugs is longer in the elderly, usually no dosage adjustment is necessary if the patient has reasonably normal renal function.

Other Medications

Because many elderly people require treatment for additional medical problems, the clinician must pay special attention to what other medications the elderly patient may be taking. This concern is necessary not only for prescription drugs but also for over-the-counter medications, especially nonsteroidal inflammatory drugs, which the elderly often need and use.

Cost and Other Barriers to Care

The astute clinician will pay attention not only to cost but also to other barriers to care, which affect elderly more than younger patients. Older patients are more likely to be dependent on others for assistance with transportation and often need help with taking medicine properly.

Mechanism of Action of Drugs and Pathophysiology of Hypertension

Many have recommended that we select therapy for hypertensive patients on the basis of the pathophysiology presumed to be respon-

sible for their elevated BP. Elderly hypertensive patients have been characterized hemodynamically as having a low plasma volume and cardiac output and elevated total peripheral resistance. Metabolically, they are likely to have low-renin hypertension, and many will be glucose intolerant and insulin resistant. But using these guidelines has not necessarily improved our ability to select proper therapy in the elderly or in any other group of patients. Few individuals fit neatly into these rubrics. Even those who do may respond well to agents that would theoretically appear likely to be ineffective.

It now appears that thiazide diuretics or CAs are the drugs of choice for elderly blacks. In whites, these agents plus ACE-Is, ARBs, or β-adrenergic receptor blockers are good alternatives. The starting dose should be half of that used in younger patients, and the clinician should increase the dose only after each dosage level has been given adequate time to be effective. As with all patients, the choice may need to be modified because of cost considerations, comorbidity, or the patient's prior experience with that drug or one in its class.

SUGGESTED READING

1. Amery A, Birkenhäger W, Brixko P, Bulpitt C, Clement D, Deruyttere M, De Schaepdryver A, Dollery C, Fagard R, Forette F, et al. Mortality and morbidity results from the European Working Party on High Blood Pressure in the Elderly trial. *Lancet.* 1985;1:1349–1354.
2. Black HR. Therapeutic considerations in the elderly hypertensive: the role of calcium channel blockers. *Am J Hypertens.* 1990;3:347S–354S.
3. Dahlöf B, Lindholm LH, Hansson L, Scherstén B, Ekbom T, Wester PO.. Morbidity and mortality in the Swedish Trial in Old Patients with Hypertension (STOP-Hypertension). *Lancet.* 1991;338:1281–1285.
4. Gottdiener JS, Reda DJ, Massie BJ, Materson BM, Williams DW, Andeerson RJ, the Department of Veterans Affairs Cooperative Study Group on Antihypertensive Agents. Effect of single-drug therapy on reduction of left ventricular mass in mild to moderate hypertension: comparison of six antihypertensive agents. *Circulation.* 1997;95:2007–2014.
5. Lever AF, Ramsay LE. Treatment of hypertension in the elderly. *J Hypertens.* 1995; 13:571–579.
6. Liebson PR, Grandits GA, Dianzumba S, Prineas RJ, Grimm RH Jr, Neaton JD, Stamler J, for the Treatment of Hypertension Study Research Group. Comparison of five antihypertensive monotherapies and placebo for change in left ventricular mass in patients receiving nutritional-hygienic therapy in the Treatment of Mild Hypertension Study (TOMHS). *Circulation.* 1995;91:698–706.
7. MRC Working Party. Medical Research Council trial of treatment of hypertension in older adults: principal results. *BMJ.* 1992;304:405–412.
8. National High Blood Pressure Education Program Working Group Report on Hypertension in the Elderly. *Hypertension.* 1994;23:275–285.
9. SHEP Cooperative Research Group. Prevention of stroke by antihypertensive drug treatment in older persons with isolated systolic hypertension: final results of the Systolic Hypertension in the Elderly Program (SHEP). *JAMA.* 1991;265: 3255–3264.
10. Staessen JA, Fagard R, Thijs L, Celis H, Arabidze GG, Birkenhäger WH, Bulpitt CJ, de Leeuw PW< dollery CT, Fletcher AE, Forette F, Leonetti G, Nachev C, O'Brien ET, Rosenfeld J, Rodicio JL, Tuomilehto J, Zanchetti A. Randomised double-blind comparison of placebo and active treatment for older patients with isolated systolic hypertension. The Systolic Hypertension in Europe (Syst-Eur) Trial Investigators. *Lancet.* 1997;350:757–764.

Chapter 150

Management of Borderline Hypertension

Stevo Julius, MD

KEY POINTS

- Patients with borderline hypertension have an increased likelihood of developing established hypertension and excess cardiovascular death.

- Patients should undergo a 6-month trial of nonpharmacological management in an effort to lower self-determined blood pressure and to modify other cardiovascular risk factors; drug therapy may be indicated if hypertension persists.

- Approximately 30% of all young men with borderline hypertension exhibit signs of increased sympathetic activity.

- There is no consistent evidence that response to cold, mental stress, isometric exercise, or tilt predicts hypertension.

See also Chapters 44, 45, 117

The term "borderline hypertension" was eliminated in the Fifth Joint National Committee Report on Prevention, Detection, Evaluation, and Treatment of Hypertension (JNC V). In the recent JNC VI report, one is either normotensive, has hypertension, or has high normal blood pressure (BP) values. Nevertheless, clinicians continue to use the term borderline hypertension.

Clinically, attention should be paid to individuals whose elevated BP does not require pharmacological treatment but who nevertheless do not have entirely normal readings. These patients have an excessive risk for future cardiovascular disease and have a complex and distinctive pathophysiology. Specific clinical measures are indicated because both borderline and white coat hypertension are distinct and important clinical conditions.

Definitions

Borderline hypertension is BP that was >140/90 mm Hg at the time of measurement, but the elevation is neither permanent nor excessive. This includes (1) subjects who, out of 3 readings taken in the previous 6 months, show 1 clinic BP >140/90 mm Hg; (2) subjects with clinic readings consistently between 140 and 150 and/or 90 and 94 mm Hg; (3) subjects with white coat hypertension, who exhibit elevated clinic BP readings but nonelevated out-of-office readings; and (4) subjects with BP readings described in (1), (2), or (3) who belong to the JNC VI risk group A or B, ie, have no signs of target-organ damage. According to this classification, ≈15% of all people 30 to 50 years old may have borderline hypertension.

Because the BP in many of these subjects is not persistently elevated, they are occasionally given the diagnosis of labile hypertension as opposed to stable or sustained hypertension. This is wrong, because all evidence indicates that BP variability (lability) in these subjects is not excessive, nor is their "reactivity" to various physical stressors increased. If needed, the term labile BP should be reserved for individuals who have "spells" of hypertension or who show wide day-to-day BP fluctuations (>30 mm Hg) irrespective of what their average BP level might be.

Borderline Hypertension as a Precursor of Cardiovascular Diseases

Since the early 1930s, life insurance company data clearly indicate that even a single elevated office BP reading carries negative prognostic connotations. The prediction from clinic BP readings is so strong that a few clinic BP readings have become the standard treatment recommendations. Nevertheless, when BP measurements are repeated, only ≈30% of subjects with borderline hypertension remain hypertensive. However, the cardiovascular prognosis for such individuals who have just an occasional BP elevation is not normal. Over a period of 20 years, they will have a 4-fold incidence of developing established hypertension and may exhibit a 300% excess of cardiovascular deaths. Recently, a study from Norway suggested that 80% of borderline hypertensive persons first seen in their third decade of life develop sustained hypertension after 20 years.

But even if the majority of patients with borderline hypertension were not to develop hypertension, they would not be free of excessive cardiovascular risk. Borderline hypertension is a complex pathophysiological condition, in which the elevated BP is only one of multiple cardiovascular risk factors.

Sympathetic Overactivity and Its Consequences in Borderline Hypertension

Approximately 30% of all young men with borderline hypertension exhibit signs of increased sympathetic activity. Their cardiac output, stroke volume, and heart rates are elevated, and this elevation can be abolished by cardiac autonomic receptor blockade. The plasma norepinephrine and norepinephrine turnover in these patients are increased, and it has recently been shown by microneurography that the baseline firing rate in their sympathetic fibers is significantly elevated. The autonomic abnormality in these patients is widespread. They frequently show high plasma renin values (due to excessive β-adrenergic stimulation of the juxtaglomerular cells), decreased plasma volume (due to excessive α-adrenergic venular constriction) and, most interestingly, diminished parasympathetic inhibitory tone to the heart.

Patients with borderline hypertension in addition to higher BP have other abnormalities (dyslipidemia, high hematocrit, insulin resistance) that put them at a higher risk for development of coronary heart disease and for complications subsequent to myocardial infarction. This association of coronary risk factors and clinical hypertension is most likely responsible for the differential effect of antihypertensive treatment on BP-related (heart failure and stroke) versus atherosclerosis-related (myocardial infarction) complications of hypertension. Antihypertensive treatment decreases the incidence of strokes and heart failure more dramatically than the incidence of myocardial infarction.

Understanding the pathophysiology of this non–BP-related excessive risk in patients with borderline hypertension may lead to better clinical and preventive practices. Acute sympathetic stimulation can cause insulin resistance. High plasma adrenaline levels, stimulating β-adrenergic receptors in the skeletal muscle as well as through α-adrenergic vasoconstriction, lead to a reduced delivery of glucose and insulin to the skeletal muscle. High insulin is predictive of the future development of atherosclerosis, most likely through the direct "trophic" effect of insulin on the blood vessel wall and the insulin-related promotion of high triglyceride and low HDL cholesterol values. Thus, high insulin and dyslipidemia may be directly related to excess sympathetic tone. Epidemiological studies have shown that a higher hematocrit, which is frequently found in patients with borderline hypertension, is also a predictor of coronary mortality, most likely through the hypercoagulability of the more viscous blood. The coronary risk factor may be associated with the enhanced sympathetic tone. Infusion of norepinephrine causes an instant increase of hematocrit through its α-adrenergic postcapillary venoconstriction.

The increased sympathetic and decreased parasympathetic tone in borderline hypertension suggests that in these patients, nonpharmacological measures such as physical conditioning and weight loss, which tend to decrease sympathetic overactivity and increase parasympathetic tone, may be particularly useful. Physical training also lowers both cardiac output and heart rate through a combination of decreased sympathetic and increased parasympathetic tone and improves insulin-mediated glucose incorporation into skeletal muscle. This, in turn, tends to lower plasma insulin levels. Physical exercise training also increases total blood volume.

Clinical Approach to Borderline Hypertension

Because the cardiovascular risk of a person with borderline hypertension is higher than normal, such an individual deserves medical attention. The absolute level of risk in borderline hypertension, however, is too small to mandate immediate antihypertensive medication. In a patient with borderline hypertension, the physician should assess the patient's risk status and the status of hypertension-related target organs and then individualize the approach.

Assessing the Risk for Hypertension

Two patients with the same average clinic BP may not have the same propensity to later development of sustained hypertension. Proven risk factors for later hypertension are average BP level, obesity and weight gain with time, tachycardia, family history of hypertension, male sex, and black race.

Subjects with higher baseline BP levels tend to have a higher increment of BP with time, but repeated elevated BP readings do not necessarily improve the prediction of future hypertension.

The effect of weight on the future development of hypertension is well documented. For example, in the Tecumseh Study of subjects whose BP at 5 years of age was in the upper quintile of the distribution and who could be categorized as overweight, 90% developed hypertension by age 35 years. In children with similar BP elevations who were not overweight, the rates of development of hypertension at age 35 were <50%. Among risk factors for the development of hypertension, fast heart rate deserves special mention. A patient with a rapid heart rate in the physician's office and reasonably normal BP readings elsewhere is usually dismissed as having "nervous BP elevation only." However, 10 years later, a person whose resting heart rate is >80 bpm has twice the chance of developing hypertension, even with normal BP readings. When this heart rate is combined with a transiently elevated office BP reading, the risk of hypertension quintuples. Family history is a significant predictive factor for future hypertension only if the parent required antihypertensive treatment before 50 years of age.

Various "reactivity" tests have been proposed to predict which individual with borderline hypertension may later develop hypertension. But there is no consistent evidence that response to cold, mental stressors, isometric exercise, or tilt predicts future hypertension. However, BP level achieved during dynamic exercise seems to be a better predictor of future BP increase than the baseline BP.

Risk for Coronary Heart Disease

A strong association between BP elevation and other coronary risk is seen even before the development of established hypertension. Compared with normotensive individuals, subjects with permanent or white coat borderline hypertension tend to be overweight; to have high cholesterol, triglycerides, plasma insulin, and hematocrit levels; and to have significantly decreased HDL cholesterol levels. It is therefore mandatory to incorporate these parameters into evaluation of borderline hypertension testing for cardiovascular risk factors. Plasma lipids ought to be determined routinely in everyone, and fasting plasma insulin value is useful to gauge the effectiveness of nonpharmacological intervention.

Assessment of BP

In the assessment of a patient with borderline hypertension, it is mandatory to obtain repeated BP readings outside of the physician's office. These can be obtained by patients or their relatives (usually 2 readings per day for 7 days) or by a BP monitoring device (daytime and when possible, nighttime readings, 2 per hour). It is important to understand the context in which these measurements are taken. Repeated out-of-office BP readings are not taken to decide whether someone is normotensive or hypertensive and whether treatment is or is not indicated. The usefulness of repeated out-of-office BP is to establish a reproducible baseline against which future intervention can be evaluated and to prevent overtreatment of borderline hypertension. This distinction is important. If repeat clinic diastolic BPs exceed 95 mm Hg, it can be said with a great deal of confidence that pharmacological treatment is indicated; at that elevation, the complication rates in the placebo group significantly exceed those in the treated group. Unfortunately, such data do not exist for self-determined or ambulatory BP readings. Furthermore, the data on distribution of ambulatory BP values have been carried out in limited populations, and age/sex-dependent criteria for limits of normality have not yet been universally agreed upon.

The absence of an established exact upper limit of normal out-of-office BP currently precludes use of ambulatory BP levels to initiate treatment. Conversely, out-of-office readings can be very useful in determining who should not be treated or who may be overtreated. If office readings are used to evaluate the efficacy of a regimen, some subjects will have lower out-of-office BP readings (≤120/70 mm Hg) and may suffer from symptoms of hypotension.

Target-Organ Assessment

The guided M-mode echocardiogram provides reliable data to assess cardiac status in borderline hypertension, but the readings must come from a reputable laboratory. A notable proportion of patients with borderline hypertension may already show left ventricular hypertrophy or concentric remodeling (relative wall thickness >0.45). Such subjects are at higher risk for later cardiovascular complications. Microalbuminuria may be an indicator of renal prognosis.

Treatment and Management Decisions in Borderline Hypertension

Home BP self-determination can be used to establish a reliable BP for long-term follow-up. The standard method is to obtain 1 reading in the morning and 1 in the afternoon on 7 consecutive days. The upper limit of normality (2 SD above the normal mean) is 142/92 mm Hg for men and 131/85 mm Hg for women; the upper limit for borderline hypertension (1 SD above the mean) is 131/83 mm Hg for men and 121/78 mm Hg for women. After home BP readings have been obtained, the following management-treatment scheme for subjects with borderline hypertension can be adopted.

Step One

All subjects should undergo a 6-month trial of lifestyle modification. As in patients with established hypertension, weight loss and physical exercise are preferred components of the treatment program. Almost all methods of weight loss yield an average loss of 3 to 4 kg and a tendency to regain the weight. However, if there is a very good correlation between the weight loss and the BP results, it becomes much easier to convince the patient to cooperate and maintain a lower weight.

Physical exercise is a practical way to improve the health of the patient with borderline hypertension. Numerous studies show that exercise lowers BP. Training also decreases heart rate, cardiac output, and plasma norepinephrine, which are elevated in this phase of the disease. The training must not be episodic, and the exercise must be isotonic ("aerobic" or dynamic) and of sufficient intensity to increase the heart rate to ≈130 bpm. Isometric exercise (bodybuilding) is not effective and, because it increases cardiac mass, may be harmful. Three 30-minute sessions per week are sufficient to achieve the maximal health benefit. Training beyond that level will not improve the BP results, but it may further increase the patient's exercise capacity. Any form of dynamic exercise (jogging, swimming, treadmill, bicycle) is acceptable.

Step Two

If therapy was successful (home BP decrease of 5 mm Hg, body weight loss of 2 kg, or cholesterol reduction of 15 mg/dL), the clinician should continue with the lifestyle modifications and recheck every 6 months.

If therapy was not successful, the clinician should consider pharmacological treatment, especially if (1) the home average BP is >140/90 mm Hg; (2) the home BP is >140/90 mm Hg, the subject is a man, and the subject has a positive family history of hypertension; (3) the home BP is >140/90 mm Hg, the subject is a woman, and the home BP actually increased; or (4) the subject, regardless of sex, has home BP readings >140/90 mm Hg and abnormal levels of cholesterol or HDL cholesterol. Continued observation toward maximization of lifestyle modification is recommended in women who do not have additional risk factors, with follow-up in 3 months. Lifestyle modification is recommended in subjects whose home BP is between 131/83 and 139/89 mm Hg. The rate of follow-up in those with additional risk factors is 3 months; in others, 6 months. Lifestyle modification is recommended in all other subjects, with 1-year follow-up.

Step Three

Excessive doses of drugs or drug combinations are usually not necessary. Quickly change to another compound if there is even the slightest side effect. All drugs have equal potential to lower BP. The choice of drug is affected by the patient's lifestyle (exercise, nervousness, sexual dysfunction), laboratory abnormalities (glucose/lipid status), and associated conditions.

The goal of treatment is to lower the home BP by 5 mm Hg of diastolic BP. If successful, treatment should be maintained for 2 years and the patient recalled on a semiannual basis. After 2 years, under a physician's supervision, treatment can be discontinued with monitoring for 3 months. If the BP returns to the hypertensive range, the patient should expect lifelong treatment of the condition. If the BP does not increase, the next visit should be at 3 months, and if still not hypertensive, then each 6 months for the next 2 years. Thereafter, annual revisits may be sufficient.

Patients who do not respond to small doses of drugs represent the biggest problem. Reiteration of lifestyle modification combined with treatment is in order. If this fails after 6 months, and particularly if the average BP increased (even a few mm Hg), combination treatment is in order.

SUGGESTED READING

1. Anderson EA, Sinkey CA, Lawton WJ, Mark AL. Elevated sympathetic nerve activity in borderline hypertensive humans: evidence from direct intraneural recordings. *Hypertension.* 1989;14:177–183.
2. Joint National Committee. The sixth report of the Joint National Committee on Prevention, Detection, Evaluation, and Treatment of High Blood Pressure. *Arch Intern Med.* 1997;157:2314–2446.
3. Julius S, Ellis CN, Pascual AV, Matice M, Hansson L, Hunyor SN, Sandler LN. Home blood pressure determination: value in borderline ("labile") hypertension. *JAMA.* 1974;229:663–666.
4. Julius S, Jamerson K, Mejia A, Krause L, Schork N, Jones K. The association of borderline hypertension with target organ changes and higher coronary risk: Tecumseh Blood Pressure Study. *JAMA.* 1990;264:354–358.
5. Julius S, Mejia A, Jones K, Krause L, Schork N, van de Ven C, Johnson E, Petrin J, Sekkarie MA, Kjeldsen SE, Schmouder R, Gupta R, Ferraro J, Nazzaro P, Weissfeld

J. "White coat" versus "sustained" borderline hypertension in Tecumseh, Michigan. *Hypertension.* 1990;16:617–623.

6. Lund-Johansen P, Omvik P. Hemodynamic patterns of untreated hypertensive disease. In: Laragh JH, Brenner BM, eds. *Hypertension: Pathophysiology, Diagnosis, and Management.* New York, NY: Raven Press Ltd; 1990:305–327.

7. Mejia Ad, Julius S, Jones KA, Schork NJ, Kneisley J. The Tecumseh Blood Pressure Study: normative data on BP self-determination. *Arch Intern Med.* 1990;150:1209–1213.

8. National High Blood Pressure Education Program. The fifth report of the Joint National Committee on Prevention, Detection, Evaluation, and Treatment of High Blood Pressure. *Arch Intern Med.* 1993;153:154–183.

Management of Hypertensive Emergencies and Urgencies

Donald G. Vidt, MD

KEY POINTS

- Patients with hypertensive emergencies usually require hospitalization for vasodilator therapy, usually in an intensive care unit where blood pressure (BP) monitoring can be maintained.

- The goal of initial treatment in the hypertensive emergency is to obtain a partial reduction in BP to a safer, noncritical level, although not necessarily to achieve normotension.

- Most hypertensive urgencies can be managed in the outpatient setting if appropriate follow-up can be provided.

- Elevated BP alone in the absence of symptoms of progressive target-organ damage rarely requires emergency therapy.

See also Chapters 45, 71

Hypertensive emergencies are those uncommon situations that require immediate blood pressure (BP) reduction (although not necessarily to normal value ranges) to limit or prevent target-organ damage. Hypertensive urgencies are associated with severely elevated BP without severe symptoms or progressive target-organ dysfunction. Adequate treatment mandates lowering BP within several to 24 hours, usually with oral agents. Examples of hypertensive emergencies and urgencies are listed in **Tables 151.1 and 151.2.**

As an example, a BP of 240/140 mm Hg in a middle-aged, asymptomatic patient with no evidence of target-organ disease may, in fact, not even require hospitalization if outpatient follow-up is available after the institution of oral medication. In contrast, a 65-year-old man with progressive aortic dissection and a BP of 160/110 mm Hg represents a hypertensive emergency and would benefit from the immediate institution of parenteral therapy. In general, severe exacerbations of hypertension are caused by excessive vasoconstriction. Affected individuals are often profoundly fluid depleted (unless they have cardiac or renal failure), often with a contraction of blood volume of 30% to 40%. Accordingly, vasodilators are preferred initial agents in most cases.

Hypertensive Emergencies

Initial management of hypertensive emergencies requires hospitalization, preferably in an intensive care unit, followed by brief but thorough initial evaluation that should focus on estimating the degree of target-organ damage and possibly identify any readily recognized secondary causes of hypertension. The goal of initial treatment is to obtain a partial reduction in BP to a safer, noncritical level, although not necessarily to achieve normotension, because precipitous decreases in BP may cause acute hypoperfusion. The heart, brain, and kidneys all have autoregulatory mechanisms that protect these organs from acute ischemia when BP is abruptly reduced. The lower limit of autoregulation in hypertensive patients is shifted upward, so that autoregulation fails and blood flow decreases at higher levels of

BP in hypertensive compared with normotensive individuals, particularly in the cerebral, renal, and possibly coronary circulations. This phenomenon is a consequence of structural changes in the arterioles of hypertensive individuals, which fail to vasodilate adequately in response to a sudden drop in BP. Aggressive treatment is appropriate, but initial therapy aimed at partial reduction in BP is probably safer for the patient with a hypertensive emergency.

The initial goal of therapy is to reduce mean arterial BP by no more than 25% (within minutes to 2 hours) or to a BP in the range of 160/100 mm Hg. In patients with an acute aortic dissection or acute pulmonary edema, an initial reduction of pressure within minutes may be appropriate. For patients with an acute cerebrovascular accident, a reduction to an initial goal pressure should be accomplished more slowly, over a period of hours, with careful attention paid to any changes in neurological status. Therapy should be initiated before the results of all initial laboratory studies are available; additional diagnostic studies may be undertaken in situations in which the cause of the hypertension remains in doubt.

A number of very effective agents are available for the treatment of a hypertensive emergency. **Table 151.3** lists those agents readily available, together with recommended dosages, route of administration, onset and duration of action, and selected precautions regarding usage.

With most parenteral agents, rapid reduction of BP is accompanied by sodium and fluid retention, which may lead to resistance to continued drug treatment. The judicious use of loop-active diuretics may be effective initially in volume-overloaded states, such as heart failure, and later in the course of therapy to maintain an adequate urine flow rate and avoid drug pseudotolerance. Loop-active diuretics are not recommended for the routine treatment of hypertensive urgencies or emergencies in the absence of fluid overload because they can cause additional reflex vasoconstriction. Furosemide (40 to 120 mg) or bumetanide (1 to 5 mg) can be given intravenously and repeated periodically to maintain an adequate urine flow rate. Alter-

Table 151.1. Hypertensive Emergencies

1. Hypertensive encephalopathy
2. Malignant hypertension (some cases)
3. Severe hypertension in association with acute complications
    A. Cerebrovascular
       Intracerebral hemorrhage
       Subarachnoid hemorrhage
       Acute atherothrombotic brain infarction (with sever hypertension)
    B. Renal
       Rapidly progressive renal failure
    C. Cardiac
       Acute aortic dissection
       Acute left ventricular failure with pulmonary edema
       Acute myocardial infarction
       Unstable angina
4. Eclampsia or severe hypertension during pregnancy
5. Catecholamine excess states
    A. Pheochromocytoma crisis
    B. Food or Drug interactions (tyramine) with monoamine oxidase inhibitors
    C. Some cases of rebound hypertension following sudden withdrawal or antihypertensive agents (ie, clonidine, guanabenz, methyldopa)
6. Drug-induced hypertension (some cases)
    A. Overdose with sympathomimetics or drugs with similar action (eg, phencyclidine, lysergic acid diethylamide [LSD], cocaine, phenylpropanolamine)
7. Head trauma
8. Post–coronary artery bypass hypertension
9. Postoperative bleeding at vascular suture lines.

Table 151.2. Hypertensive Urgencies

1. Accelerated and malignant hypertension
2. Extensive body burns*
3. Acute glomerulonephritis with sever hypertension*
4. Scleroderma crisis
5. Acute systemic vasculitis with sever hypertension*
6. Surgically related hypertension
    A. Severe hypertension in patients requiring immediate surgery*
    B. Postoperative hypertension*
    C. Severe hypertension after kidney transplantation
7. Severe epistaxis
8. Rebound hypertension after sudden withdrawal of antihypertensive agents
9. Drug-induced hypertension*
    A. Overdose with sympathomimetic agents
    B. Metoclopramide-induced hypertensive crisis
    C. Interaction between and α-adrenergic agonist and a nonselective β-adrenergic antagonist
10. Episodic and severe hypertension associated with chronic spinal cord injury: autonomic hyperreflexia syndrome*

*At times may become a true hypertensive emergency.

natively, if a history of hypersensitivity to these agents is present, ethacrynic acid (50 to 150 mg) can be used. Fenoldopam may be useful when renal insufficiency is present.

Regardless of the type of hypertensive emergency or of the antihypertensive agent used to control BP, an objective should be to start an oral regimen as soon as the patient can tolerate it. This will allow earlier tapering and discontinuation of parenteral agents. Switching abruptly from intravenous to oral therapy may result in a precipitous rise in BP.

Hypertensive Urgencies

Adequate treatment of a hypertensive urgency mandates lowering BP within several to 24 hours, usually with oral agents. Even the patient with malignant hypertension (including grade 4 hypertensive retinopathy) can be managed as a hypertensive urgency in the absence of rapidly deteriorating target-organ function. More commonly, hypertensive urgencies represent asymptomatic patients with newly diagnosed hypertension, poorly controlled BP on current regimens, or noncompliance with previous therapy. No data currently exist to show immediate benefit to acutely lowering BP in asymptomatic patients with severe hypertension, but data suggest that an aggressive approach may be harmful, especially in patients with cardiovascular risk factors.

In this regard, immediate-release nifedipine, when used in hypertensive urgencies, induces a precipitous, unpredictable fall in BP. Given the gravity of reported adverse events and the lack of clinical evidence attesting to benefit, the Food and Drug Administration (FDA) has discouraged the use of immediate-release nifedipine for treating hypertension, a use that does not have specific FDA approval. Other agents that demonstrate a rapid onset of effects are not necessarily free of potential adverse events. The risk of overly aggressive intervention in any hypertensive urgency must always be considered.

When indicated, several agents provide prompt reduction of BP from within 30 minutes to several hours (**Table 151.4**). In recommended dosages, these agents do not generally induce a sudden reduction of BP, and the duration of action may be prolonged. For many patients with severe hypertension but without symptoms or target-organ dysfunction, initiation of therapy with two agents (followed by a third if needed) is appropriate to lower BP over 24 to 48 hours. Such therapy can usually be administered in the outpatient setting, and further drug titration to optimal control can be achieved over several days to weeks as recommended in guidelines for treatment of patients with stage 2 or 3 hypertension.

Hypertensive Encephalopathy

Hypertensive encephalopathy is a potentially lethal complication of severe hypertension that occurs when an increase in BP exceeds the autoregulatory ability of the brain to maintain constant cerebral perfusion. The resulting disruption of the blood-brain barrier causes diffuse cerebral edema and neurological dysfunction. The presence of papilledema is the sine qua non of hypertensive encephalopathy, but it should be suspected when a severe elevation in BP is accompanied by other nonspecific neurological signs and symptoms. This is a diagnosis of exclusion and requires that stroke, intracranial hemorrhage, seizure disorder, mental disorder, mass lesions, vasculitis, and encephalitis be ruled out. When it is suspected, however, BP should be promptly lowered as recommended in the management of a hypertensive emergency.

Agents with a rapid onset of effect that can be titrated to a desirable, initial BP goal are preferred. Sodium nitroprusside is an agent of choice because its rapid onset of action and short half-life allow for

Table 151.3. **Management of Hypertensive Emergencies**

AGENT	DOSE	ONSET/DURATION OF ACTION (AFTER DISCONTINUATION)	PRECAUTIONS
Parenteral vasodilators			
Sodium nitroprusside	0.25–10 μg·kg^{-1}·min^{-1} as IV infusion; † maximal dose for 10 min only	Immediate/2–3 min after infusion	Nausea, vomiting, muscle twitching: with prolonged use may cause thiocyanate intoxication, methemoglobinemia acidosis, cyanide poisoning; bags, bottles, and delivery sets must be light resistant.
Glyceryl trinitrate	5–100 μg as IV infusion †	2–5 min/5–10 min	Headache, tachycardia, vomiting, flushing, methemoglobinemia; requires special delivery system due to drug binding to PVC tubing
Nicardipine	5–15 mg/h IV infusion	1–5 min/15–30 min, but may exceed 12 h after prolonged infusion	Tachycardia, nausea, vomiting, headache, increased intracranial pressure. Hypotension may be protracted after prolonged infusions.
Verapamil	5–10 mg IV; can follow with infusion of 3–25 mg/h	1–5 min/30–60 min	Heart block (1°, 2°, 3°), especially with concomitant digitalis or β-blockers, bradycardia
Diazoxide	50–150 mg as IV bolus, repeated or 15–30 mg/min by IV infusion	2–5 min/3–12h	Hypotension, tachycardia, aggravation or angina pectoris, nausea and vomiting, hyperglycemia with repeated injections
Fenoldopam mesylate	0.1–0.3 mg·kg^{-1}·min^{-1} IV infusion	<5 min/30 min	Headache, tachycardia, flushing, local phlebitis
Hydralazine	10–20 mg as IV bolus or 10–40 mg IM, repeat every 4–6 h	10 min IV/>1 hr (IV) 20–30 min IM/4–6 h (IM)	Tachycardia, headache, vomiting, aggravation of angina pectoris
Enalaprilat	0.625–1.25 mg every 6 h IV	15–60 min/12–24 h	Renal failure in patients with bilateral renal artery stenosis, hypotension
Parenteral adrenergic inhibitors			
Labetalol	20–80 mg as IV bolus every 10 min; up to 2 mg/min as IV infusion	5–10 min/2–6 h	Bronchoconstricion, heart block, orthostatic hypotension
Esmolol	500 μg/kg bolus injection IV or 25–100 μg·kg^{-1}·min^{-1} by infusion. May repeat bolus after 5 min or increase infusion rate to 300 μg·kg^{-1}·min^{-1}	1–5 min/15–30 min	First-Degree heart block, congestive heart failure, asthma
Methyldopa	250–500 mg as IV infusion every 6 h	30–60 min/4–6 h	Drowsiness
Phentolamine	5–15 mg as IV bolus	1–2 min/10–30 min	Tachycardia, orthostatic hypotension

†Requires special delivery system.

Table 151.4. **Management of Hypertensive Urgencies: Oral Agents**

AGENT	DOSE	ONSET/DURATION OF ACTION (AFTER DISCONTINUATION)	PRECAUTIONS
Captopril	25mg PO, repeat as needed SL, 25 mg	15–30 min/6–8 h SL 15–30 min/2–6 h	Hypotension, renal failure in bilateral renal artery stenosis
Clonidine	0.1–0.2 mg PO, repeat hourly as required to total dose of 0.6 mg	30–60 min/8–16 h	Hypotention, drowsiness, dry mouth
Labetalol	200–400 mg PO, repeat every 2–3 h	30 min–2 hrs/2–12 h	Bronchoconstriction, heart block, orthostatic hypotension
Prazosin	1–2 mg PO; repeat hourly, as needed	1–2 hr/8–12 h	Syncope (1st dose), palpitations, tachycardia, orthostatic hypotension

minute-by-minute control of BP and because it has minimal adverse effects on cerebral blood flow. Nicardipine and labetalol have also proved particularly effective in the management of hypertensive encephalopathy. Maintaining frequent neurological assessments during the period of BP titration is imperative. BP reduction is often associated with dramatic improvement in cerebral function. Subsequent deterioration in neurological function requires reevaluation and consideration of other possible diagnoses.

SUGGESTED READING

1. Bedoya LA, Vidt DG. Treatment of the hypertensive emergency. In: Jacobson HR, Striker GE, Klahr S, eds. *The Principles and Practice of Nephrology.* 15th ed. Philadelphia, Pa: BC Decker, Inc; 1991:547–557.

2. Furberg CD, Psaty BM, Meyer JV. Nifedipine: dose-related increase in mortality in patients with coronary heart disease. *Circulation.* 1995;92:1326–1331.

3. Gales MA. Oral antihypertensives for hypertensive urgencies. *Ann Pharmacother.* 1994;28:352–358.

4. Gifford RW Jr. Management of hypertensive crises. *JAMA.*1991;266:829–835.

5. Grossman E, Messerli FH, Grodzicki T, Kowey P. Should a moratorium be placed on sublingual nifedipine capsules given for hypertensive emergencies and pseudo-emergencies? *JAMA.* 1996;276:1328–1331.

6. Kaplan NM. Management of hypertensive emergencies. *Lancet.* 1994;344: 1335–1338.

7. Murphy C. Hypertensive emergencies. *Emerg Med Clin North Am.* 1995;13: 973–1007.

8. Thach AM, Schultz PJ. Nonemergent hypertension: new perspectives for the emergency medicine physician. *Emerg Med Clin North Am.* 1995;13:1009–1035.

Chapter 152

Workplace Management of Hypertension

Michael H. Alderman, MD

KEY POINTS

- The ability to efficiently reach many hypertensive patients in their working environment has long been an attractive opportunity to improve health.

- Isolated screening at the workplace or in any other nonmedical setting does no good and may even produce harm.

- However, experience with providing all diagnostic and therapeutic services in the occupational setting has proved acceptable, effective, and highly efficient.

- Medical cost savings over an 8-year period have more than paid for the program.

See also Chapter 121

More than 100,000,000 Americans work, most in fixed physical settings, and millions of these workers have high blood pressure. Not surprisingly, the ability to efficiently reach large numbers of hypertensive patients in their working environment has long been an attractive opportunity to improve health. Employers themselves, through their own medical departments, have exploited the occupational setting in efforts ranging from screening and case finding to the provision of diagnostic and therapeutic follow-up in the workplace.

Initially, on-site screening was popular. Frequently provided by outside vendors or volunteers, these efforts were too often isolated activities, in which blood pressure was measured and, on the basis of the numbers, employees were advised to seek further medical care. Measuring techniques were often unreliable or the diagnosis was based on single recordings that often resulted in misleading or incorrect information. Disaffection of community physicians was often coupled with frustration and confusion among patients. Indeed, this well-meaning exercise actually produced occasional adverse effects through the "labeling" phenomenon, in which inappropriately identified "hypertensive" persons suffered measurable adverse physiological, economic, and even physical consequences without a beneficial effect on the outcome. Thus, isolated screening at the workplace or in any other setting does no good and may even produce harm.

Most Americans have had their blood pressures recorded within the past 2 years, yet fully 33% of those with hypertension, defined at a single encounter as >140/90 mm Hg, are not aware of their status. Clearly, the first step toward blood pressure control is improved identification. But screening by itself, in or out of the workplace, is not the solution.

The Work-Site Program

An alternative approach is to provide all diagnostic and therapeutic services in the occupational setting. Experience has proved this approach to be acceptable, effective, and highly efficient. This initiative was stimulated by the observation that treatment in both the medical clinic of the urban teaching hospital center and the private practice setting failed to retain more than half of patients in contin-uing care for even 1 year. In the rest, blood pressure control was achieved in only about one half of all cases.

The premise tested by investigators at Cornell University Medical College was that the main impediments to achieving effective long-term blood pressure control in conventional therapeutic settings were, in large measure, logistical. The solution was to replace the conventional situation, in which patients come to therapists, by a scheme that brought all care directly to the patients.

A model program was established in New York City in 1973 for the employees of Bloomingdale's and Gimbel's department stores. The guiding principles of the program were (1) provision of all services at the workplace; (2) adherence to a formal diagnostic and therapeutic protocol; (3) a team approach to treatment, in which nurses were the primary caregivers and physicians played a supervisory, educational, and consultative role; (4) no out-of-pocket patient expenses; (5) convenience in care, which included visits on-site or nearby and delivery of medications; and (6) use of the cohesive resources of the union structure to enhance participation, persistence, and adherence to treatment.

The program began with screening ≈75% of employees at the stores. Qualifying individuals had blood pressures >160/95 mm Hg on three separate occasions, each of which involved three measurements, with the average of the final two recorded. Approximately two thirds initially opted to remain in the on-site treatment program, a remarkably high acceptance of an experimental program that depended on nurses for most direct care, because these employees retained the option for conventional health care financed by union insurance. This initial success was probably due to the overt support by the union leadership, articulated at open membership meetings at which program sponsors presented the program.

Entrants were evaluated in facilities provided by the union, thus assuring members of the comfort of receiving care in a familiar and reassuring environment. The nurse performed initial history and laboratory studies, including blood, urine, and electrocardiogram. Testing was parsimonious and limited to measures that either helped to determine appropriate drug therapy, established a basis for assessing treatment toxicity, or established overall cardiovascular disease risk. Blood tests included serum creatinine, fasting blood glucose, potassium, uric acid, and thyroid function. Urine was assessed for protein qualitatively, and an electrocardiogram was performed. The culmination of the 4- to 6-week intake process was an examination and review of all previously obtained data by the supervising physician.

At that visit, therapy was begun according to protocol. Initial drug selection was largely guided by the recommendations of sequential Joint National Commission reports (JNC I through V) and has thus varied substantially over the past 25 years. More recently, we have added determination of plasma renin and urine sodium to further estimate renin profile to further measure cardiovascular risk and to guide drug selection. In general, absent contraindications or specific indications, low-renin patients ($\approx$30%) have begun therapy with a diuretic, and high-renin subjects ($\approx$18%) begin with a β-blocker or ACE inhibitor. Demographic factors as well as coincident disease have influenced the selection of initial therapy.

Medications have been provided through a union-sponsored central delivery system and mailed directly to the patient's home. All subsequent visits, dictated by patient need, have been with the nurse. These generally total four to six per year, after an initial year of somewhat more frequent attendance with an annual revisit to the physician, who remained available for consultation as dictated by patient need.

Several medical care elements of the program are believed to be keys to its success. These include (1) systematic care delivered according to a protocol that is appropriately revised as new information or experience is gained; (2) provision of most direct patient care by a physician-supervised, specially trained hypertension nurse-expert; and (3) constant oversight of all patient data by the supervising physician. Over the years, what began as a system of paper encounter forms later entered onto computer has become a direct computer entry system in which all patient data are electronically managed, including scheduling, patient visits, laboratory tests, and consultations. This facilitates oversight and ensures that deviations from protocol can be noted and, when necessary, investigated. With increasingly sophisticated data management, patient care has benefited and outcomes have improved, largely because caregivers are freed from tedious recording responsibilities and can devote more attention to patients.

Over the 25 years of program existence, patterns of drug treatment have varied widely, both in response to emerging pharmacological innovation and to changing JNC recommendations. However, despite dramatic shifts in patterns of first-drug use, all measures of blood pressure response, including blood pressure control, adverse effects, persistence in treatment, visits, change in medication, and use of laboratory, have been constant. In other words, vastly different medication use patterns have had no discernible short-term effects.

More recently, the growing recognition of the ability to maximize cardiovascular disease prevention by comprehensive attention to all cardiovascular risk factors has led to a broadening of intervention patterns. The program has lost its initial "one size fits all" character and has evolved to an approach that uses the capacity to stratify patients according to cardiovascular risk while tailoring therapy according to need and opportunity for benefit.

Blood pressure control has been achieved and maintained by nearly 80% of patients with attrition from all causes <10%. An analysis of the program has revealed that participants, compared with those receiving conventional treatment, enjoyed a 40% reduction in cardiovascular events and reduced absenteeism. Medical cost savings over an 8-year period have more than paid for the program. A formal prospective comparison of several worksite-based approaches to care has indicated that the full onsite model was most effective in achieving blood pressure control.

Despite a quarter century of experience of safe, effective, and efficient care, this program has not been widely replicated. Clearly, a particular confluence of circumstances has been responsible for success in New York City. Perhaps a commitment to disease management within the context of accountable health care will grow in other environments. It is anticipated that suitable application of this highly structured, comprehensive approach to cardiovascular disease prevention can be found.

SUGGESTED READING

1. Alderman MH, Cohen H, Madhavan S. Distribution and determinants of cardiovascular events during twenty years of successful antihypertensive treatment. In press. J. Hypertension 1998;16, 5:761–769.

2. Alderman MH, Davis TK. Blood pressure control programs on and off the worksite. *J Occup Med.* 1980;22:167–170.

3. Alderman MH, Lamport B. Labelling of hypertensives: a review of the data. *J Clin Epidemiol.* 1990;43:195–200.

4. Alderman MH, Madhavan S, Cohen H. Antihypertensive drug therapy: the effect of JNC criteria on prescribing patterns and patient status through the first year [published correction appears in *Am J Hypertens.* 1996;9:840]. *Am J Hypertens.* 1996;9:413–418.

5. Alderman MH, Madhavan S, Davis TK. Reduction of cardiovascular disease events by worksite hypertension treatment. *Hypertension.* 1983;5(suppl V):V-138-V-143.

6. Alderman MH, Schoenbaum EE. Detection and treatment of hypertension at the worksite. *N Engl J Med.* 1975;293:65–68.

7. Alderman MH. Blood pressure management: individualized treatment based on absolute risk and the potential for benefit. *Ann Intern Med.* 1993;119:329–335.

8. Foote A, Erfurt JC. Hypertension control at the worksite: comparison of screening and referral alone, referral and follow-up, and on-site treatment. *N Engl J Med.* 1983;308:809–813.

9. Sixth report of the Joint National Committee on prevention, detection, evaluation, and treatment of high blood pressure (JNC VI). *Arch Intern Med.* 1997;157:2413–2446.

10. Stockwell DH, Madhavan S, Cohen H, Gibson G, Alderman MH. The determinants of hypertension awareness, treatment, and control in an insured population. *Am J Public Health.* 1994;84:1768–1774.

Chapter 153

Management of Renovascular Hypertension

Joseph V. Nally, Jr, MD

KEY POINTS

- The goals of therapy for renovascular hypertension (RVHT) are effective control of hypertension and preservation of renal function.

- Intolerable side effects from antihypertensive medications or nonadherence may favor intervention, but scrupulous screening for coexisting carotid and coronary artery disease as well as skilled interventionists are vital for success.

- ACE inhibitors are excellent antihypertensive agents for treating RVHT; any adverse effect on renal function is usually reversible. Calcium antagonists are also useful.

- Any class of antihypertensive therapy is capable of causing renal failure if systemic pressure is lowered excessively in the setting of "critical" high-grade renal artery stenosis.

See also Chapters 51, 112, 141

The goals of therapy for renovascular hypertension (RVHT) are effective control of blood pressure and preservation of renal function. The three therapeutic options include medical therapy, percutaneous transluminal renal angioplasty (PTRA), and surgical revascularization. PTRA (with or without renal artery stenting) or renovascular surgery usually reestablishes blood flow to an ischemic kidney, but optimal treatment for RVHT is uncertain, because there have been no prospective, randomized clinical trials comparing medical therapy, PTRA, and surgery. Earlier reports suggested the superiority of surgical intervention over medical therapy, but patients were not randomized, and older, medically unstable patients were more likely to be relegated to medical therapy. A prospective, randomized study of patients with high-grade bilateral renal artery stenosis (RAS) or atherosclerotic RAS to a solitary kidney is currently under way to compare medical versus surgical therapy. Until such definitive information is available, the clinician must individualize the therapeutic options.

The usual indications for intervention for renal artery disease are summarized in the **Table 153.1.** The traditional indication has been the inability to control blood pressure despite an appropriate antihypertensive regimen. Intolerable side effects from antihypertensive medications or noncompliance with the medical regimen may also favor intervention.

Surgical Intervention

In a subset of patients with focal, nonostial unilateral atherosclerotic renal artery stenosis, renal function is usually normal and widespread vascular disease is absent. These patients are manageable in the same manner as younger women with fibromuscular dysplasia. The lesions are usually located in the proximal to midrenal artery, and early restenosis after PTRA has not been a major problem.

Advances in medical therapy and surgical renovascular reconstruction have dramatically reduced the role of total or partial nephrectomy in the management of patients with RVHT. In the occasional patient with renal infarction or severe renal atrophy, advanced arteriolar nephrosclerosis, and noncorrectable renovascular lesions, nephrectomy may be indicated. Minimally invasive laparoscopic nephrectomy may be indicated in an elderly, "poor-surgical-risk" patient with an adequately functioning contralateral kidney or after a failed revascularization procedure.

Aortorenal bypass using autogenous saphenous vein or hypogastric artery is a common revascularization technique in patients with a nondiseased abdominal aorta. When an autogenous vascular graft is not available, a synthetic polytetrafluoroethylene graft can be used.

In elderly patients with generalized atherosclerosis, complex medical problems, and severe aortic disease including aneurysm formation, surgical approaches that avoid manipulation of the badly diseased aorta are preferable. For patients who require left or right renal revascularization, splenorenal or hepatorenal bypass, respectively, are preferred techniques. In patients who are not candidates for these procedures, an ileorenal bypass or renal autotransplantation may be used if there is no significant iliac disease. The thoracic aorta can also be used in patients with severe abdominal aortic atherosclerosis to achieve renal revascularization with an interposition saphenous vein graft.

Angioplasty and Stenting

Both surgical and nonsurgical revascularization procedures today are focused primarily on preservation of renal function, because blood pressure in most patients can be controlled with currently available antihypertensive drugs. Comparison of treatment procedures is difficult because most analyses have been uncontrolled, selection criteria varied greatly, and many were retrospective. Earlier studies suggested that surgery was more effective than PTRA in preserving kidney function, and procedural mortality rates were similar. More recent studies suggest that PTRA can also be an effective treatment for both hypertension and preservation of renal function.

Table 153.1. Indications for Surgery or Angioplasty

Inability to control blood pressure on an appropriate
antihypertensive regimen
Preservation of renal function
Intolerable side effects of medical therapy
Nonadherence with medical therapy

Factors that determine the success of PTRA include success of the initial dilatation, location of the lesion (ostial versus nonostial), and pre-PTRA renal function. A recent prospective, randomized study of PTRA versus surgical revascularization as initial therapy showed no differences with respect to technical results, primary and secondary patency, or effects on blood pressure and renal function in patients with atherosclerotic unilateral renal artery stenosis. PTRA can be recommended as initial therapy if combined with intensive follow-up and aggressive reintervention.

PTRA may be the initial choice in younger patients with a fibromuscular lesion amenable to balloon angioplasty. Results of PTRA for fibromuscular hyperplasia have been excellent and quite comparable to surgical revascularization. As many as 30% of patients with fibromuscular dysplasia have branch renal arterial involvement that may significantly increase the technical difficulty of PTRA but may not necessarily preclude this treatment modality.

Renal artery stenting has become an important adjunct to PTRA, being used to counteract elastic recoil and abolish the residual stenosis often observed after PTRA. Stenting after PTRA of ostial lesions has been associated with improved patency at 6 and 12 months. Stent placement provides the immediate advantage of preventing recoil and appears to be an attractive therapy in patients with lesions difficult to treat with PTRA, such as renal ostial lesions and restenotic lesions, as well as after a suboptimal PTRA result.

Medical Therapy

Medical therapy is often required for the short term while patients are being prepared for interventional therapy. Alternatively, chronic medical therapy may be required for medically unstable patients who cannot withstand intervention or for those who decline angioplasty or surgery. Medical therapy may be appropriate for older individuals with easily controlled hypertension and well-maintained renal function. For younger patients, use of antihypertensive medications for 30 to 40 years seems less appropriate, given the improving results of PTRA (with and without stenting) and surgery.

The approach to treatment of the renovascular hypertensive patient is similar to that for essential hypertension. However, three important distinctions from essential (primary) hypertension exist. First, hypertension with renovascular disease may be more difficult to control and often requires two or more medications of different classes. Second, vigilant attention must be given to preserving renal function during antihypertensive therapy. Finally, coexistent atherosclerotic carotid and coronary artery disease are more prevalent and may require specific intervention.

Historically, effective control of blood pressure in patients with RVHT has been difficult to achieve. Early reports of trials with diuretics, guanethidine, and hydralazine demonstrated control of hyperten-

sion in <50% of the patients. Successful early results with methyldopa were reported, but results were not sustained long-term. Success with suppression of the renin-angiotensin system by β-adrenergic blocking agents was sometimes attained but was not universal.

ACE inhibitors have proved to be excellent antihypertensive agents for treating RVHT, yet their potential for an adverse effect on renal function remains a concern. Angiotensin II (Ang II) receptor antagonists have effects similar to those of ACE inhibitors on blood pressure and renal function. The initial review of captopril therapy in 269 patients demonstrated successful short-term control of blood pressure in 74%. In a comparison of enalapril plus a diuretic with standard triple-drug therapy, control was achieved in 96% of ACE inhibitor–treated patients versus only 82% of those on triple-drug therapy. The long-term efficacy of captopril combined with a β-blocker and diuretic was reported in 90% of RVHT patients.

Use of an ACE inhibitor may cause a decrement in renal function in a kidney with hemodynamically significant stenosis, because glomerular filtration in this setting is Ang II–dependent. ACE inhibitor or angiotensin receptor blocker therapy removes Ang II–mediated vasoconstriction, particularly in the efferent arteriole, and thereby lowers glomerular pressure and filtration rate (GFR) of the affected kidney. Acute renal insufficiency with ACE inhibition has been observed in up to 23% to 38% of patients with high-grade bilateral RAS or RAS of a solitary kidney. A mild decrease in GFR has also been noted in 20% of patients with high-grade unilateral RAS treated with enalapril and a diuretic. Fortunately, the reduction in renal function is reversible when the ACE inhibitor is discontinued, but complete occlusion of high-grade unilateral stenoses has been reported with the use of an ACE inhibitor and a diuretic.

In patients with unilateral RAS or other forms of moderate renal artery disease, ACE inhibitors are preferred for short-term management. ACE inhibitors may be effectively combined with other antihypertensive agents, particularly diuretics. In patients with high-grade bilateral RAS or stenosis of a solitary kidney, ACE inhibitor therapy should probably not be used, or should be used only with caution, with attentive monitoring of renal function.

Calcium antagonists are quite effective in lowering blood pressure and induce less overall acute impairment of renal function in RVHT than ACE inhibitors. Both agents demonstrate a potent antihypertensive effect, but in two studies, nifedipine produced a much smaller decrement in GFR than captopril in patients with unilateral, bilateral, or solitary-kidney RAS. Calcium antagonists act to maintain renal blood flow and function because of their preferential preglomerular vasodilatory (afferent arteriolar) effect.

Any class of antihypertensive therapy is capable of reducing renal function if pressure is lowered excessively in the setting of "critical" high-grade RAS to all functioning renal mass. Refractory hypertension, often associated with worsening azotemia, is a common presentation of patients with RVHT due to bilateral RAS. Failure of medical therapy in such a patient may be an indication for more aggressive interventional therapy, such as PTRA (with or without stenting) or renovascular surgery.

Adjunctive Therapy

Providing optimal medical care for patients with renal artery disease secondary to atherosclerosis includes more than simply managing blood pressure. Modification of cardiovascular risk factors is extremely important, because the majority of patient deaths are due to coronary heart disease and cerebrovascular accidents. Careful attention must be given to managing coexisting hyperlipidemia and diabetes mellitus with diet, exercise, or pharmacological therapies. Patients must be strongly counseled to discontinue smoking.

SUGGESTED READING

1. Blum U, Krumme B, Flugel P, Gabelmann A, Lehnert T, Buitrago-Tellez C, Schollmeyer P, Langer M. Treatment of ostial renal-artery stenoses with vascular endoprostheses after unsuccessful balloon angioplasty. *N Engl J Med.* 1997;336: 459–465.

2. Franklin SS, Smith RD. Comparison of effects of enalapril plus hydrochlorothiazide versus standard triple therapy on renal function in renovascular hypertension. *Am J Med.* 1985;79(suppl 3C):14–23.

3. Hollenberg NK. Medical therapy for renovascular hypertension: a review. *Am J Hypertens.* 1988;1:338S–343S.

4. Novick AC, Ziegelbaum M, Vidt DG, Gifford RW Jr, Pohl MA, Goormastic M. Trends in surgical revascularization for renal artery disease: ten years' experience. *JAMA.* 1987;257:498–501.

5. Postma CT, Hoefnagels WH, Barentsz JO, de Boo T, Thien T. Occlusion of unilateral stenosed renal arteries: relation to medical treatment. *J Hum Hypertens.* 1989; 3:185–190.

6. Ribstein J, Mourad G, Mimran A. Contrasting acute effects of captopril and nifedipine on renal function in renovascular hypertension. *Am J Hypertens.* 1988; 1:239–244.

7. Rimmer JM, Gennari FJ. Atherosclerotic renovascular disease and progressive renal failure. *Ann Intern Med.* 1993;118:712–719.

8. Weibull FL, Bergqvist D, Bergentz SE, Jonsson K, Hulthen L, Manhem P. Percutaneous transluminal renal angioplasty versus surgical reconstruction of atherosclerotic renal artery stenosis: a prospective randomized study. *J Vasc Surg.* 1993;18:841–850; discussion, 850–852.

9. White CJ, Ramee SR, Collins TJ, Jenkins JS, Escobar A, Shaw D. Renal artery stent placement: utility in lesions difficult to treat with balloon angioplasty. *J Am Coll Cardiol.* 1997;30:1445–1450.

10. Zierler RE, Bergelin RO, Davidson RC, Cantwell-Gab K, Polissar NL, Strandness DE Jr. A prospective study of disease progression in patients with atherosclerotic renal artery stenosis. *Am J Hypertens.* 1996;9:1055–1061.

Chapter 154

Management of Pheochromocytoma

William F. Young, Jr, MD; Sheldon G. Sheps, MD

KEY POINTS

- The diagnosis of a catecholamine-producing tumor must be suspected and then confirmed biochemically by increased urine or plasma concentrations of catecholamines or their metabolites.

- Computer-assisted adrenal and abdominal imaging is the first localization test.

- The treatment of choice for pheochromocytomas, which are usually benign, is surgical resection after careful preoperative pharmacological preparation.

- Hypertension is usually cured by excision of the tumor.

See also Chapters 1, 2, 54

Prevalence estimates for pheochromocytoma vary from 0.01% to 0.1% of the hypertensive population, with an incidence of 2 to 8 cases per million people per year. These tumors occur equally in men and women, primarily in their third through fifth decades. Pheochromocytomas may be asymptomatic, but symptoms usually are due to the excess circulating catecholamines. Episodic symptoms include abrupt onset of throbbing headaches, generalized diaphoresis, palpitations, anxiety, chest pain, and abdominal pain. These spells can be extremely variable in their presentation and may be spontaneous or precipitated by postural changes, anxiety, exercise, or maneuvers that increase intra-abdominal pressure. The pheochromocytoma spell may last 10 to 60 minutes and may occur daily to monthly. Clinical signs include hypertension (paroxysmal in half of the patients and sustained in the other half), orthostatic hypotension, pallor, grade I to IV retinopathy, tremor, and fever.

Diagnosis

The diagnostic approach to catecholamine-producing tumors is divided into two series of studies **(Figure 154.1)**. First, the diagnosis of a catecholamine-producing tumor must be suspected and then confirmed biochemically by the presence of increased urine or plasma concentrations of catecholamines or their metabolites. Suppression testing with clonidine or provocative testing with glucagon, histamine, or metoclopramide is rarely needed. The differential diagnosis of pheochromocytoma is summarized in **Table 154.1.**

The next step is to localize the catecholamine-producing tumor to guide the surgical approach. Computer-assisted adrenal and abdominal imaging (magnetic resonance imaging or computed tomography) is the first localization test. Approximately 90% of these tumors are found in the adrenals, and 98% are in the abdomen. If the abdominal imaging is negative, then scintigraphic localization with [123I]meta-iodobenzylguanidine (123I-MIBG) is indicated. This radiopharmaceutical accumulates preferentially in catecholamine-producing tumors; however, this procedure is not as definitive as initially hoped (sensitivity, 85%; specificity, 99%). Computer-assisted chest, neck, and head imaging and octreotide scintigraphy are addi-

tional localizing procedures that can be used, although they are rarely required.

Treatment

The treatment of choice for pheochromocytoma is surgical resection. Most of these tumors are benign and can be totally excised. Hypertension is usually cured by excision of the tumor, and careful preoperative pharmacological preparation is crucial to successful treatment.

Preoperative Management

Combined α- and β-adrenergic blockade is recommended before surgery to control blood pressure and to prevent intraoperative hypertensive crises. α-Adrenergic blockade (eg, phenoxybenzamine) should be started at least 10 days before surgery to allow for expansion of the contracted blood volume. A liberal salt diet is advised during the preoperative period. Once adequate α-adrenergic blockade is achieved, β-adrenergic blockade is initiated (eg, 3 days before surgery).

α-Methyl-L-tyrosine (metyrosine) inhibits the synthesis of catecholamines by blocking the enzyme tyrosine hydroxylase. Because of the significant side-effect profile of metyrosine, it is reserved primarily for those patients who, for cardiopulmonary reasons, cannot be treated with combined α- and β-adrenergic blockade.

Anesthesia and Surgery

Extirpation of a pheochromocytoma is a high-risk surgical procedure, and an experienced surgeon/anesthesiologist team is required. The last oral doses of α- and β-adrenergic blockers can be administered early in the morning on the day of operation. Cardiovascular and hemodynamic variables must be monitored closely. Acute hypertensive crises may occur before or during operation and should be treated with nitroprusside or phentolamine administered intravenously.

In the past, an anterior midline abdominal surgical approach was usually used for adrenal pheochromocytoma. However, laparoscopic

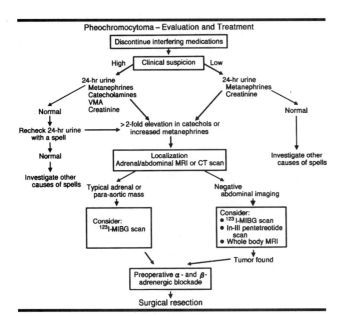

Figure 154.1. Evaluation and treatment of catecholamine-producing tumors. Clinical suspicion is triggered by the following: paroxysmal symptoms (especially hypertension); hypertension that is intermittent, unusually labile, or resistant to treatment; family history of pheochromocytoma or associated conditions; or incidentally discovered adrenal mass. For details, see text. VMA indicates vanillylmandelic acid; CT, computed tomography; MRI, magnetic resonance imaging; and ^{123}I-MIBG, [^{123}I]meta-iodobenzylguanidine. Modified and reprinted with permission from Trends in Endocrinology and Metabolism, vol 4. Young WF Jr. *Pheochromocytoma: 1926–1993.* New York, NY: Elsevier Science Inc; 1993:122.

adrenalectomy is becoming the procedure of choice in patients with solitary intra-adrenal pheochromocytomas that are <8 cm in diameter. If the pheochromocytoma is in the adrenal gland, the entire gland should be removed. If the tumor is malignant, as much tumor as possible should be removed. Paragangliomas of the neck, chest, and urinary bladder require specialized approaches. In major centers, the surgical mortality rate is <2%. The survival rate after removal of a benign pheochromocytoma is nearly that of age- and sex-matched controls.

Blood pressure usually is normal by the time of dismissal from the hospital. Approximately 2 weeks after surgery, a 24-hour urine sample should be obtained for measurement of catecholamines and metanephrines. If the levels are normal, the resection of the pheochromocytoma can be considered to have been complete. The 24-hour urinary excretion of catecholamines should be checked annually for at least 5 years as surveillance for recurrence in the adrenal bed, metastatic pheochromocytoma, or delayed appearance of multiple primary tumors. Lifelong follow-up may be indicated if tumor DNA ploidy is abnormal.

Diagnostic studies for familial disorders such as MEN II, von Hippel–Lindau syndrome, and familial pheochromocytoma should be considered during the first postoperative visit. Testing to be considered includes *RET* proto-oncogene or pentagastrin stimulation test, ophthalmology consult, head MRI scan, and 24-hour urinary metanephrines on all immediate family members.

Malignant Pheochromocytoma

The distinction between benign and malignant catecholamine-producing tumors cannot be made on clinical, biochemical, or histopathological characteristics. Malignancy is based on finding direct local invasion or disease metastatic to sites that do not have chromaffin tissue, such as lymph nodes, bone, lung, and liver. Although the 5-year survival rate is <50%, many of these patients have prolonged survival and minimal morbidity. Metastatic lesions should be resected if possible. Tumor embolization may be considered for patients with localized but unresectable tumors. Painful skeletal metastatic lesions can be treated with external radiation therapy. Local tumor irradiation with ^{131}I-MIBG has proved to be of limited therapeutic value. If the tumor is considered to be aggressive and the quality of life is affected, then combination chemotherapy may be considered. A chemotherapy program consisting of cyclophosphamide, vincristine,

Table 154.1. Differential Diagnosis of Pheochromocytoma Spells

Endocrine
  Thyrotoxicosis
  Primary hypogonadism (eg, menopausal syndrome)
  Pancreatic tumors (eg, insulinoma)
  Medullary thyroid carcinoma
  "Hyperadrenergic" spells
Cardiovascular
  Essential hypertension, labile
  Angina and cardiovascular deconditioning
  Pulmonary edema
  Dilated cardiomyopathy
  Syncope
  Orthostatic hypotension
  Paroxysmal cardiac arrhythmia
  Aortic dissection
  Renovascular hypertension
Psychological
  Anxiety and panic attacks
  Somatization disorder
  Hyperventilation
  Factitious (eg, drugs, Valsalva)
Pharmacological
  Withdrawal of adrenergic-inhibiting medication (eg, clonidine)
  Monoamine oxidase inhibitor treatment and concomitant
    ingestion of tyramine or a decongestant
  Sympathomimetic ingestion
  Illicit drug ingestion (eg, cocaine, phencyclidine, lysergic acid)
  Gold myokymia syndrome
  Acrodynia (mercury poisoning)
  Vancomycin ("red man syndrome")
Neurological
  Baroreflex failure
  Postural orthostatic tachycardia syndrome (POTS)
  Autonomic neuropathy
  Migraine headache
  Diencephalic epilepsy (autonomic seizures)
  Cerebral infarction
  Cerebrovascular insufficiency
Miscellaneous
  Mastocytosis (systemic or activation disorder)
  Carcinoid syndrome
  Recurrent idiopathic anaphylaxis
  Unexplained flushing spells

and dacarbazine given cyclically every 21 to 28 days has proved beneficial but not curative in these patients.

SUGGESTED READING

1. Averbuch SD, Steakley CS, Young RC, Gelmann EP, Goldstein DS, Stull R, Keiser HR. Malignant pheochromocytoma: effective treatment with a combination of cyclophosphamide, vincristine, and dacarbazine. *Ann Intern Med.* 1988;109: 267–273.

2. Eng C, Clayton D, Schuffenecker I, Lenoir G, Cote G, Gagel RF, von Amstel HK, Lips CJ, Nishisho I, Takai SI, Marsh DJ, Robinson BG, Frank-Raue K, Raue F, Xue F, Noll WW, Romei C, Pacini F, Fink M, Niederle B, Zendenius J, Nordenskjold M, Komminoth P, Hendy GN, Mulligan LM, et al. The relationship between specific *RET* proto-oncogene mutations and disease phenotype in multiple endocrine neoplasia type 2: international *RET* Mutation Consortium analysis. *JAMA.* 1996;276:1575–1579.

3. Lenders JW, Keiser HR, Goldstein DS, Willemsen JJ, Friberg P, Jacobs MC, Klop-penborg PW, Thien T, Eisenhofer G. Plasma metanephrines in the diagnosis of pheochromocytoma. *Ann Intern Med.* 1995;123:101–109.

4. Nativ O, Grant CS, Sheps SG, O'Fallon JR, Farrow GM, van Heerden JA, Lieber MM. The clinical significance of nuclear DNA ploidy pattern in 184 patients with pheochromocytoma. *Cancer.* 1992;69:2683–2687.

5. Sheps SG, Jiang N-S, Klee GG. Diagnostic evaluation of pheochromocytoma. *Endocrinol Metab Clin North Am.* 1988;17:397–414.

6. Stein PP, Black HR. A simplified diagnostic approach to pheochromocytoma: a review of the literature and report of one institution's experience. *Medicine.* 1991; 70:46–66.

7. Young WF Jr. Pheochromocytoma: issues in diagnosis and treatment. *Compr Ther.* 1997;23:319–326.

8. Young WF Jr. Pheochromocytoma: 1926–1993. *Trends Endocrinol Metab.* 1993;4: 122–127.

9. Young WF Jr, Maddox DE. Spells: in search of a cause. *Mayo Clin Proc.* 1995;70: 757–765.

Chapter 155

Management of Hypercortisolism and Hyperaldosteronism

Emmanuel L. Bravo, MD

KEY POINTS

- The determination of 24-hour urinary free cortisol is the best available test for documentation of endogenous hypercortisolism.

- The preferred treatment for Cushing's syndrome is surgical resection of a pituitary or ectopic source of adrenocorticotropic hormone or removal of the cortisol-producing adrenal cortical tumor.

- The recommended initial test in suspected primary aldosteronism is the determination of aldosterone excretion rate during prolonged salt loading.

- In primary aldosteronism, coupling medical therapy with sustained salt and water depletion provides effective long-term control of blood pressure.

See also Chapters 9, 10, 11, 53

Enzymatic Deficiencies
Evaluation

Deficiency of either 11-β-hydroxylase or 17-α-hydroxylase adrenocortical enzyme results in decreased cortisol production. Decreased circulating cortisol leads to enhanced release of adrenocorticotropic hormone (ACTH), which stimulates deoxycorticosterone production. The increased circulating deoxycorticosterone produces salt and water retention, hypokalemia, and ultimately, elevated arterial blood pressure.

Findings on initial physical examination provide the most important clues to the presence of an enzymatic deficiency. Virilization in female patients or precocious puberty with advanced masculinization in males (due to increased androgen production) are prominent features of 11-β-hydroxylase deficiency. Absence of secondary sex characteristics in females (due to decreased estrogen production) or failure to fully develop masculine external genitalia (male pseudohermaphroditism) in males (due to decreased androgen production) distinguishes the patient with 17-α-hydroxylase deficiency.

The diagnosis of 11-β-hydroxylase deficiency can be confirmed by demonstration of increased levels of 11-deoxycortisol in plasma and tetrahydro-*S* and 17-ketosteroids in urine. The diagnosis of 17-α-hydroxylase can be established by the demonstration of elevated deoxycorticosterone and corticosterone and decreased androgen production. In both, dexamethasone administration inhibits ACTH secretion, resulting in normalization of blood pressure and serum potassium concentration.

Treatment

The elevated arterial blood pressure that is associated with deficiencies of 11-β-hydroxylase or 17-α-hydroxylase adrenocortical enzyme is due to the excess deoxycorticosterone production caused by ACTH overdrive. Increased ACTH release results from decreased inhibitory influences by cortisol, which is lacking in both disorders. In both conditions, dexamethasone in physiological doses (0.5 to 0.75 mg/d) inhibits ACTH secretion, resulting in normalization of blood pressure and serum potassium concentration.

Cushing's Syndrome
Evaluation

The typical clinical presentation of Cushing's syndrome includes truncal obesity, moon face, hypertension, plethora, muscle weakness and fatigue, hirsutism, emotional disturbances, and typical purple skin striae. Carbohydrate intolerance or diabetes, amenorrhea, loss of libido, easy bruising, and spontaneous fractures of ribs and vertebrae may be encountered. All patients may exhibit some of these features at the time of diagnosis. However, few if any will have all of them.

For screening purposes, the overnight 1-mg dexamethasone-suppression test and the measurement of 24-hour urinary free cortisol have been used in most centers. With the overnight 1-mg dexamethasone-suppression test, reduction of basal plasma cortisol level to values <5 μg/dL is defined as normal suppression. The test is simple and has a low incidence of false-normal suppression (<3%). However, it has a high incidence of false-positive results (≈20% to 30%) and does not distinguish between hypercortisolism due to Cushing's syndrome and other non-Cushing's hypercortisolemic states (stress, pregnancy, chronic strenuous exercise, psychiatric states, malnutrition, and glucocorticoid resistance).

The determination of 24-hour urinary free cortisol is the best available test for documentation of endogenous hypercortisolism. A level >100 μg/24 h suggests excessive production of cortisol. Assuming complete collections, there are virtually no false-negative results. False-positive results, however, may be obtained in several non-Cushing's hypercortisolemic states.

The choice and success of treatment in Cushing's syndrome depend largely on accurate determination of the cause of the hypercortisolism. Spontaneous (endogenous) Cushing's syndrome can result from ACTH excess (ACTH-dependent) or from autonomous secretion of cortisol (ACTH-independent) **(Table 155.1).** Radioimmunoassay of plasma ACTH is the procedure of choice for pinpointing the basis for hypercortisolism. In cases in which differentiation between pituitary and ectopic sources of ACTH excess cannot be made on the basis of plasma levels alone, a computed tomographic (CT) scan may be very helpful. Should these tests prove to be unrevealing, pharmacological manipulation of ACTH secretion and measurement of ACTH gradients from the head and below the neck may help in differentiating pituitary from ectopic Cushing's syndrome.

The Liddle dexamethasone suppression test is regarded as one of the best to discriminate between Cushing's syndrome and other types of endogenous hypercortisolism. In normal subjects and patients with pseudo-Cushing's syndrome, ACTH release can be suppressed with low-dose administration of dexamethasone (2 mg/d divided for dosing every 6 hours, for 2 days). In patients with Cushing's syndrome, ACTH release can be inhibited only at much higher doses of dexamethasone (8 mg/d divided for every 6 hours, for 2 days). In contrast, patients with the ectopic ACTH syndrome or Cushing's syndrome due to cortisol-secreting adrenal tumors usually fail to respond to high-dose administration of dexamethasone. The diagnostic accuracy of the test is ≈85%.

Surgical Therapy

The standard of care for the majority of cases of Cushing's syndrome is surgical resection of a pituitary or an ectopic source of ACTH or removal of a cortisol-producing adrenocortical tumor. Transsphenoidal pituitary adenomectomy is the treatment of choice in most patients, but total hypophysectomy may be required in patients with diffuse hyperplasia or in patients with a large pituitary tumor. Bilateral adrenalectomy for Cushing's disease is almost universally successful in alleviating the hypercortisolemic state. However, 10% to 38% may later develop Nelson's syndrome, with hyperpigmentation and higher risk of pituitary tumor invasion.

The potential for cure of Cushing's disease (ACTH-dependent) is related to preoperative/postoperative cortisol responses to stimulation and the basal levels of cortisol achieved after surgery. The preoperative cortisol response to corticotropin-releasing hormone stimulation is greater among those cured by surgery than among surgical failures (maximal increment in serum is 18 versus 11 μg/dL). The 5% to 25% rate of recurrence at 3 to 5 years after initial surgical cure is associated with relatively higher basal cortisol levels after surgery (4.7 versus 1.5 μg/dL). The cortisol response to corticotropin-releasing hormone after surgery is also significantly greater among those who later relapse than in those who remain in remission (10.9 versus 4.3 μg/dL). Thus, cortisol levels >3.6 μg/dL after transsphenoidal adenomectomy indicate an increased risk of late recurrence.

Perioperatively, most patients undergoing selective adenomectomy are given glucocorticoid therapy to prevent postoperative hypoadrenalism that may result from the acute reduction in ACTH and cortisol production. This transient secondary insufficiency usually lasts 4 to 6 months after surgical cure. Although a number of nonsurgical treatments have been suggested, those are generally palliation and can seldom take the place of a surgical approach.

Radiotherapy

Seeding the pituitary bed with yttrium or gold has been advocated. Among patients with Cushing's disease whose radiographic studies failed to reveal sellar changes, 65% had complete remission and 16% had partial remission at 1 year after yttrium implantation therapy. In subjects with demonstrable tumors on lateral skull films, only two had similar complete remission. External pituitary irradiation has also been used, with occasionally good results. Lower doses (2000 rad given over 10 days) are described as being as effective as the conventional doses (3500 to 5000 rad) but without associated deficiencies of other pituitary hormones.

Medical Therapy

The long-acting analogue SMS 201–995 (octreotide or sandostatin) has been used with variable success to treat ectopic ACTH syndromes, but some benefit has been reported in Cushing's disease and Nelson's syndrome. Cyproheptadine, a serotonin antagonist, has demonstrated limited success in the treatment of Cushing's disease. Cyproheptadine and bromocriptine, alone or in combination, have little effect on the elevated ACTH levels after adrenalectomy for Cushing's syndrome in patients without evidence of a pituitary tumor. Ketoconazole has been advocated as an inhibitor of adrenal (and gonadal) sterol production by inhibiting several biosynthetic steps. For rapid correction of hypercortisolism awaiting definitive interven-

---

Table 155.1. Classification and Principle Diagnostic Differences in Cushing's Syndrome

TYPE	OCCURRENCE, %	PLASMA ACTH	CT SCAN
ACTH-dependent	85		
Pituitary	80	Normal	Normal size adrenals
Ectopic ACTH	20	>200 pg/mL	Bilaterally enlarged adrenals
Ectopic CRH	(rare)	>200 pg/mL	Bilaterally enlarged adrenals
ACTH-independent	15	Low/nondetectable	
Adrenal adenoma (most common)			Unilateral adrenal mass
Adrenal carcinoma			Unilateral adrenal mass
Macronodular adrenal hyperplasia			Enlarged/nodular adrenals
Primary pigmented nodular adrenal disease			Nodular adrenals

CRH indicates corticotropin-releasing hormone.

tion, ketoconazole may play a valuable role. However, hepatocellular injury and acute adrenal insufficiency are frequent complications that may necessitate discontinuation of therapy or addition of corticosteroids to the therapeutic regimen.

Mitotane (*o,p'*-DDD) is an insecticide derivative that induces destruction of the zonae reticularis and fasciculata, with relative sparing of the zona glomerulosa. Its use in Cushing's disease (associated with adrenal carcinoma) is directed toward adrenal suppression, whereas the pituitary tumor itself is not treated. Subsequent mineralocorticoid replacement is usually not needed, and several months are required for the medication to have an effect on the adrenal gland. Nausea, depression, gynecomastia, and decreased memory are common side effects. In addition, significant loss of adrenocortical reserve may ensue, requiring corticoid therapy at times of stress.

Primary Aldosteronism
Evaluation

The disorder should be considered in patients with (1) spontaneous hypokalemia (serum potassium level <3.5 mEq/L), (2) moderately severe hypokalemia (serum potassium level <3.0 mEq/L) during diuretic therapy with conventional dosages, and (3) difficulty in maintaining normal serum potassium levels during diuretic therapy despite concomitant use of oral potassium supplementation and/or potassium-sparing agents and/or ACE inhibitors.

Hypokalemia, whether spontaneous or provoked, provides an important clue to the presence of primary aldosteronism. However, serum potassium concentration is normal in 7% to 38% of reported cases. In addition, 10% to 12% of patients with proven cases may not have hypokalemia during short-term salt loading. Notable is the fact that in the "normokalemic" group, conventional diuretic therapy usually produces moderately severe hypokalemia, a finding previously considered unimportant in a hypertensive patient receiving a potassium-wasting diuretic agent.

Measurement of plasma renin activity (PRA) under conditions of stimulation (sodium restriction, diuretic administration, and upright posture) has been used as a screening test to exclude primary aldosteronism. Suppressed PRA (<1.0 ng·mL^{-1}·h^{-1}) that fails to rise above 2.0 ng·mL^{-1}·h^{-1} after salt and water depletion is considered a positive test. However, some patients with primary aldosteronism may have clearly unsuppressed values during normal dietary sodium intake, and a substantial number ($\approx$35%) may have stimulated PRA (>2.0 ng·mL^{-1}·h^{-1}). In addition, $\approx$40% of subjects with essential hypertension have suppressed PRA during normal dietary sodium intake; 15% to 20% of these patients show values <2.0 ng·mL^{-1}·h^{-1} under conditions of stimulation. The large number of false-positive and false-negative results makes PRA determinations of limited use in screening patients for the presence of primary aldosteronism.

The ratio of aldosterone to PRA is used to define the appropriateness of PRA for the circulating concentrations of aldosterone. It is assumed that the volume expansion associated with aldosteronism inhibits the synthesis of renin without affecting the autonomous production of aldosterone. One serious drawback of this test is the inherent variability of plasma levels of aldosterone, even in the presence of a tumor. Another is the use of drugs that result in either marked suppression or prolonged stimulation of renin long

after their discontinuation. Under these circumstances, both false-positives and false-negatives are likely to occur.

The single best test for identification of patients with primary aldosteronism is the measurement of aldosterone excretion rate during salt loading. A rate >14.0 μg/24 h after 3 days of salt loading (25 mL/kg of 0.9% saline over 4 hours for 3 days) distinguishes most patients with primary aldosteronism from those with essential hypertension. Only 7% of patients with primary aldosteronism have values that fall within the range for essential hypertension (**Figure 155.1**). Under the same conditions, a substantial number (39%) of patients with primary aldosteronism have plasma aldosterone values that fall within the range for essential hypertension. Thus, the measurement of aldosterone excretion rate after salt loading provides greater sensitivity and specificity than the measurement of plasma aldosterone concentration.

On the basis of the foregoing observations, the recommended initial test in suspected primary aldosteronism is the determination of aldosterone excretion rate during prolonged salt loading (**Figure 155.2**). Outpatients can be evaluated by addition of 10 to 12 g sodium chloride to the normal daily sodium intake and determination of the serum potassium concentration and the 24-hour urinary

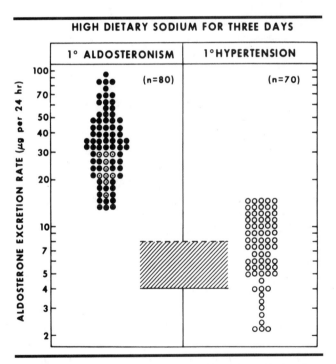

Figure 155.1. Aldosterone excretion rate after 3 days of high sodium intake. For patients with primary aldosteronism, solid circles represent adenomas (n=70) and open circles with dotted centers represent hyperplasia (n=10). The crosshatched area represents the mean (4.0 μg/24 h +2 SD (8.0 μg/24 h) of values obtained from 47 healthy subjects. No patient with primary aldosteronism had a value within the 95th percentile of the normal range. Ten patients (14%) with primary hypertension had values that fell within the range obtained in patients with primary aldosteronism. With a reference value of >14 μg/24 h after a high sodium intake for 3 days, the sensitivity and specificity of the test are 96% and 93%, respectively. Reproduced with permission from Bravo EL, Tarazi RC, Dustan HP, et al. The changing clinical spectrum of primary aldosteronism. *Am J Med.* 1983;74:641–651.

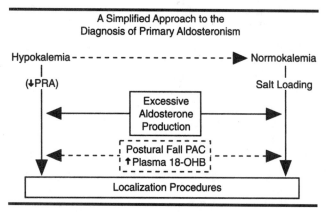

Figure 155.2. Algorithm for the diagnosis of primary aldosteronism. PAC indicates plasma aldosterone concentration; 18-OHB, plasma 18-hydroxycorticosterone concentration. Reproduced with permission from Bravo EL. Primary aldosteronism. *Urol Clin North Am.* 1989;16: 481–486.

excretion rate of sodium, potassium, and aldosterone after 5 to 7 days. Serum and urinary potassium values serve to indicate whether inappropriate kaliuresis (serum potassium ≤3.0 mEq/L, with urinary potassium excretion ≥30 mEq/L per 24 hours) occurs during salt loading. The finding of a 24-hour urinary sodium excretion rate of ≥250 mEq/L gives some assurance that the patient has ingested the prescribed amount of salt. Patients in whom aldosterone excretion rate fails to be suppressed to <14.0 μg/24 h with salt loading are prime candidates for additional studies. The presence of hypokalemia and/or suppressed PRA provides corroborative evidence of primary aldosteronism, but absence of either or both does not preclude the diagnosis.

As in Cushing's syndrome, the appropriate therapy of patients with primary aldosteronism depends on accurate determination of the cause of excessive aldosterone production. The recognizable forms of primary aldosteronism include aldosterone-producing adenoma, adrenal (glomerulosa) hyperplasia, "indeterminate hyperaldosteronism," glucocorticoid-suppressible aldosteronism, and aldosterone-producing adrenal carcinoma. Spontaneous, moderately severe hypokalemia (<3.0 mEq/L), an anomalous postural decrease in plasma aldosterone concentration, and increased plasma 18-hydroxycorticosterone values (≥100 ng/dL) distinguish an adenoma from hyperplasia. Adrenal carcinomas usually produce various adrenocorticosteroids other than aldosterone. For localization of an adenoma, an adrenal CT scan should be obtained first and is considered diagnostic if an adrenal mass is clearly identified. When the CT scan is inconclusive, adrenal venous sampling for aldosterone and cortisol levels should be done.

Medical Therapy

Medical therapy is indicated in (1) patients with adrenal hyperplasia, (2) patients with adenoma who are poor surgical risks, and (3) patients with bilateral adenomas that would otherwise require bilateral adrenalectomy. The long-standing experience has been that the hypertension associated with primary aldosteronism is salt- and water-dependent and is best treated by sustained salt and water depletion. Usual doses of diuretics are hydrochlorothiazide 25 to 50 mg/d or furosemide 80 to 160 mg/d in combination with either spironolactone 100 to 200 mg/d or amiloride 10 to 20 mg/d. This usually results in

prompt correction of hypokalemia and normalization of blood pressure within 2 to 4 weeks. In some cases, the addition of a β-adrenergic blocker, a central sympatholytic agent, or a vasodilator may be needed to normalize arterial pressure completely. Other alternatives, such as the sole use of nifedipine (40 to 60 mg/d), are not as effective as diuretic therapy and fail to correct the metabolic abnormalities. Potential side effects of spironolactone include gynecomastia, impotence, nausea, vomiting, pigmentation, and lassitude. Hyperkalemia may occur in those patients with significant impairment of renal function.

Surgical Therapy

Adrenal adenomas may now be resected through a laparoscopic approach. Operating time is similar to the conventional approach; however, there is minimal blood loss, hospital stay is short (average, 2.7 days), recovery is rapid (≈2 to 3 weeks), and cosmetic results are excellent. In the majority of cases, surgical excision of aldosterone-producing adenomas leads to normotension as well as reversal of the biochemical defects. At the very least, surgery renders arterial pressure easier to control with medications in those who have residual hypertension. Neither duration and severity of hypertension nor the degree of end-organ target involvement has any relationship to the arterial pressure response after surgery.

Patients undergoing surgery should receive drug treatment for at least 3 to 6 months, both to decrease blood pressure and to correct metabolic abnormalities. These patients have a significant potassium deficit that must be corrected before surgery because hypokalemia increases the risk of cardiac arrhythmias during anesthesia. Prolonged reduction of arterial blood pressure permits the use of intravenous fluids during surgery without producing hypertension and decreases morbidity. Administration of medications is usually continued until surgery, and glucocorticoid administration is not needed before surgery. During the immediate postoperative period, antihypertensive agents are generally not required if the patient had been normotensive for at least 3 months before surgery while receiving diuretic therapy. If hypertension becomes a problem, diuretics should be tried first and other types of antihypertensive agents later.

After the removal of an aldosterone-producing adenoma, selective hypoaldosteronism usually occurs, even in patients in whom PRA had been stimulated with chronic diuretic therapy. One likely explanation for this effect is that spironolactone may inhibit aldosterone biosynthesis by the adrenal cortex. Therefore, if indicated, potassium supplementation should be given cautiously, and serum potassium values should be monitored closely. However, sufficient residual mineralocorticoid activity is often left to prevent excessive renal retention of potassium, provided that sodium intake is adequate. If hyperkalemia does occur, all forms of potassium chloride supplementation should be discontinued, and administration of furosemide in doses of 80 to 160 mg/d should be started. Treatment with fludrocortisone is not often necessary. If it is needed, 0.1 mg/d may be used as the initial dose. Abnormalities in aldosterone production can persist for as long as 3 months.

Glucocorticoid-Remediable Aldosteronism
Evaluation

Glucocorticoid-remediable aldosteronism is an inherited autosomal-dominant disorder that mimics an aldosterone-producing adenoma. It is caused by a genetic mutation that results in a hybrid or chimeric gene product fusing nucleotide sequences of the 11-β-hydroxylase and aldosterone synthase genes. This hybrid gene allows ectopic expression of aldosterone synthase activity in the ACTH-regulated zona fasciculata, which normally produces cortisol. This enzyme thereby oxidizes the C-18 carbon of a steroid precursor, such as corticosterone or cortisol, leading to the production of aldosterone and the hybrid steroids 18-hydroxy and 18-oxocortisol. This abnormal gene duplication can readily be detected by the Southern blotting test, allowing for direct genetic screening for this disorder with a small blood sample. Administration of dexamethasone in doses of 2 mg/24 h (0.5 mg every 6 hours) usually results in remission of hypertension and hypokalemia within 7 to 10 days.

Glucocorticoid-remediable aldosteronism should be suspected in a patient with primary aldosteronism who presents with the following clinical history: first, a family history of primary aldosteronism; second, early age of onset of hypertension; and third, severe hypertension with early death of affected family members resulting from cerebrovascular accident.

Treatment

The suppression of ACTH with exogenous glucocorticoid should correct all cardiovascular and metabolic abnormalities; however, this therapy may be limited by untoward complications resulting from glucocorticoid excess. Additional treatment modalities are aimed at mineralocorticoid receptor blockade with spironolactone or inhibition of the mineralocorticoid-sensitive distal tubule sodium channel with amiloride.

SUGGESTED READING

1. Biglieri EG, Kater CE. 17 Alpha-hydroxylation deficiency. In: Nelson DH, ed. *Endocrinology and Metabolism Clinics of North America.* Philadelphia, Pa: WB Saunders Co; 1991:257–268.
2. Bravo EL. Primary aldosteronism: issues in diagnosis and management. *Endocrinol Clin N Am.* 1994;23:387–404.
3. Kaye TB, Crapo L. The Cushing syndrome: an update on diagnostic tests. *Ann Intern Med.* 1990;112:434–444.
4. Lifton RP, Dluhy RG, Powers M, et al. Hereditary hypertension caused by chimeric gene duplications and ectopic expression of aldosterone synthase. *Nat Genet.* 1992;2:66–74.
5. Melby JC. Diagnosis of hyperaldosteronism. In: Nelson DH, ed. *Endocrinology and Metabolism Clinics of North America.* Philadelphia, Pa: WB Saunders Co; 1991:247–255.
6. Miller JW, Crapo L. The medical treatment of Cushing's syndrome. *Endocrinol Rev.* 1993;14:443–458.
7. White PC, Pascoe L. Disorders of steroid 11 beta-hydroxylase isozymes. In: Bilezikian JP, ed. *Trends in Endocrinology and Metabolism, I.* New York, NY: Elsevier Science Publishing Co Inc; 1989:229–234.
8. Winfield HN, Hamilton BD, Bravo EL. Technique of laparoscopic adrenalectomy. *Urol Clin N Am.* 1997;24:459–465.

Chapter 156

Management of Thyroid and Parathyroid Disorders

William F. Young, Jr, MD

KEY POINTS

- The types of thyroid disease associated with hypertension include hyperthyroidism, hypothyroidism, and medullary thyroid carcinoma (associated with pheochromocytoma in the multiple endocrine neoplasia syndromes types IIA and IIB).

- The hypercalcemia of hyperparathyroidism is associated with an increased incidence of hypertension.

- Thyroid- and parathyroid-directed treatment in the hypertensive patient may normalize hypertension or facilitate its treatment.

See also Chapter 55

Dysfunction of the thyroid and parathyroid glands may be the sole cause of hypertension or may contribute significantly to underlying primary hypertension. The types of thyroid disease associated with hypertension include hyperthyroidism, hypothyroidism, and medullary thyroid carcinoma (MTC) (associated with pheochromocytoma in the multiple endocrine neoplasia [MEN] type IIA and IIB syndromes). Primary hyperparathyroidism is the most frequent cause of hypercalcemia, which is also associated with hypertension.

Thyroid Dysfunction

Clinical Presentation

Hyperthyroidism is the clinical syndrome that occurs when excessive amounts of circulating thyroid hormones interact with thyroid hormone receptors on peripheral tissues. This results in increased metabolic activity and increased sensitivity to circulating catecholamines. Thyrotoxic patients usually have a high cardiac output and an increased systolic blood pressure.

Hypothyroidism is the syndrome resulting from deficiency of thyroid hormones, which causes many metabolic processes to slow down. Hypothyroid patients have a 3-fold-increased prevalence of hypertension, usually diastolic.

Laboratory Diagnosis

The clinical suspicion of thyroid gland dysfunction may be confirmed with laboratory tests. Increased levels of blood thyroid hormones (thyroxine and triiodothyronine) and low serum levels of thyroid-stimulating hormone (TSH) are the hallmarks of hyperthyroidism. The diagnosis of hypothyroidism is based on low serum levels of thyroid hormone and increased serum levels of TSH.

Treatment

The initial management of the hypertensive patient with hyperthyroidism includes the use of a β-adrenergic blocker (eg, atenolol) to treat the hypertension, tachycardia, and tremor. The definitive treatment of hyperthyroidism is cause-specific. For example, patients with autoimmune hyperthyroidism (Graves' disease) should be treated with thyroid gland ablation with ^{131}I. In the patient with hyperthyroidism caused by a multinodular goiter (Plummer's disease), ^{131}I is usually not curative, and subtotal thyroidectomy is the treatment of choice. Finally, if the hyperthyroidism is associated with acute thyroid inflammation (eg, subacute thyroiditis), the temporary (eg, 3 months) use of a β-adrenergic inhibitor may be the only treatment indicated.

Treatment of thyroid hormone deficiency lowers blood pressure in most hypertensive patients. Synthetic levothyroxine is the treatment of choice for hypothyroidism. The initial dosage of levothyroxine is based on body weight ($1.6 \ \mu g \cdot kg^{-1} \cdot d^{-1}$). The daily dosage requirement may be lower in older patients (eg, $<1.0 \ \mu g \cdot kg^{-1} \cdot d^{-1}$). In patients >50 years of age or patients with cardiac disease, the initial dosage of levothyroxine should be lower (eg, 25 to 50 $\mu g/d$) and increased every 2 weeks by 25 μg until the target dosage is achieved. Clinical and biochemical reevaluations should be completed at 2-month intervals until the serum TSH concentration is normalized.

Primary Hyperparathyroidism

Clinical Presentation

Hypercalcemia is associated with an increased incidence of hypertension. Primary hyperparathyroidism is the most common cause of hypercalcemia. The prevalence of hypertension in patients with primary hyperparathyroidism varies from 10% to 60%. In the majority of cases, the disease is caused by a benign solitary parathyroid adenoma. However, when associated with the MEN syndromes, the hyperparathyroidism is usually due to hyperplasia of all four parathyroid glands.

Most patients with primary hyperparathyroidism are asymptomatic. The side effects of chronic hypercalcemia may be the focus of the presentation: polyuria and polydipsia, constipation, osteoporosis, renal lithiasis, peptic ulcer disease, and hypertension.

Laboratory Diagnosis

The hallmarks of primary hyperparathyroidism are hypercalcemia, hypophosphatemia, and increased serum concentrations of parathyroid hormone. In the patient with hypercalcemia, the measurement of serum parathyroid hormone is the most specific way of making the diagnosis of primary hyperparathyroidism. If the serum concentration of parathyroid hormone is not increased, the clinical data should be reviewed and nonparathyroid causes of hypercalcemia investigated (eg, pheochromocytoma, hyperthyroidism, cancer, multiple myeloma, vitamin D intoxication, and sarcoidosis).

Treatment

The treatment of hyperparathyroidism is surgical. This involves a neck exploration, identification of all four parathyroid glands, and removal of the single adenoma in the sporadic cases or, in the setting of MEN, subtotal parathyroid resection (3.5 glands) of the hyperplastic glands.

Medullary Thyroid Carcinoma

The occurrence of MTC may be sporadic or familial (familial MTC or MEN II). Although MTC does not cause hypertension, the close association with pheochromocytoma is recognized: MEN type IIA (MTC, pheochromocytoma, and hyperparathyroidism) and MEN type IIB (MTC, pheochromocytoma, mucosal neuromas, and marfanoid body habitus). The MEN type II syndromes are inherited as autosomal dominant traits with complete penetrance and variable expressivity.

Clinical Presentation

The usual presentation of MTC is with a thyroid nodule, a thyroid mass, or cervical lymphadenopathy. Although serum calcitonin concentrations are increased, most patients are asymptomatic. Up to 30% of patients with MTC develop watery diarrhea, presumably secondary to high circulating calcitonin levels. Serum levels of calcium and phosphorus are normal.

Laboratory Diagnosis

When the presentation is limited to a solitary thyroid nodule, the diagnosis of MTC may be made on cytological findings from a fine-needle aspirate. In other patients, MTC may be suspected and found with genetic or biochemical testing because of a family history of MEN II. All first-degree relatives of patients with MEN II should be screened with serum *RET* proto-oncogene.

Treatment

The treatment of choice of MTC is surgical resection. Most centers advocate total thyroidectomy and ^{131}I ablation of the thyroid gland remnant. After this initial treatment, patients are placed on levothyroxine replacement therapy and should be followed up on an annual basis with physical examination and serum calcitonin concentration tests. If recurrent disease is suspected on the basis of increasing serum calcitonin levels, it can usually be localized with ultrasound or computerized imaging of the neck.

SUGGESTED READING

1. Evans DB, Burgess MA, Goepfert H, Gagel RF. Medullary thyroid carcinoma. *Curr Ther Endocrinol Metab.* 1997;6:127–132.
2. Marzanol A, Porcelli A, Biondi B, Lupoli G, Delrio P, Lombardi G, Zarrilli L. Surgical management and follow-up of medullary thyroid carcinoma. *J Surg Oncol.* 1995;59:162–168.
3. Pommier RF, Brennan MF. Medullary thyroid carcinoma. *Endocrinologist.* 1992; 2:393–405.
4. Richards AM, Espiner EA, Nicholls MG, Ikram H, Hamilton EJ, Maslowski AH. Hormone, calcium and blood pressure relationships in primary hyperparathyroidism. *J Hypertens.* 1988;6:747–752.
5. Saito I, Saruta T. Hypertension in thyroid disorders. *Endocrinol Metab Clin North Am.* 1994;23:379–386.
6. Streeten DHP, Anderson GH Jr, Howland T, Chiang R, Smulyan H. Effects of thyroid function on blood pressure: recognition of hypothyroid hypertension. *Hypertension.* 1988;11:78–83.

Chapter 157

Management of Sleep Apnea

Paul D. Levinson, MD; Richard P. Millman, MD

KEY POINTS

- The transient and often marked increase in blood pressure caused by obstructive sleep apnea may contribute to the development of hypertension during waking hours.

- Obstructive sleep apnea has been associated with myocardial infarction, stroke, left ventricular hypertrophy, ventricular arrhythmias, pulmonary hypertension, and cor pulmonale.

- Patients with hypertension should be evaluated for sleep apnea if they have symptoms and/or conditions commonly associated with obstructive sleep apnea, absence of the normal blood pressure decline during sleep (as determined by ambulatory blood pressure monitoring), or resistant hypertension.

See also Chapter 57

Clinical research during the last two decades has demonstrated that the obstructive sleep apnea (OSA) syndrome is a common and potentially serious medical problem. There are at least three important reasons for considering the diagnosis of OSA in patients with hypertension. First, OSA occurs in hypertensive patients more frequently than in normotensive subjects. Second, it causes transient and often marked increases in systemic blood pressure (BP) during sleep and may contribute to the development of systemic hypertension during waking hours. Third, OSA has been associated with a variety of cardiovascular consequences, including myocardial infarction, stroke, left ventricular hypertrophy, and ventricular arrhythmias, as well as pulmonary hypertension and cor pulmonale.

Definition

OSA is generally defined by the presence of one or more characteristic symptoms in conjunction with a minimum number of obstructive apneic or hypopneic events (usually 5 to 15) per hour of sleep. The symptoms of OSA result from the recurrent but self-limited episodes of upper airway collapse that occur during sleep and result in acid-base abnormalities (hypoxia, hypercapnea, acidosis), sleep fragmentation, and other neural, hemodynamic, and hormonal alterations.

Clinical Features

Almost all persons with OSA snore, and usually very loudly. The patient's bed partner may be kept awake by loud snorts and gasps, and he or she may observe apneic episodes. Excessive sleepiness is the classic symptom associated with OSA. It may be expressed in mild form, such as dozing quietly in a chair after dinner, or in more severe forms, eg, exhaustion on awakening in the morning, uncontrollable sleepiness throughout the day, or tendency to fall asleep while driving (**Table 157.1**).

Associated Conditions

Most (60% to 80%) of the OSA patients in published clinical series are obese; that is, their body weight is >20% above ideal or their body mass index is >28 kg/(m)². While the prevalence of OSA in the adult male population has been estimated as approximately 4%, it appears to be many times greater in obese persons and probably increases with the degree of obesity. Most reports of series of patients with OSA indicate that men greatly outnumber women. As shown in the Table, several conditions in addition to obesity and male sex are associated with the development of OSA. While some, including hypothyroidism and acromegaly, cause anatomic narrowing of the pharynx, others, such as bedtime alcohol and sedative use, increase pharyngeal collapsibility during sleep. Hypothyroidism causes blunting of the ventilatory responses to hypoxia, as well as hypercapnea.

Indications for Diagnostic Testing

Even though the prevalence of OSA in hypertensive patients may be as high as 10% to 30%, complete diagnostic evaluation for OSA in all hypertensive patients does not appear to be cost effective. Patients with hypertension should be evaluated for sleep apnea if they have symptoms or conditions commonly associated with OSA, absence of the normal BP decline during sleep (as determined by ambulatory BP monitoring), or resistant hypertension (Table 157.1). The coincidence of hypertension, obesity [body mass index >30 kg/(m)²], and observed apneic episodes in snorers who complain of excessive drowsiness predicts the diagnosis of OSA.

Diagnosis

The test of choice for diagnosis of OSA is all-night polysomnography. This technique uses monitoring of the electroencephalogram, electrooculogram, and submental electromyogram to determine sleep staging and the extent of sleep fragmentation. Obstructive apneas and hypopneas are identified by using oral and nasal thermistors that detect air flow or chest/abdominal bands and intercostal electromyograms that reflect respiratory effort. Finger-pulse oximetry is used to detect the degree of oxygen desaturation, and heart rate is measured by continuous electrocardiogram monitoring. All-night polysomnography generally requires an in-patient sleep laboratory. In-home methods for assessing respiration during sleep are cur-

Table 157.1. Clinical Features Associated With Obstructive Sleep Apnea

Symptoms
  Daytime sleepiness
  Snoring, especially with choking arousals
  Apneic episodes (observed)
  Memory or attention deficits
  Personality change
  Impotence
Associated conditions
  Obesity
  Male sex
  Increasing age
  Macroglossia
  Retrognathism
  Enlarged tonsils, adenoids
  Nasal obstruction
  Evening alcohol/sedative use
  Acromegaly
  Hypothyroidism
Resistant hypertension
Blood pressures during sleep ≥ awake pressures (reverse dippers)

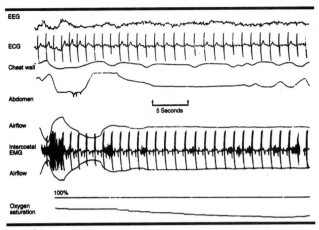

Figure 157.1. Partial output of a polysomnographic study. Channels shown from top to bottom represent electroencephalogram (EEG), electrocardiogram (ECG), chest wall movement, abdominal movement, nasal airflow, intercostal muscle electromyogram (EMG), nasal airflow (pattern inverted), and oxygen saturation. ECG complexes can be seen superimposed on the EMG tracing. At the beginning of the trace, normal airflow and movement of the chest and abdominal wall are present. Airflow then ceases, despite continued intercostal EMG activity and persistent but asynchronous chest and abdominal wall movement, typical findings of an obstructive apnea. Oxygen saturation declines progressively during the apnea.

rently undergoing evaluation and may also be useful diagnostic tools. Most investigators consider more than 5 to 15 obstructive episodes per hour of sleep, accompanied by typical symptoms, to be diagnostic of OSA **(Figure 157.1).**

Treatment

Treatment of OSA is best carried out with the help of a sleep and/or pulmonary specialist. Weight reduction and limitation of alcohol intake are essential components of the therapeutic regimen but do not always normalize the respiratory disturbances. Treatment of underlying conditions, especially hypothyroidism or acromegaly, may result in cure or improvement of the sleep apnea. Nasal continuous positive airway pressure, administered through a face mask and air pump, is currently considered the most effective noninvasive approach to treatment. Oral appliances that advance the tongue and mandible have recently been shown to be effective for mild and moderate disease. When critical anatomic abnormalities are present, surgical therapy such as uvulopalatopharyngoplasty may be indicated. Tracheostomy is indicated only when other therapeutic measures are ineffective or poorly tolerated.

While effective therapy of OSA reduces BP levels during sleep, it is not clear whether BP during waking hours also declines. If treatment of sleep apnea in a hypertensive patient is not associated with a prompt decrease in daytime BP, conventional antihypertensive therapy should be initiated.

Few studies have examined the effect of various antihypertensive agents on respiration during sleep. The findings available to date do not support a major role for antihypertensive agents as either causal or exacerbating factors for obstructive apneas.

SUGGESTED READING

1. Crocker BD, Olson LG, Saunders NA, Hensley MJ, McKeon JL, Allen KM, Gyulay SG. Estimation of the probability of disturbed breathing during sleep before a sleep study. *Am Rev Respir Dis.* 1990;142:14–18.
2. Fletcher EC, DeBehnke RD, Lovoi, MS, Gorin AB. Undiagnosed sleep apnea in patients with essential hypertension. *Ann Intern Med.* 1985;103:190–195.
3. Guilleminault C, Simmons FB, Motta J, Cummiskey J, Rosekind M, Schroeder JS. Obstructive sleep apnea syndrome and tracheostomy: long-term follow-up experience. *Arch Intern Med.* 1981;141:985–988.
4. Levinson PD, Millman RP. Causes and consequences of blood pressure alterations in obstructive sleep apnea. *Arch Intern Med.* 1991;151:455–462.
5. Noda A, Okada T, Hayashi H, Yasuma F, Yokota M. 24-Hour ambulatory blood pressure variability in obstructive sleep apnea syndrome. *Chest.* 1993;103:1343–1347.
6. Parish JM, Shepard JW Jr. Cardiovascular effects of sleep disorders. *Chest.* 1990; 97:1220–1226.
7. Partinen M, Guilleminault C. Daytime sleepiness and vascular morbidity at seven-year follow-up in obstructive sleep apnea patients. *Chest.* 1990;97:27–32.
8. Stradling JR, Crosby JH. Relation between systemic hypertension and sleep hypoxaemia or snoring: analysis in 748 men drawn from general practice. *BMJ.* 1990;300:75–78.
9. Working Group on OSA and Hypertension. Obstructive sleep apnea and blood pressure elevation: what is the relationship? *Blood Pres.* 1993;2:166–182.
10. Young T, Palta M, Dempsey J, Skatrud J, Weber S, Badr S. The occurrence of sleep-disordered breathing among middle-aged adults. *N Engl J Med.* 1993;328: 1230–1235.

Management of Drug-Induced and Iatrogenic Hypertension

Ehud Grossman, MD; Franz H. Messerli, MD

KEY POINTS

- A variety of therapeutic agents or chemical substances can induce transient or persistent hypertension, exacerbate well-controlled hypertension, or antagonize the effects of antihypertensive therapy.

- Careful evaluation of a patient's drug regimen may identify chemically induced hypertension and prevent the need for unnecessary antihypertensive therapy.

- When drug-induced or chemically induced hypertension is identified, discontinuation of the causative agent should be recommended.

- When it is not possible to discontinue agents that cause hypertension, institution of appropriate antihypertensive treatment is indicated.

See also Chapters 60, 123

Hypertension related to drugs and other substances represents an important modifiable source of secondary hypertension. An accurate and detailed medical history should include specific inquiries concerning foods, poisons, and medications, including those substances (legal and illicit) that patients do not consider to be drugs and therefore frequently omit from their history. Identification of such substances is important because their elimination can obviate the need for unnecessary, costly, and potentially dangerous evaluations or treatments. When drug-induced or chemically induced hypertension is identified, discontinuation of the causative agent should be recommended. When it is not possible to discontinue agents that cause hypertension, institution of appropriate antihypertensive treatment is indicated. In the absence of specific treatment guidelines for drug-induced hypertension, initial antihypertensive therapy should be directed at neutralizing the specific mechanism causing the hypertension **(Table 158.1).** Some of the agents discussed below are not available in the United States.

Steroids

Hypertension occurs in ≈20% of patients treated with high doses of synthetic corticosteroids. Hemodynamically, corticosteroids increase blood pressure (BP) through increasing cardiac output, with little change in peripheral resistance. Certain exogenous compounds, such as licorice, phenylbutazone, fludrocortisone, carbenoxolone, 9α-fluoroprednisolone, and 9α-fluorocortisol, have mineralocorticoid activity and, when ingested in excessive quantities, may produce arterial hypertension characterized by increased exchangeable sodium and blood volume, hypokalemia with metabolic alkalosis, and suppressed plasma renin and aldosterone levels. Prolonged use of high-dose ketoconazole may alter enzymatic degradation of steroids, leading to mineralocorticoid-related hypertension. The use of skin ointments, antihemorrhoidal preparations, ophthalmic drops,

and nasal sprays, which contain substances with mineralocorticoid activity (9α-fluoroprednisolone), as well as sympathetic amines, occasionally cause severe arterial hypertension. Discontinuation of these substances is recommended to lower BP. However, when steroid treatment is mandatory, diuretics, sympatholytic drugs, and adrenergic blockers are useful agents. Careful monitoring of potassium is also necessary.

Sex Hormones

Oral contraceptives induce hypertension in ≈5% of users of high-dose pills (>0.625 mg Premarin or equivalent). Women with a history of high BP during pregnancy, those with a family history of hypertension, black or diabetic women, and those with renal diseases may respond with a greater increase in BP. The increased pressure is usually minimal, but severe hypertensive episodes, including malignant hypertension, have been reported. Postmenopausal estrogen replacement therapy usually decreases arterial pressure slightly. Rare cases of estrogen-induced hypertension represent an idiosyncratic reaction to estrogen replacement therapy. Men receiving estrogen for the treatment of prostatic cancer may also exhibit an increase in BP.

Danazol, a semisynthetic androgen that is used in the treatment of endometriosis and hereditary angioedema, has been reported to induce hypertension because of fluid retention. Diuretic is the most logical treatment if hormones should be continued.

Anesthetics and Narcotics

Ketamine hydrochloride has been reported to severely increase arterial pressure. In one study, the central sympatholytic drug clonidine was effective in reducing the hypertensive response to ketamine. Desflurane may induce hypertension via stimulation of the sympathetic nervous system. Sympatholytic agents such as α-blockers and α,β-blockers may lower BP.

Table 158.1. **Management of Drug-Induced Hypertension**

SUBSTANCE	MANAGEMENT	COMMENTS
Steroids		
Glucocorticoids	Discontinue treatment; if not possible, start diuretics.	
Mineralocorticoids		
Sex hormones	Discontinue treatment; if not possible, start diuretics.	
Anesthetics and Narcotics		
Ketamine hydrochloride	Initial therapy: clonidine, α-blockers.	
Desflurane	Initial therapy: α-blockers, α+β-blockers.	
Naloxone	Initial therapy: α-blockers.	
Drugs affecting the sympathetic nervous system		
Opthalmic solutions	Initial therapy: α-blockers, α+β-blockers.	Avoid β-blockers.
Antimetic agents		Transient increase in BP.
Yohimbine hydrochloride	Discontinue treatment.	Avoid in hypertensive patients and in those treated with tricyclic antidepressants.
Glucagon (only in patients with pheochromocytoma)	Initial therapy: intravenous phentolamine, oral phenoxybenzamine, or α_1-blockers.	
Cocaine	Initial therapy: α-blockers.	Most patients do not require treatment.
Anorexics	Discontinue treatment.	
Nasal decongestant	Initial therapy: α+β-blockers.	
Cough medications	Discontinue treatment.	
Antidepressant agents		
MAOIs	Initial therapy: α-blockers.	
Tricyclic antidepressants	Initial therapy: α-blockers.	
Serotonin agonists	Initial therapy: α-blockers.	
Miscellaneous		
Cyclosporine	Discontinue treatment; if not possible, start calcium antagonists. Other drugs are also effective	Calcium antagonists may increase cyclosporine blood levels. Multidrug therapy may be necessary.
r-HuEPO	Lower the dose; if unsuccessful, start calcium antagonists or α-blockers. Diuretics and angiotensin-converting enzyme inhibitors may be less effective.	Dialysis with conventional antihypertensive treatment may be effective. Phlebotomy may rapidly lower BP.
Bromocriptine		Avoid use for suppression of lactation.
Alcohol	Moderate alcohol intake.	
NSAIDs		Balance the risk of an increase in BP against the expected benefit.

The simultaneous use of vasoconstrictors (felypressin) with topical cocaine can result in severe hypertension. At least one case was treated successfully with labetalol.

Hypertensive responses to naloxone (opiate antagonist), especially during attempted reversal of narcotic-induced anesthesia in hypertensive patients, have also been reported. Naloxone seems to acutely reverse the antihypertensive effects of clonidine and can thereby cause an acute hypertensive emergency.

Drugs Affecting the Sympathetic Nervous System

Phenylephrine, a sympathomimetic agent with a potent vasoconstrictor activity, has been reported to severely increase arterial pressure after its administration in an ophthalmic solution. Dipivalyl adrenaline, an adrenaline prodrug used topically in the management of chronic simple glaucoma, can also increase BP in treated hypertensive patients.

The concomitant use of sympathomimetic agents and β-blockers can severely increase arterial pressure because of unopposed α-adrenergic vasoconstriction. Theoretically, the use of α-blockers or

agents such as labetalol, which block both α- and β-adrenergic receptors, should prevent this detrimental reaction. Antiemetic agents such as metoclopramide, alizapride, and prochlorperazine have been reported to increase BP transiently in patients treated with cisplatin.

Midodrine is a prodrug that forms a potent α_1-adrenergic agonist used to treat orthostatic hypotension. It has a short half-life, and specific therapy is rarely necessary.

Yohimbine hydrochloride, an α_2-adrenergic receptor antagonist that is approved for treatment of impotence, may significantly increase BP in hypertensive patients. The drug should be avoided or used intermittently in hypertensive patients and in those undergoing concurrent treatment with tricyclic antidepressants.

Glucagon may induce severe hypertension in patients with pheochromocytoma. Blocking the α-adrenergic receptors by either intravenous phentolamine or oral agents such as phenoxybenzamine or doxazosin may prevent catastrophic cardiovascular events.

Cocaine intoxication is characterized by adrenergic overactivity associated with increased BP. Most patients with cocaine-related hypertension do not require pharmacological therapy, but if treatment is necessary, α-adrenergic receptor antagonists or nitroprusside should be chosen for initial treatment. β-Blockers can be useful in the management of cardiac dysrhythmias, but they should be used with caution owing to the possibility of exacerbating hypertension because of unopposed α-receptor activity.

Over-the-Counter Drugs

Most nonprescription anoretic agents contain combinations of an antihistamine and an adrenergic agonist (usually phenylpropanolamine, ephedrine, or pseudoephedrine). All act by potentiating presynaptic norepinephrine release and by directly activating adrenergic receptors. Prescription anorectic agents may raise BP and increase the risk of valvular heart disease and pulmonary hypertension and therefore should be used with due diligence if at all. Patients who receive sibatromine must have their BP checked frequently. α-Adrenergic intoxication induced by nasal decongestants or cough medications containing massive doses of oxymetazoline hydrochloride, phenylephrine hydrochloride, or ephedrine hydrochloride uncommonly causes severe hypertension. Labetalol may be an effective treatment in these cases.

Caffeine can acutely and transiently increase BP in caffeine-naïve individuals. Concomitant medications, such as monoamine oxidase inhibitors (MAOIs), oral contraceptives, and nonsteroidal anti-inflammatory drugs (NSAIDs), seem to increase the risk of hypertension.

Antidepressant Agents

MAOIs can induce severe hypertension when patients also consume foods containing tyramine (red wines, cheddar cheese, etc). There are some reports of MAOIs causing severe hypertensive reactions even without use of concomitant medications. Tranylcypromine is the most hazardous MAOI, whereas moclobemide and brofaromine are the least likely to induce a hypertensive reaction. These drugs exert their effects by delaying the metabolism of sympathomimetic amines and 5-hydroxytryptophan and by increasing the store of norepinephrine in postganglionic sympathetic neurons. α-Adrenergic receptor antagonists are the logical choice for initial treatment.

Tricyclic antidepressants block the reuptake of the neurotransmitters in the synapse in the central nervous system. There are some reports that these agents increase BP, mainly in patients with panic disorders.

Buspirone, a serotonin receptor type 1 α-agonist, has also been reported to increase BP. It is speculated that buspirone increases BP by its metabolite 1,2-pyrimidinyl piperazine, which is an α_2-adrenergic receptor antagonist, and therefore should not be used concomitantly with an MAOI. A small but sustained and dose-dependent increase in arterial pressure seems to occur with other serotonin agonists as well. Episodes of severe hypertension were described in patients treated with other antidepressant agents, such as fluoxetine plus selegiline and thioridazine.

Cyclosporine

Cyclosporine, a potent, orally active immunosuppressive drug, may induce arterial hypertension. The incidence of cyclosporine-associated hypertension (CAH) varies with the patient population under evaluation. The greatest experience to date has been with patients undergoing organ transplantation, with kidney recipients rep-

resenting the largest single group. CAH is also common in patients with autoimmune disease and dermatological disorders. The occurrence of CAH is unrelated to age, sex, or race. Although most patients present with mild to moderate asymptomatic BP elevation, others may rapidly develop severe hypertension and encephalopathy. BP usually falls after the withdrawal or substitution of cyclosporine immunosuppression but may not remit completely. Furthermore, it is often not possible to discontinue therapy. Calcium antagonists have been used successfully, but they can increase cyclosporine blood levels. ACE inhibitors, labetalol, β-blockers, clonidine, and diuretics are also effective in some patients. Diuretic therapy should be used with caution because of the risk of prerenal azotemia and electrolyte abnormalities. Multidrug therapy may be necessary to control CAH.

Alkylating Agents

Several alkylating agents can increase BP. In one series, 15 of 18 patients treated with multiple alkylating agents after autologous bone marrow transplantation developed hypertension.

Recombinant Human Erythropoietin

Recombinant human erythropoietin (rhEPO) is effective in correcting the anemia of patients with end-stage renal failure. The most frequent side effect of rhEPO is the development or exacerbation of hypertension due to a marked increase in peripheral resistance and a mild decrease in cardiac output. The onset of hypertension typically occurs over the first 2 to 16 weeks of therapy. The increase in BP is usually mild, however, a few cases of hypertensive crisis with encephalopathy have been reported. The increase in BP associated with rhEPO therapy appears to be dose-related or at least related to the increase in the hematocrit level. Vasodilators such as calcium antagonists and α-adrenergic receptor antagonists should be effective in lowering BP. Diuretics, ACE inhibitors, and AT_1 receptor antagonists may be less effective because blood volume has been shown to be unchanged and both plasma renin activity and angiotensin II are suppressed in rhEPO–treated patients. The hypertension associated with rhEPO has not generally been too difficult to control. In one study, 42% of the patients with rhEPO-induced hypertension were controlled with a single agent. The BP can usually be controlled with a combination of fluid removal with dialysis and conventional antihypertensive therapy. If these measures are unsuccessful, the dose of rhEPO should be lowered, or therapy should be withheld for several weeks. Phlebotomy of 500 mL of blood may rapidly lower BP in refractory patients.

Bromocriptine

Bromocriptine mesylate is commonly used for prolactin inhibition and suppression of puerperal lactation. Although bromocriptine often has a hypotensive effect, severe hypertension with subsequent stroke has been reported in the postpartum period. Patients with pregnancy-induced hypertension are at increased risk of developing hypertension. The suppression of lactation is no longer an FDA-approved use for bromocriptine.

Disulfiram

Disulfiram is commonly used as a pharmacological adjunct in the treatment of alcoholism. Administration of 500 mg/d of disulfiram for 2 to 3 weeks has been reported to increase BP slightly. A low dose of 125 mg/d may also increase BP. Changes in peripheral or central noradrenergic activity are most likely responsible for the increase in arterial pressure.

Alcohol

Excessive alcohol use has clearly been shown to raise BP and can also increase resistance to antihypertensive therapy. The BP effects of alcohol are independent of obesity, salt intake, cigarette smoking, and potassium intake. There is a dose-response relationship for the hypertensive effects of alcohol. Moderation of alcohol intake is recommended as an initial therapy for mild hypertension. A reasonable approach is to limit daily alcohol consumption to no more than ≈ 1 oz of absolute alcohol, and less in women and smaller men.

Nonsteroidal Anti-inflammatory Drugs

NSAIDs can induce an increase in BP or interfere with antihypertensive treatment, but most patients experience no problems when given these agents. Elderly patients, patients with preexisting hypertension, salt-sensitive patients, and patients with renovascular hypertension are at a higher risk of developing severe hypertension when treated with NSAIDs. NSAIDs vary considerably in their effect on BP. In one study, indomethacin and naproxen were associated with the largest increases in BP. It is wise to balance the risk of an increase in BP against the expected benefit of treatment with an NSAID. Hypertensives who appear to need NSAIDs should use them as infrequently as possible.

SUGGESTED READING

1. Bennett WM, Porter GA. Cyclosporine-associated hypertension. *Am J Med.* 1988;85:131–133.
2. Bursztyn M, Zelig O, Or R, Nagler A. Isradipine for the prevention of cyclosporine-induced hypertension in allogeneic bone marrow transplant recipients: a randomized, double-blind study. *Transplantation.* 1997;63:1034–1036.
3. Chasan-Taber L, Willett WC, Manson JE, Spiegelman D, Hunter DJ, Curhan G, Colditz GA, Stampfer MJ. Prospective study of oral contraceptives and hypertension among women in the United States. *Circulation.* 1996;94:483–489.
4. Clyburn BE, DiPette DJ. Hypertension induced by drugs and other substances. *Semin Nephrol.* 1995;15:72–86.
5. De Leeuw PW. Nonsteroidal anti-inflammatory drugs and hypertension: the risks in perspective. *Drugs.* 1996;51:179–187.
6. Grossman E, Messerli FH. High blood pressure: a side effect of drugs, poisons, and food. *Arch Intern Med.* 1995;155:450–460.
7. Levin N. Management of blood pressure changes during recombinant human erythropoietin therapy. *Semin Nephrol.* 1989;9:16–20.
8. MacMahon S. Alcohol consumption and hypertension. *Hypertension.* 1987;9:111–121.
9. Pope JE, Anderson JJ, Felson DT. A meta-analysis of the effects of nonsteroidal anti-inflammatory drugs on blood pressure. *Arch Intern Med.* 1993;153:477–484.

▌ Index

Page references in *italics* denote figures; those followed by "t" denote tables

Acetylcholine
definition of, 47
muscarinic receptor effects, 47
neurotransmitter functions of, 47
nicotinic receptor effects, 47
structure of, *48*
vasodilator responses to, 114
Acromegaly, hypertension and, 144–145
Acute stressors, hemodynamic responses to, 116–117
α-Adducin, 220
Adenosine
cardiovascular effects of, 48
composition of, 48
receptors, 48, 48t
structure of, *48*
Adenylyl cyclases
description of, 66
G protein regulation of, 66
Adhesion molecules
immunoglobulin-like, 76
in inflammatory diseases, 76–77
integrins, 76
selectins, 76
in vascular diseases, 76–77
Adipose tissue, angiotensin II production, 24
ADMA, in atherosclerosis pathogenesis, 172
Adrenal cortex
aldosterone production, 26
anatomy of, 26
Adrenal cortical hypertension, pathophysiology of, 138–140
Adrenal glands
adrenomedullin, 40
angiotensin II production, 23
proadrenomedullin N-20 terminal peptide, 40
α,β-Adrenergic blockers, 368–369, 416–417
α-Adrenergic blockers, 366–367, 416–417
β-Adrenergic blockers (*see* β-blockers)
Adrenergic receptors
coupling to G proteins, 3
function of, 3–4
pharmacology of, 3–4, 4t
regulation of, 4–5
subtypes of, 3, 4t
tissue distribution of, 4t
vascular, 113
Adrenocorticotrophin hormone
cortical synthesis by, 26
production increases, 139
Adrenomedullin, 50
Affective disorders (*see* Depression)
African-Americans, hypertension in
blood pressure control, 240
blood pressure treatment goals, 337–338
management of, 413–414
morbidity and mortality, 239–240
Alcohol consumption
blood pressure effects
clinical trials, 263–265, 264t
description of, 341, 461
epidemiology of, 263
mechanism of action, 265
detrimental effects of, 263
low intake, beneficial effects of, 263
recommendations for, 265
Aldosterone
biosynthesis of, 26
production sites of, 26
regulation of, 26
secretion of, 138
synthesis of, 138

Aldosterone-producing adenoma, 138–139, 452
Aldosteronism
glucocorticoid-remediable, 98, 452–453
primary, 451–452
Amiloride, 361t
lc.gamma-Aminobutyric acid (*see* GABA)
Androgens, 28
Androstenedione, 28
Aneurysms
abdominal aortic, 326, 411
of eye, 195
Angina pectoris
chronic, 176
description of, 175
stable, 176
unstable, 176, 318
Angiography, radionuclide, 314, 315t
Angioneurotic edema, 375
Angioplasty, for renovascular hypertension, 443–444
Angiotensin I–converting enzyme
chronic inhibition of, 21
description of, 19
distribution of, 19
in kidney, 23–24
kinin destruction by, 40
properties of, 19
structure of, 19–20, *20*
Angiotensin II
biological actions of, 11
description of, 106–107
excessive amounts, detrimental effects of, 24
in hypertension, 111, 166
oxidase activity regulation by, 165, *165*
receptor blockers, 377–378, 409, 429
tissue-generating systems for, 23–24
Angiotensin-converting enzyme inhibitors
angiotensin II receptor blockers and, comparison between, 378
antihypertensive effects of, role of kinins in, 41
blocking of kinin hydrolysis, 40
blood pressure-lowering effects of, 373–374
clinical uses
chronic renal insufficiency, 408–409
ischemic heart disease, 400
obese patients with hypertension, 417
peripheral arterial disease, 410–411
renovascular hypertension, 134, 444
systolic dysfunction, 406
concomitant therapy, 375
description of, 19
drug interactions of, 375–376
hemodynamic effects of, 373, 374t
indications, 373t
mechanism of action, 21, 372–373
in patients with concomitant disorders, 374–375
peak therapeutic levels, 347
pharmacokinetics of, 373, 374t
pregnancy contraindications, 429
side effects of, 375
therapeutic regimens, 374
treatment trials of, 282
types of, 373t
Angiotensinogen
from adipose tissue, 24
description of, 14–15
in familial aggregation of hypertension, 219–220
gene mutations, 104
salt sensitivity and, 219–220
Angiotensins
biological actions of, 11, 12t
degradation of, 21–22

description of, 11
formation of, 21–22
receptor subtypes
description of, 11
interactions among, 11, 13
regulation of, 11, 13
Anion transporters, in intracellular pH homeostasis, 53
Ankle-brachial index, for peripheral arterial disease diagnosis, 215, *324,* 326
Antidiuretic hormone (*see* Arginine vasopressin)
Antihypertensive drugs
absorption of, 343
administration routes, 343
adverse effects, 283, 284t
anti-ischemic therapy, 399–400
β-blockers (*see* β-blockers)
description of, 342
for diabetic nephropathy, 420–423
dose-effect curve of, 342–343
dose-response relationships of, 342
elimination of, 343
exercise and, 262
failure of, reasons for, 345
fixed-dose combination products, 344
gender considerations, 231–232, *232*
for hypertensive renal damage, 190, 192
mood disorders caused by, 151
pharmacogenetic considerations, 347
pharmacokinetic variations, 346–347
pseudotolerance, 346
quality of life effects, 284–285
regimen adherence, 345
side-effects of
description of, 417t
dose-related influences, 343–344
underdosing of, 346–347
vascular smooth muscle cell growth inhibition by, 159
Antihypertensive therapy
adherence to
description of, 348
factors associated with, 348
multilevel approach, 351
strategies for, 348–351, 349t–350t
algorithm, *335*
for chronic hypertension during pregnancy, 428–429
cost reductions in, 288
cost-effectiveness considerations (*see* Cost-effectiveness)
for elderly patients, 430–432
goals of, 333
historical background, 283
lifestyle modifications, 333, 334t
nonadherence to, 348, 356–357
pharmacological methods (*see also* Antihypertensive drugs)
initial regimen, 333–335
J curve, 336
regimen adherence, 336
step-down therapy, 336
for preeclampsia, 427–428
refractory hypertension and, 356
risk stratification, 334t
treatment trials of
Hypertension Detection and Follow-up Program, 279–280
Medical Research Council, 279–280
meta-analysis, 280, *281*
quality of life effects, 283–285
study design, 279

Aorta
  abdominal
    aneurysm, 326, 411
    palpation of, 324, 326
  coarctation of
    description of, 146
    diagnosis of, 146, *147, 300*
    hypertension associated with, 146–147
    management of, 146
    prognosis for, 146
  stiffness of, 177
Aortocarotid baroreflexes
  abnormalities, clinical conditions associated with, 331–332
  description of, 330
  function assessments, 330–331
  sensitivity, 330
Apnea (*see* Sleep apnea)
Apoptosis
  description of, 158
  of vascular smooth muscle cells, 171
Arachidonic acid
  cytochrome P450 and
    metabolites, 31
    oxidation, 30–31
  lipoxygenase enzymes that oxidize, 33–34
  12-lipoxygenase products of, 34
  15-lipoxygenase products of, 34
  metabolic pathways of, *32–33*
Arginine vasopressin
  description of, 38
  in hypertension, 38–39
  physiological role, 38
  receptors, 38
Arterial pressure, effect on regional blood flow regulation, 93
Arteries
  carotid, 324
  compliance of
    blood vessel damage, *328*
    definition of, 327
    estimation of, 327–328, 328t
    in hypertensive patients, 327–328
  cyclic stress of, 162
  degeneration of, 162
  peripheral disease (*see* Peripheral arterial disease)
  stiffness of
    hypertension and, 161t
    mechanisms of, 160, 161t
    peripheral pressure effects, 161
    relationship to left ventricular hypertrophy and confusion perfusion, 161–162
    therapy for, 162
    wave reflection and, 160–161
  structure of, 327
Arterioles
  abnormalities of, in hypertension, 173–174
  afferent resistance of, 191
Arteriosclerosis, 160
Asians, hypertension in, 413
Aspirin, 399
Atherogenesis
  description of, 170
  plaque formation
    characteristics of, 170
    endothelium effects on, 171–172
    nitric oxide effects on, 171–172
    pathogenesis, 170
    pathogenic consequences of, 171
  risk factors, 170
Atherosclerosis
  ADMA and, 172
  arteriosclerosis and, 160
  as cardiovascular risk factor, 199
  carotid artery, 326
  of retinal vessels, 195
  risk factors, 200–201
  in stroke etiology, 184
  symptomatic, 184

Atrial natriuretic peptide, 42–43, 88, 106–107
Atriopeptin release, 88
Autonomic nervous system
  anatomy of, 106
  cardiovascular reflexes, 330, 331t
  cardiovascular tissue effects, 107
  failure of, 330
  reflex activation, 330
  in renal parenchymal hypertension pathogenesis, 135–136
A-V nicking, 195

Baroreceptors
  arterial
    cellular events, 83
    definition of, 83
  cardiopulmonary, 87–88
  reflexes, 81
  renal, 16
Baroreflexes
  aortocarotid
    abnormalities, clinical conditions associated with, 331–332
    description of, 330
    function assessments, 330–331
    sensitivity, 330
  arterial
    during acute and chronic hypertension, 83, 85
    buffering of arterial pressure fluctuations, 83
    neural pathways, *84*
    neurohumoral modulation of, 85–86
    paracrine modulation of, 85–86
  cardiopulmonary, 87–88
  dysfunction, management of, 393–395
β-Blockers
  adverse effects of, 365
  blood pressure effects of, 365
  clinical uses
    chronic renal insufficiency, 408
    ischemic heart disease, 399
  contraindications for, 365
  elderly patient use of, 431
  elimination characteristics of, 364t
  exercise and, 262
  gender differences in effectiveness of, 231–232
  insulin resistance and, 257
  pharmacodynamic properties of, 362–363
  pharmacokinetic properties of, 363–364, 364t
  in sympathetic nervous system overactivity, 111–112
  types indicated for hypertension, 362, 363t
Blood flow
  autoregulation of, 95–97
  cerebral, 92–93, 183
  myocardial, 92
  regional
    arterial pressure in regulation of, 93
    in essential hypertension, 93–94
   regulation, 92–93, *93*
  renal, 93
  shear stress and, 96
  skeletal, 92
  skin, 92–93
Blood pressure (*see also* Hypertension)
  in African-Americans (*see* African-Americans)
  aggressive lowering of, 338
  alcohol consumption effects
    clinical trials, 263–265, 264t
    description of, 461
    epidemiology of, 263
    mechanism of action, 265
  atherosclerosis and, 199–200
  borderline hypertension and, 434–435
  brain regulation of, 80
  caffeine effects, 460
  calcium and, 253–254
  in children
    cardiovascular risk and, 233
    description of, 233–234
    elevated levels

    classification, 234–235
    definitions, 234–235
    identification of, 235
    measurement, 234, 298, 424
  determinants of, 115
  diastolic (*see* Diastolic blood pressure)
  dietary influences, 244–246
  drug-induced increases, 151
  end-stage renal disease and, 211, 212t
  estrogen effects on, 28
  ethnicity and, 239–242 (*see also specific race groups*)
  exogenous substances that increase, 355t, 355–356
  family aggregation of, 218–219
  fat intake and, 246
  gender-based differences
    antihypertensive treatment, 231
    patient awareness, 231
    treatment, 231
  gene-environment interactions of, 222–223
  high-stress jobs and, 266
  hormone replacement therapy effects on, 230
  hypercreatinemia and, 213–214
  increased levels (*see* Hypertension)
  left ventricular hypertrophy and, 210
  lifestyle change effects on, 274–277
  magnesium and, 254–255
  measurement of
    methods, 295–298
    postural considerations, 390–391
  monitoring of
    ambulatory, 303–305
    out-of-office, 302
    self-monitoring, 302–303, 305
  monogenic determinants of, 98–100
  multifactorial nature of, 222
  nutritional effects on, 274–277
  oral contraceptive effects on, 230–231
  patient age and, 218
  physical activity for reducing, 259–261
  physical inactivity and, 259
  polygenic determinants of, 101–103, 220
  potassium effects on
    clinical trials, 250–251
    epidemiology of, 250
    mechanism of action, 251–252
  prostaglandin effects on, 30
  psychosocial stress and, 266
  regulation of
    by cyclooxygenase-derived eicosanoids, 30
    by cytochrome P450-derived eicosanoids, 30–31
  serotonin effects on, 48
  sexual dimorphism of, 229
  socioeconomic status and, 240–242
  sodium intake and, 247–249, *248*, 355
  stroke and, 204–205
  sympathetic nervous system in control of, *110*
  systolic (*see* Systolic blood pressure)
  thiazide diuretic effects, 358, *359–360*
  treatment goals for, 337–338
Blood vessels
  angiotensin II production, 23
  structure of, 327
Blood volume, cardiopulmonary receptor influences on, 87–88
Blood-brain barrier disruptions, in hypertensive encephalopathy, 186
Blood-retinal barrier, 195–196
Body fat distribution, hypertension and, 118, 256
Borderline hypertension
  cardiovascular disease and, 433
  clinical approach to, 434–435
  definition of, 433
  management of, 435
  sympathetic overactivity and, 433–434
Brain
  angiotensin II production, 23
  blood pressure regulation by, 80
  cardiovascular function regulation, 80–82
  preeclamptic effects, 152

Brain attack (*see* Stroke)
Brainstem, in hypertension, 107–108
Bromocriptine, 6, 460
Bumetanide, 361t

Calcitonin gene-related peptide, 50, 106
Calcium
    absorption of, 253
    activated potassium channels, 56–57
    blood pressure and, 253–254, 340
    dietary, 126, 253
    excretion methods, 253
    intracellular, 125
        regulation of, 58
        release of, 59
        renin release inhibition by, 17
    requirements, 253
    serum levels, blood pressure and, 144
    supplementation, 126, 254, 340, 427
    in vascular smooth muscle contraction, 79
Calcium antagonists
    for chronic renal insufficiency, 408
    dihydropyridine
        administration of, 381t
        cardiac effects, 379–380, 380t
        clinical use of, 380
        dosage of, 381t
        drug interactions, 381, 381t
        mechanism of action, 379
        pharmacokinetics, 379, 380t
        safety of, 380–381
    intrarenal actions of, 422t
    for myocardial ischemia, 400
    nondihydropyridine
        administration of, 384
        adverse reactions, 384
        cardiac effects, 382–383
        cellular mechanisms of action, 382
        clinical use of, 383–384
        dosage of, 383t, 384
        pharmacokinetics and pharmacodynamics of, 382, 383t
        systemic hemodynamic effects, 382
    for obese patients with hypertension, 417
    for renovascular hypertension, 444
Calcium channel blockers, 282
Calcium channels, voltage-gated, 59
Calcium pumps, 59
Calmodulin, 58
cAMP (*see* Cyclic adenosine monophosphate)
Carbohydrates, blood pressure levels and, 246
Cardiovascular disease
    left ventricular hypertrophy and, 208–209
    mortality rates, 203
    physical activity for reducing risk of, 261–262
    physical inactivity and, 259
    risk factors, 339 (*see also specific risk factor*)
Cardiovascular system
    evaluation of
        auscultation, 311–312
        cardiac apex palpation, 311
        heart sounds, 311
        murmurs, 311–312
        physical examination, 311
    preeclampsia effects, 153
    sex steroid effects on, 28
Carotid arteries, evaluation of, 324
Carotid sinus hypersensitivity, 331–332
Carvedilol, 368
Catechol *O*-methyltransferase, in catecholamine metabolism, 9–10
Catecholamines, 111
    biosynthesis, 7, 8–9
    excess, 129, 369
    metabolism of, 9–10
    metabolites, 10
    norepinephrine (*see* Norepinephrine)
    release of, 8, 8
    reuptake of, 8, 8–9

types of, 7
    vesicular storage of, 7–8, 8
Cation transporters, in intracellular pH homeostasis, 53
Cell volume, regulation of, 53–54, 55
Cell-surface receptors
    activation of janus kinases-signal transducers and activators of transcription signaling by, 75
    coupling of, to extracellular signal–regulated kinases, 73–74
Central sympatholytics, 370, 371t
Cerebral blood flow
    in essential hypertension, 93
    reductions of, in stroke etiology, 183
Cerebral embolism, in stroke etiology, 183–184
Cerebral infarction, 309–310
Cerebral ischemia, 396
Cerebrovascular disease
    cerebral ischemia, 396, 397t
    incidence of, 203
    management of, 396–397
Cerebrum, circulation, autoregulatory mechanisms of, 95–96
CGRP (*see* Calcitonin gene–related peptide)
Chemoreceptor reflexes, 81
Children
    blood pressure in
        cardiovascular risk and, 233
        description of, 233–234
        elevated levels
            classification, 234–235
            definitions, 234–235
            identification of, 235
            measurement, 234, 298, 424
    hypertension in, management of, 424–426
Chlorthalidone, 361t
Cholesterol
    in atherosclerotic plaque formation, 170
    levels, classification of, 418, 419t
    low-density lipoprotein, 418, 419t
    renal disease and, 192
Choroidal circulation, 194–195
Choroidopathy, 194–195
Cigarette smoking
    hypertension risk and, 273
    peripheral arterial disease and, 411
    renal disease and, 192
Circulation
    cerebrum, 95–96
    choroidal, 194–195
    coronary, abnormalities of, 181
    kidney, 95
    optic nerve, 195
    retinal, 194–195
Clonidine, 343, 370, 371t
Coarctation of the aorta
    description of, 146
    diagnosis of, 146, 147, 300
    hypertension associated with, 146–147
    management of, 146
    prognosis for, 146
Cocaine use, hypertension and, 459–460
Computed tomography, electron beam, 314, 315, 315t
Congestive heart failure
    hypertension as risk factor for, 226, 406
    pathogenesis, 180–182, 181
    systemic vascular adaptations, 181–182
Contraceptives (*see* Oral contraceptives)
Coronary artery disease
    hypertension and, relationship between, 175–176
    left ventricular hypertrophy and, 209–210
    peripheral arterial disease and, 411
    treatment of, 398–399
Coronary blood flow, in essential hypertension, 93–94
Coronary heart disease
    age-adjusted annual rate of, 201
    borderline hypertension and, 434
    preventive steps, 202
    risk factors

atherosclerosis, 199
    blood pressure, 199–200
    clustering of, 200–201, 201t
    description of, 215
    global, 201
Corticosterone, 25, 27
Cortisol, 25–26, 138
Cost-effectiveness, of hypertension treatment
    analysis of, clinical practice applicability, 286–287
    calculations, 289–290
    cost and health benefits for assessing, 287t
    cost reductions, 288
    effect of patient adherence to treatment regimen, 288
    global, 286
    opportunities to improve, 286–287, 287t
Creatinine
    blood pressure and, 213–214
    clearance, 322
    elevated levels (*see* Hypercreatinemia)
Cushing's disease, 300, 449–451, 450t
Cyclic adenosine monophosphate
    protein kinase A and, nuclear signaling by, 67
    protein kinases dependent on, 67
    in renin release, 17
Cyclic guanine monophosphate, 67–68
    antiproliferative actions dependent on, 44–45
    nitric oxide mediation by, 44
    in vascular smooth muscle contraction, 79
    vasodilatory actions dependent on, 44
Cyclic nucleotide phosphodiesterases, 66–67
Cyclooxygenase
    eicosanoids derived from, 30
    inhibitors of, 30
Cyclosporin A, effect on hypertension after solid organ transplantation, 155–156
Cyclosporine, 460
Cytochrome P450
    and arachidonic acid
        metabolites, 31
        oxidation, 30–31
    eicosanoids derived from, 30–31
    forms, 31

Dehydroepiandrosterone, 28
Dementia, vascular
    clinical diagnosis, 188, 189t
    epidemiology of, 188
    hypertension and, 188
    neuroimaging of, 189
    pathophysiology of, 188–189
    treatment of, 189
Deoxycorticosterone, 26–27, 138
Depression
    anxiety disorders associated with, 150–151
    epidemiological studies of, 150
    hypertension and, 150–151
    psychopharmacology for, 151
Deserpidine, 371t
Diabetes mellitus
    β-blocker use and, 365
    description of, 115
    hypertension and, 257–258
Diabetic nephropathy, 195, 320, 421–423
Diacylglycerol
    description of, 69
    formation of, 70
Diagnostic work-up, of hypertensive patient
    establishing diagnosis, 299
    laboratory evaluation, 301
    patient history, 300
    physical examination, 300–301
    secondary hypertension, 300
    white coat hypertension considerations, 299–300
Dialysis patients, hypertension in, 409
Diastolic blood pressure
    dysfunction of, 178, 403
    J curve for, 336
    measurement of, 297
    versus systolic level, 204

Diet
  blood pressure and, 244–246
  calcium intake, 126, 253
  changes in, 340–341
  magnesium intake, 254
  sodium intake
    blood pressure and, 247–249, 248, 355
    description of, 126, 227
    hypertension risk reductions by lowering, 272, 277, 340
    restriction of, 222, 249
  vegetarian, 340
Dietary Approaches to Stop Hypertension (DASH) Trial
  description of, 244–245
  findings, 245
  food or nutrients in, 245–246
  public health applications of, 246
Dihydropyridine calcium antagonists
  administration of, 381t
  cardiac effects, 379–380, 380t
  for chronic renal insufficiency, 408
  clinical use of, 380
  dosage of, 381t
  drug interactions, 381, 381t
  mechanism of action, 379
  pharmacokinetics, 379, 380t
  safety of, 380–381
Dilated cardiomyopathy, 405–406
Diltiazem (see Nondihydropyridine calcium antagonists)
Disulfiram, 460–461
Diuretics (see Thiazide diuretics)
Divalent cation, in essential hypertension, 125, 126t
Divalent ions, in renal parenchymal hypertension pathogenesis, 136–137
Domperidone, 6
Dopamine
  agonists, 388
  receptors
    characteristics of, 5
    classification of, 5t
    description of, 5
    function of, 5–6
    pharmacology of, 5–6
Dopamine β-hydroxylase, in catecholamine biosynthesis, 7
Dose-effect curve, of antihypertensive drugs, 342–343
Dyslipidemia, 420

ECG (see Electrocardiogram)
Echocardiogram
  Doppler, 313–314
  left ventricular hypertrophy findings, 208–210, 313–314, 403
Eclampsia, 152
Eicosanoids
  cyclooxygenase-derived, 30
  cytochrome P450-derived, 30–31
Elderly
  antihypertensive therapy for, 430–432
  blood pressure measurement, 298
  hypertension in
    clinical evaluation, 237–238
    clinical trials, 236–237, 237t
    control of, 338
    epidemiology of, 236
    management of, 430–432
    mechanism of action, 432
    optimal care, 238
    pathophysiology of, 237
    pseudohypertension, 238
Electrocardiogram
  for cardiac evaluation, 312
  left ventricular hypertrophy findings, 208, 313–314, 403
  24-hour ambulatory monitoring, 312
Electrolytes (see also specific electrolyte)
  mineralocorticoid effects on, 25

Electron beam computed tomography, 314, 315, 315t
Embolism
  cardiogenic, 184, 184t
  cerebral, in stroke etiology, 183–184
Encephalopathy
  hypertensive
    clinical features, 186–187, 187t
    description of, 438
    diagnosis of, 308
    differential diagnosis, 187
    neurological investigation, 308
    pathophysiology of, 186
    treatment of, 186–187
  subcortical arteriosclerotic, 188
Endogenous ouabain (see Ouabain)
Endopeptidases, in angiotensin formation, 21
Endothelin-1
  actions of, 36
  description of, 36
  in hypertension, 37, 113–114
  receptor blockade, 389
  in renal parenchymal hypertension pathogenesis, 136
  structure of, 36
  vasorelaxant role of, 37
Endothelin-2, 36
Endothelin-3, 36
Endothelins
  antagonists, 37
  formation of, 36
  in hypertension, 37
  receptors
    antagonists, 389
    description of, 36–37
  vascular smooth muscle cells production of, 166
Endothelium
  antiatherogenic effects of, 171–172
  coronary, abnormalities of, 175–176
  dysfunction of, 167–169
  effect of fatty acids on, 35
  in renal parenchymal hypertension pathogenesis, 136
  vascular events affected by, 167t
  vasorelaxant functions of, 167, 168
Endothelium-derived relaxing factor
  description of, 44
  effect on potassium channels, 57
End-stage renal disease
  in African-Americans, 212
  blood pressure and, 211, 212t
  clinical studies of, 211–212
  diagnosis of, 322
  hypertension in, 135, 136t, 409
  prevalence of, 191
  racial predilection, 226
  socioeconomic status and, 242
Environment
  gene and, interactions between, 222–223
  risk factors, for hypertension, 222
Epoxyeicosatrienoic acids, 30
ERK (see Extracellular signal–regulated kinases)
Erythropoietin, in renal parenchymal hypertension pathogenesis, 136
Essential hypertension
  complicated, consultation for, 352–353, 353t
  description of, 101
  divalent cations in, 125–127
  genetics of, 101–103
  hemodynamic profiles in, 115–116
  regional blood flow in, 93–94
  renal manifestations of, 191
Estrogen, cardiovascular effects of, 28
Ethacrynic acid, 361t
Ethnicity, effect on hypertension incidence (see also specific race groups)
  control rates, 239–240
  description of, 239
Exercise (see Physical activity)
Exercise stress testing (see Stress testing)

Extracellular fluid volume
  altered neural control of, pathophysiologic conditions of, 91
  central-neural regulation of, 90–91
  neurogenic influences on, 89
Extracellular matrix
  mitogenic stimuli of, 159
  reactive oxygen species regulation of, 163
Extracellular signal–regulated kinases
  cascade, 74
  cell-surface receptors coupling to, 73–74
  cytosolic targets of, 74
  nuclear targets of, 74
Eye, hypertensive effects
  aneurysms, 195
  arterial changes, 195
  central vein occlusion, 195
  clinical significance, 196
  cotton wool spots, 195

Familial influences, on hypertension (see also Genetics)
  description of, 218–219
  intermediate phenotypes, 219–220
Fatty acids (see also Cholesterol; Lipids)
  blood pressure and, 246
  cardiovascular effects of, 35
  effect on vascular smooth muscle cells, 35
  endothelial function and, 35
  nonesterified, 35
  vascular α1-adrenergic receptor reactivity, 35
Fenoldopam, 388
Fiber, blood pressure levels and, 246
Fibroblasts
  angiotensin II in, 24
  angiotensinogen in, 24
Fish oil, blood pressure reductions, 246
Forebrain, in hypertension, 108
Fruits, blood pressure reductions and, 245
Furosemide, 361t

G protein (see Guanyl nucleotide binding proteins)
GABA
  description of, 48
  receptors, 61
  structure of, 48
Gender
  effect on antihypertensive treatment protocols, 231–232, 232, 282t
  hypertension and, 271
Genetics
  effect on hypertension
    description of, 218–219
    intermediate phenotypes, 219–220
  profiling, 306–307
Geographic patterns, of hypertension
  dietary difference effects, 244
  globally, 224–225, 271–272
  in United States, 226–228
Glomerular disease, 321
Glomeruli, sclerosis of, 190
Glucocorticoid receptor, 25
Glucocorticoid-remediable aldosteronism, 98, 452–453
Glucocorticoid-remediable hyperaldosteronism, 139–140
Glucocorticoids
  effect on phospholipases, 33
  hypertension, pathogenesis of, 139
Glucose
  intolerance
    diabetes mellitus and, 411–412
    thiazide diuretic use and, 360
  in regulation of intracellular ions, 126
Growth factor receptors, 61
Guanabenz, 370, 371t
Guanadrel, 371t
Guanethidine, 371t
Guanfacine, 370, 371t
Guanyl nucleotide binding proteins

activation of, 63–64, *65*
adenylyl cyclase regulation by, 66
adrenergic receptors coupling to, 3
composition of, 63
counterregulatory effects, 65
effectors, 64–65
family, 63
receptors, 62–63
α-subunits, 64t
Guanylyl cyclase, 67–68

Heart
    angiotensin II production, 23
    imaging of
        echocardiogram, 313–314, 315t
        electron beam computed tomography, 314, *315,* 315t
        magnetic resonance imaging, 314–315, 315t
        radionuclide angiography, 314, *315,* 315t
Heart disease (*see* Coronary heart disease)
Heart failure (*see* Congestive heart failure)
Heart murmur, auscultation of, 311–312
Heart rate
    dihydropyridine calcium antagonists effects on, 379
    stress testing and, 317
Heart sounds, auscultation of, 311
Hemodynamics
    acute stressor responses, 116–117
    control, patterns of, 80
    profiles, 115–116
Hemorrhage
    intracerebral, 309–310, 397
    subarachnoid, 397, 397t
High vascular resistance hypertension, 116
Hispanics, hypertension in
    control rates, 240
    management of, 413
Hormone replacement therapy
    blood pressure effects, 230
    for ischemic heart disease, 399
Hormones (*see specific hormone*)
Hydralazine, 385–386, 428
Hydrochlorothiazide, 361t
18-Hydroxydeoxycorticosterone, 26–27
Hydroxyeicosatrienoic acids, 30–31
11β-Hydroxylase
    deficiency of, 27, 140, 449
    isoforms of, 99
17-α-Hydroxylase enzyme, 449
5-Hydroxytryptamine (*see* Serotonin)
Hyperaldosteronism
    diagnosis of, 300
    glucocorticoid-remediable, 139–140
    idiopathic, 139
Hypercholesterolemia
    hypertensive patients with, treatment approaches for, 419–420, 420t
    secondary causes of, 418–419
Hypercortisolism, 139, 449–450
Hypercreatinemia, blood pressure and, 213–214
Hyperkinetic hypertension, 113
Hypermineralocorticoidism, 139–140
Hyperparathyroidism
    hypertension mechanisms in, 144
    primary, 454–455
    renin-aldosterone system in, 144
Hypertension (*see also* Blood pressure)
    accelerated, 116
    in African-Americans, 116
    after solid organ transplantation
        clinical features, 155
        incidence of, 155, *156*
        management of, 156
        pathophysiology of, 155–156, 156t
    in animal models, 107
    annual costs of, 290
    antihypertensive therapy (*see* Antihypertensive therapy)
    arginine vasopressin in, 38–39

average levels, in United States, 269t
    awareness of, 268–269
    borderline (*see* Borderline hypertension)
    cardiopulmonary baroreflexes in, 88
    as cardiovascular disease risk factor, 271
    in children, 424–426 (*see also* Children)
    chronic, during pregnancy, 428–429
    consultation for, 352–353
    definition of, 268
    drug-induced, 458–461, 459t
    dysfunctional potassium channels and, 57
    in elderly, 116
        clinical evaluation, 237–238
        clinical trials, 236–237, 237t
        epidemiology of, 236
        management of, 430–432
        mechanism of action, 432
        optimal care, 238
        pathophysiology of, 237
        pseudohypertension, 238
    estrogen use and, 28
    experimental models of, 128–130
    family history of, 218
    gender predilection, 271
    geographic patterns of
        globally, 224–225, 271–272
        in United States, 226–228, 274
    heterogeneity of, effect on antihypertensive therapy, 345–346
    high cardiac output, 115
    high vascular resistance, 116
    hyperdynamic, 115
    hyperkinetic, 113
    iatrogenic, 458–461
    insulin resistance and, 121–122, 256–257
    kallikrein-kinin system in, 40
    malignant, 116
    Mendelian forms of, 220
    in minority patients, 413–414
    monogenic, 98–100
    na⁺-H⁺ exchanger role in, 54–55
    neuropeptide Y in, 39
    nitric oxide in, 46
    nonmodulator trait, 104
    obesity and, 118, *119,* 226–227, 256, 339, 415–417
    orthostatic, 390–392
    ouabain in, *49*
    prevalence of, 268, 269t, 271, 274
    prevention of
        cigarette smoking cessation, 273
        clinical studies, 274–277
        recommendations, 277
        sodium intake reductions, 272, 277
        weight reduction, 272
    psychosocial stress and, 266
    refractory
        diagnosis of, 354
        etiology of, 354–357, 355t
    renal parenchymal (*see* Renal parenchymal hypertension)
    renovascular (*see* Renovascular hypertension)
    resistant, 352
    secondary, 300, 352, 355, 425
    steroid-induced, 116
    sympathetic nervous system in, 107, 109–112
    treatment of
        α,β-adrenergic blockers, 368–369
        α-adrenergic blockers, 367
        antihypertensive (*see* Antihypertensive drugs; Antihypertensive therapy)
        β-blockers (*see* β-Blockers)
        trends in controlling, 268–269
        vasoreactivity and, 169, *169*
        workplace management of, 441–442
    World Hypertension League studies of, 271–272
Hypertensive emergencies
    consultation for, 352
    definition of, 437
    description of, 437–438

labetalol for, 369
    management of, 437–438, 439t
    types of, 438t
Hypertensive encephalopathy
    clinical features, 186–187, 187t
    description of, 438
    diagnosis of, 308
    differential diagnosis, 187
    neurological investigation, 308
    pathophysiology of, 186
    treatment of, 186–187, 438–439
Hypertensive hypertrophic cardiomyopathy, 313
Hypertensive nephropathy, 190–191
Hypertensive nephrosclerosis, 191
Hypertensive personality, 267
Hypertensive urgencies
    treatment of, 438, 439t
    types of, 438t
Hyperthyroidism
    in children, 426
    management of, 454
Hypertrophy
    cellular signaling abnormalities in, 157
    definition of, 157
    DNA synthesis and, 157–158
    endothelium in, 157
    left ventricle (*see* Left ventricle, hypertrophy)
    vascular wall, 173
Hyperuricemia, from thiazide diuretic use, 360
Hypokalemia
    primary aldosteronism and, 451
    thiazide diuretics use and, 358–360
Hyponatremia, from thiazide diuretic use, 360
Hypotension, orthostatic, 390–392
Hypothalamus, in hypertension, 107–108
Hypothyroidism
    clinical features, 143–144
    renin in, 143

Idiopathic hyperaldosteronism, 139
Imidazolines, 389
Infarction
    cerebral, 309–310
    myocardial
        etiology of, 176
        non-Q-wave, 176
        Q-wave, 176
        in systolic hypertension, *200*
Inositol polyphosphates
    description of, 69–70
    formation of, *70*
Inositol 1,4,5-triphosphate
    description of, 69
    receptors, 69
Insulin
    α-adrenergic blockers and, 367, *367*
    receptors, 61
    in regulation of intracellular ions, 126
Insulin resistance
    β-blocker use and, 257
    description of, 121
    hypertension and, 121–122, 256–258
    for obese patients, 415
    during pregnancy, 153
Integrins, 76
Intermittent claudication, in peripheral arterial disease
    β-blockers for, 410
    description of, 215
    differential diagnosis, 323, 323t
    incidence of, 216
Interstitial renal disease, 321–322
Intracellular signaling, 71
Intracerebral hemorrhage, 309–310, 397
Intravascular volume, in renal parenchymal hypertension pathogenesis, 135
Ischemia
    border-zone, 183
    cerebral, 396

Ischemia—*Continued*
  low-flow, 183
  myocardial
    β-blockers for, 399
    etiology of, 175
    evaluation of, 398
    revascularization for, 400–401
    treatment of, 398–399
  retinal
    clinicopathological syndromes, 308
    neurological investigation of, 308–309
    transient focal cerebral, 309
  watershed, 183
Ischemic penumbra, 185

Janus kinases-signal transducers and activators of
      transcription, signaling, 75
Job, hypertension risk and, 266
Juxtaglomerular cells
  innervation of, 17
  renin synthesis in, 16, *17*

Kallikrein
  description of, 220
  in familial aggregation of hypertension, 220
Kallikrein-kinin system
  bioregulation of, 40
  excretion, 40
  in hypertension pathogenesis, 40
  renal, 40
  systemic influences of, 41
Ketamine hydrochloride, 458
Ketanserin, 48
Kidney
  angiotensin II production, 23–24
  circulation, 95
  damage to, 133–134
  disease (*see* Renal disease)
  function of, 322t
  hypertensive injury of
    antihypertensive therapy, 192
    mechanism of action, 191–192
    morphology, 191
  preeclamptic effects, 152
Kinases, 70
Kininase II (*see* Angiotensin I–converting enzyme)
Kininases, 40
Kininogenases, 40, *41*
Kininogens
  cleavage sites, *41*
  high-molecular-weight, 40
  low-molecular-weight, 40
Kinins
  in antihypertensive effect of angiotensin-converting
        enzyme inhibitors, 41
  definition of, 40
  function of, 40
Korotkoff sounds, 296t

Labetalol, 368
L-Amino acid decarboxylase, in catecholamine
      biosynthesis, 7
Left ventricle
  dilation of, 405–406
  hypertrophy
    aging effects, 177
    in congestive heart failure, 180
    coronary artery disease and, 209–210
    diagnosis of, 402–403
    echocardiographic findings, 208–210, 313–314
    in elderly, 431
    electrocardiographic findings, 208
    etiologic factors, 178t
    in general population, 208, *209*
    imaging techniques, 402–403
    mechanical forces in, 177
    myocardial blood flow effects, 177–178
    neurohumoral contributions to, 177
    regression of, 210

sequelae of, 178
severe, 178
treatment of, 403
Leukotriene A₄, 33
Leukotrienes
  description of, 33
  synthesis of, 33
Liddle's syndrome, 100, 140
Lifestyle modifications
  alcohol consumption, 341
  calcium consumption, 340
  description of, 333, 334t, 339
  diet, 340–341
  for elderly, 430
  magnesium consumption, 340
  physical activity (*see* Physical activity)
  potassium consumption, 340
  sodium chloride intake reductions, 340
  stress, 341
  weight loss, 339
Linoleic acids, 35
Lipids (*see also* Cholesterol; Fatty acids)
  abnormalities, 411
  α-adrenergic blocker effects on, 367
Lipoproteins, oxidation of, 163
Lipoxygenase enzymes, arachidonic acid oxidation by,
      33–34
12-Lipoxygenase pathway, in cardiovascular disorders,
      34t
15-Lipoxygenase pathway, in cardiovascular disorders,
      34t
5-Lipoxygenase pathway, of arachidonic acid
      metabolism, 33
Liver, preeclamptic effects on, 152–153
Low birth weight, hypertension and, 228
LVH (*see* Left ventricle, hypertrophy)

Macula densa
  description of, 16
  in renin release, 16–17
Macular degeneration, 196
Magnesium
  blood pressure and, 254–255, 340
  depletion states, 254
  dietary intake of, 254
  function of, 254
  intracellular, 125
  supplementation, 255, 340
Magnetic resonance imaging, of heart, 314–315, 315t
Medulla oblongata, circulation control functions of,
      80–81
Medullary thyroid carcinoma, 455
Menopause, effect on blood pressure, 229
Messenger ribonucleic acid, 23
Metabolic alkalosis, from thiazide diuretic use, 360
Methyldopa, 370, 371t, 428
Metolazone, 361t
Metyrosine, 446
Microvascular abnormalities
  description of, 173
  in hypertension, 173–174
  tissue and organ effects, 174
Midodrine, 459
Mineralocorticoids
  aldosterone (*see* Aldosterone)
  excess
    description of, 138–139
    syndrome of apparent, 99–100, 140
  hypertension, pathogenesis of, 138–139
  increased action of, 99–100
  overproduction of, 98
  receptors for, 25
  types of, 25
Minoxidil, 386–387
Mitogen-activated protein kinases
  description of, 71
  phosphorylation cascades, 72–74
Monoamine oxidase inhibitors, 460
Multi-infarct dementia, 188

Muscarinic receptors
  cardiovascular effects mediated by, 47
  effect on acetylcholine, 47
Myocardial infarction
  etiology of, 176
  non-Q-wave, 176
  Q-wave, 176
  in systolic hypertension, *200*
Myocardial ischemia
  β-blockers for, 399
  etiology of, 175
  evaluation of, 398
  revascularization for, 400–401
  treatment of, 398–399
Myocytes, loss of, 180

Na⁺-H⁺ exchange
  abnormalities of, 51
  in intracellular pH homeostasis, 53
Na⁺-H⁺ exchanger
  in hypertension pathogenesis, 54–55
  inactivity of, 53
  in intracellular pH homeostasis, 53
  regulation of, effect on vascular smooth muscle
        cells, 54–55, *55*
Na⁺-K⁺ (+2Cl⁻²ᴰ) cotransport, 51
Na⁺-Li⁺ countertransport, 51
Naloxone, 459
Native Americans, hypertension in, 413
Natriuresis, control of, 93
Natriuretic peptides
  biological actions of, 43t
  clinical significance of, 42–43
  physiological significance of, 42
  receptors, 42
  types of
    atrial, 42–43
    brain, 42–43
    CNP, 42
Nephrosclerosis, 322
Nervous system (*see* Autonomic nervous system; Sym-
      pathetic nervous system)
Neurohumoral factors, in modulation of arterial
      baroreflexes, 85–86
Neurons in rostral ventrolateral medulla, excitation by
      hypoxia or distortion, 81–82
Neuropeptide Y
  actions of, 39
  description of, 39
  in hypertension, 39
  receptors, 39
Neutral endopeptidase inhibitors, 389
Nicotinic receptors, effect on acetylcholine, 47
Nitrates, for myocardial ischemia, 399–400
Nitric oxide
  actions of
    biological, 44, 46t
    independent of cGMP, 46
  antiatherogenic effects of, 171–172
  biological activity, modulation of, 163–164
  and cGMP, 44–46, *45*
  definition of, 44
  effect on vascular smooth muscle cells, 44, 46
  endogenous production of, 44, *45*
  hormonal effects, 44, *45*
  in hypertension pathogenesis, 46
  metabolic interactions, 44
  physiological effects of, 44
  in vascular smooth muscle contraction, 79
  vasodilatory effects of, 46
  vasorelaxant functions of, 167, *168*
Nondihydropyridine calcium antagonists
  administration of, 384
  adverse reactions, 384
  cardiac effects, 382–383
  cellular mechanisms of action, 382
  for chronic renal insufficiency, 408
  clinical use of, 383–384
  dosage of, 383t, 384

pharmacokinetics and pharmacodynamics of, 382, 383t
systemic hemodynamic effects, 382
Nonsteroidal anti-inflammatory drugs
blood pressure increases, 355, 461
hypertension and, 460–461
19-Nordeoxycorticosterone, 27
Norepinephrine, *10, 107*

Obesity
epidemiology of, 118
hypertension and, 118, *119,* 226–227, 256, 339, 415–417
prevalence of, *119*
treatment of, 118–119
Older adults (*see* Elderly)
Oleic acid, 35
Optic nerve, circulation of, 195
Oral contraceptives
blood pressure effects, 230–231
contraindications, 230
hypertension and, 458
Orthostatic hypertension, 390–392
Orthostatic hypotension, 390–392
Ouabain
description of, 48
in hypertension pathogenesis, *49*
physiological functions of, 49
structure of, *49*
Ovaries, angiotensin II production by, 24
Oxidative stress, 163
18-Oxocortisol, 26

PAD (*see* Peripheral arterial disease)
Paracrine factors, in modulation of arterial barore-flexes, 85–86
Parathyroid hormone
hypertension and, 144
renal disease induced by, 144
in renal parenchymal hypertension pathogenesis, 136–137
Parathyroidectomy, hypertension response to, 144
Paraventricular nucleus, in hypertension, 108
Patient history, 300
P450C11β deficiency, 99
P450C17α deficiency, 99
P450C21 deficiency, 98–99
Peptides
natriuretic
biological actions of, 43t
clinical significance of, 42–43
physiological significance of, 42
receptors, 42
types of, 42–43
proadrenomedullin N-20 terminal, 50
Percutaneous transluminal coronary angioplasty, 401
Percutaneous transluminal renal angioplasty, 443–444
Peripheral arterial disease
clinical diagnosis of
angiography, 216
ankle-brachial index, 215, *324,* 326
arterial pulsation decreases, 326
blood pressure levels, 216, 216t
description of, 326
intermittent claudication, 215
noninvasive tests, 215–216
hypertension and, 216–217, 410
incidence studies of, 216–217
management of, 410–412
progression of, 217
risk factors for, 215
signs and symptoms of, 323
Peripheral circulation, physical examination of, 323–324
Peripheral sympatholytics, 370–371, 371t
pH, intracellular, 53, *54*
Phenol sulfotransferase, in catecholamine metabolism, 10

Phentolamine, 113
Phenylephrine, 459
Phenylethanolamine N-methyltransferase, in cate-cholamine biosynthesis, 7
Pheochromocytoma
clinical presentation of, 142
description of, 116
diagnosis of, 300
differential diagnosis, 447t
genetics of, 141
malignant, 447–448
management of, 446–448
pathophysiology of, 141–142
prevalence of, 141
Phosphatase, in vascular smooth muscle contraction, 79
Phosphatidylcholine signaling, 70
Phosphatidylinositol 4,5-biphosphate, 69
Phosphodiesterases
classification of, 66–67
cyclic nucleotide inactivation by, 66
Phosphoinositide kinases, 70
Phospholipase C, 69
Phosphorylation cascades
mitogen-activated protein kinase, 72–74
PI 3-kinase, 74–75
protein, 71–75
Physical activity
advice regarding, 261
blood pressure reductions, 259–260, 340
counseling, 261
hemodynamic response to, 94
national recommendations, 260–261
patient screening before starting, 261–262
peripheral arterial disease and, 411, 411t
safety issues, 261–262
Physical examination
of cardiovascular system, 311
of hypertensive patient, 300–301
of peripheral circulation, 323–324
Physical inactivity, hypertension risk and, 259
PI 3-kinase–phosphorylation cascades, 74–75
Pituitary gland, angiotensin II production by, 23
Platelets
agglutination of, by angiotensins, 11
autoregulation by, 157
Plekstrin homology domains, 70
Postmenopausal women
hormone replacement therapy, effect on blood pressure, 230
salt sensitivities of, 229
Postural adaptation, 390
Potassium
blood pressure effects
clinical trials, 250–251
description of, 340
epidemiology of, 250
mechanism of action, 251–252
cellular transport of, 56–57
current channels
ATP-sensitive, 57
calcium-activated, 56–57
dysfunctional, 57
inward rectifier, 57
openers of, 388
voltage-gated, 56
dietary intake, 227, 250
excretion of, 251t
supplementation, 340
vasuloprotective effect of, 252
Preeclampsia
antihypertensive therapy, 427–428
clinical manifestations of, 152
definition of, 152
etiology of, 153–154
genetics of, 154
immunology of, 154
management of, 427
pathology of, 152–153

pathophysiology of, 152–153
prevalence of, 152
prevention of, 427
Preganglionic sympathetic neurons, 80
Pregnancy (*see also* Preeclampsia)
chronic hypertension during, 428–429
labetalol use during, 369
Preproangiotensinogen, 14
Proadrenomedullin N-20 terminal peptide, 50
Progesterone, cardiovascular effects of, 28
Prorenin, 16
Prostacyclin, vasodilatory properties of, 30
Prostaglandins
E$_2$, 30
effect on angiotensin-converting enzyme inhibitors, 372
formation of, by cyclooxygenase pathway, *31*
I$_2$, 30
Protein
dietary, blood pressure levels and, 246
guanyl nucleotide binding (*see* Guanyl nucleotide binding proteins)
phosphorylation of, 71–75
raf, 73
translation, regulation of, 72
Protein kinase G, 44, 68
Protein kinases
cAMP-dependent, 67
mitogen-activated, 71
structure of, 71
Proteinuria, 192, 320, 423
Pseudohyperaldosteronism, 140
Pseudohypertension, in elderly, 238
Pseudotolerance, to antihypertensive drugs, 346
Psychosocial stress, hypertension caused by, 266
Pulse
palpation of, 326
popliteal, 326

Quality of life
antihypertensive drugs and, 284–285
cost-effectiveness considerations, 288
definition of, 284
lifestyle change effects on, 284

Race (*see also* Ethnicity; *specific race groups*)
hypertension incidence based on, 227t
Radiograph, chest, 312
Radionuclide angiography, 314, 315t
Raf proteins, 73
Rarefaction, 173
Rauwolfia alkaloids, 371t
Reactive oxygen species
in hypertension, 165–166
sources of, 163
vascular processes affected by, 163–165
Receptors
adenosine, 48
binding properties, 61
cell surface, 61
endothelin, 36–37
inositol 1,4,5-triphosphate, 69
with intrinsic activity, 61–62
mineralocorticoid, 25
natriuretic peptides, 42
neuropeptide Y, 39
regulation, 62
transduction mechanisms, 61
vasopressin, 38
without intrinsic activity, 62
Recombinant human erythropoietin, 460
Redox state, 163
Refractory hypertension
diagnosis of, 354
etiology of, 354–357, 355t
Renal artery stenosis, experimental models of, 128–129
Renal blood flow, in essential hypertension, 94

Renal disease
  cholesterol in, 192
  description of, 190
  end-stage, 135, 136t, *191*
    in African-Americans, 212
    blood pressure and, 211, 212t
    clinical studies of, 211–212
    diagnosis of, 322
    hypertension in, 135, 136t, 409
    prevalence of, *191*
    racial predilection, 226
    socioeconomic status and, 242
  history of, 211
  interstitial, 321–322
  progressive, 190
Renal insufficiency
  blood pressure goals for, 337–338
  chronic, management of, 407–409
  description of, 322
  thiazide diuretic contraindications, 358–359
Renal parenchymal disease
  description of, 320
  evaluation algorithm, *321*
  proteinuria and, 320
  signs and symptoms of, 320t
Renal parenchymal hypertension
  experimental models of, 129
  pathophysiology of, 135–137
Renal sympathetic nerve activity
  afferent mechanisms that control, 89
  efferent, and sodium balance control, 89–90
Renin
  in angiotensin II formation, 16–17
  essential hypertension and, 104
  in hypothyroidism, 143
  inhibitors of, 388–389
  plasma activity measurements, 451
  release, physiological regulation of, 16–18
  synthesis of, in juxtaglomerular cells, 16, *17*
Renin-angiotensin system
  divalent cations and, 125
  in renal parenchymal hypertension pathogenesis, 135
  tissue sources, 23–24
Renin-angiotensin-aldosterone system
  nonmodulation of, 220
  in preeclampsia, 153
  schematic of, *12*
Renovascular hypertension
  arterial pressure increases in, 94
  bilateral, 131–132
  diagnosis of, 300
  hemodynamic profiles in, 116
  management of, 443–445
  pathophysiology of, 131–134
  unilateral, 132–133, *133*
Reserpine, 8, 370–371, 371t
Retina
  arterial occlusion, 308
  circulation of, 194–195
  description of, 194
  ischemia
    clinicopathological syndromes, 308
    neurological investigation of, 308–309
Revascularization, for myocardial ischemia, 400–401
Risk factors, for hypertension
  atherosclerosis (*see* Atherosclerosis)
  blood pressure, 199–200
  clustering of, 200–201, 201t
Rostral ventrolateral medullary control centers
  description of, 81
  neurons, excitation by hypoxia or distortion, 81–82

Salt (*see* Sodium)
Selectins, 76
Serotonin
  agents, 388
  cardiovascular effects of, 47–48
  structure of, *48*

  synthesis of, 47
  vasodilatory effects of, 47–48
Sex steroids
  androgens, 28
  cardiovascular effects of, 28
  estrogens, 28
  progestins, 28
Shear stress
  autoregulation of blood flow and, 96–97
  blood flow and, 96
Signal transduction
  cyclic nucleotides, 66–68
  receptors, 61–62
Skeletal muscle
  blood flow, in essential hypertension, 94
  vasculature, abnormalities of, 181
Sleep apnea
  clinical features, 456, 457t
  conditions associated with, 456
  definition of, 456
  diagnosis of, 456–457
  epidemiology of, 148
  hypertension and, 148–149
  management of, 456–457
  pathophysiology of, 148, *149*
  treatment of, 457
Sleep-disordered breathing, 149
Smoking (*see* Cigarette smoking)
Smooth muscle cells, vascular (*see* Vascular smooth muscle cells)
Socioeconomic status, correlation with hypertension
  description of, 240–241
  effect on disease outcomes, 241
  prevalence, 242
  treatment effect, 242–243
Sodium
  balance of, efferent renal sympathetic nerve activity effects on, 89–90
  dietary
    blood pressure and, 247–249, *248*, 355
    description of, 126, 227
    hypertension risk reductions by lowering, 272, 277, 340
    restriction of, 222, 249
  excretion
    arterial pressure and, *132*
    factors that modulate, *90*
    in renal parenchymal hypertension pathogenesis, 135
  sensitivity
    characteristics of, 123
    clinical groups with, 124t
    clinical investigation of, 123
Sodium channels, 51
Sodium transport
  abnormalities of, *52*
  active, 51
  passive, disorders of, 51–52
  types of, 51
Sodium-lithium countertransport, 220
Solid organ transplantation, hypertension after
  clinical features, 155
  incidence of, 155, *156*
  management of, 156
  pathophysiology of, 155–156, 156t
Somatosympathetic reflexes, 81
Spironolactone, 361t
Splanchnic blood flow, in essential hypertension, 94
Spontaneously hypertensive rat, 128
Steroids
  biosynthesis disorders, 98–99
  extra-adrenal synthesis of, 27
  mineralocorticoids (*see* Mineralocorticoids)
  sex (*see* Sex steroids)
Stress
  blood pressure and, 266–267
  hypertension caused by, 266
  reduction of, 341

Stress myocardial perfusion imaging, 318–319
Stress testing
  cardiovascular responses to, 317
  contraindications for, 317–318, 318t
  description of, 317
  exaggerated pressure response to, 318
  indications, 318t
Stroke
  acute, *184*, 185
  arterial mechanisms of, 185t
  arterial occlusion in, 183
  blood pressure levels and, correlation between, 204–205, *205*
  clinical features, 183
  clinical imaging correlations, 185
  elderly predilection, 183
  etiology of, 203
  geographic predilection, 226
  high-risk populations, 203
  hypertension and, 184–185
  incidence of, 203–206
  mortality from, 205–206, *206*, 227t, 269–270
  patient education to reduce, 270
  prevention of, 206–207
  risk factors for, 204
  treatment of, 204–205
Subarachnoid hemorrhage, 397, 397t
Subcortical arteriosclerotic encephalopathy, 188
Sudden death, 176
Superoxide anion
  endothelium and, 166, 168
  vascular smooth muscle cells production of, 166
Sympathetic nervous system
  in blood pressure control, *110*
  in hypertension, 106–112
  neuromodulation of, 106–107
  overactivity of, 110–112
  sleep apnea and, 148
Sympatholytics
  central, 370, 371t
  for chronic renal insufficiency, 408
  peripheral, 370–371, 371t
Syndrome of apparent mineralocorticoid excess, 99–100, 140
Systemic vascular compliance, 327
Systolic blood pressure
  dysfunction
    in congestive heart failure etiology, 180
    management of, 405–406
  measurement of, 297
Systolic Hypertension in Elderly Program, 236–237, 334

Tachycardia, 390
Testes, angiotensin II production by, 24
Testosterone, cardiovascular effects of, 28
Thiazide diuretics
  antihypertensive agents and, concomitant therapy, 358
  blood pressure effect, mechanism of action for, 358, *359–360*
  for chronic renal insufficiency, 407–408
  complications of, 359–360
  description of, 358
  diabetes and, 257–258
  dosage guidelines for, 358–359, 361t
  for elderly patients, 432
  for obese patients with hypertension, 416
  side effects of, 359–360
  for systolic dysfunction, 406
Thromboxane A_2, 30
Thyroid
  disorders of, 144t
  dysfunction of, 454
  hypertension and, 143–144
  medullary carcinoma of, 455
Thyrotoxicosis, 143
Torsemide, 361t

Transcription factors, regulation of, 72
Transient focal cerebral ischemia, 309
Transplantation (*see* Solid organ transplantation)
Trials of Hypertension Prevention, 276–277
Triamterene, 361t
Tricyclic antidepressants, 151
Tyrosine hydroxylase, in catecholamine biosynthesis, 7
Tyrosine kinases, in mitogenic signaling, 158

Vascular dementia
    clinical diagnosis, 188, 189t
    epidemiology of, 188
    hypertension and, 188
    neuroimaging of, 189
    pathophysiology of, 188–189
    treatment of, 189
Vascular smooth muscle
    contraction of
        calcium in, 79
        cGMP in, 79
        description of, *78,* 78–79
        nitric oxide in, 79

phosphatase in, 79
phosphorylation of, *78*
Vascular smooth muscle cells
    apoptosis of, 171
    autoregulation by, 157
    effect of fatty acids on, 35
    endothelin production by, 166
    growth of, vasodilators that inhibit, 158–159
    membrane potential of, 56
    mitogenic stimuli effects, 157–158
    nitric oxide effects on, 171
    relaxation of, from nitric oxide, 44, 46
    superoxide anion production, 166
    in vessel tone maintenance, 53
    volume regulation in, 53–54
Vasoactive peptides, metabolism of, angiotensin
        I–converting enzyme involvement in, 19, *19*
Vasodilation, endothelium-dependent, 114
Vasodilators
    for chronic renal insufficiency, 408
    hydralazine, 385–386
    minoxidil, 386–387

Vasopressin (*see* Arginine vasopressin)
Vasoreactivity, hypertension and, 169, *169*
Vegetables, blood pressure reductions by,
        245
Vegetarian diet, 340–341
Verapamil (*see* Nondihydropyridine calcium antago-
        nists)
Vessels (*see* Blood vessels)
Voltage-gated channels
    calcium, 59
    potassium, 56

Weight reduction
    hypertension and, 272, 416
    physiological changes, *416*
White coat hypertension, 299–300
Workplace, hypertension treatment in, 441–442

Yohimbine hydrochloride, 459

Zona fasciculata-reticularis, 26
Zona glomerulosa, 26